Biomedical Applications of Nanoparticles

Biomedical Applications of Nanoparticles

Special Issue Editor
Nadine Millot

MDPI • Basel • Beijing • Wuhan • Barcelona • Belgrade • Manchester • Tokyo • Cluj • Tianjin

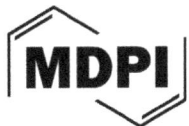

Special Issue Editor
Nadine Millot
Université Bourgogne Franche Comté/CNRS
France

Editorial Office
MDPI
St. Alban-Anlage 66
4052 Basel, Switzerland

This is a reprint of articles from the Special Issue published online in the open access journal *Nanomaterials* (ISSN 2079-4991) (available at: https://www.mdpi.com/journal/nanomaterials/special_issues/Nanoparticle_biomedic).

For citation purposes, cite each article independently as indicated on the article page online and as indicated below:

LastName, A.A.; LastName, B.B.; LastName, C.C. Article Title. *Journal Name* **Year**, *Article Number*, Page Range.

ISBN 978-3-03928-542-6 (Hbk)
ISBN 978-3-03928-543-3 (PDF)

© 2020 by the authors. Articles in this book are Open Access and distributed under the Creative Commons Attribution (CC BY) license, which allows users to download, copy and build upon published articles, as long as the author and publisher are properly credited, which ensures maximum dissemination and a wider impact of our publications.

The book as a whole is distributed by MDPI under the terms and conditions of the Creative Commons license CC BY-NC-ND.

Contents

About the Special Issue Editor ix

Preface to "Biomedical Applications of Nanoparticles" xi

Tristan Mangeolle, Ilya Yakavets, Sophie Marchal, Manon Debayle, Thomas Pons, Lina Bezdetnaya and Frédéric Marchal
Fluorescent Nanoparticles for the Guided Surgery of Ovarian Peritoneal Carcinomatosis
Reprinted from: *Nanomaterials* 2018, 8, 572, doi:10.3390/nano8080572 1

Xiaoxia Wu, Yan Peng, Xiaomei Duan, Lingyan Yang, Jinze Lan and Fu Wang
Homologous Gold Nanoparticles and Nanoclusters Composites with Enhanced Surface Raman Scattering and Metal Fluorescence for Cancer Imaging
Reprinted from: *Nanomaterials* 2018, 8, 819, doi:10.3390/nano8100819 21

Carlos Caro, Pedro Quaresma, Eulália Pereira, Jaime Franco, Manuel Pernia Leal, Maria Luisa García-Martín, Jose Luis Royo, Jose Maria Oliva-Montero, Patrick Jacques Merkling, Ana Paula Zaderenko, David Pozo and Ricardo Franco
Synthesis and Characterization of Elongated-Shaped Silver Nanoparticles as a Biocompatible Anisotropic SERS Probe for Intracellular Imaging: Theoretical Modeling and Experimental Verification
Reprinted from: *Nanomaterials* 2019, 9, 256, doi:10.3390/nano9020256 33

Sébastien Penninckx, Anne-Catherine Heuskin, Carine Michiels and Stéphane Lucas
Thioredoxin Reductase Activity Predicts Gold Nanoparticle Radiosensitization Effect
Reprinted from: *Nanomaterials* 2019, 9, 295, doi:10.3390/nano9020295 51

Cataldo Arcuri, Lorenzo Monarca, Francesco Ragonese, Carmen Mecca, Stefano Bruscoli, Stefano Giovagnoli, Rosario Donato, Oxana Bereshchenko, Bernard Fioretti and Ferdinando Costantino
Probing Internalization Effects and Biocompatibility of Ultrasmall Zirconium Metal-Organic Frameworks UiO-66 NP in U251 Glioblastoma Cancer Cells
Reprinted from: *Nanomaterials* 2018, 8, 867, doi:10.3390/nano8110867 65

Ying-Jie Hu, Jing-Ying Zhang, Qian Luo, Jia-Rui Xu, Yan Yan, Li-Min Mu, Jing Bai and Wan-Liang Lu
Nanostructured Dihydroartemisinin Plus Epirubicin Liposomes Enhance Treatment Efficacy of Breast Cancer by Inducing Autophagy and Apoptosis
Reprinted from: *Nanomaterials* 2018, 8, 804, doi:10.3390/nano8100804 79

Gibok Lee and Yong Il Park
Lanthanide-Doped Upconversion Nanocarriers for Drug and Gene Delivery
Reprinted from: *Nanomaterials* 2018, 8, 511, doi:10.3390/nano8070511 95

Romana Křivohlavá, Eva Neuhoferová, Katrine Q. Jakobsen and Veronika Benson
Knockdown of microRNA-135b in Mammary Carcinoma by Targeted Nanodiamonds: Potentials and Pitfalls of In Vivo Applications
Reprinted from: *Nanomaterials* 2019, 9, 866, doi:10.3390/nano9060866 111

Fadoua Sallem, Rihab Haji, Dominique Vervandier-Fasseur, Thomas Nury, Lionel Maurizi, Julien Boudon, Gérard Lizard and Nadine Millot
Elaboration of *Trans*-Resveratrol Derivative-Loaded Superparamagnetic Iron Oxide Nanoparticles for Glioma Treatment
Reprinted from: *Nanomaterials* **2019**, *9*, 287, doi:10.3390/nano9020287 133

Wenxing Song, Xing Su, David Alexander Gregory, Wei Li, Zhiqiang Cai and Xiubo Zhao
Magnetic Alginate/Chitosan Nanoparticles for Targeted Delivery of Curcumin into Human Breast Cancer Cells
Reprinted from: *Nanomaterials* **2018**, *8*, 907, doi:10.3390/nano8110907 153

Nimisha Singh, Fadoua Sallem, Celine Mirjolet, Thomas Nury, Suban Kumar Sahoo, Nadine Millot and Rajender Kumar
Polydopamine Modified Superparamagnetic Iron Oxide Nanoparticles as Multifunctional Nanocarrier for Targeted Prostate Cancer Treatment
Reprinted from: *Nanomaterials* **2019**, *9*, 138, doi:10.3390/nano9020138 177

Mihaela Balas, Florian Dumitrache, Madalina Andreea Badea, Claudiu Fleaca, Anca Badoi, Eugenia Tanasa and Anca Dinischiotu
Coating Dependent In Vitro Biocompatibility of New Fe-Si Nanoparticles
Reprinted from: *Nanomaterials* **2018**, *8*, 495, doi:10.3390/nano8070495 197

Yao Chen, Di Wu, Wu Zhong, Shuwen Kuang, Qian Luo, Liujiang Song, Lihua He, Xing Feng and Xiaojun Tao
Evaluation of the PEG Density in the PEGylated Chitosan Nanoparticles as a Drug Carrier for Curcumin and Mitoxantrone
Reprinted from: *Nanomaterials* **2018**, *8*, 486, doi:10.3390/nano8070486 223

Priyanka Singh, Abhroop Garg, Santosh Pandit, V.R.S.S. Mokkapati and Ivan Mijakovic
Antimicrobial Effects of Biogenic Nanoparticles
Reprinted from: *Nanomaterials* **2018**, *8*, 1009, doi:10.3390/nano8121009 239

Mohammad Jalal, Mohammad Azam Ansari, Mohammad A. Alzohairy, Syed Ghazanfar Ali, Haris M. Khan, Ahmad Almatroudi and Kashif Raees
Biosynthesis of Silver Nanoparticles from Oropharyngeal *Candida glabrata* Isolates and Their Antimicrobial Activity against Clinical Strains of Bacteria and Fungi
Reprinted from: *Nanomaterials* **2018**, *8*, 586, doi:10.3390/nano8080586 259

Eleazar Samuel Kolosovas-Machuca, Alexander Cuadrado, Hiram Joazet Ojeda-Galván, Luis Carlos Ortiz-Dosal, Aida Catalina Hernández-Arteaga, Maria del Carmen Rodríguez-Aranda, Hugo Ricardo Navarro-Contreras, Javier Alda and Francisco Javier González
Detection of Histamine Dihydrochloride at Low Concentrations Using Raman Spectroscopy Enhanced by Gold Nanostars Colloids
Reprinted from: *Nanomaterials* **2019**, *9*, 211, doi:10.3390/nano9020211 271

Xiujie Liu, Mengmeng Liu, Yudong Lu, Changji Wu, Yunchao Xu, Duo Lin, Dechan Lu, Ting Zhou and Shangyuan Feng
Facile Ag-Film Based Surface Enhanced Raman Spectroscopy Using DNA Molecular Switch for Ultra-Sensitive Mercury Ions Detection
Reprinted from: *Nanomaterials* **2018**, *8*, 596, doi:10.3390/nano8080596 283

Magdalena Ziąbka, Elżbieta Menaszek, Jacek Tarasiuk and Sebastian Wroński
Biocompatible Nanocomposite Implant with Silver Nanoparticles for Otology—In Vivo Evaluation
Reprinted from: *Nanomaterials* **2018**, *8*, 764, doi:10.3390/nano8100764 295

Maija-Liisa Mattinen, Guillaume Riviere, Alexander Henn, Robertus Wahyu N. Nugroho, Timo Leskinen, Outi Nivala, Juan José Valle-Delgado, Mauri A. Kostiainen and Monika Österberg
Colloidal Lignin Particles as Adhesives for Soft Materials
Reprinted from: *Nanomaterials* **2018**, *8*, 1001, doi:10.3390/nano8121001 313

Nagendra Kumar Kaushik, Neha Kaushik, Nguyen Nhat Linh, Bhagirath Ghimire, Anchalee Pengkit, Jirapong Sornsakdanuphap, Su-Jae Lee and Eun Ha Choi
Plasma and Nanomaterials: Fabrication and Biomedical Applications
Reprinted from: *Nanomaterials* **2019**, *9*, 98, doi:10.3390/nano9010098 333

About the Special Issue Editor

Nadine Millot is a Professor at the University of Bourgogne (Dijon, France). She is the principal investigator and founder of the BH2N ((Bio-)Hybrid Nanoparticles and Nanostructures) group in the Nanosciences Department of the Interdisciplinary laboratory Carnot de Bourgogne. Her group has extensive expertise in the field of synthesis and characterization of nanoparticles, particularly SPIONs used as bimodal contrast agents and titanate nanotubes developed for the nanovectorisation of active molecules. Nadine Millot is the author of more than 70 peer reviewed publications (h-index of 23, Scopus), 1 patent, 2 book chapters, and 1 educational book (Ed. Lavoisier, Paris, 2014). She has also given 30 invited oral presentations in the last five years and has supervised 15 Ph.D. students. She is member of the steering committee of the C'Nano France.

Preface to "Biomedical Applications of Nanoparticles"

The concept of nanomaterials that can be designed for and administered in the human body to improve health is of interest. For more than two decades, many research teams and biotechnology companies have developed different types of nanoparticles for medical purposes. Of these, some have marketing authorization such as Myocet® (carrying doxorubicin) or Abraxane® (carrying taxol). At the preclinical level, several teams combined radiotherapy with nanoparticles of gold or with gadolinium or hafnium oxides or with lipid nanocapsules of ferrociphenol. A total of 396 clinical studies implementing nanoparticles have been conducted to date and 73 are currently recruiting (March 2020). Since each nanoparticle has its own peculiarities (bioavailability, more or less important grafting capacity, internalization, etc.), developing new types and improving the properties of existing ones are essential. During the past few years, research has been increasing on the use of nanomaterials in diverse areas of biomedical research, including biological sensing, labelling, imaging, cell separation, and therapy. Nano-objects are associated with organic molecules to vectorize drugs. The objective is then to concentrate these treatments on the pathological site by limiting the side effects. Nanoparticles are also used as contrast agents in medical imaging, especially in MRI or optical imaging or intrinsically as therapeutic agents. In the latter case, the nanoparticles, via physical phenomena emanating from their composition and/or their size, lead, for example, to the destruction of cancer cells via hyperthermia or radiosensitization. For each of the new nanoparticles developed, the toxicity, efficacy, and bioavailability should be determined. The biodistribution and elimination of nanoparticles by different natural pathways, for instance, depends on many factors including the size of nanoparticle agglomerates, their surface charge, their protein ring, and so on. All these parameters must be mastered and interactions with the living world must be better understood. This book, which is a Special Issue of the Nanomaterials journal, deals with all these fields and also includes nanocomposite implant and metal detection.

Nadine Millot
Special Issue Editor

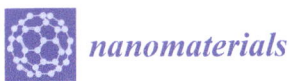

Review

Fluorescent Nanoparticles for the Guided Surgery of Ovarian Peritoneal Carcinomatosis

Tristan Mangeolle [1,2], Ilya Yakavets [1,2,3], Sophie Marchal [1,2], Manon Debayle [4], Thomas Pons [4], Lina Bezdetnaya [1,2] and Frédéric Marchal [1,5,*]

1. Centre de Recherche en Automatique de Nancy, Centre National de la Recherche Scientifique UMR 7039, Université de Lorraine, Campus Sciences, Boulevard des Aiguillette, 54506 Vandoeuvre-lès-Nancy, France; t.mangeolle@nancy.unicancer.fr (T.M.); i.yakavets@nancy.unicancer.fr (I.Y.); s.marchal@nancy.unicancer.fr (S.M.); l.bolotine@nancy.unicancer.fr (L.B.)
2. Research Department, Institut de Cancérologie de Lorraine, 6 avenue de Bourgogne, 54519 Vandoeuvre-lès-Nancy, France
3. Laboratory of Biophysics and Biotechnology, Belarusian State University, 4 Nezavisimosti Avenue, 220030 Minsk, Belarus
4. LPEM, ESPCI Paris, PSL Research University, CNRS, Sorbonne Université, 75005 Paris, France; manon.debayle@espci.fr (M.D.); thomas.pons@espci.fr (T.P.)
5. Surgical Department, Institut de Cancérologie de Lorraine, 6 avenue de Bourgogne, 54519 Vandoeuvre-lès-Nancy, France
* Correspondence: f.marchal@nancy.unicancer.fr; Tel.: +33-(0)3-83-59-84-51

Received: 6 July 2018; Accepted: 22 July 2018; Published: 26 July 2018

Abstract: Complete surgical resection is the ideal cure for ovarian peritoneal carcinomatosis, but remains challenging. Fluorescent guided surgery can be a promising approach for precise cytoreduction when appropriate fluorophore is used. In the presence paper, we review already developed near- and short-wave infrared fluorescent nanoparticles, which are currently under investigation for peritoneal carcinomatosis fluorescence imaging. We also highlight the main ways to improve the safety of nanoparticles, for fulfilling prerequisites of clinical application.

Keywords: cancer imaging; cytoreduction surgery; fluorescent nanoparticle; near-infrared; short-wave infrared

1. Introduction

1.1. Epidemiology

Some peritoneal and gastrointestinal malignancies show preferential dissemination and invasion into peritoneal cavity, leading to a peritoneal carcinomatosis with substantial consequences on survival [1]. Among these malignancies, Epithelial Ovarian cancers (EOC) remain the fifth leading cause of death with a five-year survival rate of only 46%, albeit EOCs are only the 8th most common cancer in women [2]. The poor prognosis of these cancers is mainly due to the absence of specific early symptoms, leading to late diagnosis [3]. When confined to the ovary or the regional lymph nodes, EOC provides respectively 92.5 and 73% of survival at five years but they only represent 15 and 20% of newly diagnosed EOC respectively. 65% of EOC are diagnosed at distant stage with a survival rate of 28.9% [4].

Distant stages are characterized by the presence of cancer cells in the peritoneal cavity and/or in the retroperitoneal lymph nodes, where they can induce peritoneal carcinomatosis [5]. Peritoneal carcinomatosis suggests metastases, which in turn are localized on the peritoneum and the peritoneal organs, varying in size from microscopic lesions to cancerous masses of several centimeters [6].

Ultimately, peritoneal carcinomatosis progression leads to debilitating ascites and, above all, intestinal obstruction and subsequent lethal outcomes [7].

1.2. Conventional Treatment

The frontline treatment for peritoneal carcinomatosis of ovarian origin associates extensive surgery with peri-operative chemotherapy, mainly by paclitaxel and cisplatin, to remove the whole cancerous mass.

The main objective of extensive surgery is to excise macroscopic cancerous implants from the ovary and from the entire peritoneal cavity. Initially considered as palliative treatment to alleviate abdominal pain, extensive surgery was progressively developed for a curative intent with total removal of cancerous lesions [8], and was finally standardized by Sugarbaker [9]. However, despite many improvements, this procedure remains challenging.

First, surgeons can rely only on pre-operative imaging to distinguish all cancerous lesions, mainly by position emission tomography (PET), computed tomography (CT) or magnetic resonance imaging (MRI) [10], eventually combined with ultrasound, Doppler and laparoscopic observation [11].

During surgery, surgeons must explore the whole peritoneal cavity, delineated by a serous membrane (the peritoneum), with organs such as liver, spleen, pancreas, and the whole gastrointestinal tract. Altogether, peritoneum and peritoneal organs represent an area almost equivalent to that of the body [12]. Exploration of this huge surface requires many hours and can be achieved only by experienced surgeons. The goal of primary surgery is a complete resection, without any residual disease [13]. To eliminate residual cancerous cells, several cycles of intravenous platinum-based chemotherapy combined with paclitaxel is performed [14].

To treat residual microscopic metastases and thus to achieve a complete cytoreduction initiated with the surgical procedure, it is necessary to increase the local drug concentration by intraperitoneal injections [15]. It was quickly shown that the peritoneal membrane limits the plasmatic passage in case of local injection of ionized and lipid insoluble compounds [16,17]. Therefore, hydrophilic drugs injected by intraperitoneal are maintained at higher concentrations than after intravenous injection, with a lower risk of systemic toxicity.

Although this approach was clinically validated [18–20], one limiting factor consisting of a shallow drug penetration in the tumor (no more than few millimeters) considerably reduced its clinical efficacy on gross residual colon tumors [21]. Recent studies show improved survival rate for ovarian cancer patients treated by intraperitoneal chemotherapy, with better and longer survival rate [22,23]. Combination of hyperthermy and intraperitoneal chemotherapy was recently confirmed for ovarian cancer treatment [24], showing improved survival without higher rates of side effects [25].

Irrespective of chemotherapy modalities, the residual disease after surgery remains one of the primary prognosis factors [26–28]. Survival at five years is closely related to the absence (60% of totally debulked patients) or the presence of microscopic metastases (30% for patient with "optimal" (<1 cm) residual disease) [29]. Moreover, despite complete surgery, early post-operative computerized tomography detects sub-optimal (>1 cm) residual tumors in almost half of the patients [30].

2. Fluorescence Guided Surgery

While chemotherapy has undergone adjustments and its optimization by hyperthermia is still debated, surgical debulking still depends on the extensive experience of the surgeon and his/her own ability to detect tumor deposits in the peritoneal cavity [31]. Attempts have been made to search for complementary solutions to enhance surgeon guidance. Among other options, fluorescence guided surgery (FGS) is highly demanded, especially in oncological surgery [32].

Tissue offers various autofluorescence patterns under ultraviolet illumination. Therefore, ultraviolet illumination was tested to detect cancerous tissue in the middle of the 20th century with some success [33]. Moore improved the technique by using the difference of retention between cancerous and healthy tissue of intravenous injected fluorescent dye, the fluorescein [34]. This technique was further applied with success to guide cerebral tumor resection [35]. Many improvements have been introduced since that time to FGS with fluorescein for glioblastoma surgical treatment and a similar approach to detect ovarian peritoneal carcinomatosis generated substantial improvements [36]. Van Dame and co-workers used as a target the predominant folate receptor sur-expression in ovarian cancer cells, combining fluorescein isothiocyanate (FITC) and folate. By means of filters and a fluorescence-specific camera, they increased the detection rate of residual disease four-fold [37]. The development of high-resolution cameras considerably contributed to real-time imaging of cancerous tissue with effective contrast and improved information accessible to the surgeon [32]. Another advantage provided by cameras was the possibility to use near-infrared (NIR) fluorescent dyes, invisible to human eye. Visible fluorescent dyes (fluorescein for example) are detectable mainly on the surface of tissue, no deeper than few millimeters, due to the absorption of biological chromophores (i.e., melanin, fat, hemoglobin, etc.).

By contrast, NIR fluorescence is weakly absorbed by the tissues, allowing a deeper detection (up to five millimeters) [38] and even a whole-body fluorescence imaging for small animals such as rodents [39]. From that point of view, FGS benefited from extensive development and application of NIR-fluorescent dyes [40–42]. Among other available NIR-fluorescent dyes, indocyanine green (ICG) is currently the spearhead of the probes applied for FGS purpose. This dye, developed in the middle of the 20th century, is one of the few Food and drug administration (FDA)-approved NIR dyes [43]. ICG was indicated in patients for the measurements of cardiac output, liver function, blood flow and retinal angiography, as well as tolerated and hepatic cleared dye. It has also been tested for sentinel lymph node mapping and cancer imaging [44]. Even though ICG has no specificity for cancer cells, its high affinity for plasma proteins results in a preferential accumulation of ICG-protein complex in the tumor vasculature. Tumor anarchic vasculature offers larger lumen and fenestration, facilitating both the permeability and retention of macromolecules, known as Enhanced Permeability and Retention (EPR) effect [45]. The only known exception is the hepato-cellular carcinoma, which displays specificity for ICG, probably because of their hepatic cell remnant characteristics [46].

In the case of ovarian cancer, encouraging results were obtained with intravenously injected ICG in mice, allowing the detection of few millimeters of peritoneal metastases from different origins [47]. However, the first clinical results were contradictory: high sensitivity was associated with low specificity, with a high rate (62%) of false positive non-malignant lesions being observed [48]. Another problem, raised by the hepatic clearance of ICG, was the fluorescent contamination of the gastrointestinal tract that hampers tumor implant detection [49].

From these observations, the authors identified the urgent need for targeting probes rather than passive probes. With this aim, OTL-38, the NIR folate-targeted counterpart of the FITC-folate probe, was clinically tested, showing encouraging results of a higher signal-to-background ratio (SBR) [50]. As expected, OTL-38 allows deeper tumor detection (almost one centimeter below tissue surface) than with FITC-folate. However, irrespective of the NIR-fluorescent dyes used, light excitation and emission scattering limit the detection depth to a few millimeters and the surgeon still needs a pre-operative CT/MRI scan or other intraoperative imagery modalities for precise and exhaustive tumor localization and surgery planning [38]. Thus, for ovarian peritoneal carcinomatosis and peritoneal malignancies, the ideal probe for FGS should be multimodal by associating NIR dye, targeting moiety and another imaging agent for either CT or MRI to overcome the lack of specificity and limitation of fluorescence depth of detection.

Until now, only one chemical multimodal probe has reached the phase I clinical trial for renal carcinoma. This probe consists in an antibody (girentuximab) directed against the carbonic anhydrase IX (CAIX), a common target of renal cancerous cells, bound to infrared (IR) fluorescent dye CW800 and the radioactive indium isotope ^{111}In. Early results showed better fluorescent detection of CAIX-positive tumors by using pre-operative SPECT/CT imaging and intraoperative gamma camera. However, the authors noted that the fluorescence intensity had been attenuated by the surrounding fibrous tissue and the tumor capsule [51]. Irrespective of such chemical construction of the probe and the real benefit of multimodal imaging, the intrinsic low photostability and fluorescence shared by most chemical fluorescent dyes raise at least three challenging problems for FGS application.

First, the low photostability of the chemical dye implicates either limited time for surgery, which is not recommended for achieving total peritoneal cytoreduction, or higher amount of injected dye, which seems hazardous because of the dye toxicity. Second, relatively poor fluorescence emitted by the dye decreases the contrast between labeled and unlabeled tissue. To quantify the contrast, SBR is used. SBR measures the sensitivity of imaging device, and remains "the key determinant of sensitivity, detectability, and linearity in optical imaging" [52]. The lack of brightness and weak photostability of organic dyes reduce the SBR to a value above 2 [49], while the reference research in imaging establishes that SBR must be above 5 to reliably identify the object with absolute certainty [53]. Finally, this kind of "chemical fluorophore-based" construction is obviously difficult to adapt to another probe. Third, similar to ICG, CW800 is slowly excreted through the hepatobiliary way [49], resulting in contamination of the surgical field by the remnant unbounded fluorescent dye [54].

To summarize this part of the review on clinical advances in FGS, it is obvious that future probes will require bright and photo-resistant IR fluorescent dyes adaptable to multimodality and tumor targeting. In addition, the probe must be safe and rapidly excreted from the body to avoid fluorescence "contamination" and risk of toxicity in the long term. NIR nanoparticles (NPs) constitute alternative and seductive chemical constructs with the potential to fulfill all these requirements.

3. Overview of NIR Nanoparticles

NIR-fluorescent NPs (Figure 1) possess common advantages (Table 1). First, they have higher brightness, which is the product of a far superior molar attenuation coefficient (absorption of light per mol) and very satisfying quantum yields (the ratio between emitted and absorbed photons) than any organic fluorophores, providing higher SBR [55]. In the case of long operative time such as during cytoreduction, NIR NPs maintain photostability without the production of toxic photoproducts.

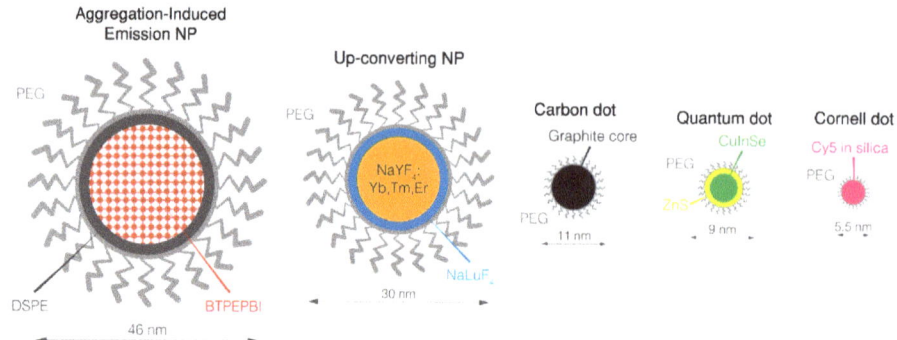

Figure 1. Overview of NIR nanoparticles. BTPEPBI: 1,7-tetraphenylethene modified 3,4:9,10-Tetracarboxylic perylene bisimide; Cy5: cyanine 5; DSPE: 1,2-distearoyl-*sn*-glycero-3-phosphoethanolamine-*N*-[amino(polyethylene glycol)]; NP: nanoparticle; PEG: poly(ethyleneglycol).

Similar to protein/ICG complexes, NPs can accumulate in tumors by EPR effect. Finally, most of them offer a versatile surface which can be easily modified for targeting and combined with another imaging modality to achieve even more effective multimodal probe.

Table 1. Fluorescent near-Infrared Dye and their characteristics.

Spectra				Near-Infrared				
Name	ICG	OTL-38	Quantum Dots	UCNP	Carbon Dot	AIE NP	Cornell Dots
Component	$C_{43}H_{47}N_2NaO_6S_2$	$C_{61}H_{63}N_9O_{17}S_4/4Na$	CuInSe/ZnS(Mn) ZnSeHg	Yb, Tm, Er doped $NaYF_4$ nanocrystal/$NaLuF_4$ shell	Graphite core	Organic core	Cyanine 5 core and silica shell
Size (nm)	–	–	9.0 (CuInSe/ZnS(Mn) 6.6 (ZnSeHg)	30	11	46	5.5
Coating	–	–	PEG	PEG	PEG	PEG	PEG
Targeting	–	Folate	iRGD	–	–	Folate	cRGD
Excretion	Hepatobiliary	Hepatobiliary	–	–	–	Hepatobiliary	Renal
Multimodality	–	–	MRI (Mn)	–	–	–	PET (^{124}I)
Photostability	Low	Low	High	High	High	High	High
Excitation (nm)	805	774	690 (CuInSe) 785 (ZnSeHg)	980 (multiphotonic)	633	635	650
Emission peak (nm)	835	794	685(CuInSe/ZnS(Mn)) >800 (ZnSeHg)	800	>710	810–815	670
SBR of i.p. tumor	2 ± 1	4.4	12	>5	–	7.2	–
Results in vivo	–	–	–	Passive accumulation in peritoneal tumors following i.p. injection	SBR ≈ 2 in subcutaneously injected matrigel	Allow the detection of sub-millimetric peritoneal tumors	–
Clinical	Low specificity	Improved cytoreduction	–	–	–	–	Preferential uptake of Cornell dots at the site of the disease, in vivo stability and safety
Reference	[47–49]	[50]	[56,57]	[58]	[59]	[60]	[61–65]

Abbreviations: AIE: aggregation-induced emission; ICG: indocyanine green; i.p.: intraperitoneal; MRI: molecular resonance imaging; NP: nanoparticle; OTL: on target laboratories incorporated (West Lafayette, USA); PEG: poly(ethyleneglycol); PET: positron emission tomography; SBR: signal-to-background ratio; UCNP: up-converting nanoparticle.

3.1. Quantum Dots

Quantum dots (QD) are small fluorescent nanocrystals composed of semiconductor compounds. Unlike organic fluorophores, QD offer broad absorption and narrow emission spectra. Their emission wavelength depends on the composition and the size of nanocrystal (e.g., 3 nm PbS QD emits around 800 nm while the increasing diameter up to 6.5 nm leads to the emission wavelength more than 1500 nm) [66].

They are mainly synthetized through colloidal chemical syntheses, under inert atmosphere, where metallic precursors are suspended in organic solvent, such as octadecene, and heated at high temperature. The precursors decompose to form monomers that nucleate, thus creating very small nanocrystals. The second step is the growing stage of the nuclei and QD increase in size until they reach the desired one. Then, the solution is cooled very quickly to stop the growth. Subsequently, hydrophobic QD are transferred into water through ligand exchange (using mercaptopropionic acid for instance) or phospholipid micelle encapsulation. These syntheses allow very high quantum yield, even in the near-infrared range. The synthesis of hydrophilic QD has also been developed through the hydrothermal process, where organic solvent is replaced by water with either stabilizer or reverse micelles. However, these last hydrothermal syntheses have a higher polydispersity and a lower quantum yield in comparison with organic synthesis.

QD are currently among the brightest known NPs. In addition, they possess longer fluorescence lifetime, from tens to hundreds of nanoseconds or even microseconds, which may be used to selectively detect QD fluorescence while eliminating autofluorescence background [67]. Therefore, QDs with variable composition and size have been developed toward their clinical applications in FGS.

Beside these attractive optical properties, the weakness of most NIR QDs comes from their composition, which is commonly based on heavy metals, such as cadmium (Cd) or lead (Pb). Despite their in vitro stability, QDs can quickly degrade in the hepatocyte cells (Hep G2) model. Following intravenous injection, QDs typically accumulate mainly in the liver and the kidney with therefore hazardous long-term consequences [68,69]. Toxicity results from Cd accumulation in the liver while Te mainly accumulates in the kidney [69,70]. The ionic leach of Cd is presumed to be the main cause of QD toxicity since the production of induced oxidative stress was proven through the role of metallothionein in cadmium retention [71]. Therefore, to protect QD from degradation, a shell constituted by different compounds such as zinc sulfide (ZnS) was placed around the QD core [72]. In addition, NIR-emitting QDs based on less toxic components, such as silver (Ag) or Indium (In), have also been developed [73]. QDs can easily be combined with other imaging modality, such as paramagnetic ion to obtain multimodal probe [56], while functionalization of their surface chemistry enables grafting of targeting moieties [74].

3.2. Up-Converting Nanoparticles (UCNP)

Up-Converting Nanoparticles (UCNPs) represent another type of solvothermal or hydrothermal made fluorescent nanocrystals, based on lanthanide atoms. The mechanism of NIR fluorescence emitted by UCNP is particular. These NPs emit in the NIR after excitation at longer wavelengths (usually 980 nm), through a multiphoton conversion process [75,76]. In addition to providing excellent penetration depth, this modality eliminates the autofluorescence background [77]. NIR UCNPs have already been used for murine peritoneal carcinomatosis imaging, showing satisfying imaging properties. The authors highlighted the good biocompatibility of UCNPs and the fact that some lanthanides, such as chelate gadolinium, are already FDA-approved for MRI imaging [58], and seem to be less concerned by toxicity issues [78]. However, gadolinium is raising safety concerns, especially due to its potential leaching in the absence of chelates [79].

Therefore, the behavior of lanthanide metals in the body through their metabolism and cell interactions remains to be elucidated to fully ensure the safety of UCNPs [80], while less toxic rare-earth elements, such yttrium, should be preferred to gadolinium [81].

3.3. Carbon Dots

Carbon dots (CD) are a new kind of NP, gaining growing interest since 2004. They are made from carbonated molecules with wide approach either from fragmented bulk material or carbonized soluble substrate.

Their synthesis mainly implicates calcination and/or solvothermal process, either at high or low temperature in acidic or basic conditions. The production of a graphene core depends on the organic precursor and the synthesis process.

To significantly enhance the photophysical properties, the carbon particle core can be doped with an inorganic salt such as ZnS before surface functionalization [82]. Similar to QD, some CDs are characterized by high quantum yields and photostability with the advantage to be purely organic [83]. CD-labeled matrigel grafted in mice can be detected in the NIR range with a SBR above 2 [59].

Therefore, low-cost CDs have been rapidly investigated in bioimaging showing high biocompatibility and acceptable fluorescence properties [84,85].

3.4. Aggregation-Induced Emission Dyes

Self-quenching is a well-known phenomenon common to many organic dyes such as ICG or fluorescein, which lose their fluorescence efficiency at high concentrations or upon aggregation. By contrast, some organic luminophores emit fluorescence only in the aggregated state. This phenomenon, namely aggregation-induced emission (AIE), takes advantage of high brightness, strong photostability and, as with most classical organic fluorophores, good biocompatibility [86].

However, their high hydrophobicity requires an encapsulation step by adding amphiphilic polymers, such as pluronic F127 in organic solvent such as chloroform or tetrahydrofuran. Solvents are eliminated through evaporation. Then, mixes of AIE luminogen and polymer are resuspended and sonicated to obtain hydrophilic AIE NP.

Intravenously injected AIE NPs accumulate in tumors by the EPR effect, and detection of sub-millimetric peritoneal tumors were achieved with the satisfying SBR of 7.2 [87]. In addition, targeting of AIE NPs can be also proposed. NIR AIE NPs with folic acid as targeting agent display enhanced fluorescence in folate receptor positive MCF7 cells and in subcutaneous tumor-bearing mice [60].

3.5. Silica-Encapsulated Dyes

Finally, silica-encapsulated dyes differ from the NPs described above by the protective confinement offered by the silica shell [61,88]. Silica surface confers the advantage to be easily adapted to various imaging modalities and targeting agents. For example, NIR dyes such as cyanine 7 encapsulated in a silica nanoparticle were investigated for sentinel lymph node mapping [88]. They demonstrated enhanced brightness and photostability, which made them interesting probes for long operative times without the need for reinjection or high initial dose.

Cornell dots (C-dots) are ultrasmall (less than 10 nm) core/shell silica NPs, which can fulfill FGS requirements with their remarkable properties. Their synthesis relies on a modified sol-gel process, where cyanine derivative is crosslinked with silica precursor, and react to form a fluorescent core. A silica shell is then added to form a core shell structure.

To date, the C-dots are the only type of silica nanoparticles to have reached clinical trial phase I. First, after encapsulation of cyanine 5 NIR-fluorescent dye, the emission of the dye remains unchanged while both photostability and brightness were greatly increased, leading to the enhancement of SBR [62]. Second, C-dots were designed to avoid the major drawbacks of the QDs as with NPs: bio-accumulation and induced toxicity [89]. Ultrasmall, to target the renal excretion windows, C-dots can be renally excreted intact from animals [61] and humans [63]. Besides the reduction of the cytotoxic risk, this fast excretion offers better imagery by rapid reduction of the remnant probe background. Third, these NIR-fluorescent NPs possess all advantages of the versatile surface chemistry of silica NPs. Appropriate coating, for example with PEG, can be easily applied and associated with a targeting agent such as cRGDY, which target $\alpha v\beta_3$-integrins and with another imaging agent such as the smallest radioactive iodine covalently linked to the cRGDY moiety. It is acknowledged that integrins play a key role during the whole metastatic process of ovarian cancer [64]. Therefore, $\alpha v\beta_3$-integrin appears to be an appropriate target for this type of cancer [90], although integrin expression may vary between patients [91]. For this purpose, Philipps et al. (2014) performed PET imaging using such a construction on patients with various types of cancer, allowing the detection of different integrin-positive lesions, from the liver to the pituitary gland, proving that intravenously injected C-dots can cross blood–brain barrier [63]. Therefore, an FGS probe should be available with different targeting to fulfill individual patient needs.

Currently, C-dots have entered early phase I clinical trials (NCT02106598) for Image-Guided Intraoperative Sentinel Lymph Node Mapping in Head and Neck Melanoma, Breast and Gynecologic Malignancies. Thus, C-dots are the first NPs to enter clinical trials for FGS. Completion of the study is expected in 2018.

Independent of fluorescence imaging, another property of C-dots was recently highlighted by showing the death of nutrient-deprived cancer cells exposed to C-dots by ferroptosis [65]. This property was confirmed in vivo in two different tumor models, thus conferring unexpected theranostic properties to C-dots.

Finally, C-dots seem able to fill all the criteria required in clinical bioimaging: high brightness, versatility, multimodality and targeting possibilities. In addition, C-dots are safe due to the fast clearance of the unbounded probe and theranostic properties. However, voluntarily made ultrasmall to target the renal clearance window, the few-nanometer size of the C-dot combined with a large-size antibody or a Super Paramagnetic Iron Oxide Nanoparticle (SPION) could hamper renal elimination, resulting in a decrease in safety.

4. Toward the Short-Wave Infrared

Another possibility to considerably improve the fluorescence imaging efficiency is to increase the infrared wavelength emission of the probe. Short-Wave InfraRed (SWIR) between 1000 and 2500 nm is gaining increasing attention in biological application, especially because of biological chromophore absorption and tissue scattering that are reduced in the 1000–1300 nm "transparent" window. Computational and in vitro simulation have long predicted that SWIR fluorescence could greatly outperform NIR fluorescence imaging, but SWIR imaging cameras have not been made widely available until recently [92]. Therefore, FGS devices were mainly focused on the NIR window and the development of FDA-approved NIR excitation sources [32].

SWIR cameras based on InGaAs sensor offer broad imaging facilities in the SWIR range [93]. Currently they are widely available in many fields of investigations including medical [94] and clinical predevelopment devices [95]. Moreover, the prediction of SWIR dye superiority as compared to NIR ones was confirmed by bioimaging [96,97]. While NIR provides a penetration depth of one or two millimeters, SWIR easily pushes the depth limit to five millimeters [98] making SWIR promising, especially for peritoneal cytoreduction.

However, SWIR dyes remain scarce and not efficient enough. The state-of-the-art dye is the IR-1050 from Nirmidas biotech (Palo Alto, CA, USA) which has several drawbacks [99]. Despite encouraging characteristics and safe renal excretion, IR-1050 displays very low SWIR fluorescence as compared to NIR dyes [100]. As with all organic dyes, IR-1050 is subjected to photobleaching and the attempt to associate it with a targeting agent and/or another imaging modality is similar to trying to square the circle. SWIR-emitting organic dyes are currently under development but their fluorescence quantum yield does not exceed a few percent [101]. Therefore, SWIR-emitting inorganic NPs (Figure 2) appear as interesting alternatives (Table 2).

Table 2. Short-Wave Infrared fluorescent nanoparticles and their characteristics.

Spectra	Short-Wave Infrared						
Name	IR-1050	ICG	Quantum Dot	Lanthanide NP	Gold NP	Phage Stabilized SWCNT	AIE NP
Component	$C_{41}H_{40}BCl_3F_4N_2$	$C_{43}H_{47}N_2NaO_6S_2$	Ag_2S InAs	$NaYF_4$ Yb:Ln core doped with rare-earth $NaYF_4$ shell	Gold	Pure carbon nanotube	Organic core
Size (nm)	–	–	3.0–4.0 (Ag_2S) 4.5 (InAs)	9.0–11	1.6	880 × 6.5 *	33
Coating	–	–	PEG	Polymeric coating by poly(ethylene oxide)	Lipoic acid-based sulfobetaine	Phage M13	Pluronic
Targeting	–	–	–	Folate	–	SPARC-Binding peptide	–
Excretion	Hepatobiliary	Hepatobiliary	Hepatobiliary (Ag_2S)	–	Renal	–	–
Multimodality	–	–	–	–	–	–	–
Photostability	Low	Low	High	High	High	High	High
Excitation (nm)	790	805	808	980	808	808	630
Emission peak (nm)	1050	835	1125 (Ag_2S) 1080–1330 (InAs)	1185 (Ho doped) 1310 (Pr doped) 1475 (Tm doped) 1525 (Er doped)	800–1400	1000 – 1300	808
SBR of i.p. tumor	–	–	14 (Ag_2Se)	>3	–	8	–
Results in vivo	–	–	i.v. injected Ag_2S QDs passively accumulate in subcutaneous murine tumor with a ratio of 10% ID/g tumors	i.p. injected lanthanide NPs accumulate, with or without targeting, in i.p. tumors from ovarian cancer OVCAR8 cell line	–	Effective imaging of peritoneal tumors after i.p. injection, with higher resection rate, especially for sub-millimetric nodules	SBR is 33 at the depth of 150 μm in mouse brain vasculature following i.v. injection
Clinical	–	–	–	–	–	–	–
Reference	[100]	[100]	[93,102,103]	[104]	[105]	[106]	[107]

*—the size of carbon nanotubes is presents as height × diameter. Abbreviations: AIE: aggregation-induced emission; ICG: indocyanine green; ID: injected dose; i.p.: intraperitoneal; i.v.: intravenously; NP: nanoparticle; PEG: Poly(ethyleneglycol); QD: quantum dot; SBR: signal-to-background ratio; SPARC: secreted protein acidic rich in cysteine; SWCNT: single-walled carbon nanotube.

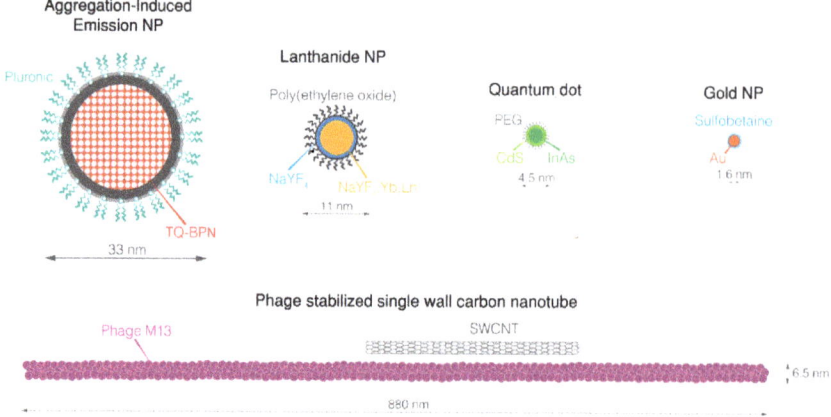

Figure 2. Overview of SWIR nanoparticles. NP, nanoparticle; PEG, poly(ethyleneglycol); SWCNT, Single-walled carbon nanotube; TQ-BNP, N,N'-((6,7-diphenyl-[1,2,5]thiadiazolo[3,4-g]quinoxaline-4,9-diyl)bis(4,1-phenylene))bis(N-phenylnaphthalen-1-amine).

4.1. SWIR QD

Similarly to NIR QDs, the main interest of SWIR QD as compared to other NPs is their outstanding photophysical properties, especially for Ag_2Se QD and InAs QD, resulting in a better signal and higher SBR [96,102,103]. Similar to NIR-emitting QDs, it will be necessary to develop bright SWIR QDs devoid of heavy metals and carefully characterize their in vivo degradation and their potential toxicity.

4.2. Lanthanide Nanoparticles

Next, by their high QY, SWIR lanthanide NPs gained attention for bioimaging. Indeed, several lanthanide NPs have been developed to be absorbed in NIR and to emit in SWIR by the doping of sodium yttrium or gadolinium tetrafluoride nanocrystals, made using a solvo- or hydrothermal process, with different rare-earth elements. These NPs, encapsulated in a 100 nm hydrodynamic diameter albumin shell, were shown to be confined in the peritoneum at least 12 h after intraperitoneal injection [104], while another group reported more than 48 h confinement for similar NPs [108]. Other SWIR fluorescent lanthanide NPs, encapsulated in 100 nm polymeric shell, led to the detection of tumor deposits up to 72 h after intraperitoneal injection in a murine ovarian peritoneal carcinomatosis model. In this case, the process by which NPs remains for a long time in the cavity is still unknown [109]. The undeniable advantage of lanthanide NPs is their relative safety, mainly because of the absence of heavy metal in their composition. For example, microparticles of radioactive yttrium were approved as radiotherapeutic agents for liver malignancies [110]. On the other hand, leaching of Gd ions from $NaGdF_4$ may present severe long-term toxicity issues. If photophysical properties remain a concern for lanthanide nanoparticles, some coatings, such as silica or $NaGdF_4$, have greatly improved it, at least in vitro for now [111].

4.3. Gold Nanoparticles

By reducing chloroauric acid in the presence of lipoic acid sulfobetaine, Chen et al. obtained SWIR fluorescent gold NPs with satisfying biocompatibility. Indeed, these NPs exhibited renal excretion and fast clearance in healthy mice, with fluorescent-observable excretion from circulation to kidney, despite a weak fluorescence. Further studies in animal tumor models could provide more interesting results [105].

4.4. Carbon Nanoparticle

Single-walled carbon nanotubes (SWCNT) are acknowledged for their SWIR emission under NIR excitation. Several synthesis methods exist to produce SWCNT, such as arc discharge, laser ablation and several chemical vapor deposition processes, which are far more productive. The nanoparticle reviewed below is a commercially available SWCNT made using a specific chemical vapor deposition process named high-pressure carbon monoxide method. In this process, carbon monoxide, which acts as carbon source, and iron carbon monoxide catalyst are continuously injected at high temperature, forming high-quality SWCNT.

Despite the low fluorescence of SWCNT, they have pure carbon composition which do not raise many concerns about QD heavy metal content [112]. Their potential toxicity can be adjusted by using appropriate length and coating. Additionally, depending on their design, they can be safely urinarily excreted or biodegraded [113].

Investigated in a murine model of ovarian peritoneal carcinomatosis, SWCNT displayed high imaging capacity upon 808 nm laser excitation. The SBR was superior to 5 in vivo, and up to 100 ex vivo [106]. Compared to unguided surgery, SWCNT guided surgery offered a significantly better detection, with ten times more sub-millimetric tumors excised through fluorescence guidance.

4.5. SWIR Fluorescent Organic Nanoparticles

Several AIE luminogens have a NIR absorption spectrum and display both NIR and weak SWIR fluorescence. Encapsulated in an organic shell such as the pluronic one, these NPs show extended photostability and allow clear visualization of tiny vessels in tissue below 0.8 mm in depth with an SBR higher than 30. They provide suitable properties to detect highly vascularized tumors when used to observe the EPR effect in the subcutaneous murine tumor model [107].

These NPs have the greatest advantage of nontoxic composition, and no adverse effects were observed after intravenous injection. However, their low photophysical properties in the SWIR region is a limiting factor for in-depth detection. Another disadvantage is related to the alteration of fluorescence and photostability upon the addition of a targeting moiety or/and another imaging agent to the NP [114].

5. NP Safety: A Major Concern

NPs are the main attractive newcomer in the field of pharmaceutics and biomedicine over the last decade. However, their exceptional properties raise major concern about safety. NP design significantly affects toxicity as well as targeting ability and biodistribution behavior of NP in vivo [115]. NPs can rely on their nanosize to cross biological barriers and to reach the most sensitive organs [116], ultrasmall NP (few nanometers) are easily endocyted, where then can disrupt cell biochemistry [117]. Therefore, these NPs are presumed more toxic than their larger counterparts [118]. It was proven that a retention for a long period in many organs such as lung and liver can be harmful, thus careful surface functionalization and passivation of NP is important for safe clinical application [119–121].

5.1. Urinary Excretion Is Mainly a Matter of Size

Safe application in clinics suggests total excretion of drugs from the organism. Therefore the main criteria to use these NPs clinically are an ultrasmall size (<5.5 nm) and/or an encapsulation in a biocompatible material likely to promote the excretion renally [122]. Additionally, NPs for FGS require appropriate photophysical properties. Considering that, inorganic NPs, especially QDs, are potent agents which could provide excellent imaging capacities if they can be excreted. Ultrasmall QDs were designed to avoid Kupfer cell endocytosis and to reach the bladder through renal filtration. Choi et al. tested cystein-coated Cd/Se QD of varying sizes and different emission wavelengths. Only the smallest QDs (less than 6 nm) were clearly removed by the renal pathway and were collected in the bladder, whereas the largest ones accumulated mainly in the liver, lungs and spleen [122].

The authors concluded that NPs should have a hydrodynamic diameter below 5.5 nm to achieve complete elimination from the body. However, the excretion rate of ultrasmall NPs is more complex than it seems. In fact, a recent study reported some differences between NPs made with varying amounts of gold atoms. Consistently, 1.7 nm NPs (201 gold atoms) are faster renally removed than 2.5 nm ones, while, surprisingly, lower excretion rate was measured with smallest NPs made of less than 20 atoms of gold. Authors also highlighted the role of the renal glycocalyx which acts like a chromatography filtration gel that allow larger NPs to pass rapidly through [123]. Therefore, it can be assumed that the ideal diameter for a NP is comprised between 1.7 nm and 6 nm to target renal excretion and to obtain an effective clearance. The clinical use of NIR Cd-based QD appears unlikely since many of them did not fit size condition.

Another approach to facilitate the renal excretion is using biocompatible coating such as silica-phosphonate for Cd-based QD. From 11.5 nm hydrodynamic diameter core, Ma et al. produced core/shell QD/silica-phosphonate NPs with a diameter of almost 30 nm. Despite its relatively large hydrodynamic diameter, the NP was mainly urinarily excreted after intravenous injection. In addition, the silica-phosphonate coating produced extended circulation time in blood to decrease liver accumulation [124].

Finally, the design of biodegradable NPs is still under investigation to reach excretion of NP after intravenous injection [125,126]. This approach can be easily applied to silica NP, AIE NP, carbon dot and SWCNT; however, its utilization for NP made of heavy metals or rare-earth elements is limited. In this context, biodegradable and heavy metal-free QDs constitute attractive alternatives. Among them, NIR silicon QDs [127] are small enough (<5 nm) [128], highly biocompatible and are able to be endocytosed by cancerous cells [129]. No toxicity was detected both in mice and monkey models even at high dose of QD (200 mg/kg). The size of silicon QDs varied from 4 to 11 nm, so they are rapidly accumulated both in the liver (the largest fraction) and in the bladder (the smallest fraction). Three months post-injection, high silica content was found in the liver and the spleen due to the retention of the largest QDs in these organs. Consistently, liver damage was histopathologically observed in mice but not in monkeys, suggesting the influence of the anatomical scale between these models exposed to identical amount of silicon QDs [130].

5.2. Rethinking of the Injection Route

Among the drawbacks in toxicity, fluorescent contamination by unbounded dye also must be considered for FGS with NPs. Evidently the biodistribution of fluorescent dye significantly depends on the injection route. For example, a large part of intravenously injected organic dye such as ICG is excreted through the liver and the intestine for a long time. The remaining part of the probe in these organs produces fluorescence contamination which can overshadow the fluorescence emitted by the cancerous tissue, decreasing SBR. Therefore, the renal excretion route is preferable for intravenously injected FGS drugs. A seen above, NPs require small size (less than 6 nm) [123] and probably a specific shape to be renally excreted [131]. This has already been shown clinically with the example of Cornell dots. However, the size of nanoparticle can be adjusted only for the limited numbers of nanomaterials. Thus, whenever possible, systemic exposition should be avoided as the simplest solution.

Additionally, intravenously injected probes demonstrated limited efficiency in the case of sub-millimetric-sized and/or small tumors which are not yet vascularized [132]. For these kind of tumors, the advantages of injection had been proved for organic NIR dyes. After intravenous injection, fluorescent contamination of many organs was observed. The appropriate SBR was displayed only for tumors larger than 5 mm. On the contrary, intraperitoneally injected dye allows detection of small tumors with reduced fluorescent contamination [133]. According to that, the use of the intraperitoneal injection route prevents systemic exposition and fluorescent contamination and provides an opportunity to safely use nanoparticle in clinics for peritoneal carcinomatosis FGS.

Biodistribution of NPs injected by the intraperitoneal route has been recently investigated in several studies reporting promising results. The intraperitoneal injection of QDs facilitated the dissection of peritoneal lymph nodes during the cytoreduction in rats due to rapid lymphatic drainage of the QDs [134]. Kato et al. (2010) monitored the biodistribution of intraperitoneally injected captopril QD by means of mass spectrometry [135]. The authors observed significant difference between QDs injected intraperitoneally and intravenously: only 2.5% of the initial dose of QDs in the liver, 1.5% in the spleen and almost 8% in the bloodstream, and almost 85% of the QDs were not detected in organs and seemed to remain confined to the peritoneal cavity six hours after intraperitoneal injection. Finally, injection of QD by intraperitoneal route showed appropriate toxicity. Adverse effects of mercaptopropionic acid coated QD were observed in mice only after 15 days of repeated intraperitoneal injection of 10 mg/kg [136]. QD induced mild toxicities in liver and lung, which they were detected by fluorescence microscopy.

Obviously intraperitoneally injected NPs can passively accumulate in ovarian peritoneal tumors e.g., lanthanide NPs [109]. However, the majority of FGS drugs possess low tumor selectivity which can be improved by using active targeting molecules. For example, SWCNTs functionalized with the secreted protein acidic and cysteine rich (SPARC)-binding peptide, actively targeting tumors with an SBR up to 5, remaining confined to peritoneal cavity at least for 24 h [106]. Indirect targeting can be also used with success in murine peritoneal carcinomatosis by injecting the peptide iRGD first, to permeate the tumor tissue before injecting NIR QDs. Then, unbounded QDs were bleached by using an etchant, and this step of the procedure allowed the detection of QD-labeled tumors [57]. To increase SBR, a peritoneal washing procedure could also be applied to any type of NPs. At the same time, the "washing" of a peritoneal cavity by etchant could enhance the safety of QDs by removing heavy metals from the organism, for example, in the case of ZnSeHg QDs [57].

6. Conclusions

Ovarian carcinomatosis FGS requires safe drugs, which selectively accumulate in the malignant tissue and provide high SBR for complete cytoreduction. NIR-fluorescent NPs possess all necessary characteristics to be potent FGS probes. To date, Cornell dots are the safest type of NIR NP, which is already in clinical trial phase I. The special design of Cornell dots results in rapid excretion renally following intravenous injection but were never applied for peritoneal carcinomatosis. By contrast, CD, UCNP and QDs were already studied using the intraperitoneal injection route, which is suggested to be the most potent for the detection of ovarian metastases. Obviously, the intraperitoneal route avoids systemic exposition, improving NP safety and providing the opportunity to use active targeting molecules to enhance selectivity and SBR of NPs. Another way to improve SBR is to use SWIR fluorescent NP, which demonstrated extended photostability and provided visualization of tiny vessels below 0.8 mm in tissue depth with an SBR higher than 30. Finally, NPs can be associated with other imaging agents in multimodal approaches to achieve pre-operative whole-body imaging, and precise tumor detection to complete cytoreduction.

Currently, NIR cameras and lasers are already FDA-approved for FGS. SWIR cameras have also become available on the market and are expected to be approved for medical use. In fact, the application of FGS in NIR and SWIR is limited by the number of FDA-approved dyes (ICG and methylene blue), therefore the investigation of NP-based FGS probes is of great interest.

Author Contributions: T.M. designed the review and drafted the manuscript, I.Y., S.M. and M.D. helped with the manuscript editing, I.Y. designed the figures, T.P., L.B. and F.M. reviewed the manuscript drafts. All authors read and approved the final manuscript.

Funding: This work was supported by the Ligue Nationale contre le Cancer, the Institut de Cancérologie de Lorraine and the Lorraine Region.

Acknowledgments: The authors thank Dominique Marius Le Prince (Nancy, France) for the proof-reading and corrections of manuscript.

Conflicts of Interest: The authors declare no conflict of interest.

References

1. Coccolini, F.; Gheza, F.; Lotti, M.; Virzi, S.; Iusco, D.; Ghermandi, C.; Melotti, R.; Baiocchi, G.; Giulini, S.M.; Ansaloni, L.; et al. Peritoneal carcinomatosis. *World J. Gastroenterol.* **2013**, *19*, 6979–6994. [CrossRef] [PubMed]
2. Siegel, R.L.; Miller, K.D.; Jemal, A. Cancer statistics, 2017. *CA Cancer J. Clin.* **2017**, *67*, 7–30. [CrossRef] [PubMed]
3. Cannistra, S.A. Cancer of the Ovary. *N. Engl. J. Med.* **2004**, *351*, 2519–2529. [CrossRef] [PubMed]
4. Baldwin, L.A.; Huang, B.; Miller, R.W.; Tucker, T.; Goodrich, S.T.; Podzielinski, I.; DeSimone, C.P.; Ueland, F.R.; van Nagell, J.R.; Seamon, L.G. Ten-year relative survival for epithelial ovarian cancer. *Obstet. Gynecol.* **2012**, *120*, 612–618. [CrossRef] [PubMed]
5. Prat, J. FIGO's staging classification for cancer of the ovary, fallopian tube, and peritoneum: Abridged republication. *J. Gynecol. Oncol.* **2015**, *26*, 87–89. [CrossRef] [PubMed]
6. Chandrashekhara, S.H.; Triveni, G.S.; Kumar, R. Imaging of peritoneal deposits in ovarian cancer: A pictorial review. *World J. Radiol.* **2016**, *8*, 513–517. [CrossRef] [PubMed]
7. Fagotti, A.; Gallotta, V.; Romano, F.; Fanfani, F.; Rossitto, C.; Naldini, A.; Vigliotta, M.; Scambia, G. Peritoneal carcinosis of ovarian origin. *World J. Gastrointest. Oncol.* **2010**, *2*, 102–108. [CrossRef] [PubMed]
8. Griffiths, C.T.; Parker, L.M.; Fuller, A.F. Role of cytoreductive surgical treatment in the management of advanced ovarian cancer. *Cancer Treat. Rep.* **1979**, *63*, 235–240. [PubMed]
9. Sugarbaker, P.H. *Peritoneal Carcinomatosis: Principles of Management*; Springer Science & Business Media: Berlin, Germany, 1996; ISBN 978-0-7923-3727-0.
10. Nougaret, S.; Addley, H.C.; Colombo, P.E.; Fujii, S.; Al Sharif, S.S.; Tirumani, S.H.; Jardon, K.; Sala, E.; Reinhold, C. Ovarian Carcinomatosis: How the Radiologist Can Help Plan the Surgical Approach. *RadioGraphics* **2012**, *32*, 1775–1800. [CrossRef] [PubMed]
11. Forstner, R.; Meissnitzer, M.; Cunha, T.M. Update on Imaging of Ovarian Cancer. *Curr. Radiol. Rep.* **2016**, *4*, 31. [CrossRef] [PubMed]
12. Albanese, A.M.; Albanese, E.F.; Miño, J.H.; Gómez, E.; Gómez, M.; Zandomeni, M.; Merlo, A.B. Peritoneal surface area: Measurements of 40 structures covered by peritoneum: Correlation between total peritoneal surface area and the surface calculated by formulas. *Surg. Radiol. Anat. SRA* **2009**, *31*, 369–377. [CrossRef] [PubMed]
13. Du Bois, A.; Reuss, A.; Pujade-Lauraine, E.; Harter, P.; Ray-Coquard, I.; Pfisterer, J. Role of surgical outcome as prognostic factor in advanced epithelial ovarian cancer: A combined exploratory analysis of 3 prospectively randomized phase 3 multicenter trials: By the Arbeitsgemeinschaft Gynaekologische Onkologie Studiengruppe Ovarialkarzin. *Cancer* **2009**, *115*, 1234–1244. [CrossRef] [PubMed]
14. Du Bois, A.; Pfisterer, J. Future options for first-line therapy of advanced ovarian cancer. *Int. J. Gynecol. Cancer Off. J. Int. Gynecol. Cancer Soc.* **2005**, *15* (Suppl. 1), 42–50. [CrossRef] [PubMed]
15. Weisberger, A.S.; Levine, B.; Storaasli, J.P. Use of Nitrogen Mustard in Treatment of Serous Effusions of Neoplastic Origin. *J. Am. Med. Assoc.* **1955**, *159*, 1704–1707. [CrossRef] [PubMed]
16. Dedrick, R.L.; Myers, C.E.; Bungay, P.M.; DeVita, V.T. Pharmacokinetic rationale for peritoneal drug administration in the treatment of ovarian cancer. *Cancer Treat. Rep.* **1978**, *62*, 1–11. [PubMed]
17. Torres, I.J.; Litterst, C.L.; Guarino, A.M. Transport of model compounds across the peritoneal membrane in the rat. *Pharmacology* **1978**, *17*, 330–340. [CrossRef] [PubMed]
18. Alberts, D.S.; Liu, P.Y.; Hannigan, E.V.; O'Toole, R.; Williams, S.D.; Young, J.A.; Franklin, E.W.; Clarke-Pearson, D.L.; Malviya, V.K.; DuBeshter, B. Intraperitoneal cisplatin plus intravenous cyclophosphamide versus intravenous cisplatin plus intravenous cyclophosphamide for stage III ovarian cancer. *N. Engl. J. Med.* **1996**, *335*, 1950–1955. [CrossRef] [PubMed]
19. Howell, S.B.; Zimm, S.; Markman, M.; Abramson, I.S.; Cleary, S.; Lucas, W.E.; Weiss, R.J. Long-term survival of advanced refractory ovarian carcinoma patients with small-volume disease treated with intraperitoneal chemotherapy. *J. Clin. Oncol.* **1987**, *5*, 1607–1612. [CrossRef] [PubMed]
20. Ozols, R.F.; Gore, M.; Tropé, C.; Grenman, S. Intraperitoneal treatment and dose-intense therapy in ovarian cancer. *Ann. Oncol.* **1999**, *10* (Suppl. 1), 59–64. [CrossRef] [PubMed]
21. Los, G.; Verdegaal, E.M.; Mutsaers, P.H.; McVie, J.G. Penetration of carboplatin and cisplatin into rat peritoneal tumor nodules after intraperitoneal chemotherapy. *Cancer Chemother. Pharmacol.* **1991**, *28*, 159–165. [CrossRef] [PubMed]

22. Eoh, K.J.; Lee, J.Y.; Nam, E.J.; Kim, S.; Kim, Y.T.; Kim, S.W. Long-Term Survival Analysis of Intraperitoneal versus Intravenous Chemotherapy for Primary Ovarian Cancer and Comparison between Carboplatin- and Cisplatin-based Intraperitoneal Chemotherapy. *J. Korean Med. Sci.* **2017**, *32*, 2021–2028. [CrossRef] [PubMed]
23. Tewari, D.; Java, J.J.; Salani, R.; Armstrong, D.K.; Markman, M.; Herzog, T.; Monk, B.J.; Chan, J.K. Long-Term Survival Advantage and Prognostic Factors Associated With Intraperitoneal Chemotherapy Treatment in Advanced Ovarian Cancer: A Gynecologic Oncology Group Study. *J. Clin. Oncol.* **2015**, *33*, 1460–1466. [CrossRef] [PubMed]
24. Elias, D.; Antoun, S.; Goharin, A.; Otmany, A.E.; Puizillout, J.M.; Lasser, P. Research on the best chemohyperthermia technique of treatment of peritoneal carcinomatosis after complete resection. *Int. J. Surg. Investig.* **2000**, *1*, 431–439. [PubMed]
25. Van Driel, W.J.; Koole, S.N.; Sikorska, K.; Schagen van Leeuwen, J.H.; Schreuder, H.W.R.; Hermans, R.H.M.; de Hingh, I.H.J.T.; van der Velden, J.; Arts, H.J.; Massuger, L.F.A.G.; et al. Hyperthermic Intraperitoneal Chemotherapy in Ovarian Cancer. *N. Engl. J. Med.* **2018**, *378*, 230–240. [CrossRef] [PubMed]
26. Elattar, A.; Bryant, A.; Winter-Roach, B.A.; Hatem, M.; Naik, R. Optimal primary surgical treatment for advanced epithelial ovarian cancer. *Cochrane Database Syst. Rev.* **2011**, CD007565. [CrossRef] [PubMed]
27. Hoskins, W.J.; Bundy, B.N.; Thigpen, J.T.; Omura, G.A. The influence of cytoreductive surgery on recurrence-free interval and survival in small-volume stage III epithelial ovarian cancer: A Gynecologic Oncology Group study. *Gynecol. Oncol.* **1992**, *47*, 159–166. [CrossRef]
28. Vermeulen, C.K.M.; Tadesse, W.; Timmermans, M.; Kruitwagen, R.F.P.M.; Walsh, T. Only complete tumour resection after neoadjuvant chemotherapy offers benefit over suboptimal debulking in advanced ovarian cancer. *Eur. J. Obstet. Gynecol. Reprod. Biol.* **2017**, *219*, 100–105. [CrossRef] [PubMed]
29. Du Bois, A.; Lück, H.-J.; Meier, W.; Adams, H.-P.; Möbus, V.; Costa, S.; Bauknecht, T.; Richter, B.; Warm, M.; Schröder, W.; et al. Arbeitsgemeinschaft Gynäkologische Onkologie Ovarian Cancer Study Group A randomized clinical trial of cisplatin/paclitaxel versus carboplatin/paclitaxel as first-line treatment of ovarian cancer. *J. Natl. Cancer Inst.* **2003**, *95*, 1320–1329. [CrossRef] [PubMed]
30. Lakhman, Y.; Akin, O.; Sohn, M.J.; Zheng, J.; Moskowitz, C.S.; Iyer, R.B.; Barakat, R.R.; Sabbatini, P.J.; Chi, D.S.; Hricak, H. Early postoperative CT as a prognostic biomarker in patients with advanced ovarian, tubal, and primary peritoneal cancer deemed optimally debulked at primary cytoreductive surgery. *AJR Am. J. Roentgenol.* **2012**, *198*, 1453–1459. [CrossRef] [PubMed]
31. Butler, J.; Gildea, C.; Poole, J.; Meechan, D.; Nordin, A. Specialist surgery for ovarian cancer in England. *Gynecol. Oncol.* **2015**, *138*, 700–706. [CrossRef] [PubMed]
32. DSouza, A.V.; Lin, H.; Henderson, E.R.; Samkoe, K.S.; Pogue, B.W. Review of fluorescence guided surgery systems: Identification of key performance capabilities beyond indocyanine green imaging. *J. Biomed. Opt.* **2016**, *21*, 080901. [CrossRef] [PubMed]
33. Herly, L. Studies in Selective Differentiation of Tissues by Means of Filtered Ultraviolet Light. *Cancer Res.* **1944**, *4*, 227–231.
34. Moore, G.E. Fluorescein as an Agent in the Differentiation of Normal and Malignant Tissues. *Science* **1947**, *106*, 130–131. [CrossRef] [PubMed]
35. Moore, G.E.; Peyton, W.T.; French, L.A.; Walker, W.W. The clinical use of fluorescein in neurosurgery. *J. Neurosurg.* **1948**, *5*, 392–398. [CrossRef] [PubMed]
36. Senders, J.T.; Muskens, I.S.; Schnoor, R.; Karhade, A.V.; Cote, D.J.; Smith, T.R.; Broekman, M.L.D. Agents for fluorescence-guided glioma surgery: A systematic review of preclinical and clinical results. *Acta Neurochir. (Wien)* **2017**, *159*, 151–167. [CrossRef] [PubMed]
37. Van Dam, G.M.; Themelis, G.; Crane, L.M.A.; Harlaar, N.J.; Pleijhuis, R.G.; Kelder, W.; Sarantopoulos, A.; de Jong, J.S.; Arts, H.J.G.; van der Zee, A.G.J.; et al. Intraoperative tumor-specific fluorescence imaging in ovarian cancer by folate receptor-α targeting: First in-human results. *Nat. Med.* **2011**, *17*, 1315–1319. [CrossRef] [PubMed]
38. Vahrmeijer, A.L.; Hutteman, M.; van der Vorst, J.R.; van de Velde, C.J.H.; Frangioni, J.V. Image-guided cancer surgery using near-infrared fluorescence. *Nat. Rev. Clin. Oncol.* **2013**, *10*, 507–518. [CrossRef] [PubMed]
39. Leblond, F.; Davis, S.C.; Valdés, P.A.; Pogue, B.W. Pre-clinical whole-body fluorescence imaging: Review of instruments, methods and applications. *J. Photochem. Photobiol. B* **2010**, *98*, 77–94. [CrossRef] [PubMed]
40. Samanta, A.; Vendrell, M.; Das, R.; Chang, Y.-T. Development of photostable near-infrared cyanine dyes. *Chem. Commun. Camb. Engl.* **2010**, *46*, 7406–7408. [CrossRef] [PubMed]

41. Umezawa, K.; Nakamura, Y.; Makino, H.; Citterio, D.; Suzuki, K. Bright, color-tunable fluorescent dyes in the visible-near-infrared region. *J. Am. Chem. Soc.* **2008**, *130*, 1550–1551. [CrossRef] [PubMed]
42. Yuan, L.; Lin, W.; Yang, Y.; Chen, H. A unique class of near-infrared functional fluorescent dyes with carboxylic-acid-modulated fluorescence ON/OFF switching: Rational design, synthesis, optical properties, theoretical calculations, and applications for fluorescence imaging in living animals. *J. Am. Chem. Soc.* **2012**, *134*, 1200–1211. [CrossRef] [PubMed]
43. Reinhart, M.B.; Huntington, C.R.; Blair, L.J.; Heniford, B.T.; Augenstein, V.A. Indocyanine Green: Historical Context, Current Applications, and Future Considerations. *Surg. Innov.* **2016**, *23*, 166–175. [CrossRef] [PubMed]
44. Zhu, B.; Sevick-Muraca, E.M. A review of performance of near-infrared fluorescence imaging devices used in clinical studies. *Br. J. Radiol.* **2014**, *88*, 20140547. [CrossRef] [PubMed]
45. Maeda, H.; Wu, J.; Sawa, T.; Matsumara, Y.; Hori, K. Tumor vascular permeability and the EPR effect in macromolecular therapeutics: A review. *J. Control. Release* **2000**, *65*, 271–284. [CrossRef]
46. Shibasaki, Y.; Morita, Y.; Sakaguchi, T.; Konno, H. Indocyanine Green-Related Transporters in Hepatocellular Carcinoma. *SpringerLink* **2016**, 351–362. [CrossRef]
47. Kosaka, N.; Mitsunaga, M.; Longmire, M.R.; Choyke, P.L.; Kobayashi, H. Near infrared fluorescence-guided real-time endoscopic detection of peritoneal ovarian cancer nodules using intravenously injected indocyanine green. *Int. J. Cancer J. Int. Cancer* **2011**, *129*, 1671–1677. [CrossRef] [PubMed]
48. Tummers, Q.R.J.G.; Hoogstins, C.E.S.; Peters, A.A.W.; de Kroon, C.D.; Trimbos, J.B.M.Z.; van de Velde, C.J.H.; Frangioni, J.V.; Vahrmeijer, A.L.; Gaarenstroom, K.N. The Value of Intraoperative Near-Infrared Fluorescence Imaging Based on Enhanced Permeability and Retention of Indocyanine Green: Feasibility and False-Positives in Ovarian Cancer. *PLoS ONE* **2015**, *10*, e0129766. [CrossRef] [PubMed]
49. Tanaka, E.; Choi, H.S.; Humblet, V.; Ohnishi, S.; Laurence, R.G.; Frangioni, J.V. Real-time intraoperative assessment of the extrahepatic bile ducts in rats and pigs using invisible near-infrared fluorescent light. *Surgery* **2008**, *144*, 39–48. [CrossRef] [PubMed]
50. Hoogstins, C.E.S.; Tummers, Q.R.J.G.; Gaarenstroom, K.N.; de Kroon, C.D.; Trimbos, J.B.M.Z.; Bosse, T.; Smit, V.T.H.B.M.; Vuyk, J.; van de Velde, C.J.H.; Cohen, A.F.; et al. A Novel Tumor-Specific Agent for Intraoperative Near-Infrared Fluorescence Imaging: A Translational Study in Healthy Volunteers and Patients with Ovarian Cancer. *Clin. Cancer Res.* **2016**, *22*, 2929–2938. [CrossRef] [PubMed]
51. Hekman, M.; Rijpkema, M.; Oosterwijk, E.; Langenhuijsen, H.; Boerman, O.; Oyen, W.; Mulders, P. Intraoperative dual-modality imaging in clear cell renal cell carcinoma using Indium-111-DOTA-girentuximab-IRDye800CW. *Eur. Urol. Suppl.* **2017**, *16*, e1831. [CrossRef]
52. Choi, H.S.; Gibbs, S.L.; Lee, J.H.; Kim, S.H.; Ashitate, Y.; Liu, F.; Hyun, H.; Park, G.; Xie, Y.; Bae, S.; et al. Targeted zwitterionic near-infrared fluorophores for improved optical imaging. *Nat. Biotechnol.* **2013**, *31*, 148–153. [CrossRef] [PubMed]
53. Rose, A. A Unified Approach to the Performance of Photographic Film, Television Pickup Tubes, and the Human Eye. *J. Soc. Motion Pict. Eng.* **1946**, *47*, 273–294. [CrossRef]
54. Kusano, M.; Kokudo, N.; Toi, M.; Kaibori, M. *ICG Fluorescence Imaging and Navigation Surgery*; Springer: Berlin, Germany, 2016; ISBN 978-4-431-55528-5.
55. Choi, H.S.; Frangioni, J.V. Nanoparticles for Biomedical Imaging: Fundamentals of Clinical Translation. *Mol. Imaging* **2010**, *9*, 291–310. [CrossRef] [PubMed]
56. Sitbon, G.; Bouccara, S.; Tasso, M.; Francois, A.; Bezdetnaya, L.; Marchal, F.; Beaumont, M.; Pons, T. Multimodal Mn-doped I-III-VI quantum dots for near infrared fluorescence and magnetic resonance imaging: From synthesis to in vivo application. *Nanoscale* **2014**, *6*, 9264–9272. [CrossRef] [PubMed]
57. Liu, X.; Braun, G.B.; Qin, M.; Ruoslahti, E.; Sugahara, K.N. In vivo cation exchange in quantum dots for tumor-specific imaging. *Nat. Commun.* **2017**, *8*, 343. [CrossRef] [PubMed]
58. Gao, Y.; Liu, L.; Shen, B.; Chen, X.; Wang, L.; Wang, L.; Feng, W.; Huang, C.; Li, F. Amphiphilic PEGylated Lanthanide-Doped Upconversion Nanoparticles for Significantly Passive Accumulation in the Peritoneal Metastatic Carcinomatosis Models Following Intraperitoneal Administration. *ACS Biomater. Sci. Eng.* **2017**, *3*, 2176–2184. [CrossRef]
59. Ko, H.Y.; Chang, Y.W.; Paramasivam, G.; Jeong, M.S.; Cho, S.; Kim, S. In vivo imaging of tumour bearing near-infrared fluorescence-emitting carbon nanodots derived from tire soot. *Chem. Commun. Camb. Engl.* **2013**, *49*, 10290–10292. [CrossRef] [PubMed]

60. Zhao, Q.; Li, K.; Chen, S.; Qin, A.; Ding, D.; Zhang, S.; Liu, Y.; Liu, B.; Sun, J.Z.; Tang, B.Z. Aggregation-induced red-NIR emission organic nanoparticles as effective and photostable fluorescent probes for bioimaging. *J. Mater. Chem.* **2012**, *22*, 15128–15135. [CrossRef]
61. Burns, A.A.; Vider, J.; Ow, H.; Herz, E.; Penate-Medina, O.; Baumgart, M.; Larson, S.M.; Wiesner, U.; Bradbury, M. Fluorescent silica nanoparticles with efficient urinary excretion for nanomedicine. *Nano Lett.* **2009**, *9*, 442–448. [CrossRef] [PubMed]
62. Burns, A.; Ow, H.; Wiesner, U. Fluorescent core–shell silica nanoparticles: Towards "Lab on a Particle" architectures for nanobiotechnology. *Chem. Soc. Rev.* **2006**, *35*, 1028–1042. [CrossRef] [PubMed]
63. Phillips, E.; Penate-Medina, O.; Zanzonico, P.B.; Carvajal, R.D.; Mohan, P.; Ye, Y.; Humm, J.; Gönen, M.; Kalaigian, H.; Schöder, H.; et al. Clinical translation of an ultrasmall inorganic optical-PET imaging nanoparticle probe. *Sci. Transl. Med.* **2014**, *6*, 260ra149. [CrossRef] [PubMed]
64. Landen, C.N.; Kim, T.-J.; Lin, Y.G.; Merritt, W.M.; Kamat, A.A.; Han, L.Y.; Spannuth, W.A.; Nick, A.M.; Jennnings, N.B.; Kinch, M.S.; et al. Tumor-Selective Response to Antibody-Mediated Targeting of αvβ3 Integrin in Ovarian Cancer. *Neoplasia* **2008**, *10*, 1259–1267. [CrossRef] [PubMed]
65. Kim, S.E.; Zhang, L.; Ma, K.; Riegman, M.; Chen, F.; Ingold, I.; Conrad, M.; Turker, M.Z.; Gao, M.; Jiang, X.; et al. Ultrasmall nanoparticles induce ferroptosis in nutrient-deprived cancer cells and suppress tumour growth. *Nat. Nanotechnol.* **2016**, *11*, 977–985. [CrossRef] [PubMed]
66. Lacroix, L.-M.; Delpech, F.; Nayral, C.; Lachaize, S.; Chaudret, B. New generation of magnetic and luminescent nanoparticles for in vivo real-time imaging. *Interface Focus* **2013**, *3*, 20120103. [CrossRef] [PubMed]
67. Damalakiene, L.; Karabanovas, V.; Bagdonas, S.; Rotomskis, R. Fluorescence-Lifetime Imaging Microscopy for Visualization of Quantum Dots' Endocytic Pathway. *Int. J. Mol. Sci.* **2016**, *17*. [CrossRef]
68. Helle, M.; Cassette, E.; Bezdetnaya, L.; Pons, T.; Leroux, A.; Plénat, F.; Guillemin, F.; Dubertret, B.; Marchal, F. Visualisation of sentinel lymph node with indium-based near infrared emitting Quantum Dots in a murine metastatic breast cancer model. *PLoS ONE* **2012**, *7*, e44433. [CrossRef] [PubMed]
69. Liu, N.; Mu, Y.; Chen, Y.; Sun, H.; Han, S.; Wang, M.; Wang, H.; Li, Y.; Xu, Q.; Huang, P.; et al. Degradation of aqueous synthesized CdTe/ZnS quantum dots in mice: Differential blood kinetics and biodistribution of cadmium and tellurium. *Part. Fibre Toxicol.* **2013**, *10*, 37. [CrossRef] [PubMed]
70. Han, Y.; Xie, G.; Sun, Z.; Mu, Y.; Han, S.; Xiao, Y.; Liu, N.; Wang, H.; Guo, C.; Shi, Z.; et al. Plasma kinetics and biodistribution of water-soluble CdTe quantum dots in mice: A comparison between Cd and Te. *J. Nanopart. Res.* **2011**, *13*, 5373. [CrossRef]
71. Lin, C.-H.; Chang, L.W.; Chang, H.; Yang, M.-H.; Yang, C.-S.; Lai, W.-H.; Chang, W.-H.; Lin, P. The chemical fate of the Cd/Se/Te-based quantum dot 705 in the biological system: Toxicity implications. *Nanotechnology* **2009**, *20*, 215101. [CrossRef] [PubMed]
72. Derfus, A.M.; Chan, W.C.W.; Bhatia, S.N. Probing the Cytotoxicity of Semiconductor Quantum Dots. *Nano Lett.* **2004**, *4*, 11–18. [CrossRef] [PubMed]
73. Cassette, E.; Helle, M.; Bezdetnaya, L.; Marchal, F.; Dubertret, B.; Pons, T. Design of new quantum dot materials for deep tissue infrared imaging. *Adv. Drug Deliv. Rev.* **2013**, *65*, 719–731. [CrossRef] [PubMed]
74. Duman, F.D.; Erkisa, M.; Khodadust, R.; Ari, F.; Ulukaya, E.; Acar, H.Y. Folic acid-conjugated cationic Ag2S quantum dots for optical imaging and selective doxorubicin delivery to HeLa cells. *Nanomedicine* **2017**, *12*, 2319–2333. [CrossRef] [PubMed]
75. Chen, G.; Qiu, H.; Prasad, P.N.; Chen, X. Upconversion Nanoparticles: Design, Nanochemistry, and Applications in Theranostics. *Chem. Rev.* **2014**, *114*, 5161–5214. [CrossRef] [PubMed]
76. Zhu, X.; Su, Q.; Feng, W.; Li, F. Anti-Stokes shift luminescent materials for bio-applications. *Chem. Soc. Rev.* **2017**, *46*, 1025–1039. [CrossRef] [PubMed]
77. González-Béjar, M.; Francés-Soriano, L.; Pérez-Prieto, J. Upconversion Nanoparticles for Bioimaging and Regenerative Medicine. *Front. Bioeng. Biotechnol.* **2016**, *4*, 47. [CrossRef] [PubMed]
78. Hirano, S.; Suzuki, K.T. Exposure, metabolism, and toxicity of rare earths and related compounds. *Environ. Health Perspect.* **1996**, *104*, 85–95. [CrossRef] [PubMed]
79. Rogosnitzky, M.; Branch, S. Gadolinium-based contrast agent toxicity: A review of known and proposed mechanisms. *Biometals* **2016**, *29*, 365–376. [CrossRef] [PubMed]

80. Chan, M.-H.; Liu, R.-S. Advanced sensing, imaging, and therapy nanoplatforms based on Nd^{3+}-doped nanoparticle composites exhibiting upconversion induced by 808 nm near-infrared light. *Nanoscale* **2017**, *9*, 18153–18168. [CrossRef] [PubMed]
81. Rim, K.T.; Koo, K.H.; Park, J.S. Toxicological Evaluations of Rare Earths and Their Health Impacts to Workers: A Literature Review. *Saf. Health Work* **2013**, *4*, 12–26. [CrossRef] [PubMed]
82. Cao, L.; Yang, S.-T.; Wang, X.; Luo, P.G.; Liu, J.-H.; Sahu, S.; Liu, Y.; Sun, Y.-P. Competitive Performance of Carbon "Quantum" Dots in Optical Bioimaging. *Theranostics* **2012**, *2*, 295–301. [CrossRef] [PubMed]
83. Zhu, S.; Meng, Q.; Wang, L.; Zhang, J.; Song, Y.; Jin, H.; Zhang, K.; Sun, H.; Wang, H.; Yang, B. Highly Photoluminescent Carbon Dots for Multicolor Patterning, Sensors, and Bioimaging. *Angew. Chem. Int. Ed.* **2013**, *52*, 3953–3957. [CrossRef] [PubMed]
84. Cao, L.; Wang, X.; Meziani, M.J.; Lu, F.; Wang, H.; Luo, P.G.; Lin, Y.; Harruff, B.A.; Veca, L.M.; Murray, D.; et al. Carbon Dots for Multiphoton Bioimaging. *J. Am. Chem. Soc.* **2007**, *129*, 11318–11319. [CrossRef] [PubMed]
85. Jaleel, J.A.; Pramod, K. Artful and multifaceted applications of carbon dot in biomedicine. *J. Control. Release* **2018**, *269*, 302–321. [CrossRef] [PubMed]
86. Hong, Y.; Lam, J.W.Y.; Tang, B.Z. Aggregation-induced emission: Phenomenon, mechanism and applications. *Chem. Commun.* **2009**, 4332–4353. [CrossRef] [PubMed]
87. Liu, J.; Chen, C.; Ji, S.; Liu, Q.; Ding, D.; Zhao, D.; Liu, B. Long wavelength excitable near-infrared fluorescent nanoparticles with aggregation-induced emission characteristics for image-guided tumor resection. *Chem. Sci.* **2017**, *8*, 2782–2789. [CrossRef] [PubMed]
88. Helle, M.; Rampazzo, E.; Monchanin, M.; Marchal, F.; Guillemin, F.; Bonacchi, S.; Salis, F.; Prodi, L.; Bezdetnaya, L. Surface Chemistry Architecture of Silica Nanoparticles Determine the Efficiency of in Vivo Fluorescence Lymph Node Mapping. *ACS Nano* **2013**, *7*, 8645–8657. [CrossRef] [PubMed]
89. Elsaesser, A.; Howard, C.V. Toxicology of nanoparticles. *Adv. Drug Deliv. Rev.* **2012**, *64*, 129–137. [CrossRef] [PubMed]
90. Kobayashi, M.; Sawada, K.; Kimura, T. Potential of Integrin Inhibitors for Treating Ovarian Cancer: A Literature Review. *Cancers* **2017**, *9*, 83. [CrossRef] [PubMed]
91. Kaur, S.; Kenny, H.A.; Jagadeeswaran, S.; Zillhardt, M.R.; Montag, A.G.; Kistner, E.; Yamada, S.D.; Mitra, A.K.; Lengyel, E. β3-Integrin Expression on Tumor Cells Inhibits Tumor Progression, Reduces Metastasis, and Is Associated with a Favorable Prognosis in Patients with Ovarian Cancer. *Am. J. Pathol.* **2009**, *175*, 2184–2196. [CrossRef] [PubMed]
92. Lim, Y.T.; Kim, S.; Nakayama, A.; Stott, N.E.; Bawendi, M.G.; Frangioni, J.V. Selection of quantum dot wavelengths for biomedical assays and imaging. *Mol. Imaging* **2003**, *2*, 50–64. [CrossRef] [PubMed]
93. Smith, A.M.; Mancini, M.C.; Nie, S. Second window for in vivo imaging. *Nat. Nanotechnol.* **2009**, *4*, 710–711. [CrossRef] [PubMed]
94. Beaulieu, R.J.; Goldstein, S.D.; Singh, J.; Safar, B.; Banerjee, A.; Ahuja, N. Automated diagnosis of colon cancer using hyperspectral sensing. *Int. J. Med. Robot. Comput. Assist. Surg.* **2018**, *14*, e1897. [CrossRef] [PubMed]
95. Hu, P.; Mingozzi, M.; Higgins, L.M.; Ganapathy, V.; Zevon, M.; Riman, R.E.; Roth, C.M.; Moghe, P.V.; Pierce, M.C. *Small Animal Imaging Platform for Quantitative Assessment of Short-Wave Infrared-Emitting Contrast Agents*; International Society for Optics and Photonics: Washington, DC, USA, 2015; Volume 9311, p. 93110T.
96. Hong, G.; Robinson, J.T.; Zhang, Y.; Diao, S.; Antaris, A.L.; Wang, Q.; Dai, H. In Vivo Fluorescence Imaging with Ag2S Quantum Dots in the Second Near-Infrared Region. *Angew. Chem. Int. Ed.* **2012**, *51*, 9818–9821. [CrossRef] [PubMed]
97. Hong, G.; Diao, S.; Chang, J.; Antaris, A.L.; Chen, C.; Zhang, B.; Zhao, S.; Atochin, D.N.; Huang, P.L.; Andreasson, K.I.; et al. Through-skull fluorescence imaging of the brain in a new near-infrared window. *Nat. Photonics* **2014**, *8*, 723. [CrossRef] [PubMed]
98. Zhang, H.; Salo, D.; Kim, D.M.; Komarov, S.; Tai, Y.-C.; Berezin, M.Y. Penetration depth of photons in biological tissues from hyperspectral imaging in shortwave infrared in transmission and reflection geometries. *J. Biomed. Opt.* **2016**, *21*, 126006. [CrossRef] [PubMed]
99. Antaris, A.L.; Chen, H.; Cheng, K.; Sun, Y.; Hong, G.; Qu, C.; Diao, S.; Deng, Z.; Hu, X.; Zhang, B.; et al. A small-molecule dye for NIR-II imaging. *Nat. Mater.* **2016**, *15*, 235. [CrossRef] [PubMed]

100. Starosolski, Z.; Bhavane, R.; Ghaghada, K.B.; Vasudevan, S.A.; Kaay, A.; Annapragada, A. Indocyanine green fluorescence in second near-infrared (NIR-II) window. *PLoS ONE* **2017**, *12*, e0187563. [CrossRef] [PubMed]
101. Yang, Q.; Hu, Z.; Zhu, S.; Ma, R.; Ma, H.; Ma, Z.; Wan, H.; Zhu, T.; Jiang, Z.; Liu, W.; et al. Donor Engineering for NIR-II Molecular Fluorophores with Enhanced Fluorescent Performance. *J. Am. Chem. Soc.* **2018**, *140*, 1715–1724. [CrossRef] [PubMed]
102. Zhu, C.-N.; Jiang, P.; Zhang, Z.-L.; Zhu, D.-L.; Tian, Z.-Q.; Pang, D.-W. Ag2Se Quantum Dots with Tunable Emission in the Second Near-Infrared Window. *ACS Appl. Mater. Interfaces* **2013**, *5*, 1186–1189. [CrossRef] [PubMed]
103. Bruns, O.T.; Bischof, T.S.; Harris, D.K.; Franke, D.; Shi, Y.; Riedemann, L.; Bartelt, A.; Jaworski, F.B.; Carr, J.A.; Rowlands, C.J.; et al. Next-generation in vivo optical imaging with short-wave infrared quantum dots. *Nat. Biomed. Eng.* **2017**, *1*, 0056. [CrossRef] [PubMed]
104. Naczynski, D.J.; Tan, M.C.; Zevon, M.; Wall, B.; Kohl, J.; Kulesa, A.; Chen, S.; Roth, C.M.; Riman, R.E.; Moghe, P.V. Rare-earth-doped biological composites as in vivo shortwave infrared reporters. *Nat. Commun.* **2013**, *4*, 2199. [CrossRef] [PubMed]
105. Chen, Y.; Montana, D.M.; Wei, H.; Cordero, J.M.; Schneider, M.; Le Guével, X.; Chen, O.; Bruns, O.T.; Bawendi, M.G. Shortwave Infrared in Vivo Imaging with Gold Nanoclusters. *Nano Lett.* **2017**, *17*, 6330–6334. [CrossRef] [PubMed]
106. Ghosh, D.; Bagley, A.F.; Na, Y.J.; Birrer, M.J.; Bhatia, S.N.; Belcher, A.M. Deep, noninvasive imaging and surgical guidance of submillimeter tumors using targeted M13-stabilized single-walled carbon nanotubes. *Proc. Natl. Acad. Sci. USA* **2014**, *111*, 13948–13953. [CrossRef] [PubMed]
107. Qi, J.; Sun, C.; Zebibula, A.; Zhang, H.; Kwok, R.T.K.; Zhao, X.; Xi, W.; Lam, J.W.Y.; Qian, J.; Tang, B.Z. Real-Time and High-Resolution Bioimaging with Bright Aggregation-Induced Emission Dots in Short-Wave Infrared Region. *Adv. Mater. Deerfield Beach Fla* **2018**, *30*, e1706856. [CrossRef] [PubMed]
108. Zevon, M.; Ganapathy, V.; Kantamneni, H.; Mingozzi, M.; Kim, P.; Adler, D.; Sheng, Y.; Tan, M.C.; Pierce, M.; Riman, R.E.; et al. CXCR-4 Targeted, Short Wave Infrared (SWIR) Emitting Nanoprobes for Enhanced Deep Tissue Imaging and Micrometastatic Lesion Detection. *Small Weinh. Bergstr. Ger.* **2015**, *11*, 6347–6357. [CrossRef] [PubMed]
109. Tao, Z.; Dang, X.; Huang, X.; Muzumdar, M.D.; Xu, E.S.; Bardhan, N.M.; Song, H.; Qi, R.; Yu, Y.; Li, T.; et al. Early tumor detection afforded by in vivo imaging of near-infrared II fluorescence. *Biomaterials* **2017**, *134*, 202–215. [CrossRef] [PubMed]
110. Murthy, R.; Nunez, R.; Szklaruk, J.; Erwin, W.; Madoff, D.C.; Gupta, S.; Ahrar, K.; Wallace, M.J.; Cohen, A.; Coldwell, D.M.; et al. Yttrium-90 microsphere therapy for hepatic malignancy: Devices, indications, technical considerations, and potential complications. *Radiogr. Rev. Publ. Radiol. Soc. N. Am. Inc* **2005**, *25* (Suppl. 1), S41–S55. [CrossRef] [PubMed]
111. Yu, X.-F.; Chen, L.-D.; Li, M.; Xie, M.-Y.; Zhou, L.; Li, Y.; Wang, Q.-Q. Highly Efficient Fluorescence of NdF3/SiO2 Core/Shell Nanoparticles and the Applications for in vivo NIR Detection. *Adv. Mater.* **2008**, *20*, 4118–4123. [CrossRef]
112. Saito, N.; Haniu, H.; Usui, Y.; Aoki, K.; Hara, K.; Takanashi, S.; Shimizu, M.; Narita, N.; Okamoto, M.; Kobayashi, S.; et al. Safe Clinical Use of Carbon Nanotubes as Innovative Biomaterials. *Chem. Rev.* **2014**, *114*, 6040–6079. [CrossRef] [PubMed]
113. Sanginario, A.; Miccoli, B.; Demarchi, D. Carbon Nanotubes as an Effective Opportunity for Cancer Diagnosis and Treatment. *Biosensors* **2017**, *7*. [CrossRef] [PubMed]
114. Caltagirone, C.; Falchi, A.M.; Lampis, S.; Lippolis, V.; Meli, V.; Monduzzi, M.; Prodi, L.; Schmidt, J.; Sgarzi, M.; Talmon, Y.; et al. Cancer-cell-targeted theranostic cubosomes. *Langmuir ACS J. Surf. Colloids* **2014**, *30*, 6228–6236. [CrossRef] [PubMed]
115. Saei, A.A.; Yazdani, M.; Lohse, S.E.; Bakhtiary, Z.; Serpooshan, V.; Ghavami, M.; Asadian, M.; Mashaghi, S.; Dreaden, E.C.; Mashaghi, A.; et al. Nanoparticle Surface Functionality Dictates Cellular and Systemic Toxicity. *Chem. Mater.* **2017**, *29*, 6578–6595. [CrossRef]
116. Pourmand, A.; Abdollahi, M. Current Opinion on Nanotoxicology. *DARU J. Pharm. Sci.* **2012**, *20*, 95. [CrossRef] [PubMed]
117. Vishwakarma, V.; Sekhar, S.; Manoharan, N. Safety and Risk Associated with Nanoparticles—A Review. *J. Miner. Mater. Charact. Eng.* **2010**, *9*, 455–459. [CrossRef]

118. Yang, L.; Watts, D.J. Particle surface characteristics may play an important role in phytotoxicity of alumina nanoparticles. *Toxicol. Lett.* **2005**, *158*, 122–132. [CrossRef] [PubMed]
119. Bahadar, H.; Maqbool, F.; Niaz, K.; Abdollahi, M. Toxicity of Nanoparticles and an Overview of Current Experimental Models. *Iran. Biomed. J.* **2016**, *20*, 1–11. [CrossRef] [PubMed]
120. Sykes, E.A.; Dai, Q.; Sarsons, C.D.; Chen, J.; Rocheleau, J.V.; Hwang, D.M.; Zheng, G.; Cramb, D.T.; Rinker, K.D.; Chan, W.C.W. Tailoring nanoparticle designs to target cancer based on tumor pathophysiology. *Proc. Natl. Acad. Sci. USA* **2016**, *113*, E1142–E1151. [CrossRef] [PubMed]
121. Polo, E.; Collado, M.; Pelaz, B.; del Pino, P. Advances toward More Efficient Targeted Delivery of Nanoparticles in Vivo: Understanding Interactions between Nanoparticles and Cells. *ACS Nano* **2017**, *11*, 2397–2402. [CrossRef] [PubMed]
122. Soo Choi, H.; Liu, W.; Misra, P.; Tanaka, E.; Zimmer, J.P.; Itty Ipe, B.; Bawendi, M.G.; Frangioni, J.V. Renal clearance of quantum dots. *Nat. Biotechnol.* **2007**, *25*, 1165–1170. [CrossRef] [PubMed]
123. Du, B.; Jiang, X.; Das, A.; Zhou, Q.; Yu, M.; Jin, R.; Zheng, J. Glomerular barrier behaves as an atomically precise bandpass filter in a sub-nanometre regime. *Nat. Nanotechnol.* **2017**, *12*, 1096–1102. [CrossRef] [PubMed]
124. Ma, N.; Marshall, A.F.; Gambhir, S.S.; Rao, J. Facile Synthesis, Silanization and Biodistribution of Biocompatible Quantum Dots. *Small Weinh. Bergstr. Ger.* **2010**, *6*, 1520–1528. [CrossRef] [PubMed]
125. Yu, S.; Xu, D.; Wan, Q.; Liu, M.; Tian, J.; Huang, Q.; Deng, F.; Wen, Y.; Zhang, X.; Wei, Y. Construction of biodegradable and biocompatible AIE-active fluorescent polymeric nanoparticles by Ce(IV)/HNO3 redox polymerization in aqueous solution. *Mater. Sci. Eng. C* **2017**, *78*, 191–197. [CrossRef] [PubMed]
126. Vlasova, I.I.; Kapralov, A.A.; Michael, Z.P.; Burkert, S.C.; Shurin, M.R.; Star, A.; Shvedova, A.A.; Kagan, V.E. Enzymatic Oxidative Biodegradation of Nanoparticles: Mechanisms, Significance and Applications. *Toxicol. Appl. Pharmacol.* **2016**, *299*, 58–69. [CrossRef] [PubMed]
127. Warner, J.H.; Hoshino, A.; Yamamoto, K.; Tilley, R.D. Water-Soluble Photoluminescent Silicon Quantum Dots. *Angew. Chem. Int. Ed.* **2005**, *44*, 4550–4554. [CrossRef] [PubMed]
128. Kang, Z.; Tsang, C.H.A.; Zhang, Z.; Zhang, M.; Wong, N.; Zapien, J.A.; Shan, Y.; Lee, S.-T. A polyoxometalate-assisted electrochemical method for silicon nanostructures preparation: From quantum dots to nanowires. *J. Am. Chem. Soc.* **2007**, *129*, 5326–5327. [CrossRef] [PubMed]
129. Erogbogbo, F.; Yong, K.-T.; Roy, I.; Xu, G.; Prasad, P.N.; Swihart, M.T. Biocompatible luminescent silicon quantum dots for imaging of cancer cells. *ACS Nano* **2008**, *2*, 873–878. [CrossRef] [PubMed]
130. Liu, J.; Erogbogbo, F.; Yong, K.-T.; Ye, L.; Liu, J.; Hu, R.; Chen, H.; Hu, Y.; Yang, Y.; Yang, J.; et al. Assessing Clinical Prospects of Silicon Quantum Dots: Studies in Mice and Monkeys. *ACS Nano* **2013**, *7*, 7303–7310. [CrossRef] [PubMed]
131. Lacerda, L.; Herrero, M.A.; Venner, K.; Bianco, A.; Prato, M.; Kostarelos, K. Carbon-Nanotube Shape and Individualization Critical for Renal Excretion. *Small* **2008**, *4*, 1130–1132. [CrossRef] [PubMed]
132. Colby, A.H.; Berry, S.M.; Moran, A.M.; Pasion, K.A.; Liu, R.; Colson, Y.L.; Ruiz-Opazo, N.; Grinstaff, M.W.; Herrera, V.L.M. Highly Specific and Sensitive Fluorescent Nanoprobes for Image-Guided Resection of Sub-Millimeter Peritoneal Tumors. *ACS Nano* **2017**, *11*, 1466–1477. [CrossRef] [PubMed]
133. Han, M.S.; Tung, C.-H. Lessons learned from imaging mouse ovarian tumors: The route of probe injection makes a difference. *Quant. Imaging Med. Surg.* **2014**, *4*, 156–162. [CrossRef] [PubMed]
134. Parungo, C.P.; Soybel, D.I.; Colson, Y.L.; Kim, S.-W.; Ohnishi, S.; De Grand, A.M.; Laurence, R.G.; Soltesz, E.G.; Chen, F.Y.; Cohn, L.H.; et al. Lymphatic Drainage of the Peritoneal Space: A Pattern Dependent on Bowel Lymphatics. *Ann. Surg. Oncol.* **2007**, *14*, 286–298. [CrossRef] [PubMed]
135. Kato, S.; Itoh, K.; Yaoi, T.; Tozawa, T.; Yoshikawa, Y.; Yasui, H.; Kanamura, N.; Hoshino, A.; Manabe, N.; Yamamoto, K.; et al. Organ distribution of quantum dots after intraperitoneal administration, with special reference to area-specific distribution in the brain. *Nanotechnology* **2010**, *21*, 335103. [CrossRef] [PubMed]
136. Haque, M.M.; Im, H.-Y.; Seo, J.-E.; Hasan, M.; Woo, K.; Kwon, O.-S. Acute toxicity and tissue distribution of CdSe/CdS-MPA quantum dots after repeated intraperitoneal injection to mice. *J. Appl. Toxicol.* **2013**, *33*, 940–950. [CrossRef] [PubMed]

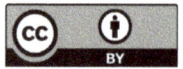

© 2018 by the authors. Licensee MDPI, Basel, Switzerland. This article is an open access article distributed under the terms and conditions of the Creative Commons Attribution (CC BY) license (http://creativecommons.org/licenses/by/4.0/).

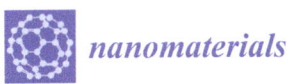

Article

Homologous Gold Nanoparticles and Nanoclusters Composites with Enhanced Surface Raman Scattering and Metal Fluorescence for Cancer Imaging

Xiaoxia Wu [1,2], Yan Peng [1], Xiaomei Duan [1], Lingyan Yang [1], Jinze Lan [1] and Fu Wang [1,*]

[1] Laboratory of Environmental Sciences and Technology, Xinjiang Technical Institute of Physics & Chemistry, Chinese Academy of Sciences, Urumqi 830011, China; wuxx@ms.xjb.ac.cn (X.W.); pengyan_15@163.com (Y.P.); duanxiaomei18@mails.ucas.edu.cn (X.D.); yanglingyan16@mails.ucas.edu.cn (L.Y.); lanjinze16@mails.ucas.edu.cn (J.L.)
[2] University of Chinese Academy of Sciences, No. 19 Yuquan Road, Beijing 100049, China
* Correspondence: wangfu@sjtu.edu.cn; Tel.: +86-021-54742824

Received: 20 September 2018; Accepted: 9 October 2018; Published: 11 October 2018

Abstract: A large number of deaths from cancer can be attributed to the lack of effective early-stage diagnostic techniques. Thus, accurate and effective early diagnosis is a major research goal worldwide. With the unique phenomenon of localized surface plasmon resonance (LSPR), plasmonic nanomaterials have attracted considerable attention for applications in surface-enhanced Raman scattering (SERS) and metal-enhanced fluorescence (MEF). Both SERS and MEF are ultra-sensitive methods for the detection and identification of early tumor at molecular level. To combine the merits of the fast and accurate imaging of MEF and the stable and clear imaging of SERS, we propose a novel dual functional imaging nanoprobe based on gold nanoparticles and gold nanocluster composites (denoted AuNPC-RGD). The gold nanoparticles are used as LSPR substrates to realized enhancement of Raman or fluorescence signal, while the gold nanoclusters serve as a fluorophore for MEF imaging, and exhibit better biocompatibility and stability. Furthermore, target molecule of cyclic Arg-Gly-Asp (cRGD) is incorporated into the composite to improve delivery efficiency, selectivity and imaging accuracy. These integrated properties endow AuNPC-RGD composites with outstanding biocompatibility and excellent imaging abilities, which could be used to achieve accurate and effective diagnosis for early cancer.

Keywords: surface-enhanced Raman scattering (SERS); metal-enhanced fluorescence (MEF); dual functional imaging nanoprobe

1. Introduction

Cancer has become one of the most serious causes of disease-related death, accounting for about 15% of total human deaths every year [1–4]. The earlier cancer is discovered, the greater the likelihood of successful treatment. Therefore, effective diagnosis for early cancer is of great importance [5]. Despite recent advances in traditional clinical diagnostic techniques (including magnetic resonance imaging, ultrasound imaging, computed tomography and positron emission tomography), the accuracy and sensitivity of diagnosis are still poor during the early stages of cancer, when the tumor is only a few cells in size [6,7]. In this context, the combination of enhanced Raman scattering and fluorescence methods, which uses nanomaterials as a probe for optical image of early-stage cancer, has come to be regarded as a promising alternative strategy, as it can achieve single-molecule imaging with excellent sensitivity and selectivity [8–12].

With the unique phenomenon of localized surface plasmon resonance (LSPR), plasmonic nanoparticles are widely used as a probe in surface-enhanced Raman scattering (SERS) and metal-enhanced fluorescence

(MEF) techniques [13–15]. SERS can provide ultra-sensitive characterization down to the single-molecular level, and a higher sensitivity (10^{10}–10^{14} times enhancement) compared to conventional Raman spectroscopy [16–18]. Jing et al. demonstrated the ability of a nanothermometer, which used a gold nanostar-indocyanine nanoprobe to realize real-time monitoring via SERS imaging [19]. However, the drawback of traditional SERS imaging is the long time required for image acquisition. MEF is capable of fluorescence enhancement via the interactions of fluorophores with metallic nanoparticles, and has attracted widespread interest as a method for developing novel nanostructures for biosensors and biomedical engineering [20–22]. Lee reported a fast and facile MEF optical method to monitor and probe bacterial interactions in three-dimensional resolution [23]. But the organic fluorophores are relatively unstable against photobleaching and can be easily degraded in microenvironments. Therefore, to achieve both more stable and faster imaging, one highly effective strategy is to combine SERS and MEF to construct a dual functional probe, which would not only obtain ultrahigh-resolution imaging in a short time, but also maintain image stability in the long term.

Herein, we designed and synthesized a novel dual functional nanoprobe combining SERS and MEF for the accurate imaging of early cancer or metastasis tissues. Specifically, gold nanoparticles (AuNPs), used as the source of plasmonic resonance, were modified with a Raman reporter molecule 4-mercaptobenzoic acid (AuNP-MBA), and encapsulated with silica (AuNP@SiO$_2$). Then, gold nanoclusters (AuNCs) were grown on surface of AuNP@SiO$_2$ (AuNPC), and functionalized with bovine serum albumin (BSA) and cyclic Arg-Gly-Asp (cRGD) to construct the final dual functional nanoprobes (AuNPC-RGD). The novel nanoprobe design combines four advantages. Firstly, the AuNPs used as plasmonic substrates to enhance the signal intensity of Raman activity or fluorescence and the AuNCs which act as a fluorophore for MEF imaging, are homologous nanomaterials possessing good biocompatibility. Secondly, compared with conventional organic dyes, AuNCs exhibit much higher stability, which improves the temporal resolution of imaging. Thirdly, the nanoprobes realize both faster and more accurate MEF imaging in the short term and more stable and clearer SERS imaging in the long term. Finally, the conjugation of the probe with the target molecule, cRGD, improves the delivery efficiency of the latter and therefore the selectivity and imaging accuracy. With these integrated properties, AuNPC-RGD is a novel dual functional imaging agent with outstanding stability and biocompatibility, and excellent SERS and MEF imaging efficiency, capabilities that are urgently needed for early cancer diagnosis and imaging.

2. Materials and Methods

2.1. Materials

Gold (III) chloride trihydrate (HAuCl$_4$·3H$_2$O), γ-mercaptopropyltrimethoxysilane (MPTES) and sodium citrate dihydrate (Na$_3$Ct·2H$_2$O) were purchased from Adamas Beta (Shanghai, China). Ammonium hydroxide (NH$_3$·H$_2$O, 25%), sodium hydroxide (NaOH) and 2-propanol were obtained from Tianjin Chemical Regent Co., Ltd. (Tianjin, China). Tetraethylorthosilicate (TEOS), bovine serum albumin (BSA) and 4-mercaptobenzoic acid (4-MBA) were purchased from Sigma-Aldrich (St. Louis, MO, USA). N-hydroxysuccinimide (NHS) and 1-ethyl-3-(3-dimethylaminopropyl) carbodiimide hydrochloride (EDC·HCl) were obtained from J&K Scientific Ltd. (Beijing, China). Cyclic Arg-Gly-Asp (cRGD) was obtained from GL Biochem Ltd. (Shanghai, China).

2.2. Synthesis of the AuNP-MBA

The AuNP-MBA was synthesized by two steps. First, HAuCl$_4$ was reduced by Na$_3$Ct to form AuNPs [24], 2 mL of HAuCl$_4$ solution (10.0 mM) was added into 60 mL of water containing 1 mL of Na$_3$Ct (1.0%) and the mixture was heated to boiling for 3.0 min. The color of solution changed to red and the resulted AuNPs dispersion were kept in 4 °C after cooled down to room temperature. Second, the modification of 4-MBA was completed according to a reported approach [25]. 20 μL of different concentration of 4-MBA (1.0–100 mM in ethanol) was mixed with AuNPs dispersion (2 mL) and reacted for 2 min. The SERS intensity of obtained AuNP-MBA1-4 were taken by Raman spectrometer.

2.3. Preparation of the AuNP@SiO$_2$ and AuNPC

AuNP@SiO$_2$ was prepared using TEOS as silicon source with a modified approach [26]. Briefly, 6 mL of AuNP-MBA and 0.75 mL of NH$_3$·H$_2$O (25%) were added into 30 mL of 2-propanol and then 10% TEOS in ethanol (21–36 µL) was added drop by drop. After the reaction of 5 h, the obtained AuNP@SiO$_2$ was washed twice with ethanol by centrifugation (11000 rpm, 10 min) and dispersed in 3 mL of ethanol. For mercapto modification, 3 mL of the above-prepared AuNP@SiO$_2$ was mixed with 1 mL of MilliQ water and 30 µL of MPTES. The mixture was kept stirring at 60 °C for 5.0 h in a constant temperature bath and the obtained nanoparticles were collected by centrifugation (11,000 rpm, 10 min) and washed with water for three times, and finally re-dispersed into 3 mL of water.

AuNPC was prepared according to a modified method [27]. 2 mL of the as-prepared mercapto functionalized AuNP@SiO$_2$ (AuNP@SiO$_2$-SH) and 0.5 mL of HAuCl$_4$ (10.0 mM) were mixed for 30 min, and 0.5 mL of BSA (50 mg/mL) was added into the solution. After 10 min, 0.2 mL of NaOH aqueous solution (1 M) was injected and the mixture was kept at 37 °C for 3 h. Subsequently, the resulting AuNPC was collected by centrifugation (12,000 rpm for 10 min) and re-dispersed into 2 mL of water. Then, the MEF intensity of AuNPC1-4 were taken by fluorescence spectrometer.

2.4. Conjugation of Targeted Molecule cRGD

Finally, the target molecule cRGD was grafted to the AuNPC nanoparticles with a modified approach [28,29]. Specifically, 2 mL of as-prepared AuNPC, 4 mg of EDC·HCl and 2.5 mg of NHS were mixed in 8 mL of PBS (pH 7.4) for the reaction of 8 h. Then, 2 mg of cRGD was added into the solution and kept stirring in the dark at room temperature. After 16 h, the resulted AuNPC-RGD was collected by centrifugal filter units (Millipore, MWCO 50.0 kDa, Darmstadt, Germany) and dispersed in 2.0 mL of water for subsequent application.

2.5. Characterization

Transmission electron microscope (TEM) images of the nanoparticles were obtained by a Tecnai G20 (FEI, Hillsboro, OR, USA), which was operated at 200 kV. The size distribution and zeta potential were measured by dynamic light scattering (DLS) with a zeta particle size analyzer (Nano-ZS, Malvern, UK). Raman spectra and imaging were taken with a confocal microprobe Raman system (LabRAM HR Evolution, Tokyo, Japan) with 633 nm laser, and scattering spectra were recorded in the range of 400–1700 cm^{-1}. The characterization of fluorescence spectra were taken on fluorescence spectrophotometer (F-7000, Hitachi, Tokyo, Japan), and fluorescence imaging was taken with a confocal laser scanning microscope (CLSM, Nikon C2 SIM, Tokyo, Japan).

2.6. Biocompatibility and Cellular Uptake of Nanoparticles

Human cervical cancer cell line HeLa cells were cultured in DMEM at 37 °C in 5% CO$_2$.

For the evaluation of in vitro cytotoxicity, the MTT assay was performed on the HeLa cells [3]. Briefly, 100 µL of HeLa cells (1 × 10^5 cells per mL) was added in 96-well plate with the incubation of 24 h. Then the culture medium was removed and 100 µL of AuNPC-RGD (0–1.0 mg/mL) in fresh culture medium was added and incubated for another 24 h. Next 10 µL of MTT (5 mg/mL) was added and incubated for 4 h, then 100 µL of DMSO was added after removing the medium and free MTT. The absorbance of the suspension was recorded by a microplate reader (Thermo MultiskanFC, Waltham, MA, USA) at a wavelength of 570 nm.

To measure the cellular uptake of nanoparticles, inductively coupled plasma (ICP) analysis was used. HeLa cells were incubated with either AuNPC or AuNPC-RGD (5 mg/mL) as described above for 2 or 4 h. Then HeLa cells were washed for three times by PBS and collected by centrifugation (1000 rpm, 5 min). Finally, the amount of Au of cell samples were measured by ICP-OES (VISTA-PRO CCD Simultaneous ICP-OES, VARIAN, Palo Alto, CA, USA).

2.7. Surface-Enhanced Raman Scattering (SERS) and Metal-Enhanced Fluorescence (MEF) Imaging

For the study of SERS imaging, 2×10^5 HeLa cells dispersed in 2 mL of culture medium were added in a 6-well plate and incubated for 24 h. Then, the culture medium was replaced with 2 mL of fresh culture containing AuNPC or AuNPC-RGD (5 mg/mL). After another 4 h, HeLa cells were washed for three times with PBS. SERS images at the Raman shift of 1065–1080 cm^{-1} were then obtained under laser excitation at 633 nm on the confocal laser Raman scanning microscopy (LabRAM HR Evolution, Tokyo, Japan).

A similar method was used to study the MEF imaging. Additionally, the HeLa cells were treated with Hoechst 33258 (0.5 μg/mL) to stain the nucleus. Hoechst and AuNPC were excited at the same wavelength of 405 nm, and the fluorescence images were taken by a CLSM (Nikon C2 SIM, Tokyo, Japan) at wavelengths of 420–480 and 600–660 nm.

3. Results and Discussion

3.1. Characterization of the Dual Functional Nanoprobes

The design, preparation and application of the SERS nanoparticles are illustrated in Scheme 1. As shown in Scheme 1a, the AuNPs are used as LSPR substrates to enhance the signal intensity of Raman scattering and fluorescence. In combination with the enhanced Raman and fluorescence signals, the novel dual functional nanoprobe is designed to simultaneously achieve SERS and MEF imaging. As shown in Scheme 1b, the LSPR substrate of AuNPs are modified with a Raman reporter molecule of 4-MBA, via an Au-S bond to realize SERS imaging. To avoid fluorescence quenching by the AuNPs, the surfaces of AuNP-MBA are encapsulated in SiO_2 shells, for which the thickness of SiO_2 is optimized with respect to fluorescence enhancement. Then, the AuNP@SiO_2 are functionalized with the –SH group to induce the growth of AuNCs on the nanoparticles. By S–Au bonds, both BSA (containing S–S) and AuNP@SiO_2 (containing –SH) could form S–Au bonds with AuNCs, which modified BSA on the surface of AuNP@SiO_2 via AuNCs. The BSA of AuNCs are attached on the surface of the dual-functional nanoparticles to improve the stability and biocompatibility of the nanoparticles and achieve MEF imaging. Then, the target molecule, cRGD, which has been demonstrated to show high binding affinity to $α_vβ_3$ integrin that are up-regulated by tumor endothelial cells, is conjugated onto the surface of the AuNPC through the amidation reaction between –COOH groups of BSA and –NH_2 groups of cRGD [29]. Scheme 1c shows the application of AuNPC-RGD for targeted imaging of cancer cells, which achieve excellent SERS and MEF imaging ability and efficiency.

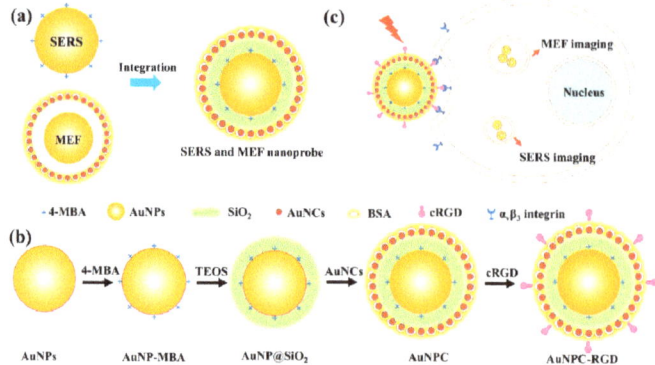

Scheme 1. The illustration for the design (**a**), preparation (**b**) and application (**c**) of the dual-functional imaging nanoprobe.

The amount of 4-MBA on the AuNPs is a very important parameter for the SERS effects of LSPR system, so that the concentration of 4-MBA during the preparation of AuNP-MBA nanoparticles were systematically optimized with respect to the stability and SERS intensity of the AuNP-MBA nanoparticles. In Table 1 and Figure 1e, the SERS intensity and spectra of preparative conditions and performances of the AuNP-MBA are presented. The major Raman peaks of AuNP-MBA1-4 at 1076 cm^{-1} are magnified and shown in Figure 1e which indicate the vibration peak of benzene ring of 4-MBA [25]. It could be found that the tendency of SERS intensity increased obviously with the increase of 4-MBA concentration from 10 to 500 µM (the magnified spectra in Figure 1e & Table 1) for AuNP-MBA1-4. On the basis of the stability and SERS intensity of the modified AuNP-MBA nanoparticles, the final concentration of 4-MBA was fixed at 500 µM in all subsequent experiments, due to the higher 4-MBA concentrations resulted in poor stability of the nanoparticles (the AuNPs was easy to agglomerate with 4-MBA at concentration of 1 mM so that its SERS intensity was not measured). To prevent fluorescence quenching, the surfaces of the AuNP-MBA (about 35 nm) were encapsulated with the SiO$_2$ shells. The thickness of the SiO$_2$ shells was optimized with respect to the MEF intensity of the nanoparticles by varying the concentration of TEOS, as shown in the TEM images of Figure 1a–d. Table 2 shows the performances of the AuNPC nanoparticles and Figure 1f shows the MEF spectra of the prepared AuNPC nanoparticles. With the increase of SiO$_2$ shell thickness (from about 6.3 to 20 nm, as shown in Table 2), the MEF intensities of the AuNPC nanoparticles first increased and then decreased. And the peak value of MEF were shown in Table 2, AuNPC2 and AuNPC3 had similar MEF intensity, but AuNPC2 had higher MEF and the thickness of SiO$_2$ in AuNPC2 was optimization condition for MEF. Therefore, SiO$_2$ shells of thickness (13 ± 1.2 nm) were chosen to maximize the fluorescence enhancement for the following application of MEF imaging.

Table 1. The conditions and results for the preparation of the AuNP-MBA.

Nomenclature	C_{Au} (mg/mL)	C_{4-MBA} (µM)	SERS Intensity [a]
AuNP-MBA1	0.05	500	964 ± 2.5
AuNP-MBA2	0.05	100	627 ± 5.2
AuNP-MBA3	0.05	50	215 ± 6.7
AuNP-MBA4	0.05	10	23 ± 4.3

[a] SERS intensity of the nanoparticles determined at 1076 cm^{-1}.

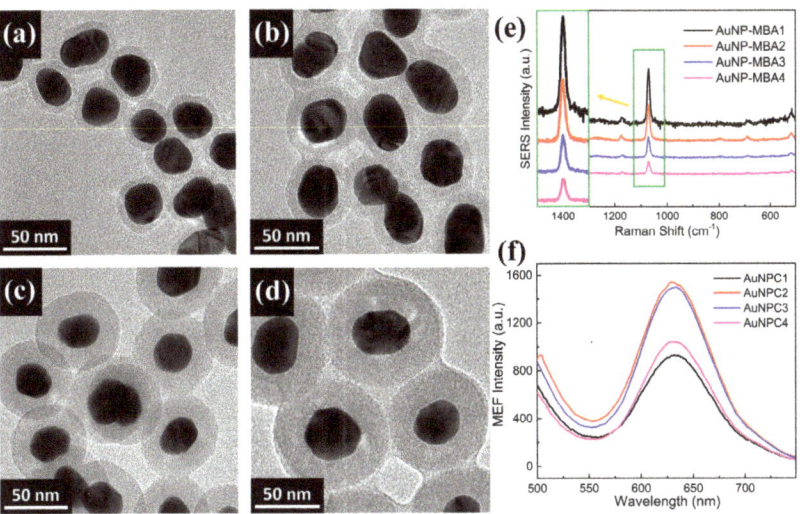

Figure 1. (**a–d**) TEM imaging of AuNP@SiO$_2$-1-4; (**e**) SERS spectra of the AuNP-MBA1-4; (**f**) MEF spectra of the AuNPC1-4.

Table 2. The conditions and results for the preparation of the AuNPC.

NO.	Size (nm)	The Thickness of Shell (nm)	MEF Intensity [a]
AuNPC1	45 ± 1.9	6.3 ± 0.8	930 ± 3.2
AuNPC2	60 ± 2.3	13 ± 1.2	1545 ± 4.2
AuNPC3	70 ± 2.9	17 ± 1.3	1480 ± 4.1
AuNPC4	78 ± 4.0	20 ± 2.0	1037 ± 5.0

[a] MEF intensity of the nanoparticles determined at 630 nm.

Figure 2a–c show TEM images of the modified AuNPs, exhibiting their core-shell structure. It can be seen that the AuNP@SiO$_2$, AuNPC and AuNPC-RGD are all well dispersed. The SiO$_2$ was modified with –SH groups which could link AuNCs by S–Au bonds and anchored in the surface of SiO$_2$ shell. The size of AuNCs was below 2 nm which was too small to be seen [27]. When it was enlarged (the insert image of Figure 2b), AuNCs could be found on the SiO$_2$ shell in AuNPC nanoparticles, indicating that the AuNCs were modified on AuNPC successfully. Figure 2d shows the size distributions of the AuNPs, AuNP-MBA, AuNP@SiO$_2$, AuNPC and AuNPC-RGD in MilliQ water. The hydrodynamic diameters of the nanoparticles increase in the order AuNPs < AuNP-MBA < AuNP@SiO$_2$ < AuNPC < AuNPC-RGD, i.e., the nanoparticles have successively larger diameters after each modification step. Both the TEM and DLS results indicate that the size of the AuNPC-RGD nanoparticles is less than 200 nm, which is sufficiently small to allow enhanced permeability and retention effect for targeting tumor cells [7]. As shown in Figure 2e, the zeta potentials of the AuNPs, AuNP-MBA, AuNP@SiO$_2$, AuNPC and AuNPC-RGD are −4.2 mV, 9.7 mV, −42.3 mV, −41.5 mV and −29.8 mV, respectively. All of the nanoparticles are therefore negatively charged, which can be expected to suppress their non-specific interaction with cells [24,25]. Figure 2f shows the UV-Vis spectra of the AuNPs, AuNP-MBA, AuNP@SiO$_2$, AuNPC and AuNPC-RGD. It could be found that the absorbance peak of AuNPs at 525 nm with the wavelength range of 460–700 nm, indicating that AuNPs had a strong plasmonic absorption peak in LSPR [14]. And strong resonance effect was induced with the incident light of 525 nm which could produce high SERS effect [17]. In consideration of fluorescence interference of cells, long wavelength of 633 nm laser was used to excite SERS imaging. The absorption peak shifts from 525 nm for the AuNPs to 550 nm for the AuNPC-RGD. This red shift of surface plasmon band can be ascribed to modification of 4-MBA, SiO$_2$ shell, AuNCs and cRGD which changed the refractive index surrounding the AuNPs [30]. The modification of 4-MBA on AuNPs does not change the plasmonic absorption of AuNPs due to the low concentration of 4-MBA encoded on AuNPs. When encapsulated with AuNCs and cRGD, the absorption at range of long wavelength (650–800 nm) increased obviously, which resulted from the interaction between the LSPR effects of AuNPs and AuNCs [31]. Figure 2g shows SERS spectra of 4-MBA, AuNP-MBA, AuNP@SiO$_2$, AuNPC and AuNPC-RGD. The peaks of 1076 cm^{-1} associated with vibration peak of benzene ring, and 1581 cm^{-1} were identified along with the band at 1422 cm^{-1} corresponding to deformation and stretching vibrations of carboxylate groups [32]. It is clear that Raman intensity of 4-MBA increases due to the SERS of AuNPs, and the enhancement factor (EF) of SERS for AuNPC-RGD is calculated according to the equation (EF = [I_{SERS}]/[I_{Raman}] × [N_{Raman}]/[N_{SERS}]) [18,33]. The Raman intensity of 4-MBA or AuNPC-RGD are I_{Raman} or I_{SERS}, and N_{Raman} or N_{SERS} indicated molecular weight of 4-MBA in dispersion or on AuNPC-RGD. The EF is calculated to be 500, suggesting that the intensity of AuNP-MBA is 500 times greater than that of 4-MBA without AuNPs substrates. Figure 2h exhibits MEF spectra of AuNPC, AuNPC-RGD and silica nanospheres (~70 nm) without AuNPs core that grow gold nanoclusters on the surface (abbreviated as SNPC). The fluorescence property of AuNCs mostly relate to ligands with Au atoms, which influence the emission wavelength and intensity of AuNCs [21]. The fluorescence peak of AuNCs shifted when modified cRGD, it could be ascribed to the ligand molecule of BSA changed to BSA-cRGD which had great influence on luminous properties of AuNCs. Moreover, the AuNPs could also influence the emission property of AuNCs induced the difference of AuNPC and SNPC. AuNPC-RGD had higher MEF intensity due to the enrichment of

AuNPC-RGD after centrifugation. The silica nanoparticles with similar size of AuNP@SiO$_2$ (about 70 nm), was prepared by hydrolysis of tetraethylorthosilicate (TEOS) [26]. SNPC (silica nanoparticles modified with AuNCs with the same preparation method with AuNPC) was used as control to calculate EF of MEF for AuNPC. There was no AuNPs core in silica nanoparticles but AuNCs were conjugated on their surfaces. Comparing the fluorescence spectra of AuNPC and SNPC, we can find that the fluorescence intensity is approximately doubled than AuNPC.

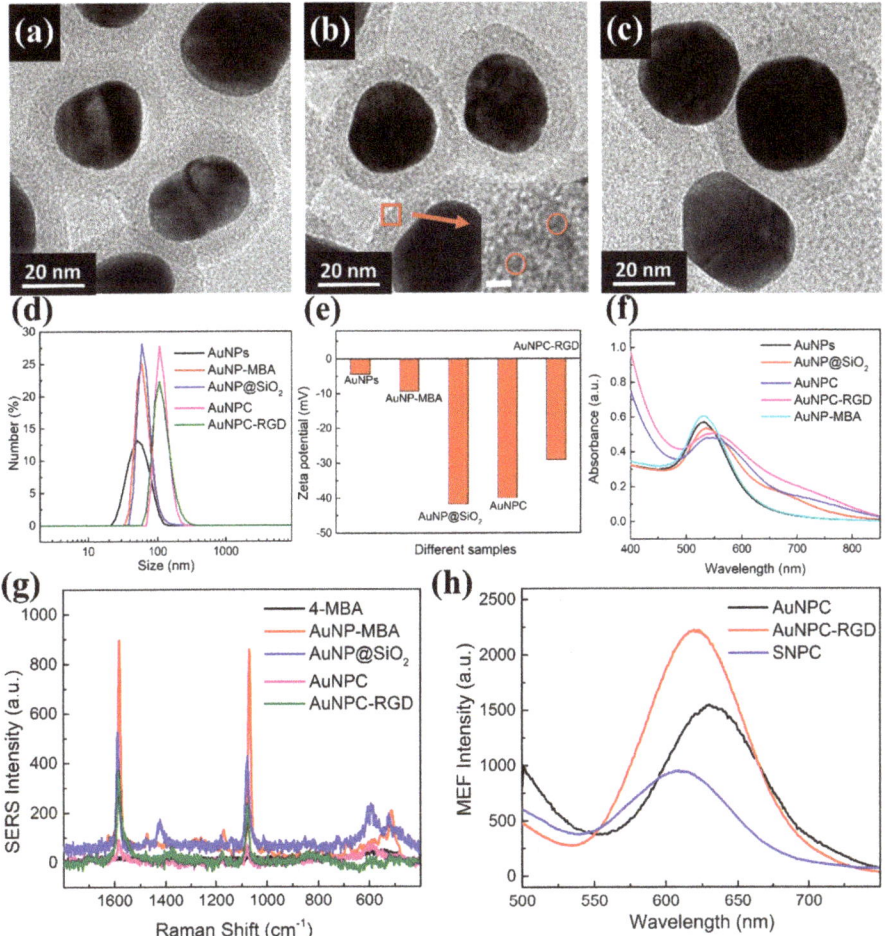

Figure 2. Characterization of the bifunctional nanoprobes. (**a–c**) TEM images of the AuNP@SiO$_2$, AuNPC and AuNPC-RGD; (**d–e**) Size distributions and zeta potentials of the AuNPs, AuNP-MBA, AuNP@SiO$_2$, AuNPC and AuNPC-RGD in water; (**f**) UV-Vis spectra of the AuNPs, AuNP-MBA, AuNP@SiO$_2$, AuNPC and AuNPC-RGD in aqueous solution; (**g**) SERS spectra of the 4-MBA, AuNPs, AuNP@SiO$_2$, AuNPC and AuNPC-RGD; (**h**) MEF spectra of the AuNPC, AuNPC-RGD and SNPC in aqueous solution.

3.2. Biocompatibility and Cellular Uptake of Nanoparticles

It is well known that biocompatibility is an important factor for any nanoplatforms in a drug delivery system, as it determines whether a nanomaterial can be used in vivo [34]. AuNPC and AuNPC-RGD were modified with BSA, which not only increases the stability and biocompatibility of the nanomaterials, but also provides a large number of functional groups of –COOH and –NH$_2$. Through the amidation reaction between –COOH and –NH$_2$, the target molecule cRGD was grafted onto the nanoparticles. In preparation of AuNPC-RGD, a tiny amount of cRGD reacted with a high amount of BSA, suggesting most of cRGD reacted with BSA and conjugated on AuNPC. The amount of AuNCs and BSA were all the same, and then cRGD was modified on AuNPC, which could not interfere the amount of cRGD on AuNPC-RGD. cRGD is a typical target molecule possessing high binding affinity to $α_vβ_3$ integrin, which are highly expressed in tumor endothelial cells (such as lung adenocarcinoma, cervical cancer and breast cancer cells) [29].

The in vitro cytotoxicity and cellular uptake of nanoparticles must be evaluated before their application to ensure that the biocompatibility of nanoparticles could be applied for cell imaging [24]. Firstly, the cytotoxicity of the as-prepared different nanoparticles were evaluated via MTT assay, in which HeLa cells were separately incubated with AuNPs@SiO$_2$, AuNPC and AuNPC-RGD. From Figure 3a, it can be observed that AuNPs@SiO$_2$ had the most severe cytotoxicity (survival rates of 74.7% for 0.1 mg/mL and 57.1% for 1 mg/mL), while the other nanoparticles had excellent biocompatibility (survival rates higher than 85.0% for 0.1 mg/mL and 83.3% for 0.8 mg/mL for both materials). Nonetheless, the cell viability in the presence of AuNPC-RGD, in which cRGD was conjugated onto the nanoparticles, was reduced (compared with 92.65% for 1 mg/mL of AuNPC), because the cellular uptake of the former was higher than the latter, as shown in Figure 3b. Figure 3b shows the quantitative ICP measurement of AuNPC and AuNPC-RGD accumulated in cells. The cellular uptake of the nanoparticles increased with the increase of incubation time from 2 h to 4 h. And the cellular uptake of AuNPC-RGD increased compared with AuNPC, which indicates that it could realize active targeting for AuNPC-RGD delivery to tumor cells.

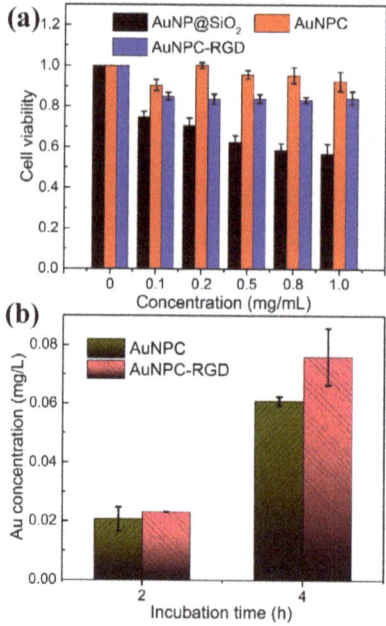

Figure 3. In vitro cytotoxicity and cellular uptake of different nanoparticles. (**a**) Viabilities of HeLa cells incubated with different nanoparticles; (**b**) Cellular uptake performance of AuNPC and AuNPC-RGD with incubation for 2 and 4 h.

3.3. Application of SERS and MEF Imaging

As is widely known, AuNPs have strong plasmonic properties through their long electronic relaxation time, which provide powerful enhancement for Raman scattering and fluorescence signals [18]. As the SERS and MEF techniques possess ultrahigh-sensitivity that can reach single molecule detection, the prepared AuNPC-RGD has the potential to be used in single cell imaging.

To investigate the performance of the nanoprobe for SERS imaging, HeLa cells were incubated with AuNPC or AuNPC-RGD. Figure 4a shows the bright field cell imaging of HeLa cells incubated with AuNPC, and Figure 4b,c are the corresponding SERS images, in which the Raman signals were collected in the range of 1065–1080 cm^{-1} and the excitation wavelength was chosen as 633 nm to avoid fluorescence interference [19]. The SERS images of Figure 4b,c are enlarged views of the cells in the green boxes in Figure 4a, which are well matched with the corresponding bright field images. SERS images of HeLa cells incubated with AuNPC-RGD are exhibited in Figure 4d–f. Similar to AuNPC, Figure 4d shows the bright field imaging of the cells and Figure 4e,f are the SERS images under the same conditions as mentioned above, and both the bright field and SERS images are again completely matched. Compared with Figure 4b,c, the SERS intensities of Figure 4e,f are much brighter, which can be ascribed to the higher cellular uptake of AuNPC-RGD than AuNPC. The very close matching of the SERS images with the bright field images indicates that the SERS nanoprobes can achieve single-cell imaging.

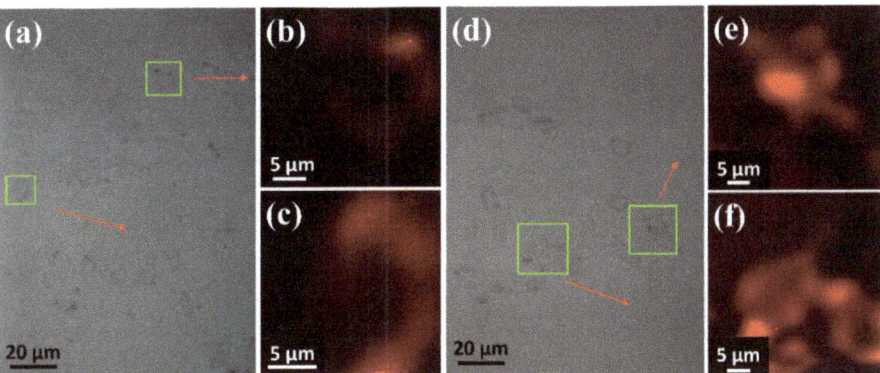

Figure 4. SERS images of HeLa cells incubated with nanoprobes. (**a**–**c**) AuNPC; (**d**–**f**) AuNPC-RGD. SERS images at the Raman shift of 1065–1080 cm^{-1} were obtained under the laser of 633 nm.

Compared with Raman scattering signals, fluorescence signals are stronger and more sensitive [35]. By utilizing the MEF effect, fluorescence intensity and photostability can be further increased [18]. As presented in Figure 5, the as-prepared nanoparticles show excellent MEF performance. Figure 5a–d show the HeLa cells incubated without nanoparticles as a control for comparison with AuNPC and AuNPC-RGD. The bright field and MEF images of HeLa cells incubated with AuNPC or AuNPC-RGD are as shown in Figure 5e–l, respectively. The images of bright field were shown clearly in Figure S1–S3 (Supplementary Materials). The images of the second columns (Figure 5b,f,j) and third columns (Figure 5c,g,k) are fluorescence images of Hoechst 33258 (blue) and AuNPC (red) under single-wavelength 405 nm excitation. The MEF image of AuNPC-RGD displays stronger fluorescence than the image of AuNPC, as a result of the active-targeting effect of AuNPC-RGD. From the merged images (Figure 5d,h,l), the cell nucleus (blue) and cytoplasm (red) are matched accurately, indicating that the MEF nanoprobes can achieve single-cell fluorescence imaging. The results of SERS and MEF imaging demonstrate that AuNPC-RGD as a dual-functional imaging agent shows outstanding biocompatibility and excellent SERS and MEF imaging efficiency, and is expected to be applied for effective cancer imaging.

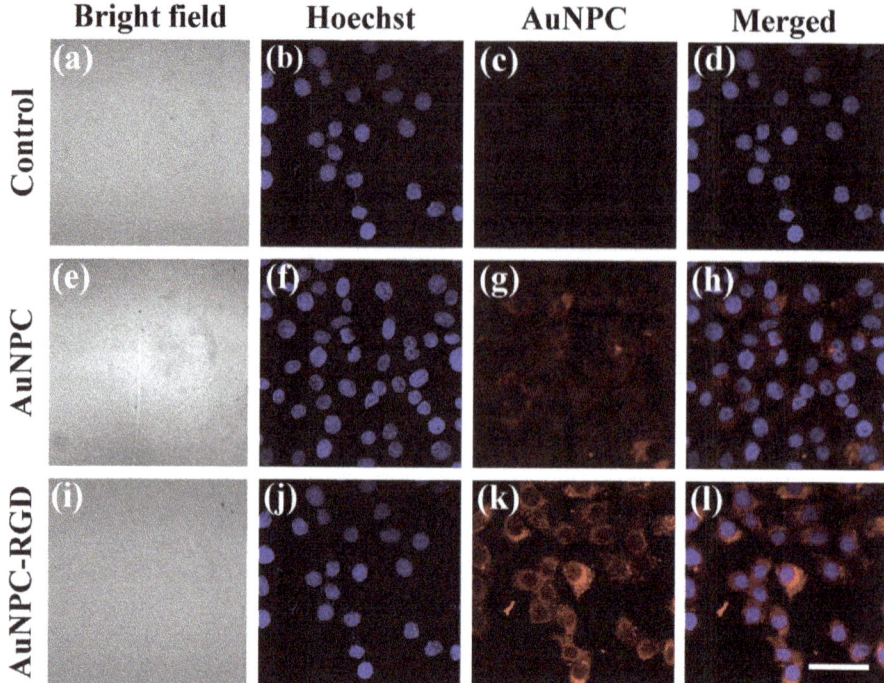

Figure 5. Laser confocal microscopy images of HeLa cells incubated with/without nanoparticles. (**a–d**) Without nanoparticles; (**e–h**) with AuNPC; (**i–l**) with AuNPC-RGD (**i–l**). Hoechst and AuNPC were excited at the same wavelength of 405 nm, and the fluorescence images were taken at 420–480 and 600–660 nm, respectively. Scale bar: 50 μm.

4. Conclusions

In summary, we have developed new nanoprobe for SERS and MEF dual functional imaging to achieve fast and long-lasting imaging for early cancer. AuNPs of about 35 nm in size are modified with a Raman reporter molecule of 4-MBA, encapsulated with SiO_2, grown AuNCs on the surface, and functionalized with BSA and cRGD to construct the dual functional (i.e., SERS and MEF) probes, denoted AuNPC-RGD. To maximize the stability, SERS intensity and MEF intensity of the AuNPC-RGD nanoparticles, the concentration of 4-MBA was optimized to be 500 μM, and the thickness of SiO_2 was optimized to be about 13 nm. The TEM and DLS results indicate the monodisperse AuNPC-RGD, with a negative surface charge that suppresses the non-specific interaction with cells. From the SERS and MEF spectra, the calculated EFs of AuNPC-RGD are 500 and 2, respectively. Moreover, cell viability in the presence of 1 mg/mL AuNPC-RGD is 84.3%, indicating the outstanding biocompatibility of the nanoprobe. For application in SERS and MEF imaging, our AuNPC-RGD nanoparticles exhibit excellent imaging abilities, which suggest that the AuNPC-RGD composite is a powerful probe for accurate and effective cancer imaging.

Supplementary Materials: The following are available online at http://www.mdpi.com/2079-4991/8/10/819/s1.

Author Contributions: F.W. conceived and designed the experiments; X.W. performed the major experiments; Y.P., X.D., L.Y. and J.L. performed a part of the measurements; F.W. and X.W. analyzed the data and wrote the manuscript.

Funding: This work is financially supported by National Natural Science Foundation of China (Grant No. 21503271) and The National Key Research and Development Program of China, (Grant No. 2017YFC0110202).

Acknowledgments: We sincerely appreciate Yuanhao Wang (Xinjiang Technical Institute of Physics & Chemistry, Chinese Academy of Sciences) for his effective suggestions.

Conflicts of Interest: The authors declare no conflict of interest.

References

1. Siegel, R.L.; Miller, K.D.; Jemal, A. Cancer statistics, 2017. *CA-Cancer J. Clin.* **2017**, *67*, 7–30. [CrossRef] [PubMed]
2. Kalluru, P.; Vankayala, R.; Chiang, C.S.; Hwang, K.C. Nano-graphene oxide-mediated in vivo fluorescence imaging and bimodal photodynamic and photothermal destruction of tumors. *Biomaterials* **2016**, *95*, 1–10. [CrossRef] [PubMed]
3. Pan, Y.; Zhang, L.; Zeng, L.; Ren, W.; Xiao, X.; Zhang, J.; Zhang, L.; Li, A.; Lu, G.; Wu, A. Gd-based upconversion nanocarriers with yolk-shell structure for dual-modal imaging and enhanced chemotherapy to overcome multidrug resistance in breast cancer. *Nanoscale* **2016**, *8*, 878–888. [CrossRef] [PubMed]
4. Cao, H.; Dan, Z.; He, X.; Zhang, Z.; Yu, H.; Yin, Q.; Li, Y. Liposomes coated with isolated macrophage membrane can target lung metastasis of breast cancer. *ACS Nano* **2016**, *10*, 7738–7748. [CrossRef] [PubMed]
5. Li, S.; Hu, R.; Yang, C.; Zhang, X.; Zeng, Y.; Wang, S.; Guo, X.; Li, Y.; Cai, X.; Li, S.; et al. An ultrasensitive bioluminogenic probe of γ-glutamyltranspeptidase in vivo and in human serum for tumor diagnosis. *Biosens. Bioelectron.* **2017**, *98*, 325–329. [CrossRef] [PubMed]
6. Aerts, H.J.W.L.; Velazquez, E.R.; Leijenaar, R.T.H.; Parmar, C.; Grossmann, P.; Carvalho, S.; Bussink, J.; Monshouwer, R.; Haibe-Kains, B.; Rietveld, D.; et al. Decoding tumour phenotype by noninvasive imaging using a quantitative radiomics approach. *Nat. Commun.* **2014**, *5*, 4006. [CrossRef] [PubMed]
7. Thaxton, C.S.; Rink, J.S.; Naha, P.C.; Cormode, D.P. Lipoproteins and lipoprotein mimetics for imaging and drug delivery. *Adv. Drug Deliv. Rev.* **2016**, *106*, 116–131. [CrossRef] [PubMed]
8. Erami, R.; Ovejero, K.; Meghdadi, S.; Filice, M.; Amirnasr, M.; Rodríguez-Diéguez, A.; De La Orden, M.; Gómez-Ruiz, S. Applications of nanomaterials based on magnetite and mesoporous silica on the selective detection of zinc ion in live cell imaging. *Nanomaterials* **2018**, *8*, 434. [CrossRef] [PubMed]
9. Luo, Y.; Zhang, W.; Liao, Z.; Yang, S.; Yang, S.; Li, X.; Zuo, F.; Luo, J. Role of Mn^{2+} doping in the preparation of core-shell structured Fe_3O_4@upconversion nanoparticles and their applications in T_1/T_2-weighted magnetic resonance imaging, upconversion luminescent imaging and near-infrared activated photodynamic therapy. *Nanomaterials* **2018**, *8*, 466. [CrossRef] [PubMed]
10. Zhang, Z.Y.; Liu, Q.H.; Gao, D.L.; Luo, D.; Niu, Y.; Yang, J.; Li, Y. Graphene oxide as a multifunctional platform for Raman and fluorescence imaging of cells. *Small* **2015**, *11*, 3000–3005. [CrossRef] [PubMed]
11. Lim, E.-K.; Kim, T.; Paik, S.; Haam, S.; Huh, Y.-M.; Lee, K. Nanomaterials for theranostics: Recent advances and future challenges. *Chem. Rev.* **2015**, *115*, 327–394. [CrossRef] [PubMed]
12. Lim, E.-K.; Chung, B.H. Preparation of pyrenyl-based multifunctional nanocomposites for biomedical applications. *Nat. Protoc.* **2016**, *11*, 236–251. [CrossRef] [PubMed]
13. Ju, K.Y.; Lee, S.; Pyo, J.; Choo, J.; Lee, J.K. Bio-inspired development of a dual-mode nanoprobe for MRI and Raman imaging. *Small* **2015**, *11*, 84–89. [CrossRef] [PubMed]
14. Sanz-Ortiz, M.N.; Sentosun, K.; Bals, S.; Liz-Marzán, L.M. Templated growth of surface enhanced Raman scattering-active branched gold nanoparticles within radial mesoporous silica shells. *ACS Nano* **2015**, *9*, 10489–10497. [CrossRef] [PubMed]
15. Jin, X.; Khlebtsov, B.N.; Khanadeev, V.A.; Khlebtsov, N.G.; Ye, J. Rational design of ultrabright SERS probes with embedded reporters for bioimaging and photothermal therapy. *ACS Appl. Mater. Interfaces* **2017**, *9*, 30387–30397. [CrossRef] [PubMed]
16. Chen, Y.; Zhang, Y.; Pan, F.; Liu, J.; Wang, K.; Zhang, C.; Cheng, S.; Lu, L.; Zhang, W.; Zhang, Z.; et al. Breath analysis based on surface-enhanced Raman scattering sensors distinguishes early and advanced gastric cancer patients from healthy persons. *ACS Nano* **2016**, *10*, 8169–8179. [CrossRef] [PubMed]
17. Lee, S.; Chon, H.; Yoon, S.Y.; Lee, E.K.; Chang, S.I.; Lim, D.W.; Choo, J. Fabrication of SERS-fluorescence dual modal nanoprobes and application to multiplex cancer cell imaging. *Nanoscale* **2012**, *4*, 124–129. [CrossRef] [PubMed]

18. Tong, L.; Zhu, T.; Liu, Z. Approaching the electromagnetic mechanism of surface-enhanced Raman scattering: From self-assembled arrays to individual gold nanoparticles. *Chem. Soc. Rev.* **2011**, *40*, 1296–1304. [CrossRef] [PubMed]
19. Chen, J.; Sheng, Z.; Li, P.; Wu, M.; Zhang, N.; Yu, X.F.; Wang, Y.; Hu, D.; Zheng, H.; Wang, G.P. Indocyanine green-loaded gold nanostars for sensitive SERS imaging and subcellular monitoring of photothermal therapy. *Nanoscale* **2017**, *9*, 11888–11901. [CrossRef] [PubMed]
20. Zhang, L.; Song, Y.K.; Fujita, T.; Zhang, Y.; Chen, M.W.; Wang, T.H. Large enhancement of quantum dot Fluorescence by highly scalable nanoporous gold. *Adv. Mater.* **2014**, *26*, 1289–1294. [CrossRef] [PubMed]
21. Ji, X.; Xiao, C.; Lau, W.-F.; Li, J.; Fu, J. Metal enhanced fluorescence improved protein and DNA detection by zigzag Ag nanorod arrays. *Biosens. Bioelectron.* **2016**, *82*, 240–247. [CrossRef] [PubMed]
22. Zhang, T.S.; Gao, N.Y.; Li, S.; Lang, M.J.; Xu, Q.H. Single-particle spectroscopic study on fluorescence enhancement by plasmon doupled gold nanorod dimers assembled on DNA origami. *J. Phys. Chem. Lett.* **2015**, *6*, 2043–2049. [CrossRef] [PubMed]
23. Lee, K.; Hahn, L.D.; Yuen, W.W.; Vlamakis, H.; Kolter, R.; Mooney, D.J. Metal-enhanced fluorescence to quantify bacterial adhesion. *Adv. Mater.* **2011**, *23*, H101–H104. [CrossRef] [PubMed]
24. Wu, X.; Xia, Y.; Huang, Y.; Li, J.; Ruan, H.; Chen, T.; Luo, L.; Shen, Z.; Wu, A. Improved SERS-active nanoparticles with various shapes for CTC detection without enrichment process with supersensitivity and high specificity. *ACS Appl. Mater. Interfaces* **2016**, *8*, 19928–19938. [CrossRef] [PubMed]
25. Wu, X.; Luo, L.; Yang, S.; Ma, X.; Li, Y.; Dong, C.; Tian, Y.; Zhang, L.E.; Shen, Z.; Wu, A. Improved SERS nanoparticles for direct detection of circulating tumor cells in the blood. *ACS Appl. Mater. Interfaces* **2015**, *7*, 9965–9971. [CrossRef] [PubMed]
26. Stober, W.; Fink, A.; Bohn, E. Controlled growth of monodisperse silica spheres in micron size range. *J. Colloid Interface Sci.* **1968**, *26*, 62–69. [CrossRef]
27. Xie, J.P.; Zheng, Y.G.; Ying, J.Y. Protein-directed synthesis of highly fluorescent gold nanoclusters. *J. Am. Chem. Soc.* **2009**, *131*, 888–889. [CrossRef] [PubMed]
28. Qiu, M.; Ouyang, J.; Sun, H.; Meng, F.; Cheng, R.; Zhang, J.; Cheng, L.; Lan, Q.; Deng, C.; Zhong, Z. Biodegradable micelles based on poly(ethylene glycol)-b-polylipopeptide copolymer: A robust and versatile nanoplatform for anticancer drug delivery. *ACS Appl. Mater. Interfaces* **2017**, *9*, 27587–27595. [CrossRef] [PubMed]
29. Chen, D.; Li, B.; Cai, S.; Wang, P.; Peng, S.; Sheng, Y.; He, Y.; Gu, Y.; Chen, H. Dual targeting luminescent gold nanoclusters for tumor imaging and deep tissue therapy. *Biomaterials* **2016**, *100*, 1–16. [CrossRef] [PubMed]
30. Yuan, J.; Hajebifard, A.; George, C.; Berini, P.; Zou, S. Ordered gold nanoparticle arrays on glass and their characterization. *J. Colloid Interface Sci.* **2013**, *410*, 1–10. [CrossRef] [PubMed]
31. Mishra, Y.K.; Chakravadhanula, V.S.K.; Hrkac, V.; Jebril, S.; Agarwal, D.C.; Mohapatra, S.; Avasthi, D.K.; Kienle, L.; Adelung, R. Crystal growth behaviour in Au-ZnO nanocomposite under different annealing environments and photoswitchability. *J. Appl. Phys.* **2012**, *112*, 064308. [CrossRef]
32. Indrasekara, A.S.D.S.; Meyers, S.; Shubeita, S.; Feldman, L.C.; Gustafsson, T.; Fabris, L. Gold nanostar substrates for SERS-based chemical sensing in the femtomolar regime. *Nanoscale* **2014**, *6*, 8891–8899. [CrossRef] [PubMed]
33. Mishra, Y.K.; Adelung, R.; Kumar, G.; Elbahri, M.; Mohapatra, S.; Singhal, R.; Tripathi, A.; Avasthi, D.K. Formation of Self-organized Silver Nanocup-Type Structures and Their Plasmonic Absorption. *Plasmonics* **2013**, *8*, 811–815. [CrossRef]
34. Yanamala, N.; Kagan, V.E.; Shvedova, A.A. Molecular modeling in structural nano-toxicology: Interactions of nano-particles with nano-machinery of cells. *Adv. Drug Deliv. Rev.* **2013**, *65*, 2070–2077. [CrossRef] [PubMed]
35. Aslan, K.; Wu, M.; Lakowicz, J.R.; Geddes, C.D. Fluorescent core-shell Ag@SiO$_2$ nanocomposites for metal-enhanced fluorescence and single nanoparticle sensing platforms. *J. Am. Chem. Soc.* **2007**, *129*, 1524–1525. [CrossRef] [PubMed]

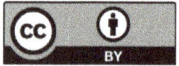

© 2018 by the authors. Licensee MDPI, Basel, Switzerland. This article is an open access article distributed under the terms and conditions of the Creative Commons Attribution (CC BY) license (http://creativecommons.org/licenses/by/4.0/).

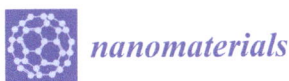

Article

Synthesis and Characterization of Elongated-Shaped Silver Nanoparticles as a Biocompatible Anisotropic SERS Probe for Intracellular Imaging: Theoretical Modeling and Experimental Verification

Carlos Caro [1,2,3,4,*,†], Pedro Quaresma [5,†], Eulália Pereira [5], Jaime Franco [3,6], Manuel Pernia Leal [4,7], Maria Luisa García-Martín [4], Jose Luis Royo [8], Jose Maria Oliva-Montero [1], Patrick Jacques Merkling [1], Ana Paula Zaderenko [1], David Pozo [3,6,*] and Ricardo Franco [2,*]

1. Department of Physical, Chemical and Natural Systems, Universidad Pablo de Olavide, Carretera de Utrera Km 1, 41013 Seville, Spain; josolimon@gmail.com (J.M.O.-M.); pjmerx@upo.es (P.J.M.); apzadpar@upo.es (A.P.Z.)
2. Departamento de Química, UCIBIO, REQUIMTE, Faculdade de Ciências, Universidade NOVA de Lisboa, 2829-516 Caparica, Portugal
3. CABIMER, Andalusian Center for Molecular Biology and Regenerative Medicine, Av. Americo Vespucio, 24, 41092 Sevilla, Spain; jaime.munoz@cabimer.es
4. BIONAND, Andalusian Centre for Nanomedicine and Biotechnology, Junta de Andalucía, Universidad de Málaga, 29590 Málaga, Spain; mpernia@us.es (M.P.L.); mlgarcia@bionand.es (M.L.G.-M.)
5. Departamento de Química e Bioquímica, LAQV-REQUIMTE, Faculdade de Ciências, Universidade do Porto, 4169-007 Porto, Portugal; pedro.cq1@gmail.com (P.Q.); efpereir@fc.up.pt (E.P.)
6. Department of Medical Biochemistry, Molecular Biology and Immunology, Universidad de Sevilla, Av. Sanchez Pizjuan, 4, 41009 Sevilla, Spain
7. Department of Organic and Pharmaceutical Chemistry, Universidad de Sevilla, 41012 Seville, Spain
8. Department of Biochemistry, Molecular Biology and Immunology, Universidad de Málaga, 29071 Málaga, Spain; joseluisroyo@uma.es
* Correspondence: ccaro@bionand.es (C.C.); david.pozo@cabimer.es (D.P.); rft@fct.unl.pt (R.F.); Tel.: +34-954-467-841 (D.P.)
† These authors contributed equally to this work.

Received: 27 December 2018; Accepted: 9 February 2019; Published: 13 February 2019

Abstract: Progress in the field of biocompatible SERS nanoparticles has promising prospects for biomedical applications. In this work, we have developed a biocompatible Raman probe by combining anisotropic silver nanoparticles with the dye rhodamine 6G followed by subsequent coating with bovine serum albumin. This nanosystem presents strong SERS capabilities in the near infrared (NIR) with a very high (2.7×10^7) analytical enhancement factor. Theoretical calculations reveal the effects of the electromagnetic and chemical mechanisms in the observed SERS effect for this nanosystem. Finite element method (FEM) calculations showed a considerable near field enhancement in NIR. Using density functional quantum chemical calculations, the chemical enhancement mechanism of rhodamine 6G by interaction with the nanoparticles was probed, allowing us to calculate spectra that closely reproduce the experimental results. The nanosystem was tested in cell culture experiments, showing cell internalization and also proving to be completely biocompatible, as no cell death was observed. Using a NIR laser, SERS signals could be detected even from inside cells, proving the applicability of this nanosystem as a biocompatible SERS probe.

Keywords: surface enhanced Raman scattering; SERS; finite element method; density functional theory calculations; cell labeling; cancer

1. Introduction

In recent years, Raman spectroscopy has been studied extensively, given its wide range of applications especially those based on the Surface Enhanced Raman Scattering (SERS) effect [1–8], by which Raman-active compounds can be detected at very low concentrations. This approach is especially valuable since Raman scattering is a very inefficient spectroscopic process and its use for detection purposes is limited. In SERS, to obtain an efficient amplification, the organic compound should be near the surface of metallic nanoparticles (NPs), especially those based on the reduced form of metals such as copper, gold or silver, where the Raman signals can be amplified by factors as high as 10^{14}–10^{15} [9–11]. In this manner, the ultimate detection limit could be a single analyte molecule [12–14]. The net SERS effect is the outcome of two mechanisms, which can act simultaneously or separately. These have come to be called electromagnetic (EM) and chemical (CM), respectively [15,16]. The EM is a consequence of the local increase of electric field in the vicinity of the NPs, due to surface plasmon excitation. This increase leads to a more intense absorption of electromagnetic radiation in molecules in the vicinity of the NPs, and therefore to enhanced Raman scattering [17]. The CM arises from changes in the polarizability of a given molecule, owing to charge transfer interaction between electronic states of the molecule and the NPs surface, leading also to increased Raman signals [18]. The CM depends exclusively on the Raman-active molecule and its interaction with the surface of NPs, while the EM depends on the surface plasmon resonance (SPR) [19–21]. SPR can be defined as a quantized collective oscillation of electrons confined within a metal/dielectric boundary that strongly interact with electromagnetic fields. According to the latest findings, Raman spectroscopy parallel to the SERS effect can be considered as one of the most powerful techniques currently available for sensing applications [22–27].

Rhodamine 6G (R6G) is a rigid molecule composed of a xanthene ring, an ethoxycarbonylphenyl group, and two ethylamino groups. Rhodamine 6G exhibits a high Raman cross-section and has been extensively studied experimentally, and so it represents a suitable benchmark molecule for SERS studies. Specifically, R6G has been shown to exhibit SERS effect on films composed of aggregates of thiol-immobilized silver-based NPs (AgNPs) [28]. In this sense, it is worth to mention that detailed data analysis from computational studies have been useful and valuable to understand SERS experimental-based phenomena, including the vibrational analysis of the R6G cation [29–31], the SERS effect on AgNPs to characterize the highest occupied molecular orbital (HOMO) and lowest unoccupied molecular orbital (LUMO) states [32], the effect of geometry on SERS of minimal silver clusters [33], as well as the spectroscopic states involved in the transition in resonance Raman [34].

Since SERS is able to detect Raman-active compounds at picomolar concentration, it could be used as a powerful tool for diagnosis and/or monitoring disease progression through tracking of specific biomarkers [35]. Typically, NPs used as SERS nanotags are obtained by interaction or anchoring of a Raman dye onto the surface of metallic NPs such as gold- or silver-based NPs. Subsequently, these NPs-dye conjugates are coated with a biocompatible, protective layer such as polymers or proteins [36,37]. For instance, gold nanoparticles (GNPs) conjugated with bovine serum albumin (BSA) have been used with encouraging results for *in vivo* multiplexing SERS [38].

Development of new non-spherical nanoparticles is becoming an option to increase SERS amplification for intracellular applications [39], since this type of anisotropic nanoparticles produce a high confinement of electromagnetic energy at sharp-nanostructured corners and edges [40]. Among them, of particular interest are star-shaped [6,41] or elongated/rod-shaped nanoparticles [42] which show considerable field amplifications near the tips, i.e., at the extremities of the particle long axis. In addition, another advantage of these nanoparticles is the possibility of using lasers in the near-IR, due to a shifting of the SPR, which is a particularly interesting feature for their usage in biological systems. Thus, an evaluation of the suitability of these nanoparticles for SERS applications can be made by using the finite element method to determine the near field around the particle, followed by comparison of the intensity of the electromagnetic field enhancement for different nanoparticle shapes and laser wavelengths [43,44]. In this sense, it has been shown that in general AgNPs have an intrinsically higher enhanced factor (EF) compared to GNPs [45]. However, Yuan et al. [46] demonstrated that EF of gold nanostars and silver spheres are similar, and both are considerably higher than gold spheres, making those particular NPs suitable for cellular SERS labelling. Remarkably, recent studies have been reported the use of AgNPs in cellular SERS labelling [39,47,48], suggesting that these could discriminate between different cell compartments for *in vitro* experimental approaches.

Nevertheless, for *in vivo* purposes, SERS-based nanoparticles should be compatible with the use of lasers with wavelengths within the so-called biological window, in order to minimize the absorption from living tissues [49,50].

Based on the above, the aim of this work was to obtain a biocompatible nanosystem that allows sensitive intracellular SERS probing. For that purpose, anisotropic AgNPs with an elongated shape were conjugated with the R6G Raman active dye and BSA. These elongated shape AgNPs show a SPR band in the near-IR region. The BSA coating entraps the Raman active dye and confers colloidal stability as well as biocompatibility to the nanosystem. To the best of our knowledge, this is the first time that analytical enhanced factor (AEF) is analyzed both by density functional theory (DFT) and finite element method (FEM) calculations. Remarkably, our results are in good agreement with SERS experimental findings. In this sense, FEM calculations show a significant field enhancement at 785 nm, making the elongated AgNPs excellent SERS probes. Finally, we were able to label by intracellular SERS a carcinoma cell line (A431), using a laser in the near-IR region and without any detectable toxicity to cells.

2. Materials and Methods

2.1. Materials

All chemicals were of reagent grade and have been used without further purification: tetraethylrhodamine hydrochloride (Rhodamine 6G) and BSA from Sigma Aldrich (Madrid, Spain), silver nitrate, sodium citrate, ascorbic acid and hydroxylamine hydrochloride from Panreac (Barcelona, Spain). Water was purified using a Milli-Q (18.2 MΩ) water system from Millipore (Madrid, Spain).

2.2. Synthesis of Silver Nanoparticles (AgNPs)

A solution containing silver nitrate (3.06 mM) and sodium citrate (6.2 mM) was prepared in 25 mL of Milli-Q water in a round bottom flask dipped in an ice bath and was stirred at 700 rpm. Upon complete dissolution of both salts, 0.5 mL of a 56.7 mM solution of ascorbic acid was quickly added and the reaction was allowed to proceed for additional 5 min. After this, the dispersion was centrifuged at 4000 rpm for 20 min and the resulting pellet was redispersed in Milli-Q water. This process was repeated 3 times to remove unreacted reagents, resulting in a final dispersion of AgNPs.

2.3. Transmission Electron Microscopy (TEM)

TEM measurements were performed in a 200 kV Philips CM-200 microscope (Philips, Amsterdam, Netherlands) with a supertwin objective lens, a LaB6 filament and side-entry specimen holder (point resolution 0.24 nm). To prepare the TEM samples, ~5 µL of solution containing the sample were removed from the bottom of the vial, followed by the removal of ~5 µL of the supernatant into the same pipette tip. Two drops of this suspension were deposited on a carbon-coated copper TEM grid (Ted Pella, Redding, CA, USA). The instrument is equipped with an energy-dispersive X-ray spectroscopy (EDX) detector (EDAX Inc., Tilburg, Netherlands). Signals from the elements Si, Cu and C are originated from carbon-coated copper TEM grid. Taking into consideration that EDX is based on the principle that each element has a unique atomic structure (with a unique set of peaks on its electromagnetic emission spectrum), we can discriminate between silver NPs and the TEM grid. The size histogram was prepared using Image-Pro Plus software (Media Cybernetics, Rockville, MD, USA), based on the measurements obtained from more the 150 nanoparticles.

2.4. Preparation of AgNPs@R6G@BSA

AgNPs concentration was determined by direct weighing of a sample after drying. A volume of 0.65 mL of the AgNPs suspension (2.84 mg/mL) was incubated with 120 µL of R6G 10^{-3} M. After two hours of incubation, 2 mL of a 50 µM BSA solution in phosphate buffer saline (PBS) was added and allowed to incubate overnight, followed by centrifugation at 4000 rpm for 30 min and re-suspension in Milli-Q water. The amount of bound R6G was determined using the UV-Vis spectrum (Ocean Optic, Largo, FL, USA) of a R6G blank solution (mixing 120 µL R6G and 0.65 mL of Milli-Q water) as a standard and comparing with the supernatant obtained after incubation with the particles and centrifugation. The remaining concentration of R6G in AgNPs was calculated to be 9.8×10^{-7} M (4.1×10^{-10} mol R6G/mg AgNPs).

2.5. UV-Vis Spectroscopy

The UV-Vis spectra were recorded with an Ocean Optic spectrometer (Ocean Optic, Largo, FL, USA) equipped with a HR4000 detector with a quartz tray with a light path of 1 cm.

2.6. Dynamic Light Scattering (DLS)

The size distribution measurements of the nanoparticles were performed on a Zetasizer Nano ZS90 (Malvern, UK). The nanoparticles were dispersed in milli-Q water or PBS at a concentration of 50 mg/L of Ag. The measurements were done on a cell type: ZEN0118-low volume disposable sizing cuvette, with 173° Backscatter (NIBS default) as angle of detection. The measurement duration was set to automatic and three measurement repeats. The analysis model was set to general purpose (normal resolution). The polydispersity index (PDI) is determined using a Malvern software (Malvern, UK), based on a cumulants analysis that performs a single fit to the correlogram.

2.7. Raman Spectroscopy

Raman IR spectra were measured on a Bruker Senterra Confocal Raman Microscope (Bruker, Hamburg, Germany) equipped with a 785 nm Ne laser and a DU420A-OE-152 detector (Oxford Instruments, Abingdon, UK). A 50× objective was used for all measurements, with a slit aperture fixed to 50 µm and an integration time of 100 s with a laser power of 50 mW. All spectra were recorded with a 3 cm^{-1} resolution. In order to calculate the analytical enhanced factor (AEF), measurements were carried out on a Labram 300 Jobin Yvon spectrometer (Horiba Jobin Yvon, Bensheim, Germany) equipped with a 17 mW HeNe laser operating at 632.8 nm and with an air-cooled CCD detector. Spectra were recorded as extended scans. The laser beam was focused with a 50× Olympus objective lens (Olympus, Tokyo, Japan). The laser power at the surface of the samples was fixed with the aid of a neutral density filter (optical density 0.3). All measurements were performed using 5 scans with 25 s of laser exposure.

2.8. Density Functional Theory (DFT) Calculations

DFT calculations were performed with the Gaussian 2009 program [51], using B3LYP exchange and correlation functional as a well-established and robust method along with DGDZVP as basis set (Gaussian, Wallingford, CT, USA). Structure optimizations of the R6G molecule and of the metal/R6G complex were carried out in vacuum with a very tight convergence criterion. All the presented spectra lacked imaginary frequencies, indicating that the minimization yielded true (at least local) minima. Calculated spectra were broadened by a 5 cm^{-1} convolution to facilitate comparison with experimental spectra. No shifting or scaling of wavenumbers was performed in any of the represented spectra. Raman spectra were obtained according to the methodology known from the literature [29], calculation of Raman intensities was based on Placzeks polarizability theory. It should be noted that the theoretical values were obtained within the double harmonic approximation, i.e., the force constants were assumed to be harmonic, and only the linear terms were retained in the series expansion of the polarizability tensor components with respect to a normal mode [51]. Spectra were calculated at room temperature and for a 785 nm wavelength. The basis set DGDZVP was applied to the silver-R6G conjugates. DGDZVP, as a full electron basis set, provides roughly 50% more basis functions than other basis set such as LANL2DZ and spectra obtained were found to compare more favorably in preliminary calculations. This has also been reported for related systems [52,53]. Although it is customary to apply a scaling factor of 0.975 to all computed frequencies due to the finite size of the basis set employed, this has not been done in this work.

2.9. Finite Element Method (FEM) Calculations

FEM calculations were performed using a commercial software package, Comsol Multiphysics 4.4 (Comsol, Burlington, MA, USA) to obtain the near field enhancement around the nanoparticle at the wavelengths of the Raman lasers used (633 and 785 nm). A particle geometry similar to the most elongated structures visualized by TEM was simulated using an ellipsoid shape with dimensions of $30 \times 13 \times 5$ nm. A single particle aligned along the y-axis of the simulation was used to calculate electric field intensities. The complex dielectric functions for silver were calculated from Johnson and Christy's data [54]. Nanoparticles were enveloped in water simulated as an isotropic dielectric medium with a refractive index of 1.33. The meshing of the geometry was performed using a minimum element size of 1.2 nm and a total of 73,208 mesh elements. An incident electromagnetic field was applied along the y-axis direction and the simulation was solved using a direct solver for a scattered field formalism.

2.10. Cell Culture

Epidermoid (squamous cell) carcinoma cell line (A431) (from CLS Cell LinesServiceGmbH, Eppelheim, Germany) were cultured in Dulbecco's Modified Eagle Medium (DMEM) supplemented with 4.5 g/L glucose, 2 mM L-glutamine, 10% fetal bovine serum (FBS) and 1% penicillin/streptomycin (ATCC, Manassas, VA, USA) at 37 °C in an incubator with a humidified atmosphere with 5% CO_2 for 24 h at different experimental conditions.

2.11. Cytotoxicity Assays

Epidermoid A431 cells were seeded overnight in 96-well plates at a density of 10.000 cells per well, in a final volume of 200 µL. For 3-[4,5-dimethylthiazol-2-yl]-2,5-diphenyl tetrazolium bromide (MTT) and lactate dehydrogenase (LDH) determination, the medium was replaced the day after with fresh media containing AgNPs@R6G@BSA at concentrations ranging from 0.5 µg/mL to 140 µg/mL for 24 h. As a negative control, cells without exposure to NPs have been used while positive controls for cell death were obtained by exposing cells to 20% ethanol in the media culture. After treatment, the supernatant of each well was saved for LDH measurements and replaced by 100 µL of media containing the MTT labelling reagent (Roche Diagnostics GmbH, Mannheim, Germany) at a final concentration of 0.5 mg/mL. After further incubation for 4 h under a humidified atmosphere (37 °C, 5% CO_2), 100 µL of the solubilization solution was added to each well. The plates were kept overnight in the incubator under a humidified atmosphere after complete solubilization of the formazan crystals. Then, spectrophotometric absorbances were measured using a microplate (ELISA) reader (Dynatech, Burlington, MA, USA) at 570 nm with 660 nm as the reference wavelength. LDH release after 24 h incubation with AgNPs@R6G@BSA was determined in the saved supernatant according to manufacturer's instructions (Roche Diagnostics GmbH, Mannheim, Germany). Data were obtained from three independent experiments. Measurements were made in five replicas for each experimental condition.

The relative cell viability (%) and its error related to control wells were calculated by the equations:

$$\mathrm{Relative Cell Viability}(RCV)(\%) = \left(\frac{[Abs]test - [Abs]Negative\ control}{[Abs]Negative\ control - [Abs]Positive\ control} \right) \times 100 \quad (1)$$

$$\text{Error}(\%) = \text{RCVtest} \times \sqrt{\left(\frac{[\sigma]\text{test}}{[\text{Abs}]\text{test}}\right)^2 + \left(\frac{[\sigma]\text{control}}{[\text{Abs}]\text{control}}\right)^2} \qquad (2)$$

Non-parametric tests were used for statistical analyses using IBM SPSS package v22 (SPSS, Chicago, IL, USA).

2.12. Flow Cytometry

For detection of apoptotic cells by flow cytometry, A431 cells were seeded overnight in 12-well plates at a density of 120,000 cells per well, in a final volume of 1 mL, and treated for 24 h at different nanoparticle concentrations. At the end of the experiment, the cells were fixed in an ice-cold solution of 70% (*v/v*) ethanol for at least 24 h, incubated for 10 min in DNA extraction buffer (0.2 MNa_2HPO_4, pH 7.8) and then incubated with 0.1% (*w/v*) RNAse (Thermofisher, Waltham, MA, USA) and 50 µg/mL propidium iodide at 37 °C for 30 min before analysis of the DNA content by flow cytometry using cell quest software (BD Biosciences, San Jose, CA, USA).

2.13. Dark Field Microscopy (DFM)

Epidermoid (squamous cell) carcinoma cell line (A431) (from CLS) were cultured on 1 mm thick and 1 cm in diameter (Goldseal number 1) glass coverslips for 48 h in Dulbecco's Modified Eagle Medium (DMEM) supplemented with 4.5 g/L glucose, 2 mM L-glutamine, 10% fetal bovine serum (FBS) and 1% penicillin/streptomycin (ATCC) at 37 °C in an incubator with a humidified atmosphere with 5% CO_2. AgNPs@R6G@BSA resuspended in DMEM (15 µg/mL final concentration) were added to the cell culture and kept under the same incubation conditions for 24 h. These assays were performed in duplicate. In order to ensure that only internalized nanoparticles are present in cell preparations, the cell culture was washed repeatedly with PBS 1×. After that, cells were fixed with paraformaldehyde and treated with Hoechst dye (dye with affinity for cell nuclei). Finally, the coverslips were mounted onto microscope slides using Vectashield Mounting Medium (Vector Laboratories, Burlingame, CA, USA) and analyzed using an upright fluorescence microscope Leica DM 2500 (Leica, Wetzlar, Germany), 100 W quartz halogen light and an external light source EL6000 for fluorescence images. Microscope was equipped with a dark field condenser without lens and a condenser upper lens DF D 0.80–0.95. Overlay fluorescence and DFM images were recorded using a Leica DFC 450 C camera and an HCX PL APO 100×/1.40–0.70 oil immersion objective.

3. Results and Discussion

Anisotropic silver nanoparticles were easily produced by a one-pot method, using non-toxic reagents and water as solvent. The conditions of low temperature and mild reducing agent that were used favour a kinetic-driven process and thus the formation of anisotropic nanoparticles [55]. TEM images of the nanoparticles are shown in Figure 1.

The TEM picture depicts a representative field in which the majority of particles exhibit an anisotropic and elongated irregular shape (Figure 1A). Energy-dispersive X-ray spectroscopy (EDX) results show a clear peak for Ag, Cu and C elements corresponding to the grid, while Si and O indicate are related to minor associated impurities (Figure 1B). The particle size distribution is shown in histograms (Figure 1C,D). The long-axis of the nanoparticles has an average distribution of lengths around 19 ± 5 nm, with more elongated populations reaching up to 30 nm, while the short-axis has dimensions of 13 ± 5 nm.

The UV-Vis spectrum of the AgNPs in solution shows a strong, broad SPR band with a maximum intensity in the range of 650–950 nm (Figure 1E). In addition, this SPR band makes these nanoparticles particularly suitable for studies in cells and tissues, due to the limited absorption of biological materials in the NIR region, which implies deeper penetration of radiation energy. In this sense, the laser wavelength used in this work (see details below) for *in vitro* experiments (785 nm) is within the high extinction range of the surface plasmon resonance of AgNPs, which favors the EM component of the SERS effect.

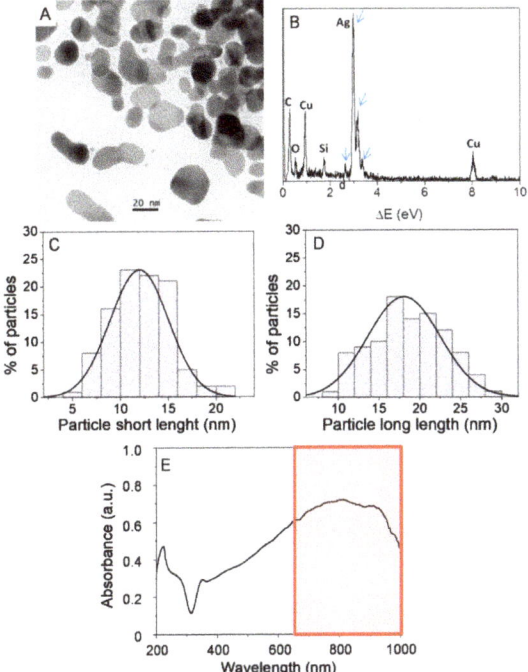

Figure 1. Microstructural characterization of AgNPs by TEM (**A**), EDX analysis of AgNPs (**B**), in which arrows indicate silver peaks. Particles short-length (**C**) and long-length (**D**) histograms-based on the measurements of over 150 nanoparticles. UV-Vis spectrum of AgNPs in solution (**E**) showing a maximum absorption in the NIR region (650–1350 nm in a red box). Signals from the elements Si, Cu and C are originated from carbon-coated copper TEM grid.

The particles have a high degree of stability, as DLS determinations in PBS (pH = 7.4) shown immediately after and one month after the synthesis procedure (Figure S1). Synthesized AgNPs showed a hydrodynamic diameter by DLS of 153.6 ± 0.9 nm. This high value might be explained by some degree of sample aggregation, especially because DLS is more sensitive to aggregates and large nanoparticles compared to small ones.

This partial sample aggregation is also reflected in the high value of the polydispersity index (PDI) of 0.184 ± 0.006. The large variety of shapes and sizes of the AgNPs could also contribute to this PDI value. After R6G physical adsorption procedure to AgNPs, the AgNP@R6G obtained showed an increase in size up to 269.2 ± 26 nm and due to some aggregation, the PDI was increased to 0.410 ± 0.098. In order to minimize this aggregation, BSA was used as a stabilization agent, yielding AgNP@R6G@BSA with smaller sizes (214.6 ± 0.5 nm) and PDI values (0.212 ± 0.007) compared to AgNP@R6G.

The suitability of these AgNPs for SERS using a NIR laser was further confirmed by finite element method (FEM) calculations of the near field enhancement, assuming excitation lasers at 633 and 785 nm. FEM calculations were performed on a model particle of greater than average dimensions and with a high aspect ratio (shape similar to a rice grain) based on the results observed by TEM. This shape was chosen since the bigger and most elongated particles will have a greater contribution to the overall hotspots formed. The results from FEM calculations were mapped as color-coded field enhancements around the particle (Figure 2A).

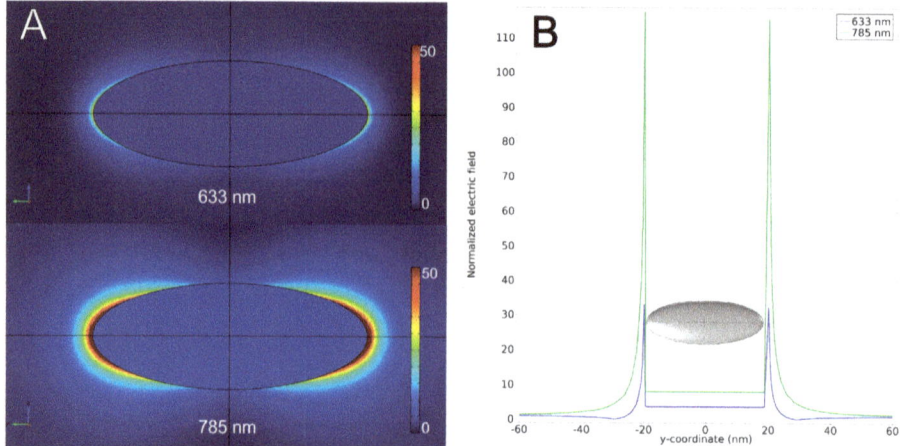

Figure 2. Local electric field enhancement (**A**) in the vicinity of one AgNP for incident radiation at 633 nm (**A**, top scheme) and at 785 nm (**A**, bottom scheme). Graphical representation of the electric field strength (**B**) (normalized to the incident field) along the y-axis of the simulation crossing the points of greater electric field intensity around the apexes of the AgNP.

The numerical values for the calculated electric field strength were extracted along a line through the y-axis of the simulation that crosses the points of greatest electric field intensity around the apexes of the AgNPs. The electric field enhancement was then calculated by dividing these values by the incident electric field and was plotted against the distance on this line (Figure 2B). This allowed a numerical comparison to the maximum electric field enhancements for the two considered wavelengths. For the 633 nm laser, a moderate increase in the near field electromagnetic enhancement could be obtained, with a maximum of ca. 30-fold at a point near the particle surface.

However, for the 785 nm laser, we calculated a considerable field enhancement of 110–120-fold, and near points close to the surface of AgNPs corresponding to the apexes of a rice shape (Figure 2).

This considerable increase in the local field intensity stresses the potential usefulness of these particles as NIR capable Raman probes.

Once we have previously obtained an estimation of the EM component and in order to have a comprehensive understanding of our nanostructured system, we performed a computational study of R6G in Ag clusters to estimate the CM component of the SERS effect.

We chose a flat surface of 10 atoms of Ag to compare it with the computational Raman spectrum of isolated R6G. In Figure 3, we show the results from DFT calculations for the SERS effect on a flat surface composed of 10 atoms of Ag.

Notably, the Raman intensity is 1 order of magnitude higher when compared to isolated R6G (area under the curve for the peak 1545 cm^{-1}; calculated SERS = 429,898/isolated R6G = 39,682). These calculations demonstrate that Ag atoms themselves are very significant in SERS effect and are in good agreement with previous work modelling a flat surface of 6 atoms [56].

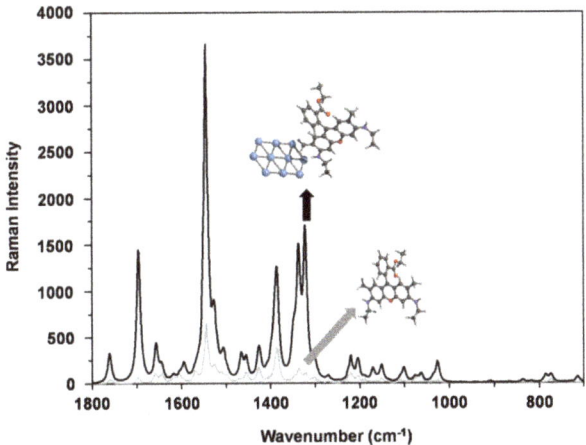

Figure 3. DFT calculation of R6G alone (grey line) and R6G interacting with a thin layer of 10 atoms of Ag (black line). The Ag layer causes a SERS effect leading to an increase in Raman signal intensity of one order of magnitude.

DFT calculations have some limitations, such as that calculated Raman spectra only take into account the interaction of the R6G with a single Ag atom of the thin layer. Actually, the nanoparticle has multiple Ag atoms interacting with the chemical compound, but the electronic structure of the nanoparticle is not considered in the previous estimation (Figure 3). Comparing computational enhanced and non-enhanced spectra, changes in the relative intensities of the signals are mainly in the lines appearing at 1695, 1335 and 1322 cm^{-1}. These vibrations are primarily assigned to aromatic C–C stretching vibrations (Table S1) [57]. Another limitation using DFT to predict SERS spectra is that the calculation invariably gives rise to peaks that are not experimentally detected. Experimentally, some of the adjacent Raman lines in the SERS spectra will merge into a new and stronger line, and these adjacent lines will become difficult to distinguish due to limitations in instrumental resolution. In addition, a phenomenon that plays a dominant role in SERS enhancement, i.e., the local enhancement of the electromagnetic field due to the localized surface plasmon resonance (LSPR) is not taken into account in DFT [58]. Experimentally, the similarity of the spectra of pure R6G and AgNP@R6G@BSA (A and B in Figure S2) is useful for the identification of the adsorbed compound. The computational spectrum is similar to both experimental condensed phase spectra. This confirms that computational methods are in good agreement for this system (Figure S1C). It should be mentioned that all computationally-obtained vibrations have higher wavenumbers, as explained in the methods section. The peak positions and intensities are shown in Table S1. After adding the Raman indicator R6G to the AgNP solution, the next step in the synthesis was the incorporation of BSA to complete our design for the nanosystem.

This protein not only provides colloidal stability to the particles, but also prevents desorption of the Raman active dye and provides a biocompatible outer surface to the nanosystem. Furthermore, our AgNP@R6G@BSA platform opens the possibility for additional binding of antibodies which could ultimately lead to smart-targeted delivery approaches.

Pure solid R6G crystals and AgNP@R6G@BSA have very similar spectra (Figure 4A,E, respectively) indicating that BSA does not replace the R6G on the nanoparticle surface nor mask the R6G vibrations, allowing its detection by Raman.

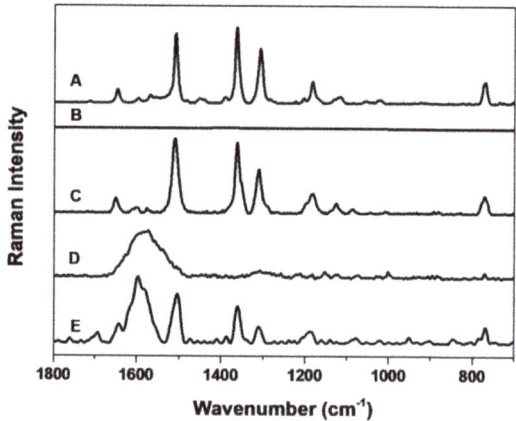

Figure 4. Raman and SERS spectra from different steps in the nanosystem synthesis. Raman spectra of pure R6G solution (**A**) and R6G at the same concentration used in the AgNP@R6G@BSA nanosystem (**B**). No spectrum is obtained from (**B**) because of the very low concentration of R6G. SERS spectra of AgNP@R6G (**C**), which is Raman active but has a very limited colloidal stability. AgNP@BSA is not Raman active (**D**). Raman spectra of AgNP@R6G@BSA nanosystem (**E**).

Furthermore, AgNP@R6G (Figure 4C) also has a very similar spectrum to pure R6G (Figure 4A) and to AgNP@R6G@BSA (Figure 4E). However, AgNP@R6G displays a very low colloidal stability in cell culture medium, and therefore it is not suitable as an *in vitro* Raman probe. In the spectrum of AgNP@R6G@BSA (Figure 4E), a broad line between 1550 and 1650 cm^{-1} can be assigned to BSA, since the spectrum of AgNP@BSA presents the same signal (Figure 4D). A hypothesis for the absence of changes in vibrations upon encapsulation with BSA could be that R6G interacts with the surface of the nanoparticle by one of the lateral amino groups, so that the main vibrations of xanthene and the aromatic ring are not affected. In Figure 4, the intensities of the spectra have been scaled for comparison. Moreover, it is noticeable that the R6G spectrum (Figure 4B), at the same concentration that the estimated for nanoparticles (AgNP@R6G and AgNP@R6G@BSA) shows no measurable signals.

A parameter which is widely used for a more accurate measurement of the SERS effect, other than just the Raman Intensity, is the AEF [59]. The AEF value can be defined by equation 1 in which the Raman intensity (I_{SERS}) obtained at a particular concentration of analyte (C_{SERS}) for the SERS experiment is related to the Raman intensity (I_{NR}) for a concentration of analyte (C_{NR}) obtained under normal conditions.

$$\text{AEF} = \frac{I_{SERS}/C_{SERS}}{I_{NR}/C_{NR}} \tag{3}$$

All measurements for calculating the AEF were performed with a 633 nm laser since both the R6G control and AgNPs@R6G@BSA can be measured with the same time and laser power experimental conditions. Conversely, for the 785 nm laser measurement, the R6G control have to be measured under different acquisition conditions in comparison to the AgNP@R6G@BSA nanosystem, rendering non-comparable results and thus making it impossible to calculate a reliable AEF. The control Raman spectrum was measured on glass without silver nanoparticles, in a drop of R6G solution with a concentration of 10^{-3} M (data not shown). All intensities were calculated by using the area under the signal at 1360 cm^{-1}, for both normal Raman intensity and SERS intensity. The AEF for the AgNP@R6G@BSA nanosystem was thus calculated as 2.7×10^7. Although this is a remarkably high AEF, it should be noted that this calculation is done based on a Raman spectrum obtained with a 633 nm laser. As AgNPs show a higher near field enhancement as well as a much closer absorption maximum for the 785 nm wavelength than for the 633 nm (as shown in FEM calculations), it is possible that the AEF value for the 785 nm laser might be even higher. To estimate AEF for the 785 nm wavelength, we can first make an approximation to the EM contribution in this system for both lasers using the values for field enhancement obtained in the FEM simulations. The EM contribution to the SERS effect can be expressed, in a first approximation, by the fourth power of the ratio between the total electric field $E(r_m, \nu)$ at the location of the molecule (r_m) and the incident field with $E_{inc}(\nu)$ with ν being the frequency of the laser Equation (4) [60].

$$EM_{SERS}(r_m, \nu) = \left| \frac{E(r_m, \nu)}{E_{inc}(\nu)} \right|^4 \qquad (4)$$

Using the ratios between the total and incident electric field that was determined in the FEM calculations, we can estimate the magnitude of the EM component in our system. For the 633 nm laser and assuming the R6G to be near the spot with the highest near field enhancement, the EM contribution would be of the order of 8×10^5. However, using equation 2 and the field enhancements obtained from the FEM calculations for the 785 nm laser under the same conditions, we can estimate that the EM contribution in this case could be as high as 2×10^8. Therefore, the EM component for the 785 nm laser could be almost 3 orders of magnitude higher than at 633 nm, leading us to expect a much higher AEF at 785 nm. Regarding the EM component calculated for the 633 nm laser, this is a value consistent to the experimentally determined AEF of 2.7×10^7 since the AEF depends on both the EM component and the CM contribution.

Finally, intracellular SERS measurements were performed on cells (A431 human carcinoma cell line), taking advantage of the very large SERS effect shown by the nanosystem even for extremely low levels of adsorbed R6G. For this purpose, we used a laser at 785 nm which takes advantage of the so-called biological window. Also, these AgNPs are particularly suited for use with this laser wavelength since the SPR maximum is in this region and the FEM calculations yielded a much higher near field enhancement for the 785 nm laser over the 633 nm laser. After the exposure of AgNP@R6G@BSA with A431 cells, the R6G spectrum could be clearly identified (Figure 5A).

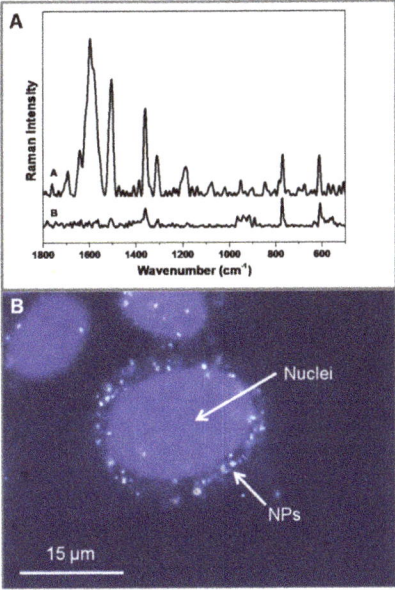

Figure 5. SERS spectra of AgNP@R6G@BSA (**A**. Inset A) and AgNP@R6G@BSA-treated human carcinoma cell line (A431) (**B**. Inset B). Overlay images of blue fluorescence channel (Hoechst dye labelling cell nuclei) and dark field microscopy (DFM) reveal nanoparticle internalization.

This proof-of-concept experiment demonstrates the possibility of using this AgNP@R6G@BSA nanosystem as a highly sensitive intracellular SERS label. Furthermore, the biocompatible BSA-covered surface in these AgNPs opens the possibility for further conjugation with recognition biomolecules (e.g., antibodies or DNA-BSA adducts) leading to different targeted delivery strategies.

In addition, to demonstrate an efficient internalization of the AgNP@R6G@BSA, A431 cells were labelled in order to identify the nuclei (Hoechst). Cells were then observed at the same time with a microscope both under fluorescence and dark field experimental settings. A perinuclear accumulation of AgNPs was clearly observed in merge images (Figure 5B).

Key factors that influence further development of engineered nanoparticles for biological applications are firstly related to cellular biocompatibility. To this aim, we used three different experimental settings to assess cell metabolic activity, cell membrane integrity and cell cycle as readouts of cell viability after exposure of AgNP@R6G@BSA (Figure 6).

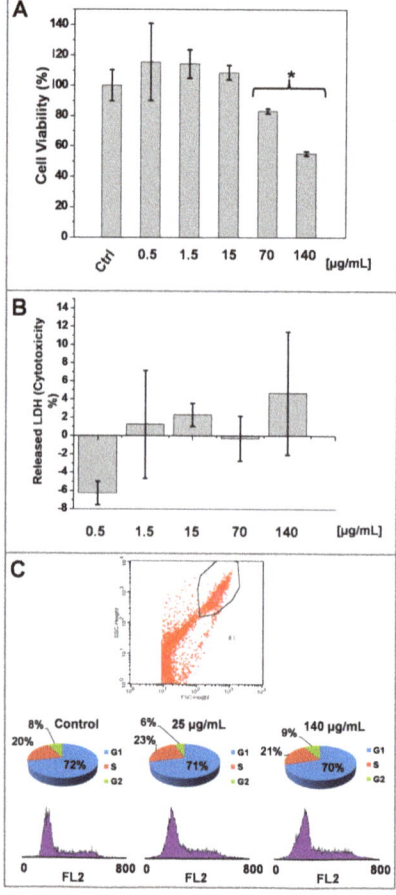

Figure 6. Effect of AgNP@R6G@BSA on A431 human epidermoid carcinoma cell line biocompatibility. Mitochondrial function (MTT reduction) after 24 h of treatment with increasing concentrations of AgNPs (**A**). Lactate dehydrogenase release assay (LDH) after 24 h of treatment with increasing concentrations of AgNP@R6G@BSA (**B**). Flow cytometry analysis of cell cycle after 24 h of treatment with increasing concentrations of AgNP@R6G@BSA (**C**). Data represented the mean ± SD. Measurements were made in three replicas for each experimental condition.

A431 human carcinoma cells exposure to increasing concentrations of AgNP@R6G@BSA from 0.3 µg/mL up to 140 µg/mL (referred also as 'nanoparticle concentration' farther ahead in the text) for 24 h was shown not to be detrimental to mitochondrial activity up to 70 µg/mL, ($p < 0.05$ U Mann-Whitney Test), as the MTT activity was maintained around or above 80% at all concentrations tested within this range. However, in the case of 140 µg/mL, cell viability decreased to 50%, implying an interference with the normal function of the mitochondria (Figure 6A). When we determined the extracellular LDH activity in A431 treated cells as a surrogate marker of cell death, mainly due to necrosis processes, we did not observe a substantial effect at any concentration tested (Figure 6B). The latter MTT reduction is inconsistent with the modest LDH values obtained in A431 cells treated at the highest concentration of AgNP@R6G@BSA, suggesting that AgNPs might drive apoptotic processes, characterized by a high degree of cell membrane integrity during the first 24 h.

The LDH results are in close agreement with the flow cytometry analysis obtained at the highest dose of nanoparticles. As shown in the scatter plot, A431 treated cells were not necrotic and the analysis of the subG1 cell cycle revealed no features of apoptosis, without differences respect to the untreated A431 cells (Figure 6C). Thus, AgNP@R6G@BSA seems to be compatible with key parameters related to cell viability at concentrations below 70 µg/mL.

4. Conclusions

Novel silver nanoparticles with elongated-shaped (AgNPs) and a size of about 13 ± 5 nm have been synthesized and characterized. With an SPR band in the near-IR zone (~800 nm) and BSA capping for biocompatibility, the newly synthesized AgNPs have potential uses as bioprobes, since living tissues do not absorb light energy in near-IR-zone.

The AgNP@R6G@BSA bioprobe has shown an extraordinary capacity to amplify the Raman signal of the R6G dye, reaching an AEF of 2.7×10^7 at 633 nm and possibly even higher at 785 nm. This high AEF might be attributed to the joint contributions of the EM and CM components for the Raman signal enhancement as demonstrated in both the DFT calculations for the CM component and FEM calculations for the EM component.

The AgNP@R6G@BSA bioprobes have been exposed to cells in culture, and demonstrated a very low toxicity, despite their high degree of internalization. A proof-of-concept experiment is also shown, in which an intracellular SERS spectrum is obtained. For future directions, we will use different NIR Raman dyes with this nanosystem platform and a wider variety of Raman-active dyes suitable for multiplex analysis. Additionally, detailed single-cell analysis of microRaman reconstructed imaging of our NPs might help to better understand the cell fate and internalization processes. Further antibody conjugation of the nanosystem will allow a more detailed molecular imaging of cancer cells.

Supplementary Materials: The following are available online at http://www.mdpi.com/2079-4991/9/2/256/s1, Figure S1: Stability determinations by DLS in PBS (pH = 7.4) up to one month after synthesis procedure, Figure S2: Experimental and computational SERS spectra and main assignments for R6G, Table S1: Correspondence between the main peaks in the experimental and the calculated (DFT) spectra

Author Contributions: C.C., P.Q., D.P. and R.F. designed and discussed the experimental work. C.C. also carried out most of the experimental procedures. P.Q. and E.P. carried out the FEM experiments. D.P. and J.F. performed flow cytometry experiments and part of the cell culture studies. M.P.L. and M.L.G.-M. carried out, with C.C., part of the in vitro experiments. J.L.R. performed the statistical analysis. J.M.O.-M. assisted C.C. in the synthesis of nanoparticles. P.J.M. and P.Z. performed the DFT experiment, with the assistance of C.C. All the authors helped in the discussion of the work. C.C., P.Q., R.F. and D.P. wrote the manuscript.

Funding: This work was supported by the following grants: In Spain: P07-FQM-02595 (to CC), P10-FQM-06615 (to JMOM), P10-CTS-6928 (to DP) and PAIDI2020 Program (FQM319 to RFM and CTS677 to DP) from the Regional Ministry of Economy, Junta de Andalucía, Spain. PI-0070/2008 (to PZ) and PI-0068/2008 (to DP) from the Regional Ministry of Health, Junta de Andalucía, Spain. PI-14-1600 from the Spanish Ministry of Economy-Instituto de Salud Carlos III (to DP), and in Portugal: (a) Unidade de Ciências Biomoleculares Aplicadas-UCIBIO which is financed by Portuguese national funds from FCT/MEC (UID/Multi/04378/2013) and co-financed by the ERDF under the PT2020 Partnership Agreement (POCI-01-0145-FEDER-007728); (b) European Union (FEDER funds through COMPETE) and National Funds (FCT, Fundação para a Ciência e Tecnologia), under the Partnership Agreement PT2020 through project UID/QUI/50006/2013-POCI/01/0145/FEDER/007265 (LAQV/REQUIMTE),

Programa Operacional Regional do Norte (ON.2 - O Novo Norte), under the Quadro de Referência Estratégico Nacional (QREN) and funded by Fundo Europeu de Desenvolvimento Regional NORTE-01-0145-FEDER-000011; and (c) Grants EXPL/CTM-NAN/0754/2013 and PTDC/CTM-NAN/2912/2014, and post-doctoral fellowship (SFRH/BPD/84018/2012) to PQ, all financed by Fundação para a Ciência e a Tecnologia, Portugal.

Acknowledgments: The authors thank the Conservation and Restoration Department, FCT/UNL and LAQV, REQUIMTE for the use of the Jobin-Yvon Raman spectrometer. Special thanks to Maria Jesús Sayagues for TEM images and useful discussion. In remembrance of Jose Antonio Mejías Romero on the 10th anniversary of his death.

Conflicts of Interest: The authors declare no conflict of interest.

References

1. Sánchez-Iglesias, A.; Aldeanueva-Potel, P.; Ni, W.; Pérez-Juste, J.; Pastoriza-Santos, I.; Alvarez-Puebla, R.A.; Mbenkum, B.N.; Liz-Marzán, L.M. Chemical seeded growth of Ag nanoparticle arrays and their application as reproducible SERS substrates. *Nano Today* **2010**, *5*, 21–27. [CrossRef]
2. Alvarez-Puebla, R.A.; Liz-Marzán, L.M. SERS-Based Diagnosis and Biodetection. *Small* **2010**, *6*, 604–610. [CrossRef] [PubMed]
3. Leopold, N.; Lendl, B. A New Method for Fast Preparation of Highly Surface-Enhanced Raman Scattering (SERS) Active Silver Colloids at Room Temperature by Reduction of Silver Nitrate with Hydroxylamine Hydrochloride. *J. Phys. Chem. B* **2003**, *107*, 5723–5727. [CrossRef]
4. Abalde-Cela, S.; Abell, C.; Alvarez-Puebla, R.A.; Liz-Marzán, L.M. Real Time Dual-Channel Multiplex SERS Ultradetection. *J. Phys. Chem. Lett.* **2014**, *5*, 73–79. [CrossRef] [PubMed]
5. Piorek, B.D.; Andreou, C.; Moskovits, M.; Meinhart, C.D. Discrete Free-Surface Millifluidics for Rapid Capture and Analysis of Airborne Molecules Using Surface-Enhanced Raman Spectroscopy. *Anal. Chem.* **2014**, *86*, 1061–1066. [CrossRef] [PubMed]
6. Quaresma, P.; Osório, I.; Dória, G.; Carvalho, P.A.; Pereira, A.; Langer, J.; Araújo, J.P.; Pastoriza-Santos, I.; Liz-Marzán, L.M.; Franco, R.; et al. Star-shaped magnetite@gold nanoparticles for protein magnetic separation and SERS detection. *RSC Adv.* **2014**, *4*, 3659–3667. [CrossRef]
7. Caro, C.; Sayagues, M.J.; Franco, V.; Conde, A.; Zaderenko, P.; Gámez, F. A hybrid silver-magnetite detector based on surface enhanced Raman scattering for differentiating organic compounds. *Sens. Actuator B Chem.* **2016**, *228*, 124–133. [CrossRef]
8. Caro, C.; Gámez, F.; Zaderenko, P. Preparation of Surface-Enhanced Raman Scattering Substrates Based on Immobilized Silver-Capped Nanoparticles. *J. Spectrosc.* **2018**, *2018*, 4127108. [CrossRef]
9. Kneipp, K.; Wang, Y.; Kneipp, H.; Perelman, L.T.; Itzkan, I.; Dasari, R.R.; Feld, M.S. Single Molecule Detection Using Surface-Enhanced Raman Scattering (SERS). *Phys. Rev. Lett.* **1997**, *78*, 1667–1670. [CrossRef]
10. Xu, H.; Bjerneld, E.J.; Käll, M.; Börjesson, L. Spectroscopy of Single Hemoglobin Molecules by Surface Enhanced Raman Scattering. *Phys. Rev. Lett.* **1999**, *83*, 4357–4360. [CrossRef]
11. Futamata, M.; Maruyama, Y.; Ishikawa, M. Microscopic morphology and SERS activity of Ag colloidal particles. *Vib. Spectrosc.* **2002**, *30*, 17–23. [CrossRef]
12. Lee, S.J.; Guan, Z.; Xu, H.; Moskovits, M. Surface-Enhanced Raman Spectroscopy and Nanogeometry: The Plasmonic Origin of SERS. *J. Phys. Chem. C* **2007**, *111*, 17985–17988. [CrossRef]
13. Kneipp, J.; Kneipp, H.; Kneipp, K. SERS—A single-molecule and nanoscale tool for bioanalytics. *Chem. Soc. Rev.* **2008**, *37*, 1052–1060. [CrossRef] [PubMed]
14. Kneipp, J.; Wittig, B.; Bohr, H.; Kneipp, K. Surface-enhanced Raman scattering: A new optical probe in molecular biophysics and biomedicine. *Theor. Chem. Acc.* **2010**, *125*, 319–327. [CrossRef]
15. Lombardi, J.R.; Birke, R.L. A Unified Approach to Surface-Enhanced Raman Spectroscopy. *J. Phys. Chem. C* **2008**, *112*, 5605–5617. [CrossRef]
16. Malek, K.; Brzózka, A.; Rygula, A.; Sulka, G.D. SERS imaging of silver coated nanostructured Al and Al2O3 substrates. The effect of nanostructure. *J. Raman Spectrosc.* **2014**, *45*, 281–291. [CrossRef]
17. Schatz, G.C.; Young, M.A.; Van Duyne, R.P. Electromagnetic Mechanism of SERS. In *Surface-Enhanced Raman Scattering Physics and Applications. Topics in Applied Physics*; Kneipp, K., Moskovits, M., Kneipp, H., Eds.; Springer: Berlin, Germany, 2006.

18. Otto, A.; Futamata, M. Electronic Mechanisms of SERS. In *Surface-Enhanced Raman Scattering Physics and Applications. Topics in Applied Physics*; Kneipp, K., Moskovits, M., Kneipp, H., Eds.; Springer: Berlin, Germany, 2006.
19. El-Sayed, M.A. Some Interesting Properties of Metals Confined in Time and Nanometer Space of Different Shapes. *Acc. Chem. Res.* **2001**, *34*, 257–264. [CrossRef]
20. Jain, P.K.; Huang, X.; El-Sayed, I.H.; El-Sayed, M.A. Review of Some Interesting Surface Plasmon Resonance-enhanced Properties of Noble Metal Nanoparticles and Their Applications to Biosystems. *Plasmonics* **2007**, *2*, 107–118. [CrossRef]
21. Sepúlveda, B.; González-Díaz, J.B.; García-Martín, A.; Lechuga, L.M.; Armelles, G. Plasmon-Induced Magneto-Optical Activity in Nanosized Gold Disks. *Phys. Rev. Lett.* **2010**, *104*, 147401. [CrossRef] [PubMed]
22. Guerrini, L.; Garcia-Ramos, J.V.; Domingo, C.; Sánchez-Cortés, S. Nanosensors Based on Viologen Functionalized Silver Nanoparticles: Few Molecules Surface-Enhanced Raman Spectroscopy Detection of Polycyclic Aromatic Hydrocarbons in Interparticle Hot Spots. *Anal. Chem.* **2009**, *81*, 1418–1425. [CrossRef] [PubMed]
23. Abalde-Cela, S.; Ho, S.; Rodríguez-González, B.; Correa-Duarte, M.A.; Alvarez-Puebla, R.A.; Liz-Marzán, L.M.; Kotov, N.A. Loading of Exponentially Grown LBL Films with Silver Nanoparticles and Their Application to Generalized SERS Detection. *Angew. Chem. Int. Ed.* **2009**, *48*, 5326–5329. [CrossRef] [PubMed]
24. Das, A.; Zhao, J.; Schatz, G.C.; Sligar, S.G.; Van Duyne, R.P. Screening of Type I and II Drug Binding to Human Cytochrome P450-3A4 in Nanodiscs by Localized Surface Plasmon Resonance Spectroscopy. *Anal. Chem.* **2009**, *81*, 3754–3759. [CrossRef]
25. Castillo, P.M.; Herrera, J.L.; Fernandez-Montesinos, R.; Caro, C.; Zaderenko, A.P.; Mejías, J.A.; Pozo, D. Tiopronin monolayer-protected silver nanoparticles modulate IL-6 secretion mediated by Toll-like receptor ligands. *Nanomedicine* **2008**, *3*, 627–635. [CrossRef] [PubMed]
26. Araújo, A.; Caro, C.; Mendes, M.J.; Nunes, D.; Fortunato, E.; Franco, R.; Aguas, H.; Martins, R. Highly efficient nanoplasmonic SERS on cardboard packaging substrates. *Nanotechnology* **2014**, *25*, 415202. [CrossRef] [PubMed]
27. Caro, C.; Castillo, P.M.; Klippstein, R.; Pozo, D.; Zaderenko, A.P. Silver nanoparticles: Sensing and imaging applications. In *Silver Nanoparticles*; Pozo, D., Ed.; IntechOpen: Vienna, Italy, 2010; pp. 201–210, ISBN 9789533070285.
28. Caro, C.; Lopez-Cartes, C.; Zaderenko, A.P.; Mejías, J.A. Thiol-immobilized silver nanoparticle aggregate films for surface enhanced Raman scattering. *J. Raman Spectrosc.* **2008**, *39*, 1162–1169. [CrossRef]
29. Watanabe, H.; Hayazawa, N.; Inouye, Y.; Kawata, S. DFT Vibrational Calculations of Rhodamine 6G Adsorbed on Silver: Analysis of Tip-Enhanced Raman Spectroscopy. *J. Phys. Chem. B* **2005**, *109*, 5012–5020. [CrossRef] [PubMed]
30. Saini, G.S.S.; Sharma, A.; Kaur, S.; Bindra, K.S.; Sathe, V.; Tripathi, S.K.; Mhahajan, C.G. Rhodamine 6G interaction with solvents studied by vibrational spectroscopy and density functional theory. *J. Molec. Struct.* **2009**, *931*, 10–19. [CrossRef]
31. Jensen, L.; Schatz, G.C. Resonance Raman Scattering of Rhodamine 6G as Calculated Using Time-Dependent Density Functional Theory. *J. Phys. Chem. A* **2006**, *110*, 5973–5977. [CrossRef]
32. Morton, S.M.; Jensen, L. Understanding the Molecule−Surface Chemical Coupling in SERS. *J. Am. Chem. Soc.* **2009**, *131*, 4090–4098. [CrossRef]
33. Pagliai, M.; Muniz-Miranda, M.; Cardini, G.; Schettino, V. Solvation Dynamics and Adsorption on Ag Hydrosols of Oxazole: A Raman and Computational Study. *J. Phys. Chem. A* **2009**, *113*, 15198–15205. [CrossRef]
34. Avila, F.; Soto, J.; Arenas, J.F.; Rodríguez, J.A.; Peláez, D.; Otero, J.C. Outstanding Role of Silver Nanoparticles in the Surface-Enhanced Resonance Raman Scattering of p-Benzosemiquinone. *J. Phys. Chem. C* **2009**, *113*, 105–108. [CrossRef]
35. Xie, W.; Qiu, P.; Mao, C. Bio-imaging, detection and analysis by using nanostructures as SERS substrates. *J. Mater. Chem.* **2011**, *21*, 5190–5202. [CrossRef] [PubMed]
36. Murshid, N.; Kitaev, V. Role of poly(vinylpyrrolidone) (PVP) and other sterically protecting polymers in selective stabilization of {111} and {100} facets in pentagonally twinned silver nanoparticles. *Chem. Commun.* **2014**, *50*, 1247–1249.

37. Jiang, X.; Foldbjerg, R.; Miclaus, T.; Wang, L.; Singh, R.; Hayashi, Y.; Sutherland, D.; Chen, C.; Autrup, H.; Beer, C. Multi-platform genotoxicity analysis of silver nanoparticles in the model cell line CHO-K1. *Tox. Lett.* **2013**, *222*, 55–63. [CrossRef] [PubMed]
38. Maiti, K.K.; Dinishm, U.S.; Samanta, A.; Vendrell, M.; Soh, K.S.; Park, S.J.; Olivo, M.M.; Chang, Y.T. Multiplex targeted in vivo cancer detection using sensitive near-infrared SERS nanotags. *Nano Today* **2012**, *7*, 85–93. [CrossRef]
39. Potara, M.; Boca, S.; Licarete, E.; Damert, A.; Alupei, M.C.; Chiriac, M.T.; Popescu, O.; Schmidt, U.; Astilean, S. Chitosan-coated triangular silver nanoparticles as a novel class of biocompatible, highly sensitive plasmonic platforms for intracellular SERS sensing and imaging. *Nanoscale* **2013**, *5*, 6013–6022. [CrossRef] [PubMed]
40. Rodríguez-Lorenzo, L.; Álvarez-Puebla, R.A.; Pastoriza-Santos, I.; Mazzucco, S.; Stéphan, O.; Kociak, M.; Liz-Marzán, L.M.; De Abajo, F.J.G. Zeptomol Detection Through Controlled Ultrasensitive Surface-Enhanced Raman Scattering. *J. Am. Chem. Soc.* **2009**, *131*, 4616–4618. [CrossRef]
41. Barbosa, S.; Agrawal, A.; Rodriguez-Lorenzo, L.; Pastoriza-Santos, I.; Alvarez-Puebla, R.A.; Kornowski, A.; Weller, H.; Liz-Marzan, L.M. Tuning Size and Sensing Properties in Colloidal Gold Nanostars. *Langmuir* **2010**, *26*, 14943–14950. [CrossRef]
42. Khlebtsoy, B.N.; Khanadeev, V.A.; Tsvetkov, M.Y.; Bagratashvili, V.N.; Khlebtsoy, N.G. Surface-Enhanced Raman Scattering Substrates Based on Self-Assembled PEGylated Gold and Gold–Silver Core–Shell Nanorods. *J. Phys. Chem. C* **2013**, *117*, 23162–23171. [CrossRef]
43. Sivapalan, S.T.; DeVetter, B.M.; Yang, T.K.; Schulmerich, M.V.; Bhargava, R.; Murphy, C.J. Surface-Enhanced Raman Spectroscopy of Polyelectrolyte-Wrapped Gold Nanoparticles in Colloidal Suspension. *J. Phys. Chem. C* **2013**, *117*, 10677–10682. [CrossRef]
44. McMahon, J.M.; Henry, A.I.; Wustholz, K.L.; Natan, M.J.; Freeman, R.G.; Van Duyne, R.P.; Schatz, G.C. Gold nanoparticle dimer plasmonics: Finite element method calculations of the electromagnetic enhancement to surface-enhanced raman spectroscopy. *Anal. Bioanal. Chem.* **2009**, *394*, 1819–1825. [CrossRef] [PubMed]
45. Banholzer, M.J.; Millstone, J.E.; Qin, L.; Mirkin, C.A. Rationally designed nanostructures for surface-enhanced Raman spectroscopy. *Chem. Soc. Rev.* **2008**, *37*, 885–897. [CrossRef] [PubMed]
46. Yuan, H.; Fales, A.M.; Khoury, C.G.; Liu, J.; Vo-Dinh, T. Spectral characterization and intracellular detection of Surface-Enhanced Raman Scattering (SERS)-encoded plasmonic gold nanostars. *J. Raman Spectrosc.* **2013**, *44*, 234–239. [CrossRef] [PubMed]
47. Palonpon, A.F.; Ando, J.; Yamakoshi, H.; Dodo, K.; Sodeoka, M.; Kawata, S.; Fujita, K. Raman and SERS microscopy for molecular imaging of live cells. *Nat. Protoc.* **2013**, *8*, 677–692. [CrossRef] [PubMed]
48. Potara, M.; Bawaskar, M.; Simona, T.; Gaikwad, S.; Licaretem, E.; Ingle, A.; Banciu, M.; Vulpoi, A.; Astilean, S.; Rai, M. Biosynthesized silver nanoparticles performing as biogenic SERS-nanotags for investigation of C26 colon carcinoma cells. *Colloids Surf. B* **2015**, *133*, 296–303. [CrossRef] [PubMed]
49. Bardhan, M.; Satpati, B.; Ghosh, T.; Senapati, D. Synergistically controlled nano-templated growth of tunable gold bud-to-blossom nanostructures: A pragmatic growth mechanism. *J. Mater. Chem. C* **2014**, *2*, 3795–3804. [CrossRef]
50. Ferber, S.; Baabur-Cohen, H.; Blau, R.; Epshtein, Y.; Kisin-Finfer, E.; Redy, O.; Shabat, D.; Satchi-Fainaro, R. Polymeric nanotheranostics for real-time non-invasive optical imaging of breast cancer progression and drug release. *Cancer Lett.* **2014**, *352*, 81–89. [CrossRef]
51. Frisch, M.J.; Trucksm, G.W.; Schlegel, H.B.; Scuseria, G.E.; Robb, M.A.; Cheeseman, J.R.; Scalmani, G.; Barone, V.; Mennucci, B.; Petersson, G.A.; et al. *Wallingford CT Gaussian 09, Revision A.02*; Gaussian, Inc.: Wallingford, CT, USA, 2009.
52. Michalska, D.; Wysokinski, R. The prediction of Raman spectra of platinum(II) anticancer drugs by density functional theory. *Chem. Phys. Lett.* **2005**, *403*, 211–217. [CrossRef]
53. Kaczor, A.; Malek, K.; Baranska, M. Pyridine on Colloidal Silver. Polarization of Surface Studied by Surface-Enhanced Raman Scattering and Density Functional Theory Methods. *J. Phys. Chem. C* **2010**, *114*, 3909–3917. [CrossRef]
54. Johnson, P.B.; Christy, R.W. Optical Constants of the Noble Metals. *Phys. Rev. B* **1972**, *6*, 4370–4379. [CrossRef]
55. Grzelczak, M.; Pérez-Juste, J.; Mulvaney, P.; Liz-Marzán, L.M. Shape control in gold nanoparticle synthesis. *Chem. Soc. Rev.* **2008**, *37*, 1783–1791. [CrossRef] [PubMed]
56. Caro, C.; Zaderenko, A.P.; Merkling, P.J. *Advanced Structured Materials*; Springer: Berlin/Heidelberg, Germany, 2012.

57. He, X.N.; Gao, Y.; Mahjouri-Samani, M.; Black, P.N.; Allen, J.; Mitchell, M.; Xiong, W.; Zhou, Y.S.; Jiang, L.; Lu, Y.F. Surface-enhanced Raman spectroscopy using gold-coated horizontally aligned carbon nanotubes. *Nanotechnology* **2012**, *23*, 205702. [CrossRef] [PubMed]
58. Wu, X.; Gao, S.; Wang, J.S.; Wang, H.; Huang, Y.W.; Zhao, Y. The surface-enhanced Raman spectra of aflatoxins: Spectral analysis, density functional theory calculation, detection and differentiation. *Analyst* **2012**, *137*, 4226–4234. [CrossRef] [PubMed]
59. Le Ru, E.C.; Blackie, E.; Meyer, M.; Etchegoin, P.G. Surface Enhanced Raman Scattering Enhancement Factors: A Comprehensive Study. *J. Phys. Chem. C* **2007**, *111*, 13794–13803. [CrossRef]
60. Garcia-Vidal, F.J.; Pendry, J.B. Collective Theory for Surface Enhanced Raman Scattering. *Phys. Rev. Lett.* **1996**, *77*, 1163–1166. [CrossRef] [PubMed]

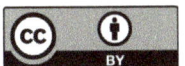

© 2019 by the authors. Licensee MDPI, Basel, Switzerland. This article is an open access article distributed under the terms and conditions of the Creative Commons Attribution (CC BY) license (http://creativecommons.org/licenses/by/4.0/).

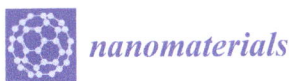

Article

Thioredoxin Reductase Activity Predicts Gold Nanoparticle Radiosensitization Effect

Sébastien Penninckx [1], Anne-Catherine Heuskin [1], Carine Michiels [2],* and Stéphane Lucas [1]

1. Research Center for the Physics of Matter and Radiation (PMR-LARN), Namur Research Institute for Life Sciences (NARILIS), University of Namur, Rue de Bruxelles 61, B-5000 Namur, Belgium; sebastien.penninckx@unamur.be (S.P.); anne-catherine.heuskin@unamur.be (A.-C.H.); stephane.lucas@unamur.be (S.L.)
2. Unité de Recherche en Biologie Cellulaire (URBC), Namur Research Institute for Life Sciences (NARILIS), University of Namur, Rue de Bruxelles 61, B-5000 Namur, Belgium
* Correspondence: carine.michiels@unamur.be; Tel.: +32-81-724131; Fax: +32-81-724135

Received: 30 January 2019; Accepted: 15 February 2019; Published: 19 February 2019

Abstract: Gold nanoparticles (GNPs) have been shown to be effective contrast agents for imaging and emerge as powerful radiosensitizers, constituting a promising theranostic agent for cancer. Although the radiosensitization effect was initially attributed to a physical mechanism, an increasing number of studies challenge this mechanistic hypothesis and evidence the importance of oxidative stress in this process. This work evidences the central role played by thioredoxin reductase (TrxR) in the GNP-induced radiosensitization. A cell type-dependent reduction in TrxR activity was measured in five different cell lines incubated with GNPs leading to differences in cell response to X-ray irradiation. Correlation analyses demonstrated that GNP uptake and TrxR activity inhibition are associated to a GNP radiosensitization effect. Finally, Kaplan-Meier analyses suggested that high TrxR expression is correlated to low patient survival in four different types of cancer. Altogether, these results enable a better understanding of the GNP radiosensitization mechanism, which remains a mandatory step towards further use in clinic. Moreover, they highlight the potential application of this new treatment in a personalized medicine context.

Keywords: gold nanoparticles; radiosensitization; thioredoxin reductase; radiation; prognosis; biochemical mechanism

1. Introduction

Over the past century, radiotherapy has emerged as the main treatment modality for cancer [1]. This powerful technique is based on the induction of lethal cellular damages caused by ionizing radiation delivered to tumors. Even if successful, this approach is still limited by dose distribution heterogeneity causing side effects to healthy tissues surrounding the tumor. In this way, the research on new strategies to achieve a better tumor targeting and enhance the biological effectiveness of radiation is growing [2,3]. Pushed by the development of nanotechnology, the scientific community takes advantage of nanoscale materials as sensitizers for therapeutic applications. It was suggested that the strong difference in energy absorption between high Z nanoparticles and water could be used to increase the local dose deposition in cells [4–6]. The proof-of-concept was demonstrated by Hainfeld et al. [7] who evidence that injections of 1.9 nm gold nanoparticles (GNPs) increased the survival of tumor-bearing mice in combination with 250 kVp X-rays compared to X-rays alone. Since this pioneering work, the development of new high-Z radiosensitizers (including silver [8,9], gadolinium [10–12], hafnium [13,14], platinum [15,16], gold [6,17,18] or bismuth [19,20] nanoparticles) has accelerated and many studies have shown their ability, when injected into the tumor, to amplify the X-ray radiation treatment efficacy. While evidencing this potential use as a radiosensitizer, the large variations in all these experimental settings revealed the high variability of GNP effects according to different physico-chemical parameters including GNP size, shape and coating agent. Zhang et al. [21] performed radiosensitization experiments using four distinct polyethylene glycol (PEG)-coated GNP (5 nm, 12 nm, 27 nm, 46 nm). Although they showed that all GNP sizes caused a decrease in cancer cell survival after irradiation, they reported a stronger effect using the 12 nm and 27 nm GNPs due to a more important tumor accumulation. Moreover, other groups demonstrated the influence of coating agent and GNP shape in the cell uptake process and so, in their involvement in the radiosensitization effect [22,23].

Despite the increasing amount of data regarding GNP-induced radiosensitization, it is still difficult to draw conclusions regarding this radiosensitization effect due to the diversity of parameters and conditions (nanoparticle size, cell lines, radiation source, administration route, ...) used in literature [2]. This leads to important open questions regarding the mechanism(s) responsible for this effect, which remains a mandatory step towards the clinical use of metallic radiosensitizers. In this context, the present work aims at shedding light on non-physical mechanisms responsible for the GNP-induced radiosensitization based on preliminary results described in our previous study [24]. In the present work, we focused on the effect of homemade 10 nm amino-PEG functionalized GNPs in five different cell lines (A431 epidermoid carcinoma, A549 lung adenocarcinoma, MDA-MB-231 breast adenocarcinoma, PANC-1 pancreatic epithelioid carcinoma and T98G glioblastoma cell lines). We evidenced correlations between GNP uptake, residual thioredoxin reductase (TrxR) activity and radiosensitization effect.

2. Material and Methods

2.1. GNP Synthesis

10 nm amino-PEG functionalized GNPs were synthesized according to reference [24]. Briefly, $HAuCl_4$ (Sigma Aldrich, Overijse, Belgium) and TA-PEG_{550}-OCH_3 (Biochempeg Scientific Inc., Watertown, MA, USA) were mixed at a 2000:1 Au: PEG molar ratio in deionized water and stirred at room temperature for 1 h. $NaBH_4$ (Sigma Aldrich) was then added to the mixture under vigorous stirring and the solution was left stirring for 3 h. Then, TA-PEG_{400}-NH_2 (Biochempeg Scientific Inc., Watertown, MA, USA) was added to the solution for extra passivation. After 3 h of stirring, the colloidal suspension was purified using a membrane filtration device (Vivaspin, Millipore, Darmstadt, Germany).

GNPs were lyophilized with a freeze-drying system (Alpha 2-4 LD Plus; Analis, Rhisnes, Belgium) and stored at 4 °C for further use. In all experiments, cells were incubated with 50 µg of gold per mL of medium, which corresponds to 8.22 nM of GNPs.

2.2. Cell Culture

Human lung carcinoma A549 cells were grown in Eagle's Minimum Essential Medium (MEM Glutamax; Gibco® by Life Technologies, Merelbeke, Belgium) supplemented with 10% (v/v) fetal bovine serum (FBS; Gibco® by Life Technologies). Epidermoid carcinoma A431 cells, mammary gland adenocarcinoma MDA-MB-231 cells, glioblastoma T98G cells and pancreas epithelioid carcinoma PANC-1 cells were grown in Dulbecco's Modified Eagle's medium (DMEM 4.5 g/L glucose; Gibco® by Life Technologies) supplemented with 10% (v/v) FBS. All cell lines were incubated at 37 °C in a humidified atmosphere incubator containing 5% CO_2.

2.3. GNP Uptake

Gold content quantification was performed by atomic absorption spectroscopy (AAS, AA-7000F from Shimadzu, Kyoto, Japan). After a 24 h incubation with GNPs, the cells were washed twice with PBS at 37 °C and then harvested using trypsin. Detached cells were then washed twice with culture medium by successive centrifugation. The actual number of cells in each sample was determined using a cell counter (Countess Automated Cell Counter, Invitrogen, Merelbeke, Belgium). After the third centrifugation, the medium was discarded, and the pellets were digested using 2 mL of aqua regia (37% HCl, 65% HNO_3 Sigma-Aldrich) overnight. The gold content was quantified using an atomic absorption spectrophotometer (AA-7000F from Shimadzu, Kyoto, Japan) by plotting the calibration curve with known concentrations of a gold standard solution (Merck Chemicals, Overijse, Belgium) in aqua regia-solubilized cells used for external calibration. Triplicate readings were analyzed for each sample. The amount of gold detected in the cells was expressed as an gold quantity (pg) per cell. Using the theoretical mass of a 10 nm GNP (=1.01×10^{-17} g), results were expressed as a number of GNPs per cell.

2.4. X-ray Irradiation

48 h before irradiation, 5×10^4 cells were seeded as 50 µL drops in 24-well plates and placed in an incubator at 37 °C with 5% CO_2. 2 h after seeding, the wells were filled with corresponding medium and placed in the incubator overnight. The medium was then removed and the wells were filled with medium + 10% FBS without (control cells) or with 50 µg Au·mL^{-1} of GNPs and incubated at 37 °C until irradiation (24 h of incubation). Prior to irradiation, the medium was discarded from the wells, the plate was rinsed with PBS and filled with CO_2-independent medium (Gibco® by Life Technologies) without FBS. The cell monolayer was irradiated with a homogenous X-ray beam produced by an X-Rad 225 XL (PXi Precision X-ray, North Branford, CT, USA) at 225 kV. The dose rate was fixed to 3 Gy·min^{-1} and the dose to 2 Gy.

2.5. Clonogenic Assay

Immediately after irradiation, the cells were detached using 0.25% trypsin and counted. In order to obtain countable colony numbers, the cells were seeded in 6-well plates containing medium supplemented with 10% FBS, penicillin/streptomycin and incubated at 37 °C. In parallel, cells were also seeded in separate dishes. 2 h after seeding, they were fixed with 4% paraformaldehyde (Merck Chemicals) for 10 min and washed with PBS 3 times. The cells attached to the dish were counted manually under an optical microscope to obtain the precise number of cells seeded. Eleven days post-irradiation, the colonies were stained with violet crystal in 2% ethanol. The number of visible colonies (containing 50 or more cells) was considered to represent the surviving cells, which were counted manually. The plating efficiency (PE) was calculated by dividing the number of colonies by the initial numbers of seeded cells. The survival fraction was obtained as the PE ratio for irradiated cells to the PE for control cells. The control cells underwent the same procedure except the irradiation step. At least three independent experiments were performed and the errors were evaluated as standard error of mean (SEM). In order to quantify the GNP ability to enhance cell death, the amplification factor (AF) was calculated as previously described [6].

2.6. TrxR Activity Assay

The TrxR activity was measured with a commercially available kit (Sigma Aldrich). The assay is based on the catalytic reduction of 5,5′-dithiobis(2-nitrobenzoic) acid to 5-thio-2-nitrobenzoic acid by TrxR. This reduction generates a yellow colored product. Its absorbance is measurable at 412 nm by spectrophotometry. The cells were incubated 24h with or without 50 µg Au.mL^{-1} of GNPs before to being detached with 0.25% trypsin. The cells were pelleted by centrifugation (1000 rpm, 5 min, 4 °C) and the medium was discarded. The pellet was resuspended in a homemade lysis buffer (9% *w/w* sucrose; 5% *v/v* aprotinin (Sigma-Aldrich), in deionized water) and disrupted by a dounce homogenizer. Then, the TrxR activity was measured according to the manufacturer's instructions. The linear increase in absorbance at 412 nm was measured during 10 min using a spectrophotometer (Ultrospec 8000; GE Healthcare, Chicago, IL, USA). The TrxR activity rate was calculated from the slope of absorbance at 412 nm versus time. Data are plotted as mean absorbance values normalized by the total protein in the sample.

2.7. Patient Survival Analysis

The online SurvExpress gene expression database (http://bioinformatica.mty.itesm.mx:8080/Biomatec/SurvivaX.jsp) [25] was used for the analysis of overall survival in different cancer types (1296 samples in total). Patients were classified into two risk groups according to their TXNRD1 gene expression. The median in gene expression was used as the cutoff. The association between TXNRD1 expression and overall patient survival was assessed by using the Kaplan-Meier method and the significance was analyzed using the log-rank test. $p < 0.05$ was considered to indicate a statistically significant difference.

2.8. Statistical Analysis

All experiments were repeated at least three times on separate days. A one-way analysis of variance (ANOVA) was performed using Origin 8 (OriginLab, Northampton, MA, USA) in order to compare the differences between groups. The number of asterisks in the figures indicates the level of statistical significance as follows: * $p < 0.05$, ** $p < 0.01$, *** $p < 0.001$.

3. Results

3.1. GNP Uptake

To assess the GNP uptake in each cell type after a 24 h incubation, AAS measurements were performed. As illustrated in Figure 1, a gold content of 0.51 ± 0.07, 0.71 ± 0.18, 0.84 ± 0.17, 0.97 ± 0.08 and 2.0 ± 0.4 pg Au/cell was measured for PANC-1, A431, MDA-MB-231, T98G and A549 cells respectively, revealing a cell type-dependent uptake. Moreover, no significant toxicity was observed in any studied cell lines (Figure S1).

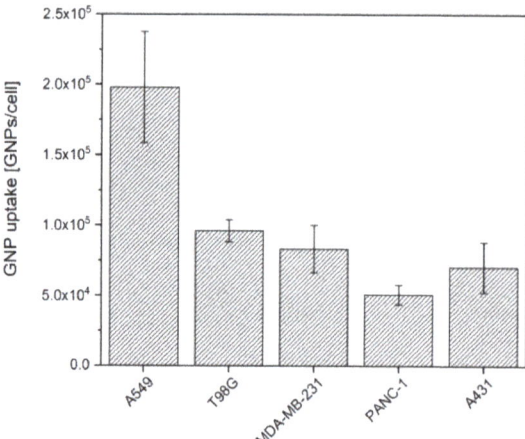

Figure 1. Cellular uptake of 10 nm GNPs in different cancer cell lines. Cells were incubated during 24 h with 50 µg·mL^{-1} of GNPs and the gold content was assessed by atomic absorption spectroscopy. Results are expressed as means ± SD for three independent experiments.

3.2. GNPs Decrease the TrxR Activity in Different Cell Lines

The enzymatic activity of TrxR was evaluated in the different cell lines incubated with or without 50 µg·mL^{-1} of GNPs during 24 h. As shown in Figure 2, a decrease in TrxR activity was observed in all the cell lines when incubated with GNPs. Moreover, results demonstrated that the level of this enzymatic inhibition is cell type-dependent with a $49 \pm 7\%$, $64 \pm 5\%$, $75 \pm 4\%$ and $88 \pm 7\%$ of residual TrxR activity for A431, T98G, MDA-MB-231 and PANC-1 cells respectively. However, one-way

ANOVA (Tukey test) evidenced that this inhibition was not significant for PANC-1 and MDA-MB-231 cells. It must be noted that a 28 ± 3% residual activity was previously measured in A549 cells incubated with the same GNPs [24].

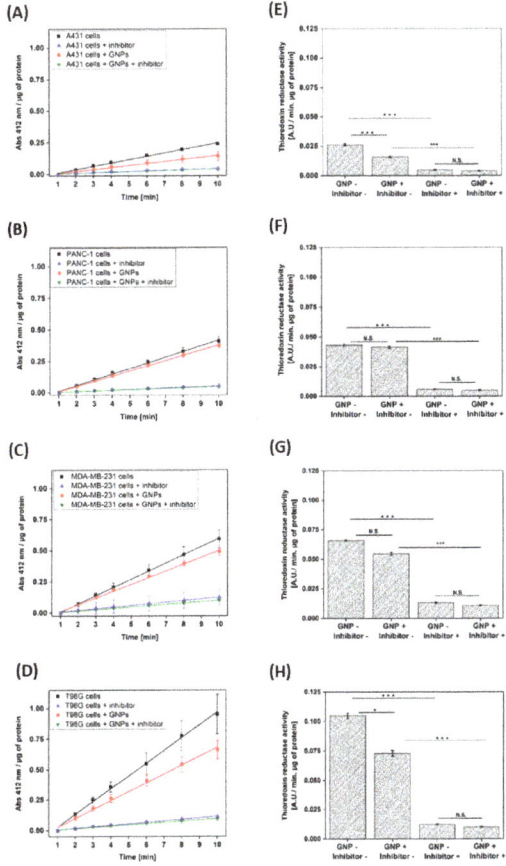

Figure 2. TrxR activity in cells incubated with or without 50 µg Au·mL^{-1} GNPs during 24 h. The activity was measured by the absorption at 412 nm over time in cell lysate of (**A**) A431, (**B**) PANC-1, (**C**) MDA-MB-231 and (**D**) T98G. Data are plotted as mean values of absorbance normalized by the total protein content ± S.D. of 3 independent experiments. Slopes of these TrxR activity curves were used to calculate the TrxR activity rate in (**E**) A431, (**F**) PANC-1, (**G**) MDA-MB-231 and (**H**) T98G cell lines. Data are plotted as mean values ± S.D. of 3 independent experiments. All results were statistically analyzed using a one-way ANOVA (Tukey test, * $p < 0.05$, *** $p < 0.001$, N.S. = not significant).

3.3. GNPs Enhance the Cell Death upon Irradiation

The five cancer cell lines were pre-incubated during 24 h with or without 50 µg·mL^{-1} of GNPs prior to be irradiated using 225 kVp X-rays. Cell survival fractions were assessed by standard clonogenic assays. As shown in Figure 3, survival fraction decreased in all cell lines when they were pre-incubated with GNPs. To quantify this decrease in survival fraction, we calculated the amplification factor (AF) which indicates the enhanced proportion of dead cells in the presence of GNPs compared with irradiation alone for a given dose. At 2 Gy, a clinically relevant dose per fraction, a 13 ± 4%, 23 ± 1%, 7 ± 4%, 14 ± 3% and 2 ± 1% AF was calculated for, respectively, A431, A549, MDA-MB-231, T98G and PANC-1 cells.

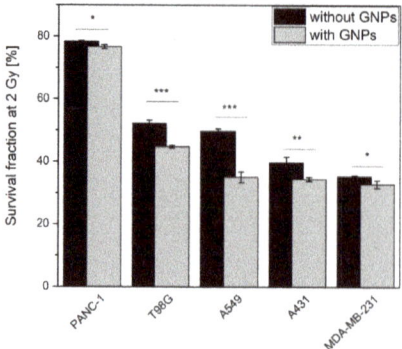

Figure 3. GNPs enhance cell death upon irradiation. Survival fractions were determined by colony forming assay for cells pre-incubated with 50 µg·mL^{-1} GNPs. After a 24 h incubation with GNPs, cells were irradiated with 225 kVp X-rays. Results are expressed as mean values of at least three independent experiments ± SEM. Data were statistically analyzed using a one-way ANOVA (Tukey test, * $p < 0.05$, ** $p < 0.01$; ** $p < 0.001$).

3.4. Correlation between Cell Response to Radiation, TrxR Activity and GNP Uptake

To better understand the relationship between survival fractions, gold content in cells and the GNP-induced TrxR inhibition, correlation studies were performed. Results highlighted a strong correlation between GNP uptake and the amount of inhibited TrxR (Figure 4A, Pearson's r = 0.991), between the AF at 2 Gy and the residual level of TrxR activity (Figure 4B, Pearson's r = −0.978) and between the AF at 2 Gy and the GNP uptake (Figure 4C, Pearson's r = 0.872).

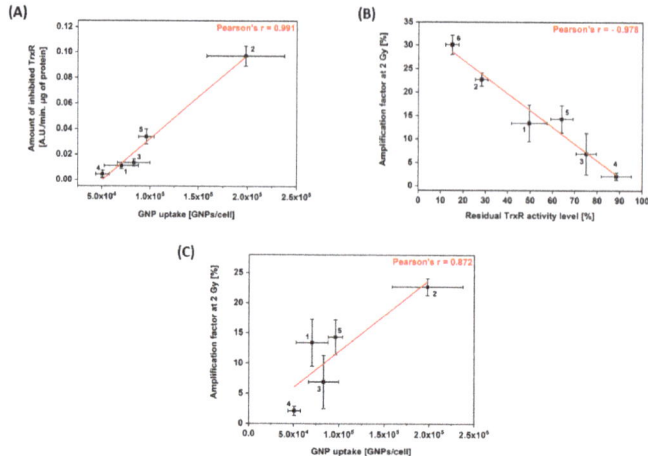

Figure 4. Correlation analysis showing the relation between (**A**) the amount of inhibited TrxR in cells and gold content; (**B**) the AF at 2 Gy and the residual TrxR activity level at irradiation time; (**C**) the AF at 2 Gy and the GNPs uptake. Data are presented as means of at least three independent experiments ± SEM (for AF) or ± SD (for TrxR activity and GNP uptake). 1 = A431 cells; 2 = A549 cells; 3 = MDA-MB-231 cells; 4 = PANC-1 cells; 5 = T98G cells; 6 = A549 cells invalidated for TrxR [24].

3.5. TXNRD1 Is an Unfavorable Prognostic Factor

To investigate the possible involvement of TXNRD1 (gene coding for TrxR) expression in patient survival, we retrospectively analyzed microarray datasets of different types of cancer. A total of 1,296 samples with TXNRD1 status from five datasets were taken into account in this study.

Five independent clinical cohort datasets were used: GSE-42669 [26] and GSE-30219 [27] cohorts for glioblastoma and lung adenocarcinoma respectively, TCGA-BRCA and TCGA-HNSC cohorts for invasive breast and squamous cell carcinomas respectively as well as PACA-AU for pancreatic ductal adenocarcinoma. The characteristics of these different cohorts are described in Table 1. Using SurvExpress tools, overall patient survival was analyzed according to TXNRD1 mRNA expression. Figure 5 shows the Kaplan-Meier curves for different cancer types while a box plot across the groups is shown in Figure S2. The results showed that high expression of TXNRD1 gene was significantly associated with poor overall patient survival in brain, breast, lung and head & neck. The effect was the most pronounced for lung adenocarcinoma, for which the median survival time decreased from 102 months (low TXNRD1 expression) to 44 months (high TXNRD1 expression).

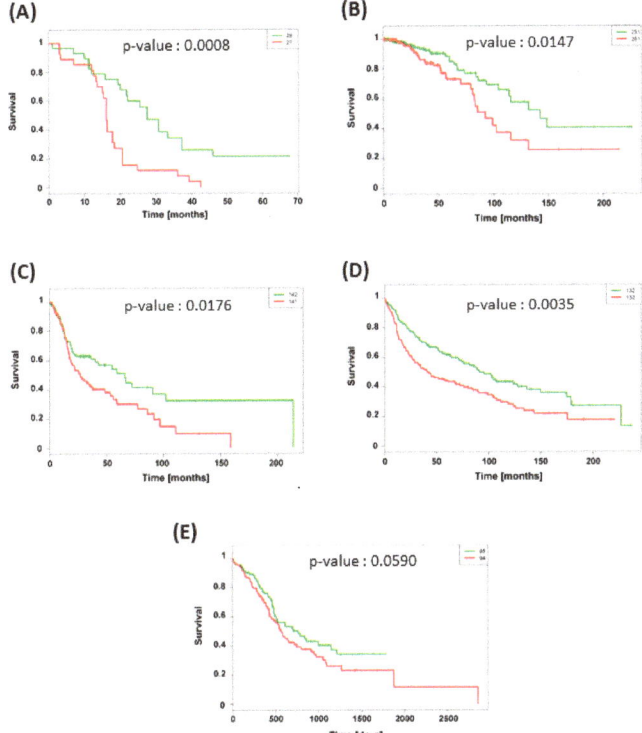

Figure 5. Kaplan-Meier analysis for overall patient survival according to TXRND1 mRNA expression in (**A**) brain (GSE42669), (**B**) breast (TCGA-BRCA), (**C**) head & neck (TCGA-HNSC), (**D**) lung (GSE 30219) and (**E**) pancreas (PACA-AU) cancer datasets. Green and red curves mean low and high TXNRD1 expression groups respectively. Log-rank equal curves p-values were calculated using the SurvExpress tools and were considered to be significant when $p < 0.05$.

Table 1. Overall characteristics of the five datasets used in this study.

Organ	Cancer Type	Number of Patients	Median Survival Time (Months)		Database
			Low TXNRD1 Expression	High TXNRD1 Expression	
Brain	Glioblastoma	58	27	16	GSE 42669 [26]
Breast	Invasive carcinoma	502	142	92	TCGA-BRCA
Head & Neck	Squamous cell carcinoma	283	66	27	TCGA-HNSC
Lung	Adenocarcinoma	264	102	44	GSE 30219 [27]
Pancreas	Ductal adenocarcinoma	189	26	19	PACA-AU

4. Discussion

For the past several decades, oncology has been shifting towards a personalized medicine approach where the treatment selection for each cancer patient is becoming individualized [28]. This medical field is rapidly evolving driven by networks such as "The Cancer Genome Atlas" (TCGA) or "Gene Expression Omnibus" (GEO) that enable to catalogue genetic changes in key genes associated to cancer. These datasets permit the scientific community to identify new potential biomarkers and therapeutic targets [28,29]. In this study, Kaplan-Meier survival plots generated from cohort data demonstrated that higher expression of TXNRD1 gene is significantly correlated with poor survival outcome, identifying this gene as an unfavorable prognostic factor for cancer patients. The protein encoded by TXNRD1 belongs to the pyridine nucleotide-disulfide oxidoreductase family and is a member of the thioredoxin (Trx) system. This system is a major redox regulator and comprises an oxido-reductase enzyme (TrxR) which catalyzes the reduction of oxidized Trx by coupling with the oxidation of NADPH to $NADP^+$ [30]. Since TrxR is also involved in tumor growth and DNA replication [31,32], it is not surprising that TXNRD1 overexpression has been evidenced in many aggressive tumors [30,33]. Moreover, breast cancer resistance to docetaxel has been demonstrated in tumor expressing high mRNA TrxR level [34,35].

In the context of personalized medicine, a therapeutic strategy to treat overexpressing TXNRD1 tumors could involve the use of Trx system inhibitors such as auranofin. Several studies have shown the ability of auranofin to trigger ROS overproduction and apoptosis in different cell lines [36–38] and to exert an antitumor activity in mice bearing breast or lung xenografts [38,39]. These works paved the way to ongoing lung cancer [40], leukemia [41] or ovarian cancer [42] clinical trials. Although auranofin was already FDA approved for the treatment of rheumatoid arthritis, its use is associated to cytotoxicity in vitro as demonstrated by Wang et al. (IC_{50} values of 19 and 11 µM for 4T1 and EMT6 cells respectively) [38]. One less toxic alternative could be GNPs. This study reported a cell type-dependent TrxR inhibition that may be explained by differences in cell capacity to internalize GNPs as well as in basal TrxR expression in each cell line. Indeed, we showed that even if we measured a similar gold content in A431 and MDA-MB-231 cells, we observed differences in TrxR inhibition (49% of residual TrxR activity level in A431 cells versus 75% in MDA-MB-231 cells). These differences may be due to a lower TrxR expression in A431 cells compared to MDA-MB-231 cells as suggested by activity measurement in Figure 2 (0.026 versus 0.066 A.U./min. µg of protein for A431 and MDA-MB-231 cells respectively).

Our work highlighted a cell-dependent radiosensitization effect with 225 kVp X-ray photons enabling to eradicate up to 23% more cells (in case of A549 cells) at 2 Gy compared to irradiation without GNPs. Although various works evidenced the GNP ability to enhance the biological effectiveness of radiation [6,24,43,44], the mechanism responsible for this effect remains poorly understood. Currently, two theories have been suggested. On one hand, a physico-chemical mechanism coming from the difference in energy absorption between gold and the surrounding soft tissues enables a dose enhancement in cells containing GNPs [5]. The interaction between the ionizing particles and high Z atoms can lead to the emission of low-energy electrons (LEE) from the nanoparticle [11,45] and the production of ROS [46,47]. This "ballistic" approach which predicts that the cell response would be directly correlated to the gold content, requires a direct interaction between the incident beam and the GNPs. However, a growing amount of simulation works evidenced that the number of hits in a cell containing GNPs is very low, especially in case of charged particles [48,49]. Consequently, the calculated physical enhancement effects of GNPs are very low compared to the radiosensitization effect observed in in vitro studies. Moreover, various studies have reported significant radiosensitization effect with megavoltage X-rays where little or no increase in overall dose deposition would be expected according to the theory [50–52]. This suggests that other mechanisms have greater contribution than physical interaction to the radiosensitization effect [48,49,53,54]. On the other hand, we previously demonstrated the involvement of the Trx system in GNP-induced radiosensitzation, suggesting a biological mechanism [24]. We performed an invalidation of the TrxR expression in A549 cells using siRNA technology leading to a residual 15% TrxR protein level. These invalidated A549 cells were irradiated without GNPs, evidencing a significant radiosensitization effect (AF of 30% at 2 Gy) [24]. Therefore, we suggested a new mechanism: following cell uptake through a receptor-mediated endocytosis, endosomes containing GNPs fuse with lysosomes. By decreasing pH inside the vesicle, lysosomes trigger a GNP degradation leading to the release of gold ions, well-known TrxR inhibitors. This inhibition induces various dysfunctions of pathways leading to a cytoplasmic ROS accumulation, a decrease in ATP production and DNA damage repair alterations. Irradiation of these weakened cells will cause DNA damage and an extra oxidative stress in cells with limited ATP stocks and detoxification systems [24]. Although this link between TrxR and GNP-induced radiosensitization was previously hypothesized to explain lung carcinoma cells radiosensitization, the present study validated it in four other cell lines. Indeed, correlation analyses (Figure 4) demonstrated that the radiosensitization effect is strongly correlated to the residual TrxR level. The aforementioned suggested mechanism is in agreement with an increasing number of works that have started to take nanoparticle impacts on cellular processes into account. By comparing a large amount of studies describing GNP-induced radiosensitization, Butterworth et al. [54] concluded that oxidative stress plays a central role in the radiosensitization effect. This hypothesis was confirmed by various groups which evidenced a reduction in radiosensitization effect when DMSO, a ROS scavenger was present upon irradiation [6,15,55,56]. Recently, protein disulphide isomerase, an enzyme catalyzing the formation and breakage of disulfide bonds in cysteine residues, was suspected to be a key mediator of the cellular response to GNPs [57]. Interestingly, some studies have showed that oxide nanoparticles have the ability to decrease DNA repair efficiency without any ROS production enhancement, on the opposite effect to metallic NPs [58,59]. This highlights the need to consider biological impacts of nanoparticles in further studies in order to rationalize reported differences in literature and to progress in our global understanding of the phenomenon.

It must be noted that all the results in this work are based on in vitro cell culture studies. Hence, this experimental set up displays some limitations. We evidenced that the TrxR inhibition increases with the gold uptake in the cells. However, the GNP delivery to tumors in vivo at similar concentrations is much more challenging. This will require tumor cell targeting strategies such as GNP surface modifications with antibodies [60]. Moreover, in vivo studies are required to investigate if similar metabolic changes occur in tumor than the ones described in cells, when GNPs are injected into mice. Lastly, irradiations of cell monolayers performed in this study may not accurately represent the 3-dimensional in vivo setting.

5. Conclusions

This work highlights the importance of nanoparticle - cell interactions to fully understand the radiosensitization mechanism. It evidences that the implication of TrxR, previously reported in GNP-induced lung cancer cell radiosensitization, seemingly confirmed in other cancer types since a good correlation between cell response to radiation and residual TrxR activity level is highlighted. Overall, this would suggest that GNPs play a radiosensitizer role by weakening detoxification system in addition to the radioenhancer role widely described in literature. To progress in the development of nanotechnology for oncology applications, the capacity of nanomaterials to inhibit the thiol-reductases protein family (such as TrxR) and their impact on antioxidants need to be assessed. A deep understanding of the mechanism responsible for this enhancement effect still remains a mandatory step towards the optimized clinical use of nanomaterials as radiosensitizers.

Supplementary Materials: The following are available online at http://www.mdpi.com/2079-4991/9/2/295/s1, Figure S1: Toxicity of GNPs across the cell lines. All cells were incubated 24 h with 50 µg/mL GNPs prior the clonogenic assay. Results were reported as mean plating efficiency ± SEM, Figure S2: Box plot of TXNRD1 expression levels in (A) brain (GSE42669), (B) breast (TCGA-BRCA), (C) head & neck (TCGA-HNSC), (D) lung (GSE 30219) and (E) pancreas (PACA-AU) tumors.

Author Contributions: S.P. performed the experiment and wrote the paper. A.-C.H., C.M. and S.L. conceived and designed the studies.

Funding: This research received no external funding.

Acknowledgments: We are grateful to Tijani Tabarrant for its skillful assistance with the irradiation facilities. The authors acknowledge the TCGA Research Network as well as the technical support of the SIAM technological platform of UNamur. The X-ray irradiator was purchased thanks to the financial support from Oncobeth ASBL and Fonds Anciaux de Solidarité-Espoir ASBL. Sébastien Penninckx is a fellow funded by the Belgian Funds for Scientific Research (FRS-FNRS, Belgium).

Conflicts of Interest: The authors declare no conflict of interest.

References

1. Delaney, G.; Jacob, S.; Featherstone, C.; Barton, M. The role of radiotherapy in cancer treatment: Estimating optimal utilization from a review of evidence-based clinical guidelines. *Cancer* **2005**, *104*, 1129–1137. [CrossRef] [PubMed]
2. Laprise-Pelletier, M.; Simao, T.; Fortin, M.A. Gold Nanoparticles in Radiotherapy and Recent Progress in Nanobrachytherapy. *Adv. Healthc. Mater.* **2018**, *7*, e1701460. [CrossRef] [PubMed]
3. Genard, G.; Wera, A.C.; Huart, C.; le Calve, B.; Penninckx, S.; Fattaccioli, A.; Tabarrant, T.; Demazy, C.; Ninane, N.; Heuskin, A.C.; et al. Proton irradiation orchestrates macrophage reprogramming through NFkappaB signaling. *Cell Death Dis.* **2018**, *9*, 728. [CrossRef] [PubMed]
4. Kobayashi, K.; Usami, N.; Porcel, E.; Lacombe, S.; le Sech, C. Enhancement of radiation effect by heavy elements. *Mutat. Res.* **2010**, *704*, 123–131. [CrossRef] [PubMed]
5. Currell, F.; Villagomez-Bernabe, B. Physical and Chemical Processes for Gold Nanoparticles and Ionising Radiation in Medical Contexts. In *Gold Nanoparticles for Physics, Chemistry and Biology*; World Scientific: Singapore, 2017; pp. 509–536.
6. Li, S.; Penninckx, S.; Karmani, L.; Heuskin, A.C.; Watillon, K.; Marega, R.; Zola, J.; Corvaglia, V.; Genard, G.; Gallez, B.; et al. LET-dependent radiosensitization effects of gold nanoparticles for proton irradiation. *Nanotechnology* **2016**, *27*, 455101. [CrossRef] [PubMed]
7. Hainfeld, J.F.; Slatkin, D.N.; Smilowitz, H.M. The use of gold nanoparticles to enhance radiotherapy in mice. *Phys. Med. Biol.* **2004**, *49*, N309–N315. [CrossRef] [PubMed]
8. Xu, R.; Ma, J.; Sun, X.; Chen, Z.; Jiang, X.; Guo, Z.; Huang, L.; Li, Y.; Wang, M.; Wang, C.; et al. Ag nanoparticles sensitize IR-induced killing of cancer cells. *Cell Res.* **2009**, *19*, 1031–1034. [CrossRef]
9. Liu, P.; Jin, H.; Guo, Z.; Ma, J.; Zhao, J.; Li, D.; Wu, H.; Gu, N. Silver nanoparticles outperform gold nanoparticles in radiosensitizing U251 cells in vitro and in an intracranial mouse model of glioma. *Int. J. Nanomed.* **2016**, *11*, 5003–5014. [CrossRef]
10. Miladi, I.; Aloy, M.T.; Armandy, E.; Mowat, P.; Kryza, D.; Magne, N.; Tillement, O.; Lux, F.; Billotey, C.; Janier, M.; et al. Combining ultrasmall gadolinium-based nanoparticles with photon irradiation overcomes radioresistance of head and neck squamous cell carcinoma. *Nanomed. Nanotechnol. Biol. Med.* **2015**, *11*, 247–257. [CrossRef]
11. Porcel, E.; Tillement, O.; Lux, F.; Mowat, P.; Usami, N.; Kobayashi, K.; Furusawa, Y.; le Sech, C.; Li, S.; Lacombe, S. Gadolinium-based nanoparticles to improve the hadrontherapy performances. *Nanomed. Nanotechnol. Biol. Med.* **2014**, *10*, 1601–1608. [CrossRef]
12. Detappe, A.; Kunjachan, S.; Rottmann, J.; Robar, J.; Tsiamas, P.; Korideck, H.; Tillement, O.; Berbeco, R. AGuIX nanoparticles as a promising platform for image-guided radiation therapy. *Cancer Nanotechnol.* **2015**, *6*, 4. [CrossRef] [PubMed]
13. McGinnity, T.L.; Dominguez, O.; Curtis, T.E.; Nallathamby, P.D.; Hoffman, A.J.; Roeder, R.K. Hafnia (HfO2) nanoparticles as an X-ray contrast agent and mid-infrared biosensor. *Nanoscale* **2016**, *8*, 13627–13637. [CrossRef] [PubMed]
14. Pottier, A.; Borghi, E.; Levy, L. New use of metals as nanosized radioenhancers. *Anticancer Res.* **2014**, *34*, 443–453. [PubMed]
15. Li, S.; Porcel, E.; Remita, H.; Marco, S.; Réfrégiers, M.; Dutertre, M.; Confalonieri, F.; Lacombe, S. Platinum nanoparticles: An exquisite tool to overcome radioresistance. *Cancer Nanotechnol.* **2017**, *8*, 4. [CrossRef]

16. Porcel, E.; Liehn, S.; Remita, H.; Usami, N.; Kobayashi, K.; Furusawa, Y.; le Sech, C.; Lacombe, S. Platinum nanoparticles: A promising material for future cancer therapy? *Nanotechnology* **2010**, *21*, 085103. [CrossRef] [PubMed]
17. Zhang, X.-D.; Luo, Z.; Chen, J.; Song, S.; Yuan, X.; Shen, X.; Wang, H.; Sun, Y.; Gao, K.; Zhang, L. Ultrasmall glutathione-protected gold nanoclusters as next generation radiotherapy sensitizers with high tumor uptake and high renal clearance. *Sci. Rep.* **2015**, *5*, 8669. [CrossRef] [PubMed]
18. Liu, Y.; Liu, X.; Jin, X.; He, P.; Zheng, X.; Dai, Z.; Ye, F.; Zhao, T.; Chen, W.; Li, Q. The dependence of radiation enhancement effect on the concentration of gold nanoparticles exposed to low- and high-LET radiations. *Phys. Med.* **2015**, *31*, 210–218. [CrossRef] [PubMed]
19. Hossain, M.; Luo, Y.; Sun, Z.; Wang, C.; Zhang, M.; Fu, H.; Qiao, Y.; Su, M. X-ray enabled detection and eradication of circulating tumor cells with nanoparticles. *Biosens. Bioelectron.* **2012**, *38*, 348–354. [CrossRef] [PubMed]
20. Huang, Y.; Ma, M.; Chen, S.; Dai, J.; Chen, F.; Wang, Z. Construction of multifunctional organic–inorganic hybrid Bi2S3–PLGA capsules for highly efficient ultrasound-guided radiosensitization of brachytherapy. *RSC Adv.* **2014**, *4*, 26861–26865. [CrossRef]
21. Zhang, X.D.; Wu, D.; Shen, X.; Chen, J.; Sun, Y.M.; Liu, P.X.; Liang, X.J. Size-dependent radiosensitization of PEG-coated gold nanoparticles for cancer radiation therapy. *Biomaterials* **2012**, *33*, 6408–6419. [CrossRef] [PubMed]
22. Villanueva, A.; Canete, M.; Roca, A.G.; Calero, M.; Veintemillas-Verdaguer, S.; Serna, C.J.; Mdel, P.M.; Miranda, R. The influence of surface functionalization on the enhanced internalization of magnetic nanoparticles in cancer cells. *Nanotechnology* **2009**, *20*, 115103. [CrossRef] [PubMed]
23. Ma, N.; Wu, F.-G.; Zhang, X.; Jiang, Y.-W.; Jia, H.-R.; Wang, H.-Y.; Li, Y.-H.; Liu, P.; Gu, N.; Chen, Z. Shape-Dependent Radiosensitization Effect of Gold Nanostructures in Cancer Radiotherapy: Comparison of Gold Nanoparticles, Nanospikes, and Nanorods. *ACS Appl. Mater. Interfaces* **2017**, *9*, 13037–13048. [CrossRef] [PubMed]
24. Penninckx, S.; Heuskin, A.C.; Michiels, C.; Lucas, S. The role of thioredoxin reductase in gold nanoparticle radiosensitization effects. *Nanomedicine (Lond. Engl.)* **2018**. [CrossRef] [PubMed]
25. Aguirre-Gamboa, R.; Gomez-Rueda, H.; Martinez-Ledesma, E.; Martinez-Torteya, A.; Chacolla-Huaringa, R.; Rodriguez-Barrientos, A.; Tamez-Pena, J.G.; Trevino, V. SurvExpress: An online biomarker validation tool and database for cancer gene expression data using survival analysis. *PLoS ONE* **2013**, *8*, e74250. [CrossRef] [PubMed]
26. Joo, K.M.; Kim, J.; Jin, J.; Kim, M.; Seol, H.J.; Muradov, J.; Yang, H.; Choi, Y.L.; Park, W.Y.; Kong, D.S.; et al. Patient-specific orthotopic glioblastoma xenograft models recapitulate the histopathology and biology of human glioblastomas in situ. *Cell Rep.* **2013**, *3*, 260–273. [CrossRef] [PubMed]
27. Rousseaux, S.; Debernardi, A.; Jacquiau, B.; Vitte, A.L.; Vesin, A.; Nagy-Mignotte, H.; Moro-Sibilot, D.; Brichon, P.Y.; Lantuejoul, S.; Hainaut, P.; et al. Ectopic activation of germline and placental genes identifies aggressive metastasis-prone lung cancers. *Sci. Transl. Med.* **2013**, *5*, 186ra166. [CrossRef] [PubMed]
28. La Thangue, N.B.; Kerr, D.J. Predictive biomarkers: A paradigm shift towards personalized cancer medicine. *Nat. Rev. Clin. Oncol.* **2011**, *8*, 587–596. [CrossRef]
29. Leone, A.; Roca, M.S.; Ciardiello, C.; Costantini, S.; Budillon, A. Oxidative Stress Gene Expression Profile Correlates with Cancer Patient Poor Prognosis: Identification of Crucial Pathways Might Select Novel Therapeutic Approaches. *Oxid. Med. Cell. Longev.* **2017**, *2017*, 2597581. [CrossRef]
30. Arner, E.S.; Holmgren, A. The thioredoxin system in cancer, Seminars in cancer biology. **2006**, *16*, 420–426.
31. Dunn, L.L.; Buckle, A.M.; Cooke, J.P.; Ng, M.K. The emerging role of the thioredoxin system in angiogenesis. *Arterioscler. Thromb. Vasc. Biol.* **2010**, *30*, 2089–2098. [CrossRef]
32. Yoo, M.H.; Xu, X.M.; Carlson, B.A.; Patterson, A.D.; Gladyshev, V.N.; Hatfield, D.L. Targeting thioredoxin reductase 1 reduction in cancer cells inhibits self-sufficient growth and DNA replication. *PLoS ONE* **2007**, *2*, e1112. [CrossRef] [PubMed]
33. Yoo, M.H.; Xu, X.M.; Carlson, B.A.; Gladyshev, V.N.; Hatfield, D.L. Thioredoxin reductase 1 deficiency reverses tumor phenotype and tumorigenicity of lung carcinoma cells. *J. Biol. Chem.* **2006**, *281*, 13005–13008. [CrossRef] [PubMed]

34. Kim, S.J.; Miyoshi, Y.; Taguchi, T.; Tamaki, Y.; Nakamura, H.; Yodoi, J.; Kato, K.; Noguchi, S. High thioredoxin expression is associated with resistance to docetaxel in primary breast cancer. *Clin. Cancer Res.* **2005**, *11*, 8425–8430. [CrossRef] [PubMed]
35. Iwao-Koizumi, K.; Matoba, R.; Ueno, N.; Kim, S.J.; Ando, A.; Miyoshi, Y.; Maeda, E.; Noguchi, S.; Kato, K. Prediction of docetaxel response in human breast cancer by gene expression profiling. *J. Clin. Oncol. Off. J. Am. Soc. Clin. Oncol.* **2005**, *23*, 422–431. [CrossRef] [PubMed]
36. Fiskus, W.; Saba, N.; Shen, M.; Ghias, M.; Liu, J.; Gupta, S.D.; Chauhan, L.; Rao, R.; Gunewardena, S.; Schorno, K.; et al. Auranofin induces lethal oxidative and endoplasmic reticulum stress and exerts potent preclinical activity against chronic lymphocytic leukemia. *Cancer Res.* **2014**, *74*, 2520–2532. [CrossRef] [PubMed]
37. Zou, P.; Chen, M.; Ji, J.; Chen, W.; Chen, X.; Ying, S.; Zhang, J.; Zhang, Z.; Liu, Z.; Yang, S.; et al. Auranofin induces apoptosis by ROS-mediated ER stress and mitochondrial dysfunction and displayed synergistic lethality with piperlongumine in gastric cancer. *Oncotarget* **2015**, *6*, 36505–36521. [CrossRef] [PubMed]
38. Wang, H.; Bouzakoura, S.; de Mey, S.; Jiang, H.; Law, K.; Dufait, I.; Corbet, C.; Verovski, V.; Gevaert, T.; Feron, O.; et al. Auranofin radiosensitizes tumor cells through targeting thioredoxin reductase and resulting overproduction of reactive oxygen species. *Oncotarget* **2017**, *8*, 35728–35742. [CrossRef]
39. Fan, C.; Zheng, W.; Fu, X.; Li, X.; Wong, Y.S.; Chen, T. Enhancement of auranofin-induced lung cancer cell apoptosis by selenocystine, a natural inhibitor of TrxR1 in vitro and in vivo. *Cell Death Dis.* **2014**, *5*, e1191. [CrossRef] [PubMed]
40. Sirolimus and Auranofin in Treating Patients with Advanced or Recurrent Non-Small Cell Lung Cancer or Small Cell Lung Cancer. Available online: Clinicaltrials.org (accessed on 19 February 2019).
41. Phase I and II Study of Auranofin in Chronic Lymphocytic Leukemia (CLL). Available online: Clinicaltrials.org (accessed on 19 February 2019).
42. Auranofin in Treating Patients with Recurrent Epithelial Ovarian, Primary Peritoneal, or Fallopian Tube Cancer. Available online: Clinicaltrials.org (accessed on 19 February 2019).
43. Butterworth, K.T.; Coulter, J.A.; Jain, S.; Forker, J.; McMahon, S.J.; Schettino, G.; Prise, K.M.; Currell, F.J.; Hirst, D.G. Evaluation of cytotoxicity and radiation enhancement using 1.9 nm gold particles: Potential application for cancer therapy. *Nanotechnology* **2010**, *21*, 295101. [CrossRef] [PubMed]
44. Polf, J.C.; Bronk, L.F.; Driessen, W.H.; Arap, W.; Pasqualini, R.; Gillin, M. Enhanced relative biological effectiveness of proton radiotherapy in tumor cells with internalized gold nanoparticles. *Appl. Phys. Lett.* **2011**, *98*, 193702. [CrossRef] [PubMed]
45. Hespeels, F.; Heuskin, A.C.; Scifoni, E.; Kraemer, M.; Lucas, S. Backscattered electron emission after proton impact on carbon and gold films: Experiments and simulations. *Nucl. Instrum. Methods Phys. Res. Sect. B Beam Interact. Mater. Atmos* **2017**, *401*, 8–17. [CrossRef]
46. Misawa, M.; Takahashi, J. Generation of reactive oxygen species induced by gold nanoparticles under x-ray and UV Irradiations. *Nanomed. Nanotechnol. Biol. Med.* **2011**, *7*, 604–614. [CrossRef] [PubMed]
47. Sicard-Roselli, C.; Brun, E.; Gilles, M.; Baldacchino, G.; Kelsey, C.; McQuaid, H.; Polin, C.; Wardlow, N.; Currell, F. A new mechanism for hydroxyl radical production in irradiated nanoparticle solutions. *Small* **2014**, *10*, 3338–3346. [CrossRef] [PubMed]
48. Sotiropoulos, M.; Henthorn, N.T.; Warmenhoven, J.W.; Mackay, R.I.; Kirkby, K.J.; Merchant, M.J. Modelling direct DNA damage for gold nanoparticle enhanced proton therapy. *Nanoscale* **2017**, *9*, 18413–18422. [CrossRef] [PubMed]
49. Heuskin, A.C.; Gallez, B.; Feron, O.; Martinive, P.; Michiels, C.; Lucas, S. Metallic nanoparticles irradiated by low-energy protons for radiation therapy: Are there significant physical effects to enhance the dose delivery? *Med. Phys.* **2017**, *44*, 4299–4312. [CrossRef] [PubMed]
50. Wang, C.; Li, X.; Wang, Y.; Liu, Z.; Fu, L.; Hu, L. Enhancement of radiation effect and increase of apoptosis in lung cancer cells by thio-glucose-bound gold nanoparticles at megavoltage radiation energies. *J. Nanopart. Res.* **2013**, *15*, 1642. [CrossRef]
51. Saberi, A.; Shahbazi-Gahrouei, D.; Abbasian, M.; Fesharaki, M.; Baharlouei, A.; Arab-Bafrani, Z. Gold nanoparticles in combination with megavoltage radiation energy increased radiosensitization and apoptosis in colon cancer HT-29 cells. *Int. J. Radiat. Biol.* **2017**, *93*, 315–323. [CrossRef]
52. Liu, C.J.; Wang, C.H.; Chien, C.C.; Yang, T.Y.; Chen, S.T.; Leng, W.H.; Lee, C.F.; Lee, K.H.; Hwu, Y.; Lee, Y.C.; et al. Enhanced x-ray irradiation-induced cancer cell damage by gold nanoparticles treated by a new synthesis method of polyethylene glycol modification. *Nanotechnology* **2008**, *19*, 295104. [CrossRef]

53. Liu, Y.; Zhang, P.; Li, F.; Jin, X.; Li, J.; Chen, W.; Li, Q. Metal-based NanoEnhancers for Future Radiotherapy: Radiosensitizing and Synergistic Effects on Tumor Cells. *Theranostics* **2018**, *8*, 1824–1849. [CrossRef] [PubMed]
54. Butterworth, K.T.; McMahon, S.J.; Taggart, L.E.; Prise, K.M. Radiosensitization by gold nanoparticles: Effective at megavoltage energies and potential role of oxidative stress. *Transl. Cancer Res.* **2013**, *2*, 269–279.
55. Jeynes, J.C.; Merchant, M.J.; Spindler, A.; Wera, A.C.; Kirkby, K.J. Investigation of gold nanoparticle radiosensitization mechanisms using a free radical scavenger and protons of different energies. *Phys. Med. Biol.* **2014**, *59*, 6431–6443. [CrossRef] [PubMed]
56. Schlathölter, T.; Eustache, P.; Porcel, E.; Salado, D.; Stefancikova, L.; Tillement, O.; Lux, F.; Mowat, P.; Biegun, A.K.; van Goethem, M.J.; et al. Improving proton therapy by metal-containing nanoparticles: Nanoscale insights. *Int. J. Nanomed.* **2016**, *11*, 1549–1556. [CrossRef] [PubMed]
57. Taggart, L.E.; McMahon, S.J.; Butterworth, K.T.; Currell, F.J.; Schettino, G.; Prise, K.M. Protein disulphide isomerase as a target for nanoparticle-mediated sensitisation of cancer cells to radiation. *Nanotechnology* **2016**, *27*, 215101. [CrossRef] [PubMed]
58. Chiu, S.J.; Lee, M.Y.; Chou, W.G.; Lin, L.Y. Germanium oxide enhances the radiosensitivity of cells. *Radiat. Res.* **2003**, *159*, 391–400. [CrossRef]
59. Mirjolet, C.; Papa, A.L.; Créhange, G.; Raguin, O.; Seignez, C.; Paul, C.; Truc, G.; Maingon, P.; Millot, N. The radiosensitization effect of titanate nanotubes as a new tool in radiation therapy for glioblastoma: A proof-of-concept. *Radiother. Oncol.* **2013**, *108*, 136–142. [CrossRef] [PubMed]
60. Li, S.; Bouchy, S.; Penninckx, S.; Marega, R.; Fichera, O.; Gallez, B.; Feron, O.; Martinive, P.; Heuskin, A.C.; Michiels, C.; et al. Antibody-functionalized gold nanoparticles as tumor targeting radiosensitizers for proton therapy. *Nanomedicine (Lond. Engl.)* **2019**. [CrossRef]

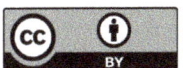

© 2019 by the authors. Licensee MDPI, Basel, Switzerland. This article is an open access article distributed under the terms and conditions of the Creative Commons Attribution (CC BY) license (http://creativecommons.org/licenses/by/4.0/).

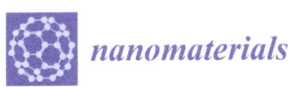

Article

Probing Internalization Effects and Biocompatibility of Ultrasmall Zirconium Metal-Organic Frameworks UiO-66 NP in U251 Glioblastoma Cancer Cells

Cataldo Arcuri [1,*], Lorenzo Monarca [2], Francesco Ragonese [2], Carmen Mecca [1], Stefano Bruscoli [3], Stefano Giovagnoli [4], Rosario Donato [1], Oxana Bereshchenko [3], Bernard Fioretti [2] and Ferdinando Costantino [2,*]

1. Department of Experimental Medicine, Perugia Medical School, University of Perugia, Piazza Lucio Severi 1, 06132 Perugia, Italy; carmen.mecca@unipg.it (C.M.); rosario.donato@unipg.it (R.D.)
2. Department of Chemistry, Biology and Biotechnologies, University of Perugia, Via Elce di Sotto 8, 06123 Perugia, Italy; lorenzomonarca.92@gmail.com (L.M.); francescoragonese85@gmail.com (F.R.); bernard.fioretti@unipg.it (B.F.)
3. Department of Medicine, Perugia Medical School, University of Perugia, Piazza Lucio Severi 1, 06132 Perugia, Italy; stefano.bruscoli@unipg.it (S.B.); oxana.bereshchenko@unipg.it (O.B.)
4. Department of Pharmaceutical Sciences, University of Perugia, Via A. Fabretti 48, 06123, Perugia, Italy; stefano.giovagnoli@unipg.it
* Correspondence: cataldo.arcuri@unipg.it (C.A.); ferdinando.costantino@unipg.it (F.C.); Tel.: +39-0750-585-5563 (F.C.)

Received: 28 September 2018; Accepted: 19 October 2018; Published: 23 October 2018

Abstract: The synthesis of ultrasmall UiO-66 nanoparticles (NPs) with an average size of 25 nm, determined by X-ray powder diffraction and electron microscopies analysis, is reported. The NPs were stabilized in water by dialyzing the NP from the DMF used for the synthesis. DLS measurements confirmed the presence of particles of 100 nm, which are spherical aggregates of smaller particles of 20–30 nm size. The NP have a BET surface area of 700 m^2/g with an external surface area of 300 m^2/g. UiO-66_N (UiO-66 nanoparticles) were loaded with acridine orange as fluorescent probe. UV-vis spectroscopy analysis revealed no acridine loss after 48 h of agitation in simulated body fluid. The biocompatibility of UiO-66_N was evaluated in human glioblastoma (GBM) cell line U251, the most malignant (IV grade of WHO classification) among brain tumors. In U251 cells, UiO-66_N are inert since they do not alter the cell cycle, the viability, migration properties, and the expression of kinases involved in cancer cell growth. The internalization process was evident after a few hours of incubation. After 24 h, UiO-66_N@Acr (UiO-66_N loaded with acridine orange) were detectable around the nuclei of the cells. These data suggest that small UiO-66 are biocompatible NP and could represent a potential carrier for drug delivery in glioblastoma therapies.

Keywords: UiO-66; nanoparticles; glioblastoma; biocompatibility; drug delivery

1. Introduction

In the recent past, nanomedicine has become an attractive approach for targeted drug delivery and for new therapeutic strategies able to overcome the traditional limitations due to toxicity, healthy tissue damage, or other undesired side effects of direct drug administration [1–3]. The synthesis and application of nano-objects to be employed for therapeutic, pharmacological and diagnostic purposes has been rapidly growing [4,5]. Metallic nanoparticles (NPs), (i.e., plasmonic gold nanoclusters, silver NP, ferrite or magnetite superparamagnetic NP) of very small size are currently used as theranostic agents in living cells for a large number of diseases [6–8]. Nanomaterials are able to offer an efficient drug delivery by means of cellular internalization after encapsulation or surface attachment of the drugs. The use of nanocarriers such as lyposomes and dendrimers to be used in physiological conditions for drug delivery is also of great interest [9]. Among the mentioned compounds commonly used for these purposes, there is a class of materials called metal-organic frameworks (MOF) which has already been used for several application as drug delivery carriers and for imaging in living cells [10–13]. MOF are inorganic–organic hybrid compounds with porous crystalline structure and they are constituted of polynuclear metal clusters (also called nodes) linked each other by organic ligands such as carboxylate, phosphonates, heterocycles, and so on. The regular arrangement of nodes and ligands designs porous cages, normally filled by solvent molecules that make these materials suitable for transportation of bioactive molecules to be released in living cells [14–16]. Therapeutic agents and drugs—such as antibacterial and antiviral [17], as well as anticancer drugs like cisplatin [18]—have been successfully included in MOF NP and tested in living cells. In light of their low cytotoxicity, Zn and Fe based MOF are still the most employed. However, Zr based MOF are today considered the benchmark MOF materials in many fields [19]. UiO-66, which structure was first published by Lillerud et al. in 2008, has formula $((Zr_6O_4(OH)_4(O_2C-C_6H_4-CO_2)_6)$ and it is composed of hexa-zirconium(IV) oxo hydroxyl clusters, which are 12-connected by means of linear terephthalate linkers to form a cubic network with small tetrahedral and large octahedral cavities connected through narrow triangular pore windows about 1 nm wide [20]. It is well known that this structure is highly defective and the internal terephtalate linker can be replaced by monocarboxylic groups like acetate, benzoate, and formiate, thus increasing the internal pore volume [21]. Depending on the crystallinity degree the internal surface area can vary from 900 to 1300 m^2/g and the pore volume from 0.35 to 0.5 cm^3/g. Generally, UiO-66 crystals with 200 to 500 nm size can be obtained by conventional hydrothermal synthesis. However, crystals of ultrasmall size of 20–30 nm can be fabricated by properly changing synthetic conditions (amount of water, crystallinity modulator, and aging of the Zr(IV) solutions) [22,23]. Despite the ultrasmall size, the structure of UiO-66 is preserved at the expenses of a reduction of the internal surface area (400 m^2/g, pore volume 0.16 cm^3/g). On the other hand, the small size of the NP strongly increases the external surface area of about 5 to 10 times with respect to large crystals (up to 400 m^2/g for 15 nm average size crystals) [23]. The use of such a small particles could be of potential interest for their potential capacity to easily pass the blood-brain barrier. Recently, surface modified UiO-66 nanocrystals have been used as luminescent sensors for cysteine and GHS detection [24] to unveil the endocytosis mechanism in He-La cells [25], for pH responsive drug delivery after surface PEGylation [26], as anticancer drug carriers after modification with ε-polycaprolactone [17], folic acid, and fluorescent markers (BODYPI) for enhanced cellular uptake [27]. UiO-66 NP have been recently employed after mechanical amorphization for studying the release of fluorescent dye calcein and α-cyano-4-hydroxycinnamic acid (α-CHC) [28,29] and also for miRNA detection [30]. Herein, we report the synthesis of ultrasmall UiO-66_N, their stabilization in water dispersion through dialysis, the loading with fluorescent acridine orange and the study of internalization and biocompatibility on U251 Glioblastoma cells line. Glioblastoma multiforme (GBM) is the most malignant (IV grade of WHO classification) and the most frequent among brain tumors of neuroepithelial origin [31]. The incidence in the United States is 2.96 cases/1,000,000 population/year with a higher peak in males older than 40 years of age [32]. The therapeutic approach to this tumor is complicated primarily by the proximity to the brain parenchyma, but also by the high infiltration capacity and low radio-sensitivity. Standard treatments include surgery, whenever possible, chemotherapy and radiotherapy, according to the Stupp's protocol [33]. Nonetheless, the median survival remains 6 months after surgery alone, while surgery plus radiotherapy extends median survival to 12 months [34]. Moreover, recent experimental evidences have shown that, like other tumors, also GBM harbor a subpopulation of cancer stem cells, namely glioblastoma stem cells (GSCs) that are quiescent and thus evade radio and chemotherapy, causing tumor relapse [35]. To date, numerous genetic alterations of oncogene or tumor suppressor genes have been identified in GBM, including EGFR, PDGFRA, PIK3C2B, p16INK4a/p14ARF, PTEN, and RB1 [36], considering that many of these mutations result in an uncontrolled activation of tyrosine kinase receptors (TKR) and their downstream pathways, many efforts have been made to inhibit these deregulated pathways without significant result. The MOF incorporation in U251 cells was evaluated by flow cytometry after loading of the NP with acridine orange (UiO-66_N@Acr). Cytotoxicity studies, cell cycle evaluation, migration tests were also performed. Moreover, two major signaling pathways were also considered: ERK1/2 and PTEN/PI3K/Akt. The results obtained show that U251 cells internalize UiO-66_N without altering their physiology. These observations suggest that UiO-66_N may represent suitable nanocarriers to target drugs and/or active molecules to glioblastoma cells.

2. Materials and Methods

2.1. Chemicals

$ZrCl_4$, acetic acid (99.5%), terephtalic acid, N,N-dimethylformamide were purchased from Sigma-Aldrich® (St. Louis, MO, USA). The biological reagents are described along the experimental section.

2.2. Synthesis of Nanometric UiO-66_N (Average Crystal Size 25 nm)

UiO-66_N was prepared by dissolving 0.35 g of $ZrCl_4$ (1.5 mmol) in 15 mL of DMF in a 50 mL Teflon vial. Then 0.635 mL of water (0.035 mmol) were added to the mixture. 1.4 mL (0.024 mmol) of acetic acid was added. The mixture was aged for 2 days at room temperature (RT). After that, 5 mL of 0.3 M 1,4 benzenedicarboxylic acid (BDC) solution in DMF was then added to the mixture. The Teflon vial was put in an oven at 120 °C for 24 h. After this time, a gel was recovered, washed twice with acetone and once with water. Then the solid was dried at 60 °C for two days and then soaked in chloroform.

2.3. Dialysis of UiO-66_N from DMF to Water.

In order to avoid the formation of big aggregates during the separation of the solid from DMF, UiO-66_N were purified by dialysis. Specifically, the reaction solution of UiO-66_N in DMF was withdrawn from the reaction vial and put in a dialysis tubing. The tubing was then closed at both sides and put into a beaker with deionized water, stirring for one week. The water in the beaker was changed every day. UiO-66_N dispersion appeared as a milky and homogeneous suspension that remains stable for week at RT. SEM analysis revealed that most of the UiO-66_N were aggregated in spherical clusters of 100–200 nm average diameter, as confirmed by DLS analysis.

2.4. Synthesis of Acridine Orange Loaded UiO-66_N (UiO-66_N@Acr)

50 mg of UiO-66_N (0.06 mmol) were first degassed overnight under vacuum and then dispersed in 5 mL of water. Then 5 mg of acridine orange (0.02 mmol) were added. The suspension was stirred at RT for three days. Then the solid was separated for centrifugation and washed three times with methanol. The amount of acridine orange absorbed by the MOF was evaluated from TGA analysis resulting in about 10 wt % of acridine orange absorbed from the MOF.

2.5. Gas Sorption Measurements

A Micromeritics 2010 apparatus (Micromeritics, Norcross, GA, USA) was used to obtain the adsorption and desorption isotherms with nitrogen at 77 K. Before the adsorption analysis the samples were first soaked in chloroform for two days. Then they were outgassed at 100 °C under vacuum overnight.

2.6. TGA Analysis

Thermogravimetric (TG) measurements were performed using a Netzsch STA490C thermoanalyser (NETZSCH Group, Selb, Germany) under a 20 mL min^{-1} air flux with a heating rate of 10 °C min^{-1}.

2.7. Powder X-ray Diffraction

The PXRD patterns were collected in the 3°–60° 2θ range and with a 40 s/step counting time with the CuKα radiation on a PANalytical X'PERT PRO diffractometer (Malvern Panalytical Ltd., Malvern, UK), PW3050 goniometer (Malvern Panalytical Ltd., Malvern, UK), equipped with an X'Celerator detector (Malvern Panalytical Ltd., Malvern, UK). The long fine focus (LFF) ceramic tube operated at 40 kV and 40 mA.

2.8. DLS and Zeta Potential

Size of UiO-66_N was investigated by dynamic light scattering (DLS) measurements in pure water at 20 °C. Briefly, dialyzed suspensions of UiO-66_N with or without acridine orange, prepared as reported above, were analyzed in ultrapure water at 20 °C. Analyses were performed using a Nicomp 380 ZLS photocorrelator (PSS, Santa Barbara, CA, USA) equipped with a 35 mWHe/Ne laser (λ = 658 nm) and an Avalanche photodiode detector. In the same conditions, zeta potential (ζ) was determined by measuring the electrophoretic mobility of particles at 20 °C. The scattering intensity was measured at 14° scattering angle over a time course of 180 s. The applied potential was 0.5 V cm^{-1}.

2.9. Cell Culture Conditions

The U251 cell line was grown in DMEM with high glucose (EuroClone S.p.A., Milano, Italy) supplemented with 10% FBS (EuroClone S.p.A., Milano, Italy), 100 IU/mL penicillin G, 100 µg/mL streptomycin (EuroClone S.p.A., Milano, Italy) in an H$_2$O-saturated 5% CO$_2$ atmosphere at 37 °C.

2.10. Western Blotting

Cells were cultivated as detailed in the legends of the pertinent figure, washed twice with phosphate-buffered saline (PBS) and solubilized with 20% SDS, 1M Tris-HCl pH 7,4, 1M dithiothreitol, 200 mM PMSF, 10 mg/mL aprotinin (Gold Biotecnology, St. Louis, MO, USA), 1 mg/mL pepstatin (EuroClone S.p.A., Milano, Italy) and 5 mg/mL leupeptin (SERVA Electrophoresis GmbH, Heidelberg, Germany). Equal amounts of cell lysates were separated through 10% SDS page. The following antibodies were used: polyclonal anti phosphorylated (serine 473) Akt (1:1000), polyclonal anti Akt (1:1000), polyclonal anti phosphorylated (Thr202/Tyr204) Erk1/2 (1:1000), polyclonal anti total Erk1/2 (1:1000) (all from Cell Signaling Technology, Leiden, The Netherlands). The immune reaction was developed by SuperSignal West Pico Luminol/Enhancer Solution (Thermo Fisher Scientific, Waltham, MD, USA). Filters were subjected to densitometric analysis of the pertinent immune bands and their relative standard references using the software Image Studio Digit (LI-COR, Lincoln, NE, USA).

2.11. Measurement of Cell Cycle and Apoptosis

Cells were treated with Ethanol and UiO-66_N at 1 µg for 24 h and 48 h respectively; then the culture medium was collected and centrifuged (400× g, 7 min) in order to recover cells in suspension and cells were washed two times with PBS and processed for cell cycle analysis by propidium iodide staining and flow cytometry. Briefly, the cells were resuspended in 0.4 mL of hypotonic fluorochrome solution (50 µg/mL propidium iodide in 0.1% sodium citrate plus 0.1% Triton X-100) in 12 × 75-mm polypropylene tubes (BD Biosciences Italy, Milano, Italy). The tubes were kept at 4 °C for at least 30 min before flow cytometric analysis. The propidium iodide fluorescence of individual nuclei was measured using a FACScan flow cytometer (BD Biosciences Italy, Milano, Italy) at 488 nm. The percentages of cells in G0/G1, S, and G2/M phases and apoptotic cells were calculated using Cell FIT cell cycle analysis version 2.0.2 software.

2.12. Scratch/Wound Healing Assay

Cells were grown to confluent monolayer and, when the confluence reached the 100%, the surface was scratched as uniformly as possible with a pipette tip forming a wound. This initial scratch and the movement of the cells into the wound area were photographed using the Olympus IX51 microscope (Olympus, Tokyo, Japan) with a 4× magnification until the wound area of the control sample was definitively closed. The size of the wound's area of all samples was calculated at each time point using the open source software ImageJ (National Institutes of Health, Bethesda, MD, USA). Two independent series of experiments were performed for each cell line.

2.13. Internalization of UiO-66_N by U251 Glioblastoma Cell Line

One hundred thousand cells were seeded into 35 mm Petri dish plates (Thermo Fisher Scientific, Waltham, MD, USA) in complete medium. After 24 h the medium was renewed and ethanol and UiO-66_N@Acr at the final concentration of 30 µg/mL were added. After 24 h and 48 h, the culture medium was discharged, cells washed five times with PBS, detached with trypsin/EDTA (0.1%), collected and centrifuged (400× g, 7 min). The cells were resuspended in 0.4 mL of PBS and tubes were kept at 4 °C for at least 30 min before flow cytometric analysis. The UiO-66_N@Acr fluorescence of individual cells was detected with Coulter Epics XL-MCL flow cytometer (Beckman Coulter, Brea, CA, USA) and data were analyzed using FlowJo software (TreeStar, Ashland, OR, USA).

2.14. MTT Viability Assay

Cells were seeded in 96 well plates with a cell density of 4×10^3 and after 24 h in culture were treated with UiO-66_N in pure water at the final concentrations of 0.1, 0.5, 1, 5 and 10 µg/mL. 24 and 48 h later, cells were incubated with the 3-(4,5-Dimethylthiazol-2-yl)-2,5-Diphenyltetrazolium Bromide (MTT) solution (Sigma Aldrich®, St. Louis, MO, USA) for four hours and after this incubation period, a water-insoluble formazan dye was formed. After solubilisation, the formazan dye was quantified using a LabSystems Multiskan MS spectrophotometer at 550 nm (Artisan Technology Group ®, Champaign, IL, USA). Each experiment was performed in triplicate.

2.15. FURA-2 Calcium Imaging Assay

U251 cells were plated at the concentration of 1.5×10^3 cells/mL and used on the third day of culture. Before experiments, cells were incubated with FURA-2 AM (3 µM; Sigma-Aldrich, Sigma Aldrich®, St. Louis, MO, USA) for 45 min and extensively washed with a Ringer solution of the following composition (in mM): NaCl 106.5, KCl 5, $CaCl_2$ 2, $MgCl_2$ 2, MOPS 5, glucose 20, Na gluconate 30, at pH 7.25 (all from Sigma Aldrich®, St. Louis, MO, USA). Cells were continuously perfused using a gravity-drive perfusion system, with tubing connected to a final tip of 100 to 200-µm diameter focally oriented onto the field of interest. UiO-66_N were added at the concentration of 1 µg/mL after 9 min of perfusion for 8 min. A standard control pressure perfused the cells for about 20 min with only the Ringer solution. A positive control pressure perfused a solution of ionomycin calcium salt (Tocris Bioscience, Bristol, UK) for about 7 min. The estimation of intracellular free Ca^{2+} concentration was reported as change of the ratio between fluorescence emission at 510 nm, obtained with 340 and 380-nm excitation wavelengths (optical filters and dichroic beam splitter were from Lambda DG4, Shutter Instruments, Novato, CA, USA). Ratiometric data was randomly acquired from 30 cells every 3 s.

2.16. Microscopic Fluorescence Observation and Analysis

All the imaging analyses have been conducted with an upright fluorescence microscope (Axiozoom V16, Zeiss, Oberkochen, Germania); all the images are snapped with a digital camera (Axiocam 502 mono, Zeiss, Oberkochen, Germania) and elaborated with ZEN 2 software (Zeiss, Oberkochen, Germania).

2.17. Statistical Analysis

Each experiment was performed at least three times and data are expressed as mean values ± SEM. Data were subjected variance (ANOVA) analysis using a statistical GraphPad Prism, version 7.00 software package (GraphPad Software, La Jolla, CA, USA).

3. Results

UiO-66_N was synthesized in a nanometric form according to a modified synthetic procedure [22]. This synthesis produced UiO-66_N nanocrystals in the low nanometric range with an average size around 25 nm. To the best of our knowledge, this is the first report on ultrasmall MOFs being investigated for their cell internalization capacity.

Figure 1A displays the XRPD patterns of UiO-66_N with 100 nm average particle size (1); showed for comparison, of UiO-66_N (25 nm average particle size) (2); UiO-66_N soaked overnight in chloroform (3); and UiO-66_N loaded with acridine-orange (4). The average crystal size was estimated by applying the Scherrer formula on the 111, 200 and 220 peaks after analytical deconvolution and by correcting the instrumental broadening with a line profile standard (LaB_6), according to a procedure already applied for similar materials [36]. For the nanometric samples the average crystalline domain size obtained, after the application of the Scherrer formula, was 15 nm. A drastic broadening of the peaks, in agreement with very small crystalline domains, was indeed observed. From the comparison of patterns (1) and (2), it can be seen that the structure of UiO-66-N is fully retained although an important peak broadening is observed. The soaking in chloroform was used in order to remove the residual DMF solvent molecules, the successive acridine inclusion did not change the X-ray pattern. The amount of acridine loaded is about 10 wt % as calculated from the TGA analysis (Figure S1). The nitrogen adsorption isotherm of UiO-66_N is shown in Figure 1B and the BET surface area is 736 m^2/g. The hysteresis of the desorption curve is indicative of the presence of mesopores probably due to interparticle contacts. The micropore surface area is 411 m^2/g (pore volume of 0.17 cm^3/g), whereas the external surface area is about 325 m^2/g. These results are in good agreement with those recently reported on UiO-66 nanocrystals with size around 20 nm [22,23]. The value of the external surface area is about 5 to 10 times higher than that normally measured for UiO-66_N samples with average crystalline size > 100 nm. However, an important reduction of the internal surface area (more than a half) compared to that normally measured for crystalline UiO-66_N (around 1000 m^2/g) was observed.

Figure 2a,b show the TEM and FE-SEM images of UiO-66_N obtained by direct synthesis. They appear to be strongly aggregated but their size has a homogeneous distribution centered around 30 nm, which is a value slightly higher than that found by XRPD data (see Figure S2). However, the broadening of the X-ray peaks also takes into account the presence of defects resulting in a larger broadening than that only related to the crystal size. Another SEM image of UiO-66N is placed in Supporting Information (Figure S7) Figure 2c shows the UiO-66_N separated from DMF by dialysis and loaded with acridine. The picture was taken from the sample dried from the water dispersion after dialysis. The small particles are aggregated into spherical structures of 100 to 200 nm size. These spherical structures are also aggregated in larger clusters being attached each other. Photo correlation spectroscopy (Figure 2d) confirmed the observed formation of large aggregates especially for UiO-66_N@Acr. The dialyzed suspensions showed populations with mean hydrodynamic diameters of 65 nm and 345 nm with large aggregates at size > 5000 nm and 1000 nm for UiO-66_N@Acr and UiO-66_N, respectively. Such findings clearly highlight once more the tendency of UiO-66_N to aggregate in water, matching the TEM observations on the non-dialyzed sample. Even though more dispersed than UiO-66_N, the presence of a smaller particle population for UiO-66_N@Acr particles may suggest that a change in surface properties due to acridine orange adsorption could prevent to some extent aggregation. Such a modification is proved by the change measured in the ξ value that changed from negative (−14.8 mV) for UiO-66_N to slightly positive

(+4.1 mV) for UiO-66_N@acr as a result of the presence of acridine on the surface of the particles. Therefore, acridine may produce some small repulsion able to partially reduce particle agglomeration.

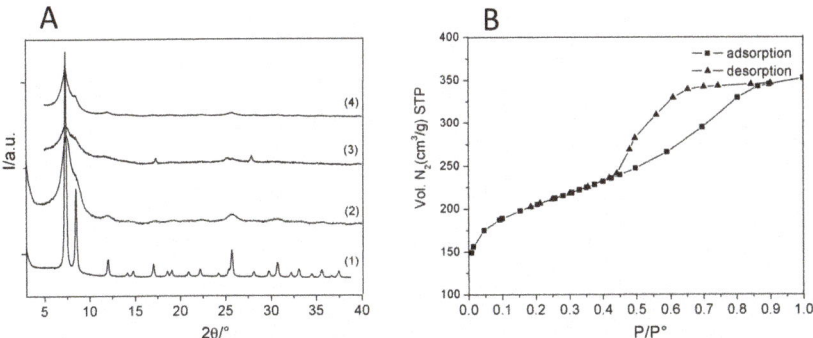

Figure 1. (**A**) XRPD patterns for UiO-66_N 100 (1), UiO-66_N (2), UiO-66_N soaked overnight in chloroform (3), and UiO-66_N@Acr (4); (**B**) N_2 adsorption-desorption isotherms for sample UiO-66_N measured at 100 K.

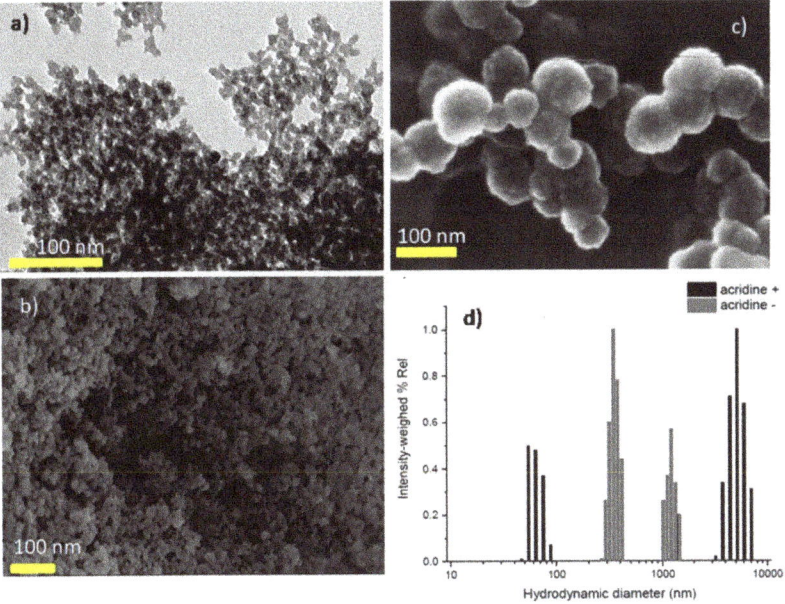

Figure 2. (**a**) TEM and (**b**) FE-SEM images of UiO-66_N obtained by hydrothermal synthesis; (**c**) spherical particles aggregates of smaller UiO-66_N@Acr obtained by dialysis; and (**d**) photo correlation spectroscopy measurements depicting hydrodynamic populations for UiO-66_N (grey) and UiO-66_N@Acr (black) in pure water at 20 °C.

In order to check the acridine adsorption/inclusion degree inside the MOF structure, the effective release of such a dye in PBS (which simulate the cell culture conditions) was studied by UV-vis spectroscopy. UV-vis spectra of UiO-66_N@Acr dispersed in PBS (about 2 mg/mL) are shown in Figure S3. After 24 h and 48 h, no acridine absorption signal could be detected suggesting that no molecules were released from the MOFs. This experimental evidence excludes the presence of free acridine molecules into the cells over the entire incubation timeframe. As our main interest is directed toward pharmaceutical applications, the biological inertness of our MOFs must be a pivotal feature. Since no acridine molecules are released from the MOF, we have evaluated the UiO-66_N@Acr incorporation in U251 cells. After 48 h of 30 µg/mL UiO-66_N@Acr treatment, the 97.9% of the cells showed fluorescence assessed by cytofluorimetry (Figure 3B) compared to untreated cells (Figure 3A) that did not show fluorescence. The same percentage of U251 fluorescent cells was shown after 24 and 72 h of treatment (data not shown). These results demonstrate that UiO-66_N are quickly incorporated by U251 cells and held permanently inside them for at least 72 h.

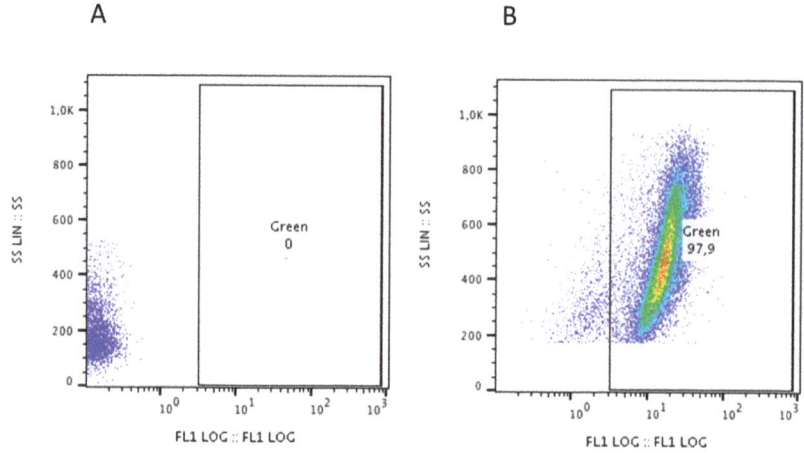

Figure 3. UiO-66_N internalization by U251 cells. (**A**) Not treated cells showed no fluorescence. (**B**) UiO-66_N@Acr treated cells showed fluorescence after 48 h of treatment. Fluorescent cells accounts for 97.9% of total cells.

In order to confirm UiO-66_N internalization, U251 cells were treated with UiO-66_N@Acr at the final concentration of 1 µg/mL for 48 h and observed by immunofluorescence. Before observation, excess of MOFs in the cell medium was removed by extensive washes in PBS; nuclei of cells have been marked with DAPI. Cells were observed alive in PBS. Results of fluorescence imaging are shown in Figure 4: UiO-66_N@Acr are detectable inside U251 glioblastoma cells after 2 h from the incubation and they are still detectable after 48 h. The accumulation of MOFs seems to concentrate around the nuclei of the cells (Figure 4).

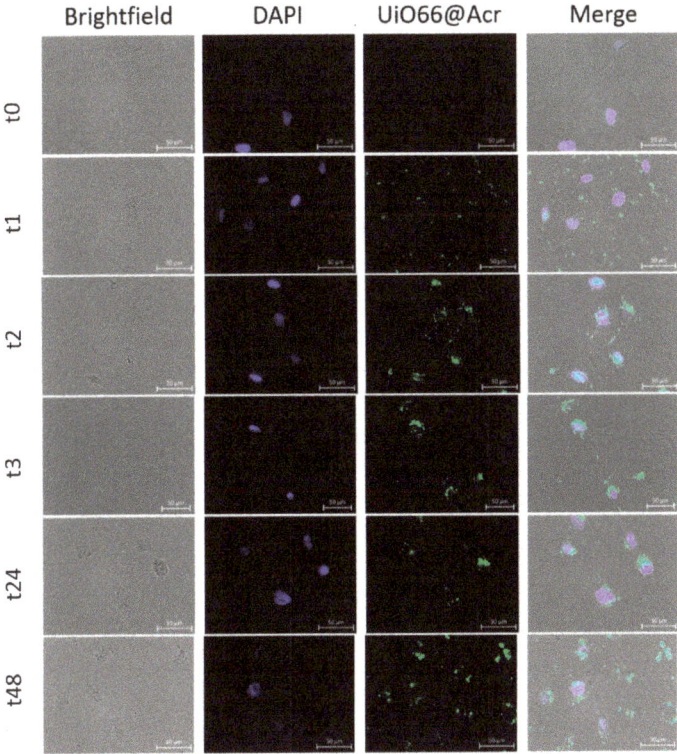

Figure 4. Fluorescence imaging of cells treated with UiO-66_N@Acr at the final concentration of 1 μg/mL at different times (0, 1, 2, 3, 24, and 48 h) of treatment. Bar 50 μm

Cells have been washed with PBS and incubated with DAPI for three minutes, in order to stain cellular nuclei. Cells have been washed again before observation. Figure 5 displays the biocompatibility of UiO-66_N in terms of viability: MTT assay shows no significant changes in U251 cells viability compared to control after 24 and 48 h of exposition at different concentrations (Figure 5). MTT assay uses tetrazolium salt 3-(4,5-dimethyl-2-thia-zolyl)-2,5-diphenyl-2H-tetrazolium bromide) as a biological tool to measure cell viability. Reduction of MTT is associated with flavin-containing enzymes, which are well-known mitochondrial enzymes, and this demonstrates that mitochondria are the main site of MTT reduction. Thus, UiO-66_N do not alter cell viability and do not interfere with the mitochondrial activity of the cells.

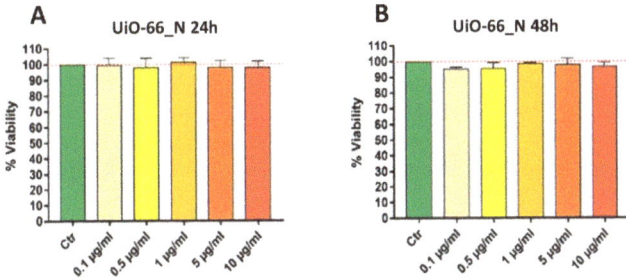

Figure 5. U251 cells viability by MTT assay, after 24 (**A**) and 48 (**B**) hours of incubation with UiO-66_N at various concentrations.

As calcium plays an important role in cell physiology, a ratiometric intracellular calcium concentration measurement with the FURA-2 assay following acute treatment with UiO-66_N was performed. Data shown in Figure S4, displays no significant changes in the intracellular calcium concentration following the application of 1 µg/mL on UiO-66_N; Similar results were obtained with the higher concentration of 10 µg/mL UiO-66_N (Figure S5). The FURA2 assay was conducted even without MOF perfusing, as an assay control showing no differences with the previously described experiment. Such data support further MOF biocompatibility.

Having demonstrated that UiO-66_N are quickly incorporated, the cell cycle of U251 cells to exclude UiO-66_N effects on cell cycle machinery was evaluated. Propidium iodide staining shows no significant differences between not treated and MOF-treated cells (Figure 6), further confirming that they are a biocompatible and an inert nanomaterial. In accordance with these findings, the percentage of cell distribution in G0/G1, S, and G2/M phases was not modified between not treated and MOF-treated cells (data not shown).

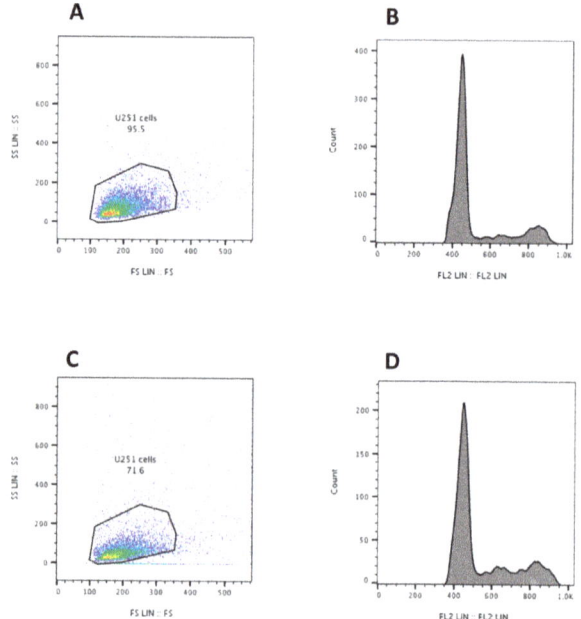

Figure 6. Flow cytometry analysis of not treated (**A**,**B**) or treated (**C**,**D**) U251 cells with UiO-66_N (30 µg/mL) for 48 h. Left panels represent dot plot of not treated (**A**) and UiO-66_N treated (**C**) live U251 cells (gated inside the dot plot). Events outside the gate of U251 cells in UiO-66_N-treated group are mostly MOF aggregates. Right panels represent propidium iodide staining showing cell cycle profiles. No significant differences between not treated (**B**) and UiO-66_N treated (**D**) cells were detected.

Moreover, by FACS analysis, we measured the percentage of apoptotic cells in UiO-66_N (20 or 50 µg/mL) treated U251 cells compared to not treated cells (Figure 7). After 48 h of treatment, the percentage of apoptotic U251 cells in treated and not treated cells was similar, with slight not statistically significant differences. These results demonstrate that in U251 cells UiO-66_N does not affect apoptosis.

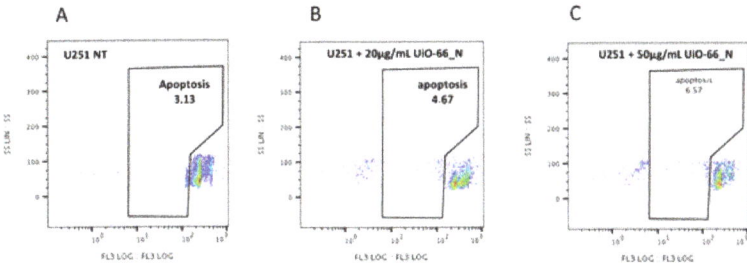

Figure 7. UiO-66_N administration does not induce apoptosis in U251 cells. Flow cytometry analysis of not treated (**A**) or treated U251 cells with 20 (**B**) or 50 (**C**) µg/mL UiO-66_N for 48 h. Numbers inside the gates represent percentage of apoptotic U251 cells assessed by propidium iodide staining.

In GBM, high level of phosphorylated AKT has been reported to correlate with a poor prognosis [36]. Epidermal growth factor receptor (EGFR) amplification and/or overexpression occurs in 40–50 % of GBM [30] and leads to the activation of PI3K/AKT signaling pathway. [36]. Thus, inhibition of this pathway seems to be a promising target for developing more effective GBM therapies. However, the modest efficacy of these approaches observed in the clinical trials conducted so far, suggests that they might be more effective in combination with other agents. [37] In GBM, EGFR overexpression also activates the extracellular signal-regulated kinases 1 and 2 (ERK1/2), [32] proteins belonging to the mitogen-activated protein kinase (MAPK) family contributing to the highly altered phenotype of this tumor cells. UiO-66_N did not affect Akt and ERK1/2 phosphorylation level in U251 glioblastoma cells. From a metabolic point of view UiO-66_N showed a completely inert behavior (Figure 8).

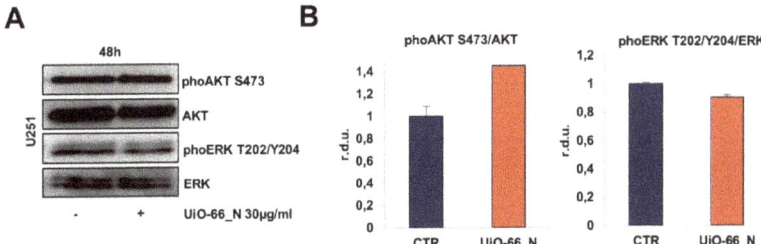

Figure 8. UiO-66_N do not affect Akt and ERK1/2 phosphorylation in U251 glioblastoma cells. Western blots (**A**) and densitometric quantification of Akt and ERK1/2 phosphorylation levels (**B**). The cells were treated with 30 µg/mL UiO-66_N for 48 h. Blots are representative of at least three experiments. The difference in phoAkt level is not statistically significant.

Invasiveness is considered as a major determinant for malignant behavior in human gliomas and U251 cells represent a highly invasive tumor [38]. For this reason, the involvement of UiO-66_N in influencing migration properties was investigated. In order to avoid filling up of the wound by proliferating rather than migrating cells, these tests were conducted under non-proliferative conditions. As expected, UiO-66_N did not affect U251 cell migration evaluated by wound healing assay, compared to not treated cells (Figure S6). It is noteworthy that glioblastoma infiltration is an extremely complex phenomenon that also requires the steady support of extracellular cues [39]. Our preliminary data demonstrate that UiO-66_N do not affect this phenomenon.

4. Conclusions

UiO-66 nanocrystals of ultrasmall size were synthesized and tested for the first time on glioblastoma U251 cells in order to evaluate their biocompatibility and internalization mechanism.

The UiO-66_N were used without any surface modification. The particles separated from the mother liquors tend to strongly aggregate and they cannot be easily stabilized in water dispersion. However, dialysis of the NPs from the DMF solution to water allows to obtain stable dispersion of 100 nm spherical aggregates. Despite the absence of surface modification, nude UiO-66_N are avidly internalized by GBM cells and retained within them. No morphological changes or decrease in cell viability were highlighted. Similarly, the cell cycle, the apoptosis as well as the migration capacity were not altered. From a metabolic point of view, neither changes in mitochondrial activity nor alterations of fundamental transduction pathways were evidenced. Ultimately UiO-66_N are ideal for drug and active molecule delivery towards GBM cells. The treatment of GBM represents a very complex challenge and new strategies must be put into place. Nanomedicine can provide new opportunity for this disease. To date, different NPs have been utilized for drug delivery in GBM, through different administration routes [40]. Various criticisms, such as restricted passage across the blood–brain barrier, have been highlighted. Moreover, GBM are characterized by high infiltrative ability and the potential therapeutics should not only be able to pass through the blood–brain barrier but also should be able to diffuse within the brain. In this context, future studies will have to address not only the brain accumulation and infiltration capacity of these NP but also strategies to grant selectivity with respect to GBM. If successful, ultrasmall UiO-66_N may lead to new treatment approaches for GBM treatment.

Supplementary Materials: The following are available online at http://www.mdpi.com/2079-4991/8/11/867/s1, Figure S1: TGA curves of UiO-66_N (blue line) and UiO-66_N@Acr (orange line); Figure S2: Size distribution of UiO-66_N obtained by direct synthesis; Figure S3: UV-vis spectra in simulated body fluids (SBF) of acridine orange (orange line), UiO-66_N@Acr (red line) and SBF surnatant after 24 h and 48 h; Figure S4: Calcium channels activation in untreated cells; Figure S5: Calcium channels activation during treatment with UiO-66_N; Figure S6: Wound healing assay of U251 cells; Figure S7: High magnification FE-SEM image of UiO-66_N.

Author Contributions: Conceptualization, C.A., S.B., S.G., R.D., and F.C.; Data curation, S.B., S.G., O.B. and B.F.; Funding acquisition, B.F.; Investigation, L.M., F.R., C.M., and O.B.; Writing—original draft, C.A. and F.C.

Funding: This work was funded by Ministero dell'Istruzione, dell'Università e della Ricerca, Italy (SIR RBSI144EUA) to B.F., Fondazione Cassa di Risparmio di Perugia (2014.0254.021) to C.A.

Acknowledgments: The authors thank Fabio Marmottini for the gas-sorption measurements.

Conflicts of Interest: The authors declare no conflict of interest.

References

1. Cho, K.; Wang, X.; Nie, S.; Chen, Z.G.; Shin, D.M. Therapeutic nanoparticles for drug delivery in cancer. *Clin. Cancer. Res.* **2008**, *14*, 1310–1316. [CrossRef] [PubMed]
2. Poljaková, J.; Eckschlager, T.; Hřebačková, J.; Hraběta, J.; Stiborová, M. The comparison of cytotoxicity of the anticancer drugs doxorubicin and ellipticine to human neuroblastoma cells. *Interdiscip. Toxicol.* **2008**, *1*, 186–189. [CrossRef] [PubMed]
3. Chen, G.; Roy, I.; Yang, C.; Prasad, P.N. Nanochemistry and Nanomedicine for Nanoparticle-based Diagnostics and Therapy. *Chem. Rev.* **2016**, *116*, 2826–2885. [CrossRef] [PubMed]
4. Wicki, A.; Witzigmann, D.; Balasubramanian, V.; Huwyler, J. Nanomedicine in cancer therapy: Challenges, opportunities, and clinical applications. *J. Control. Release* **2015**, *200*, 138–157. [CrossRef] [PubMed]
5. Janib, S.M.; Moses, A.S.; MacKay, J.A. Imaging and drug delivery using theranostic nanoparticles. *Adv. Drug. Deliv. Rev.* **2010**, *62*, 1052–1063. [CrossRef] [PubMed]
6. Zhang, J.; Atay, T.; Nurmikko, A.V. Optical detection of brain cell activity using plasmonic gold nanoparticles. *Nano Lett.* **2009**, *9*, 519–524. [CrossRef] [PubMed]
7. Lengert, E.; Saveleva, M.; Abalymov, A.; Atkin, V.; Wuytens, P.C.; Kamyshinsky, R.; Vasiliev, A.L.; Gorin, D.A.; Sukhorukov, G.B.; Skirtach, A.G.; et al. Silver Alginate Hydrogel Micro- and Nanocontainers for Theranostics: Synthesis, Encapsulation, Remote Release, and Detection. *ACS. Appl. Mater. Interfaces* **2017**, *9*, 21949–21958. [CrossRef] [PubMed]
8. Filippousi, M.; Altantzis, T.; Stefanou, G.; Betsiou, M.; Bikiaris, D.N.; Angelakeris, M.; Pavlidou, E.; Zamboulis, D.; Van Tendeloo, G. Polyhedral iron oxide core-shell nanoparticles in a biodegradable polymeric

matrix: Preparation, characterization and application in magnetic particle hyperthermia and drug delivery. *RSC Adv.* **2013**, *3*, 24367–24377. [CrossRef]
9. Blanco, E.; Shen, H.; Ferrari, M. Principles of nanoparticle design for overcoming biological barriers to drug delivery. *Nat. Biotechnol.* **2015**, *33*, 941–951. [CrossRef] [PubMed]
10. Della Rocca, J.; Liu, D.; Lin, W. Nanoscale metal-organic frameworks for biomedical imaging and drug delivery. *Acc. Chem. Res.* **2011**, *44*, 957–968. [CrossRef] [PubMed]
11. Wu, M.X.; Yang, Y.W. Metal-organic Framework (MOF)-Based Drug/Cargo Delivery and Cancer Therapy. *Adv. Mater.* **2017**, *29*, 1606134. [CrossRef] [PubMed]
12. Horcajada, P.; Serre, C.; Vallet-Regí, M.; Sebban, M.; Taulelle, F.; Férey, G. Metal-organic frameworks as efficient materials for drug delivery. *Angew. Chem. Int. Ed.* **2006**, *45*, 5974–5978. [CrossRef] [PubMed]
13. Horcajada, P.; Gref, R.; Baati, T.; Allan, P.K.; Maurin, G.; Couvreur, P.; Férey, G.; Morris, R.E.; Serre, C. Metal-organic frameworks in biomedicine. *Chem. Rev.* **2012**, *112*, 1232–1268. [CrossRef] [PubMed]
14. Yaghi, O.M.; O'Keeffe, M.; Ockwig, N.W.; Chae, H.K.; Eddaoudi, M.; Kim, J. Reticular synthesis and the design of new materials. *Nature* **2003**, *423*, 705–714. [CrossRef] [PubMed]
15. Kitagawa, S.; Kitaura, R.; Noro, S. Functional porous coordination polymers. *Angew. Chem. Int. Ed.* **2004**, *43*, 2334–2375. [CrossRef] [PubMed]
16. Férey, G. Hybrid, porous solids: Past, present, future. *Chem. Soc. Rev.* **2008**, *37*, 191–214. [CrossRef] [PubMed]
17. Tamames-Tabar, C.; Imbuluzqueta, E.; Guillou, N.; Serre, C.; Miller, S.R.; Elkaïm, E.; Horcajada, P.; Blanco-Prieto, M.J. A Zn azelate MOF: Combining antibacterial effect. *Cryst. Eng. Comm.* **2015**, *17*, 456–462. [CrossRef]
18. Filippousi, M.; Turner, S.; Leus, K.; Siafaka, P.I.; Tseligka, E.D.; Vandichel, M.; Nanaki, S.G.; Vizirianakis, I.S.; Bikiaris, D.N.; Van Der Voort, P.; et al. Biocompatible Zr-based nanoscale MOFs coated with modified poly(ε-caprolactone) as anticancerdrug carriers. *Int. J. Pharm.* **2016**, *509*, 208–218. [CrossRef] [PubMed]
19. Bai, Y.; Dou, Y.; Xie, L.H.; Rutledge, W.; Li, J.R.; Zhou, H.C. Zr-based metal–organic frameworks: Design, synthesis, structure, and applications. *Chem. Soc. Rev.* **2016**, *45*, 2327–2367. [CrossRef] [PubMed]
20. Cavka, J.H.; Jakobsen, S.; Olsbye, U.; Guillou, N.; Lamberti, C.; Bordiga, S.; Lillerud, K.P. A new zirconium inorganic building brick forming metal organic frameworks with exceptional stability. *J. Am. Chem. Soc.* **2008**, *130*, 13850–13851. [CrossRef] [PubMed]
21. Wu, H.; Chua, Y.S.; Krungleviciute, V.; Tyagi, M.; Chen, P.; Yildirim, T.; Zhou, W. Unusual and highly tunable missing-linker defects in zirconium metal–organic framework UiO-66 and their important effects on gas adsorption. *J. Am. Chem. Soc.* **2013**, *135*, 10525–10532. [CrossRef] [PubMed]
22. Taddei, M.; Dümbgen, K.C.; van Bokhoven, J.A.; Ranocchiari, M. Aging of the reaction mixture as a tool to modulate the crystallite size of UiO-66 into the low nanometer range. *Chem. Commun.* **2016**, *52*, 6411–6414. [CrossRef] [PubMed]
23. Donnadio, A.; Narducci, R.; Casciola, M.; Marmottini, F.; D'Amato, R.; Jazestani, M.; Chiniforoshan, H.; Costantino, F. Mixed Membrane Matrices Based on Nafion/UiO-66/SO$_3$H-UiO-66 Nano-MOFs: Revealing the Effect of Crystal Size, Sulfonation, and Filler Loading on the Mechanical and Conductivity Properties. *ACS. Appl. Mater. Interfaces* **2017**, *9*, 42239–42246. [CrossRef] [PubMed]
24. Li, Y.A.; Zhao, C.W.; Zhu, N.X.; Liu, Q.K.; Chen, G.J.; Liu, J.B.; Zhao, X.D.; Ma, J.P.; Zhang, S.; Dong, Y.B. Nanoscale UiO-MOF-based luminescent sensors for highly selective detection of cysteine and glutathione and their application in bioimaging. *Chem. Commun.* **2015**, *51*, 17672–17675. [CrossRef] [PubMed]
25. Orellana-Tavra, C.; Mercado, S.A.; Fairen-Jimenez, D. Endocytosis Mechanism of Nano Metal-organic Frameworks for Drug Delivery. *Adv. Healthc. Mater.* **2016**, *5*, 2261–2270. [CrossRef] [PubMed]
26. Abánades Lázaro, I.; Haddad, S.; Sacca, S.; Orellana-Tavra, C.; Fairen-Jimenez, D.; Forgan, R.S. Selective Surface PEGylation of UiO-66 Nanoparticles for Enhanced Stability, Cell Uptake, and pH-Responsive Drug Delivery. *Chem* **2017**, *2*, 561–578. [CrossRef] [PubMed]
27. Wang, L.; Wang, W.; Zheng, X.; Li, Z.; Xie, Z. Nanoscale Fluorescent Metal-organic Framework@Microporous Organic Polymer Composites for Enhanced Intracellular Uptake and Bioimaging. *Chem. Eur. J.* **2017**, *23*, 1379–1385. [CrossRef] [PubMed]
28. Orellana-Tavra, C.; Baxter, E.F.; Tian, T.; Bennett, T.D.; Slater, N.K.; Cheetham, A.K.; Fairen-Jimenez, D. Amorphous metal-organic frameworks for drug delivery. *Chem. Commun.* **2015**, *51*, 13878–13881. [CrossRef] [PubMed]

29. Orellana-Tavra, C.; Marshall, R.J.; Baxter, E.F.; Lázaro, I.A.; Tao, A.; Cheetham, A.K.; Forgan, R.S.; Fairen-Jimenez, D. Drug delivery and controlled release from biocompatible metal–organic frameworks using mechanical amorphization. *J. Mater. Chem. B.* **2016**, *4*, 7697–7707. [CrossRef]
30. Wu, Y.; Han, J.; Xue, P.; Xu, R.; Kang, Y. Nano metal-organic framework (NMOF)-based strategies for multiplexed microRNA detection in solution and living cancer cells. *Nanoscale* **2015**, *7*, 1753–1759. [CrossRef] [PubMed]
31. Arcuri, C.; Fioretti, B.; Bianchi, R.; Mecca, C.; Tubaro, C.; Beccari, T.; Franciolini, F.; Giambanco, I.; Donato, R. Microglia-glioma cross-talk: A two way approach to new strategies against glioma. *Front. Biosci.* **2017**, *22*, 268–309. [CrossRef]
32. Ostrom, Q.T.; Gittleman, H.; Liao, P.; Vecchione-Koval, T.; Wolinsky, Y.; Kruchko, C.; Barnholtz-Sloan, J.S. CBTRUS Statistical Report: Primary brain and other central nervous system tumors diagnosed in the United States in 2010–2014. *Neuro-Oncology* **2017**, *19*, v1–v88. [CrossRef] [PubMed]
33. Stupp, R.; Mason, W.P.; van den Bent, M.J.; Weller, M.; Fisher, B.; Taphoorn, M.J.; Belanger, K.; Brandes, A.A.; Marosi, C.; Bogdahn, U.; et al. Radiotherapy plus concomitant and adjuvant temozolomide for glioblastoma. *N. Engl. J. Med.* **2005**, *352*, 987–996. [CrossRef] [PubMed]
34. Jhanwar-Uniyal, M.; Labagnara, M.; Friedman, M.; Kwasnicki, A.; Murali, R. Glioblastoma: Molecular pathways, stem cells and therapeutic targets. *Cancers* **2015**, *7*, 538–555. [CrossRef] [PubMed]
35. Taddei, M.; Donnadio, A.; Costantino, F.; Vivani, R.; Casciola, M. Synthesis, crystal structure, and proton conductivity of one-dimensional, two-dimensional, and three-dimensional zirconium phosphonates based on glyphosate and glyphosine. *Inorg. Chem.* **2013**, *52*, 12131–12139. [CrossRef] [PubMed]
36. Suzuki, Y.; Shirai, K.; Oka, K.; Mobaraki, A.; Yoshida, Y.; Noda, S.E.; Okamoto, M.; Suzuki, Y.; Itoh, J.; Itoh, H.; et al. Higher pAkt expression predicts a significant worse prognosis in glioblastomas. *J. Radiat. Res.* **2010**, *51*, 343–348. [CrossRef] [PubMed]
37. Li, X.; Wu, C.; Chen, N.; Gu, H.; Yen, A.; Cao, L.; Wang, E.; Wang, L. PI3K/Akt/mTOR signaling pathway and targeted therapy for glioblastoma. *Oncotarget* **2016**, *7*, 33440–33450. [CrossRef] [PubMed]
38. Mecca, C.; Giambanco, I.; Bruscoli, S.; Bereshchenko, O.; Fioretti, B.; Riccardi, C.; Donato, R.; Arcuri, C. PP242 Counteracts Glioblastoma Cell Proliferation, Migration, Invasiveness and Stemness Properties by Inhibiting mTORC2/AKT. *Front. Cell. Neurosci.* **2018**, *12*, 99. [CrossRef] [PubMed]
39. Ortensi, B.; Setti, M.; Osti, D.; Pelicci, G. Cancer stem cell contribution to glioblastoma invasiveness. *Stem Cell Res. Ther.* **2013**, *4*, 18. [CrossRef] [PubMed]
40. Gutkin, A.; Cohen, Z.R.; Peer, D. Harnessing nanomedicine for therapeutic intervention in glioblastoma. *Expert Opin. Drug. Deliv.* **2016**, *13*, 1573–1582. [CrossRef] [PubMed]

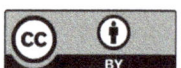

© 2018 by the authors. Licensee MDPI, Basel, Switzerland. This article is an open access article distributed under the terms and conditions of the Creative Commons Attribution (CC BY) license (http://creativecommons.org/licenses/by/4.0/).

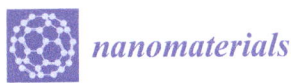

Article

Nanostructured Dihydroartemisinin Plus Epirubicin Liposomes Enhance Treatment Efficacy of Breast Cancer by Inducing Autophagy and Apoptosis

Ying-Jie Hu, Jing-Ying Zhang, Qian Luo, Jia-Rui Xu, Yan Yan, Li-Min Mu, Jing Bai and Wan-Liang Lu *

State Key Laboratory of Natural and Biomimetic Drugs, Beijing Key Laboratory of Molecular Pharmaceutics and New Drug System, School of Pharmaceutical Sciences, Peking University, Beijing 100191, China; yingjie.hu93@gmail.com (Y.-J.H.); zhangjingying1995@126.com (J.-Y.Z.); Luoqian7777@126.com (Q.L.); xujiarui228@foxmail.com (J.-R.X.); yanyan1992111@163.com (Y.Y.); liminmu@163.com (L.-M.M.); vivalajing@163.com (J.B.)
* Correspondence: luwl@bjmu.edu.cn; Tel.: +86-10-8280-2683

Received: 12 September 2018; Accepted: 5 October 2018; Published: 9 October 2018

Abstract: The heterogeneity of breast cancer and the development of drug resistance are the relapse reasons of disease after chemotherapy. To address this issue, a combined therapeutic strategy was developed by building the nanostructured dihydroartemisinin plus epirubicin liposomes. Investigations were performed on human breast cancer cells in vitro and xenografts in nude mice. The results indicated that dihydroartemisinin could significantly enhance the efficacy of epirubicin in killing different breast cancer cells in vitro and in vivo. We found that the combined use of dihydroartemisinin with epirubicin could efficiently inhibit the activity of Bcl-2, facilitate release of Beclin 1, and further activate Bax. Besides, Bax activated apoptosis which led to the type I programmed death of breast cancer cells while Beclin 1 initiated the excessive autophagy that resulted in the type II programmed death of breast cancer cells. In addition, the nanostructured dihydroartemisinin plus epirubicin liposomes prolonged circulation of drugs, and were beneficial for simultaneously delivering drugs into breast cancer tissues. Hence, the nanostructured dihydroartemisinin plus epirubicin liposomes could provide a new therapeutic strategy for treatment of breast cancer.

Keywords: dihydroartemisinin; liposomes; autophagy; apoptosis; breast cancer

1. Introduction

Breast cancer is the most common malignancy and the leading cause of cancer-related mortality among women worldwide. In 2012 alone, there were an estimated 1.7 million cases diagnosed, and 521,900 breast cancer-related deaths [1]. The high morbidity of breast cancer is associated with the genetic heterogeneity of tumors [2]. In the last few decades, five different molecular subtypes of breast cancer have been identified, termed luminal A, luminal B, HER2-enriched, basal-like, and claudin-low [3]. Each subtype displays varying sensitivity to different cancer drugs [4]. If a universal drug formulation could treat varying subtypes of breast cancer cells, it would be useful for improving clinical treatment.

One emerging therapeutic strategy to overcome this obstacle has focused on drugs that preferentially induce autophagy and apoptosis in otherwise resistant cancer cells [5]. Induction of apoptosis is used as a cancer treatment strategy by triggering type I programmed death of refractory cancer cells. This is typically achieved through a combinational chemotherapy treatment. However, this approach tends to be ineffective in the case of heterogeneous breast cancers. In contrast, accumulating evidence suggests that autophagy, which triggers type II programmed cell death, could significantly enhance the efficacy of cancer treatments [6]. Autophagy (or "self-eating") is a stress-induced process involving lysosomal degradation, which conserves cellular energy and maintains cytoplasmic homeostasis by eliminating protein aggregates and damaged organelles [7]. Autophagy is initiated by double-membraned autophagosomes that engulf portions of the cytoplasm. These autophagosomes ultimately fuse with lysosomes where the cytoplasmic contents are degraded [8,9].

Interestingly, autophagy plays a paradoxical role in cancer cells, and it can either promote or inhibit tumor formation depending upon the circumstances [10–13]. For example, defects in autophagy can lead to chronic tissue damage and inflammation, which may create an environment that promotes tumorigenesis. Moderate induction of autophagy also promotes the growth of cancer cells by limiting the stress response and supporting the metabolism and survival of cancer cells [14]. In contrast, excessive autophagy can also trigger type II programmed death in cancer cells due to the overconsumption of cytoplasmic proteins and organelles.

The relationship between these two types of programmed cell death is complicated. On one hand, apoptosis can lead to the activation or suppression of autophagy [15,16]. On the other hand, inhibition of apoptosis can result in either suppression or activation of autophagy [15,17]. The exact mechanisms underpinning these contradictory interactions remain unclear. Therefore, exploring the interaction between autophagy and apoptosis is an important avenue of research for developing treatments for heterogeneous breast cancers.

Dihydroartemisinin is a derivative of artemisinin, which is a naturally occurring sesquiterpene extracted from the traditional Chinese medicinal herb Qing Hao (*Artemesia annua*) [18]. Because the chemical structure has been optimized by modifying carbonyl groups into hydroxyl groups, dihydroartemisinin exhibits stronger antimalarial effect. Hence, it has become one of the first alternative antimalarial drugs recommended by the World Health Organization in the case where *Plasmodium falciparum* is resistant to traditional therapy. Further studies showed that dihydroartemisinin also exhibits strong antibacterial, antiviral, and anticancer activities [19–22]. In particular, dihydroartemisinin enables the induction of apoptosis in cancer cells through different mechanisms, such as by targeting JAK2/STAT3, NF-kB, JNK1/2, and p38 MAPK signaling pathways [23–25]. Besides, dihydroartemisinin also induces autophagy in ovarian cancer cells, pancreatic cancer cells, gliomas, and breast cancer cells [26–29]. Therefore, dihydroartemisinin was included in this study as a potential anticancer enhancer and epirubicin was used as an anticancer agent. Because drugs can distribute differentially in tissues, the two agents were incorporated into liposome vesicles to simultaneously deliver both drugs to cancer cells. The efficacy of this treatment approach was examined both in vitro (in human breast cancer cell lines) and in vivo (using mouse xenografts).

2. Materials and Methods

2.1. Preparation of Liposomes

Three types of liposomes were fabricated, including dihydroartemisinin plus epirubicin liposomes, dihydroartemisinin only liposomes, and epirubicin only liposomes.

To construct dihydroartemisinin liposomes, egg phosphatidylcholine (EPC), cholesterol, polyethylene glycol-distearoylphosphosphatidylethanolamine (PEG$_{2000}$-DSPE, NOF Corporation, Tokyo, Japan) (EPC:CHOL:PEG$_{2000}$-DSPE = 65:30:5, μmol/μmol), and dihydroartemisinin (Tokyo Chemical Industry Co., Ltd., Tokyo, Japan) were dissolved in chloroform in a pear-shaped flask. Chloroform was evaporated under a vacuum with a rotary evaporator. The remaining lipid film was hydrated with 250 mM ammonium sulfate in a water bath sonicator for 3 min followed by probe-type sonication for 10 min. The suspensions were then serially filtered through polycarbonate membranes (pore sizes 400 and 200 nm) 3 times each to yield dihydroartemisinin liposomes.

To construct dihydroartemisinin plus epirubicin liposomes, above dihydroartemisinin liposomes were dialyzed (12,000–14,000 molecular mass cutoff) against HEPES-buffered saline (25 mM HEPES, 150 mM NaCl) twice for 12 h each. Dihydroartemisinin liposomes were then added to epirubicin hydrochloride (R&D systems, Minneapolis, MN, USA). After mixing, the suspensions were incubated at 40 °C in a water bath and intermittently shaken for 30 min to produce liposomes containing both drugs.

To construct epirubicin liposomes, the same method for synthesizing the dihydroartemisinin and epirubicin liposomes was used, except that there was no addition of dihydroartemisinin.

The mean particle sizes, polydispersity indexes (PDI), and zeta potential values of all liposomes were measured using the Nano Series Zenith 4003 Zetasizer (Malvern Instruments Ltd., Malvern, UK).

2.2. Cell Culture

Human breast cancer cell lines (*MDA-MB-435S*, *MDA-MB-231*, and *MCF-7*) were purchased from the Institute of Basic Medical Science, Chinese Academy of Medical Science (Beijing, China) and used below passage 10. *MDA-MB-435S* and *MDA-MB-231* cells were grown in Leibovitz's L15 medium (Macgene Biotech Co., Ltd., Beijing, China) supplemented with 10% fetal bovine serum (FBS, PAN, Adenbach, Germany) in a 37 °C humidified incubator. *MCF-7* cells were cultured in RPMI 1640 (Macgene Biotech Co., Ltd., Beijing, China) supplemented with 10% FBS in a humidified incubator at 37 °C under 5% CO_2.

2.3. Cellular Uptake and Mitochondrial Co-Localization

To measure cellular uptake of liposomes, cancer cells were seeded at a density of 2×10^5 cells/well in 6-well culture plates for 24 h. The cells were treated with free epirubicin (10 µM), epirubicin liposomes (10 µM), or dihydroartemisinin plus epirubicin liposomes (20 µM dihydroartemisinin, 10 µM epirubicin) for 8, 12, or 16 h. Culture medium was used as a blank control. After incubation, cells were harvested and washed twice with cold phosphate-buffered saline (PBS, pH 7.4, 137 mM NaCl, 2.7 mM KCl, 8 mM Na_2HPO_4, and 2 mM KH_2PO_4). Cells (1×10^4) were collected and fluorescence intensity was measured using a flow cytometer (FACSCalibur, Becton Dickinson, Franklin Lakes, NJ, USA) according to the manufacturer's instructions. Each assay was repeated in triplicate.

Coumarin was used as a fluorescent probe to assess mitochondrial co-localization. Briefly, cancer cells were seeded into chambered cover slides at a density of 2×10^5 cells/dish. After 24 h of incubation, cells were treated with free coumarin (1 µM), coumarin liposomes (1 µM), or coumarin plus dihydroartemisinin liposomes (1 µM coumarin, 10 µM dihydroartemisinin) for 16 h. Culture medium was used as a blank control. The cells were then washed with PBS, and mitochondria were stained with Mitotracker Deep Red (20 nM, Life Technologies Corporation, Carlsbad, NM, USA) at 37 °C for 30 min. Nuclei were stained with Hoechst 33342 (5 µg/mL) for 10 min. Finally, the cells were imaged using confocal microscopy (Leica, Oskar-Barnack, Germany). Each assay was repeated in triplicate.

2.4. Induction of Autophagy

Autophagy was quantified using a monodansylcadaverine (MDC) staining kit (Leagene, China). Cancer cells were seeded into 6-well culture plates at a density of 2×10^5 cells/well for 24 h at 37 °C. Cells were treated with free dihydroartemisinin (10 µM), free epirubicin (5 µM), free dihydroartemisinin plus free epirubicin (10 µM dihydroartemisinin, 5 µM epirubicin), dihydroartemisinin liposomes (10 µM), epirubicin liposomes (5 µM), or dihydroartemisinin plus epirubicin liposomes (10 µM dihydroartemisinin, 5 µM epirubicin). The molar ratio of dihydroartemisinin to epirubicin was 2:1 in the liposomal formulation when they were simultaneously incorporated into one liposomal vesicle. Culture medium was used as a blank control. After incubation for 10 h, the cells were washed with a buffer provided in the kit, and incubated with the MDC stain at room temperature for 15 min in the dark. Subsequently, the cells were washed and suspended in a collection buffer provided in the kit. Both buffers were properly diluted according to the manufacturer's instructions. Extent of autophagy in the cancer cells was determined by the fluorescence intensity measured on a flow cytometer (FACSCalibur, Becton Dickinson, Franklin Lakes, NJ, USA).

Direct observation of autophagy was performed on cancer cells seeded into 6-well culture plates for 24 h, followed by treatment with the same drug formulations as above. After MDC staining as described previously, cell suspensions were dripped onto a glass slide and imaged using confocal microscopy (Nikon, Tokyo, Japan).

2.5. Induction of Apoptosis

Apoptosis was assayed using an Annexin V-kFluor647 staining kit (Nanjing Keygen Biotech. Co., Ltd., Nanjing, China) and the nuclear dye SYTOX Green (Nanjing Keygen Biotech. Co., Ltd., Nanjing, China). Cancer cells were seeded at a density of 2×10^5 cells/well in 6-well culture plates for 24 h at 37 °C. Cells were treated with free dihydroartemisinin (10 µM), free epirubicin (5 µM), free dihydroartemisinin plus free epirubicin (10 µM dihydroartemisinin, 5 µM epirubicin), dihydroartemisinin liposomes (10 µM), epirubicin liposomes (5 µM), or dihydroartemisinin plus epirubicin liposomes (10 µM dihydroartemisinin, 5 µM epirubicin). Culture medium was used as a blank control. After incubation for 12 h, the cells were collected, resuspended in the binding buffer provided in the kit, and 10 µL Annexin V-kFluor647 was added. The suspensions were incubated at room temperature for 15 min in the dark. Finally, 5 µL of SYTOX Green was added to each sample for 5 min before analysis on a flow cytometer (Gallios, Beckman Coulter, Brea, CA, USA). Each assay was repeated in triplicate.

2.6. Mechanisms of Autophagy and Apoptosis

To evaluate mechanisms of autophagy and apoptosis, cells were seeded into 96-well plates and incubated for 24 h. Cells were then treated with free dihydroartemisinin (10 µM), free epirubicin (5 µM), free dihydroartemisinin plus free epirubicin (10 µM dihydroartemisinin, 5 µM epirubicin), dihydroartemisinin liposomes (10 µM), epirubicin liposomes (5 µM), or dihydroartemisinin plus epirubicin liposomes (10 µM dihydroartemisinin, 5 µM epirubicin). Culture medium was used as a blank control. After incubation for 12 h, cells were fixed with 4% formaldehyde for 15 min, permeabilized with 0.5% Triton X-100 for 15 min, and blocked with 10% goat serum supplemented with 0.3 M glycine for 2 h at room temperature. Cells were then incubated at 4 °C overnight with the following primary antibodies: anti-Beclin 1 (Bioss, Beijing, China), anti-LC3B (Beyotime, Shanghai, China), anti-Bcl-2, anti-Bax, anti-Caspase 3, or anti-Caspase 9 (Sangon, Shanghai, China). Cells were then incubated with the appropriate secondary antibody conjugated to Alexa Fluor-488 (OriGene Local Agent, Beijing, China) at room temperature for 2 h. Both primary and secondary antibodies were diluted according to the manufacturer's instructions. Nuclei were stained with Hoechst 33342 (5 µg/mL) for 10 min at room temperature. The fluorescence intensity of each well was measured using the Operetta High-Content Screening System (Perkin Elmer, Waltham, MA, USA) and calculated with the Columbus system (Waltham, MA, USA).

2.7. Morphological Changes

Changes in cell morphology following drug treatments were assessed by seeding cancer cells into a 96-well plate at a density of 6×10^3 cells/well and culturing for 24 h. The cells were treated for 12 h with free dihydroartemisinin (10 µM), free epirubicin (5 µM), free dihydroartemisinin plus free epirubicin (10 µM dihydroartemisinin, 5 µM epirubicin), dihydroartemisinin liposomes (10 µM), epirubicin liposomes (5 µM), or dihydroartemisinin plus epirubicin liposomes (10 µM dihydroartemisinin, 5 µM epirubicin). Culture medium was used as a blank control. After incubation, cells were harvested and washed twice with cold PBS (pH 7.4), and mitochondria were stained with Mitotracker Deep Red (20 nM, Life Technologies Corporation, Carlsbad, NM, USA) at 37 °C for 30 min. Afterwards, nuclei were stained with Hoechst 33342 (5 µg/mL) for 10 min. Finally, cells were imaged using the Operetta High-Content Screening System (Perkin Elmer, Waltham, MA, USA), and calculations were performed using the Columbus system (Waltham, MA, USA).

2.8. Inhibitory Effects In Vitro

Cancer cells were seeded into a 96-well plate at a density of 6×10^3 cells/well and cultured for 24 h. Fresh medium containing the free drug or drug formulation was added to each well, including free epirubicin (0–2.5 µM), a fixed concentration of free dihydroartemisinin (1, 2.5, or 5 µM) plus free epirubicin (0–2.5 µM), dihydroartemisinin liposomes (0–5 µM), epirubicin liposomes (0–5 µM), or dihydroartemisinin plus epirubicin liposomes (0–10 µM for dihydroartemisinin, 0–5 µM for epirubicin). Culture medium was used as a blank control. After incubation for 48 h, cytotoxicity was determined by sulforhodamine B staining assay based on absorbance measurements at a wavelength of 540 nm using a microplate reader (Infinite F50, Tecan Group Ltd., Shanghai, China). The survival rate was calculated using the following formula: Cell survival % = (A_{540nm} for the treated cells/A_{540nm} for the control cells) × 100%, where A_{540nm} is the absorbance value.

2.9. Anticancer Efficacy in Cancer-Bearing Mice

Female BALB/c nude mice (weighing 15–17 g) were obtained from Peking University Health Science Center. All animal experiments were performed in accordance with the principles of care and use of laboratory animals, and were approved by the Institutional Animal Care and Use Committee of Peking University. Briefly, approximately 1×10^7 *MDA-MB-435S* cells were resuspended in 200 µL of serum-free medium and injected subcutaneously into the right flanks of nude mice. When tumors reached 100–150 mm^3 in volume, mice were randomly divided into five treatment groups ($N = 5$ per group). At the 10th, 12th, 14th, and 16th day after inoculation, physiological saline, free epirubicin (4 mg/kg), dihydroartemisinin liposomes (4 mg/kg), epirubicin liposomes (4 mg/kg), or dihydroartemisinin plus epirubicin liposomes (4 mg/kg for both drugs) were administered to mice via tail vein injection. The mice were then monitored and the tumor volume was calculated according to the following formula: the tumor volume (mm^3) on the nth day = length × width^2/2. A routine blood analysis of the mice was also conducted using a MEK-6318K Hematology Analyzer (Nihon Kohden, Tokyo, Japan).

2.10. In Vivo Imaging

Noninvasive optical imaging systems were used to observe the real-time distribution and tumor accumulation of DiR (1,10-dioctadecyl-3,3,30,30 tetramethyl indotricarbocyanine iodide) plus dihydroartemisinin liposomes in breast cancer-bearing xenografts in BALB/c nude mice. DiR was used as fluorescence probe to replace epirubicin for indicating the distribution of nanostructured epirubicin plus dihydroartemisinin liposomes. Female mice were divided into four groups ($N = 3$ per group). After inoculation with *MDA-MB-435S* cells at day 19, the tumor volumes reached approximately 300 mm^3. These mice were then injected with physiological saline, free DiR, DiR liposomes, or DiR plus dihydroartemisinin liposomes via the tail vein. Mice were scanned at 0.5, 1, 3, 6, 9, 12, and 24 h using an IVIS Spectrum system (Xenogen Corporation, Alameda, CA, USA) under anesthesia with isoflurane.

To visualize the distribution status in tumors and in major organs, the tumor-bearing mice were sacrificed at 36 h after drug administration, and the tumor masses, heart, liver, spleen, lungs, and kidneys were immediately removed. The fluorescent signal intensities in different tissues were imaged and analyzed.

2.11. Statistical Analysis

Data are presented as the means ± standard deviation. One-way analysis of variance was used to determine significance among the groups. Post hoc tests with a Bonferroni correction were used to make comparisons between individual groups. $p < 0.05$ was considered statistically significant.

3. Results

3.1. Characterization of Liposome Formulations

The various liposome formulations were characterized before performing experiments on the cells and mice (Table S1). To summarize, the average particle sizes of the liposomes ranged from 90 to 100 nm with a narrow PDI (approximately 0.2). Zeta potential values were approximately electrically neutral. The encapsulation efficiencies of both dihydroartemisinin and epirubicin were about 90% for all liposomes.

3.2. Cellular Uptake and Co-Localization Effect

Cellular uptake was indicated by the fluorescence intensity in *MDA-MB-435S* cells after treatment with varying drug formulations (Figure 1A). Results showed that the rank of cellular uptake was free epirubicin > dihydroartemisinin plus epirubicin liposomes > epirubicin liposomes > blank control after treatment at 16 h. Among treatment groups, the cellular uptakes between liposomes exhibited less distinction patterns at 8 h or 12h.

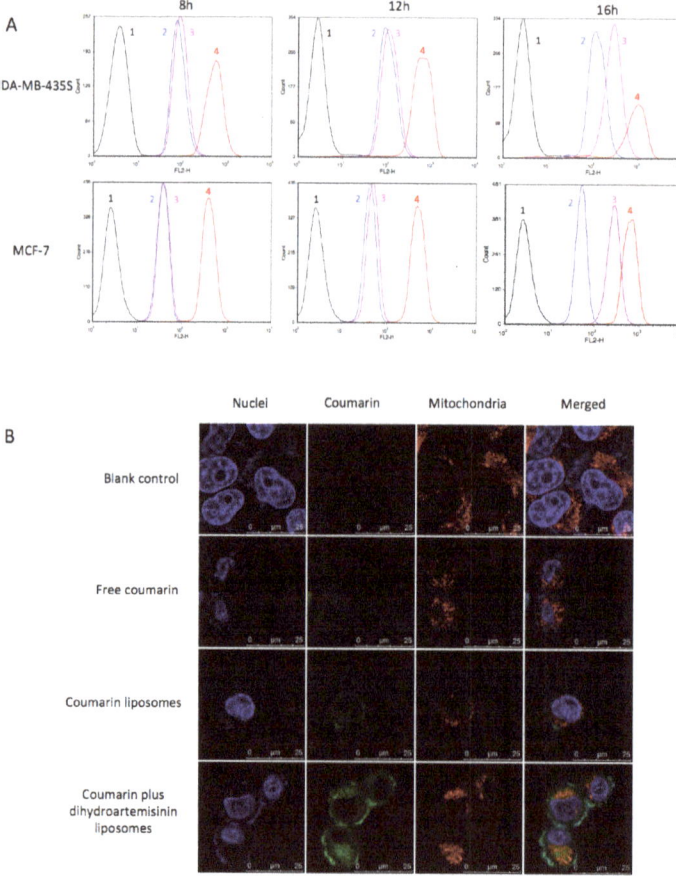

Figure 1. Cellular uptake and co-localization effects in breast cancer cells. (**A**) drug uptake measured by flow cytometry in breast cancer *MDA-MB-435S* and *MCF-7* cells; (**B**) co-localization effect of fluorescent indicator coumarin with mitochondria observed by confocal microscope in breast cancer *MCF-7* cells (scale bar = 25 μm). 1, blank medium; 2, epirubicin liposomes; 3, dihydroartemisinin plus epirubicin liposomes; 4, free epirubicin.

The fluorescence probe coumarin was used to label the liposomes for evaluating the co-localization effect with mitochondria (Figure 1B). In the confocal images, coumarin exhibited green fluorescence, mitochondria exhibited red fluorescence, whereas the nuclei were stained in blue. Bright yellow fluorescence was a composite image of green and red fluorescence, and used to indicate the co-localization effect of drug formulations with mitochondria in MCF-7 cells. Results demonstrated that the coumarin plus dihydroartemisinin liposomes were co-localized with mitochondria, and exhibited the highest green fluorescence intensity in the cells as compared to other drug formulations.

3.3. Induction of Autophagy

Induction of autophagy in MDA-MB-435S cells was evaluated by the MDC staining assay (Figure 2A). Using confocal microscopy, the MDC dye (green) was observed to enter autophagosomes. Cells treated with dihydroartemisinin plus epirubicin liposomes or with free dihydroartemisinin plus free epirubicin had stronger fluorescence intensity compared to other drug groups. The autophagy ratios for cancer cells were also measured by flow cytometry (Figure 2B). The results showed that the rank of autophagy ratios was free dihydroartemisinin plus free epirubicin (6.50 ± 0.72) ≈ dihydroartemisinin plus epirubicin liposomes (6.28 ± 0.33) > epirubicin liposomes (4.96 ± 0.12) > free epirubicin (4.35 ± 0.26) > free dihydroartemisinin (1.73 ± 0.27) > dihydroartemisinin liposomes (1.41 ± 0.07) > blank medium (1.00 ± 0.06).

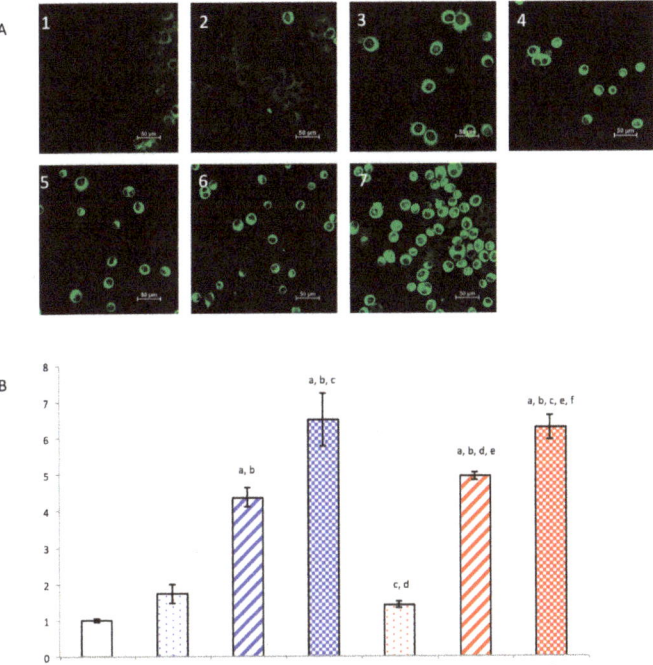

Figure 2. Autophagy induced in breast cancer breast cancer MDA-MB-435S cells. (**A**) qualitative confocal observation on the induced autophagy of breast cancer after processing with monodansylcadaverine kit; (**B**) quantitative flow cytometric estimation on the induced autophagy of breast cancer cells after processing with monodansylcadaverine. 1, blank control; 2, free dihydroartemisinin; 3, free epirubicin; 4, free dihydroartemisinin plus epirubicin (mole ratio = 2:1); 5, dihydroartemisinin liposomes; 6, epirubicin liposomes; 7, dihydroartemisinin plus epirubicin liposomes. Data are presented as the mean ± standard deviation ($n = 3$). $p < 0.05$; a, vs. 1; b, vs. 2; c, vs. 3; d, vs. 4; e, vs. 5; f, vs. 6.

3.4. Induction of Apoptosis

Induction of apoptosis in MDA-MB-435S cells was evaluated by flow cytometry (Figure 3). The results showed that the rank of apoptotic percentage in breast cancer cells was dihydroartemisinin plus epirubicin liposomes (45.9 ± 3.8) ≥ free dihydroartemisinin plus free epirubicin (43.1 ± 2.5) > dihydroartemisinin liposomes (35.9 ± 8.8) > free epirubicin (35.3 ± 0.3) > epirubicin liposomes (22.4 ± 5.1) > free dihydroartemisinin (7.7 ± 1.0) > blank medium (1.5 ± 0.4) (Figure 3B). No significant difference was observed between free drug and the corresponding liposomes (e.g., "free epirubicin" vs. "epirubicin liposomes"; "free dihydroartemisinin plus free epirubicin" vs. dihydroartemisinin plus epirubicin liposomes), demonstrating that the nanostructured dihydroartemisinin plus epirubicin liposomes significantly enhancing the apoptotic effects although the liposome vesicle itself did not alter the apoptosis-inducing capability of free drugs.

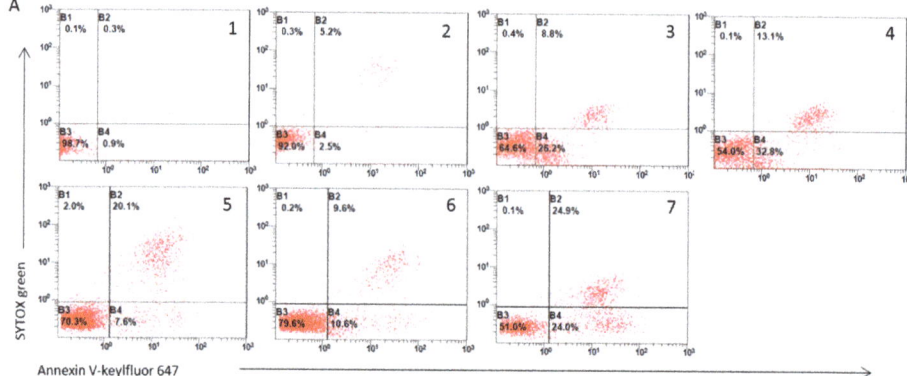

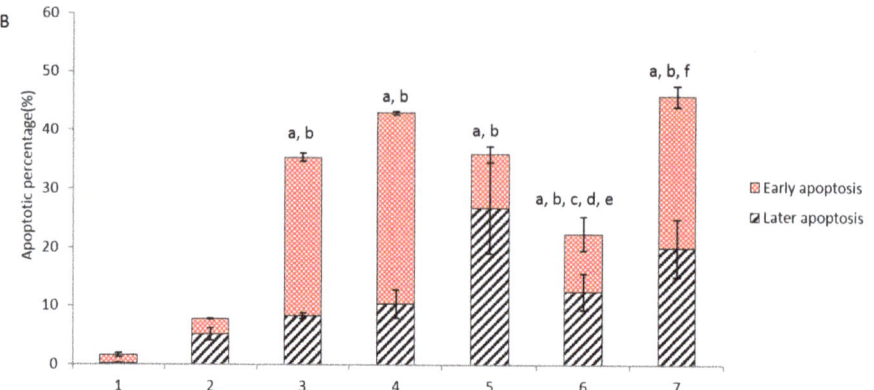

Figure 3. Apoptosis induced in breast cancer MDA-MB-435S cells. (**A**) Flow cytometry plot of breast cancer cells after treatment with varying formulations; (**B**) apoptotic percentage in breast cancer cells after the treatment. 1, blank control; 2, free dihydroartemisinin; 3, free epirubicin; 4, free dihydroartemisinin plus epirubicin (mole ratio = 2:1); 5, dihydroartemisinin liposomes; 6, epirubicin liposomes; 7, dihydroartemisinin plus epirubicin liposomes. Data are presented as the mean ± standard deviation (n = 3). $p < 0.05$; a, vs. 1; b, vs. 2; c, vs. 3; d, vs. 4; e, vs. 5; f, vs. 6.

3.5. Mechanism of Autophagy and Apoptosis

The mechanisms of autophagy and apoptosis were evaluated by measuring autophagy- and apoptosis-related proteins in *MDA-MB-436S* cells (Figure 4). After incubation with the blank medium, free dihydroartemisinin, free epirubicin, or free dihydroartemisinin plus free epirubicin, the expression levels of the anti-apoptotic protein Bcl-2, the pro-apoptotic protein Bax, the apoptotic enzymes Caspase-9 and -3, and autophagy-related proteins Beclin 1 and LC3B were assessed. The activity ratios of Bcl-2 were 1.00 ± 0.01, 0.89 ± 0.01, 0.93 ± 0.01, 0.88 ± 0.02, 0.91 ± 0.00, 0.93 ± 0.01, and 0.87 ± 0.01; the activity ratios of Bax were 1.00 ± 0.02, 1.05 ± 0.01, 1.07 ± 0.01, 1.11 ± 0.01, 1.11 ± 0.01, 1.13 ± 0.01, and 1.21 ± 0.01; the activity ratios of Caspase-9 were 1.00 ± 0.01, 1.17 ± 0.03, 1.15 ± 0.02, 1.33 ± 0.04, 1.25 ± 0.02, 1.21 ± 0.01, and 1.40 ± 0.03; the activity ratios of Caspase-3 were 1.00 ± 0.01, 1.13 ± 0.02, 1.23 ± 0.01, 1.28 ± 0.01, 1.12 ± 0.01, 1.21 ± 0.01, and 1.46 ± 0.01; the activity ratios of Beclin 1 were 1.00 ± 0.04, 1.07 ± 0.03, 1.68 ± 0.04, 2.10 ± 0.06, 1.26 ± 0.01, 1.67 ± 0.04, and 2.37 ± 0.06; the activity ratios of LC3B were 1.00 ± 0.02, 1.17 ± 0.01, 1.20 ± 0.00, 1.36 ± 0.03, 1.12 ± 0.01, 1.19 ± 0.02, and 1.33 ± 0.03, respectively. Compared to control groups, dihydroartemisinin plus epirubicin liposomes significantly increased the expressions of Caspase-9, Caspase-3, Bax, Beclin 1, and LC3B, while evidently suppressing the expression of Bcl-2. In addition, the levels of reactive oxygen species (ROS) in the cells treated with dihydroartemisinin plus epirubicin liposomes were significantly higher compared to the controls (Figure S1).

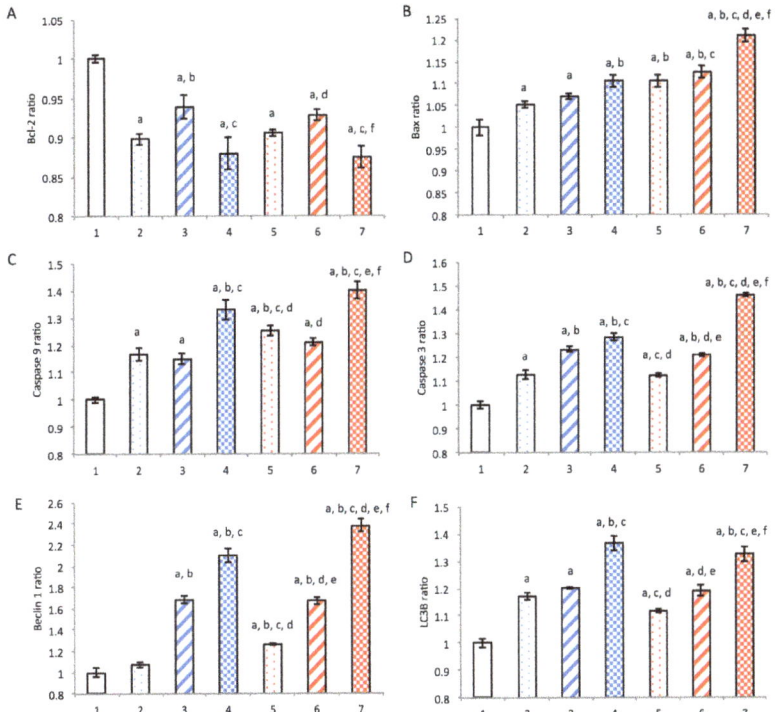

Figure 4. Mechanisms of autophagy and apoptosis in breast cancer MDA-MB-435S cells. 1, blank control; 2, free dihydroartemisinin; 3, free epirubicin; 4, free dihydroartemisinin plus epirubicin (mole ratio = 2:1); 5, dihydroartemisinin liposomes; 6, epirubicin liposomes; 7, dihydroartemisinin plus epirubicin liposomes. Data are presented as the mean $\pm$ standard deviation (n = 3). $p < 0.05$; a, vs. 1; b, vs. 2; c, vs. 3; d, vs. 4; e, vs. 5; f, vs. 6.

3.6. Morphological Changes

Morphological changes in the cells treated with the various formulations were evaluated with a high-content screening system to visualize the mitochondria (red) and nuclei (blue) (Figure S2). Both qualitative (Figure S2A) and quantitative (Figure S2B) measurements showed that mitochondria were disrupted, and they displayed an obvious decrease in fluorescence after drug treatments. Changes in the spherical morphology of the nuclei were also observed (Figure S2C). Specifically, after treatment with the blank medium, free dihydroartemisinin, free epirubicin, free dihydroartemisinin plus free epirubicin, dihydroartemisinin liposomes, epirubicin liposomes, or dihydroartemisinin plus epirubicin liposomes, the fluorescence intensities of the mitochondria were 384.13 ± 7.54, 312.51 ± 8.11, 285.90 ± 11.15, 228.08 ± 8.50, 315.40 ± 6.70, 289.96 ± 14.12, and 219.21 ± 12.86; the nuclear roundness was 0.96 ± 0.00, 0.92 ± 0.01, 0.86 ± 0.01, 0.81 ± 0.01, 0.93 ± 0.01, 0.84 ± 0.01, and 0.80 ± 0.01, respectively. These results indicated that the integrity of the mitochondria and nuclei of the cancer cells were disrupted by treatment with dihydroartemisinin plus epirubicin liposomes, respectively.

3.7. Cytotoxic Effects In Vitro

In vitro cytotoxicity was evaluated in the MDA-MB-435S, MDA-MB-231, and MCF-7 cells (Figure S3). Results indicated that a single free epirubicin treatment caused limited cytotoxicity in cancer cells, while co-treatment of free dihydroartemisinin with free epirubicin significantly enhanced this effect in a concentration-dependent manner for dihydroartemisinin (Figure S3A–C). Furthermore, dihydroartemisinin plus epirubicin liposomes exhibited the strongest cytotoxicity at various dosages. In addition, dihydroartemisinin liposomes displayed a moderately cytotoxic effect (Figure S3D–F).

3.8. Anticancer Efficacy and In Vivo Imaging

Anticancer efficacy was evaluated with respect to tumor volume in xenografts of MDA-MB-435S cells in mice (Figure 5). After treatment with the various formulations, the ranking for tumor volumes was as follows: physiological saline > dihydroartemisinin liposomes > free epirubicin > epirubicin liposomes > dihydroartemisinin plus epirubicin liposomes. These results indicated that the dihydroartemisinin plus epirubicin liposomes had the strongest overall anticancer efficacy. In addition, the body weights of tumor-bearing mice did not differ among the experimental groups (Figure S4). After treatment with free epirubicin, white blood cells of the mice significantly decreased. In contrast, liposomal drug formulations did not cause obvious changes in blood indices (Figure S5, Table S2).

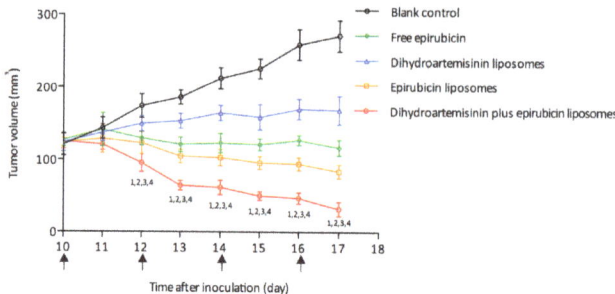

Figure 5. Antitumor efficacy in breast cancer MDA-MB-435S xenografts in nude mice. The arrows indicate the day of drug administration. Data are presented as the mean ± standard deviation ($n = 5$). $p < 0.05$; 1, vs. blank control; 2, vs. free epirubicin; 3, vs. dihydroartemisinin liposomes; 4, vs. epirubicin liposomes.

Real-time imaging of fluorescently labeled liposomes was also performed on the xenografts of MDA-MB-435S cells in these mice (Figure S6A). After treatment with free DiR, the fluorescent signal rapidly accumulated in the liver. In contrast, after treatment with DiR plus dihydroartemisinin liposomes or DiR liposomes, the fluorescent signal remained predominantly in the blood system and tumor tissues. Ex vivo imaging similarly showed that the fluorescent signal for DiR plus dihydroartemisinin liposomes remained in the tumor tissues, while those of control formulations were only weakly visible or invisible (Figure S6B). In addition, the fluorescent signal was detected in the livers and spleens of these mice after treatment with all DiR formulations.

4. Discussion

In a comprehensive treatment strategy for breast cancer, chemotherapy is an important tool used to eliminate cancer cells. However, breast cancer is a typically heterogeneous malignancy, which leads to poor clinical outcomes. Most current treatment strategies rely on inducing necrosis and type I programmed cell death (apoptosis). Nevertheless, this approach is often inefficient at eradicating heterogeneous cancer cells. In this study, we propose a new strategy for overcoming this clinical problem by initiating cross-talk between autophagy and apoptosis in cancer cells, which may help increase the efficacy of heterogeneous breast cancer therapies.

In the dihydroartemisinin plus epirubicin liposomes, dihydroartemisinin incorporated into the lipid bilayer, while epirubicin was encapsulated in the inner vesicle of the liposome. The liposomes were coated with DSPE-PEG$_{2000}$ and exhibited a homogeneously distributed nanoscale particle size (Table S1). This prolonged the circulation of the drugs in the blood stream by avoiding rapid clearance by the reticuloendothelial system [30]. Thus, the drugs accumulation in tumor tissues as a result of enhanced permeability and retention effects [31–33]. Meanwhile, the liposomal drug formulation also reduced the systemic cytotoxicity of epirubicin by decreasing concentrations in healthy tissues. This is because anthracyclines have cardiotoxic side effects that can lead to myocardial damage. As a typical example of anthracyclines, the cardiotoxicity of doxorubicin could be reduced by liposomal encapsulation [34]. Epirubicin has the same mechanism of myocardial damage as doxorubicin, therefore, the liposome encapsulation has the potential to reduce the distribution of epirubicin in heart tissue, thereby reducing cardiotoxicity.

The evaluation of cellular uptake of liposomes revealed that both dihydroartemisinin and epirubicin were efficiently internalized by cancer cells. Moreover, dihydroartemisinin significantly enhanced the co-uptake of epirubicin (Figure 1). This effect was time-dependent, and could be due to the disruption of the cell membrane of the cancer cells exposed to dihydroartemisinin.

Under normal conditions, autophagy allows the orderly degradation and recycling of unnecessary or dysfunctional cellular components to maintain cytoplasmic homeostasis. In the case of a diseased cell, moderate autophagy facilitates an adaptive response to stress that promotes cancer cell survival and metastasis. However, excessive autophagy can ultimately result in type II programmed death of cancer cells [35]. In this study, we found that dihydroartemisinin induced excessive autophagy in cancer cells, and the co-treatment of dihydroartemisinin and epirubicin in liposomes caused significant autophagy that resulted in type II programmed death of breast cancer cells (Figure 2).

In the initiation of autophagy, dihydroartemisinin alone and dihydroartemisinin plus epirubicin released from liposomes activated Beclin 1, which played an essential role in autophagosome formation as a core component of the Class III phosphatidylinositol 3-kinase (PI3K) complex. The Class III PI3K complex utilized PtdIns as a substrate to generate PtdIns3P, which mediated the recruitment of other autophagy proteins onto the pre-autophagosomal membrane [36]. This resulted in excessive autophagy. These effects were demonstrated using the enhanced expression of LC3B, which was the most commonly used autophagy-related marker [37].

Apoptosis is a highly regulated process of cell death and helps maintain survival/death homeostasis in multicellular organisms [38]. It can be initiated through two signaling pathways: the intrinsic mitochondrial pathway and the extrinsic death receptor signaling pathway [39]. Because multidrug resistance exists in heterogeneous cancer cells, the induction of apoptosis is a common approach for improving the efficacy of chemotherapy treatments. In this study, we found that the dihydroartemisinin plus epirubicin formulation significantly enhanced apoptosis in breast cancer cells (Figure 3).

In the initiation of apoptosis, the liposomal release of dihydroartemisinin alone and the combination of dihydroartemisinin plus epirubicin activated the pro-apoptotic protein Bax, which was attached into mitochondria to permeabilize the mitochondrial outer membrane. This process initiated a cascade of apoptotic reactions by activating the upstream initiator Caspase-9 and the downstream effector Caspase-3. This ultimately led to type I programmed death in the cancer cells.

A study of the literature indicates that ROS mediates the mitochondrial permeability transition and increases expression of apoptosis-related proteins, such as Bax and Caspase-9. Therefore, in our study, the generated ROS might be involved in damaging the mitochondrial membrane, upregulating Bax, and activating Caspase-9, thereby promoting apoptosis via the mitochondrial pathway [40].

The present study also found that dihydroartemisinin induced cross-talk between autophagy and apoptosis. In this process, Bcl-2 likely interacted with Beclin 1 or Bax, since it was known to be an anti-apoptotic protein that can bind to Bax to block mitochondrial depolarization [41]. Previous studies demonstrated that Bcl-2 prevented autophagy by binding Beclin 1 [42]. In this study, the released dihydroartemisinin or dihydroartemisinin plus epirubicin from liposomes significantly inhibited the activity of Bcl-2, further destabilizing the binding of Bcl-2 with Beclin 1 and Bax. This disaggregation likely resulted in the release of Beclin 1 from the Bcl-2/Beclin 1 complex, and activated the Class III PI3K complex. This would cause excessive autophagy and induce type II programmed death of cancer cells. Meanwhile, this suppression likely promoted the release of Bax from the Bcl-2/Bax complex, allowing Bax to participate in apoptosis. In addition, epirubicin intercalated into DNA, which could have caused the observed necrosis of cancer cells (Figures 4 and 6). Morphological changes in the mitochondria and nuclei (Figure S2) provided additional evidence that dihydroartemisinin or dihydroartemisinin plus epirubicin liposomes destroyed mitochondria and disrupted the integrity of DNA, which also could have contributed to the observed apoptosis and necrosis.

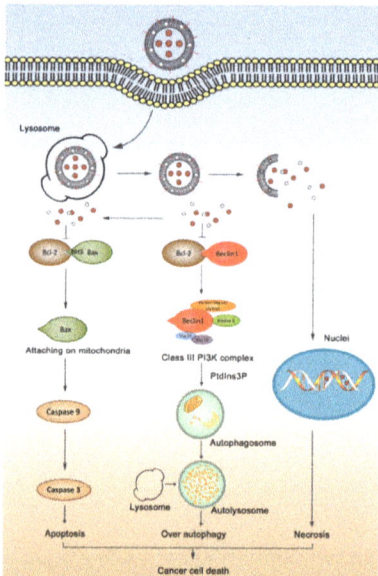

Figure 6. Illustration of heterogeneous cancer death induced by dihydroartemisinin plus epirubicin liposomes through autophagy, apoptosis and necrosis. The nanostructured dihydroartemisinin plus epirubicin liposomes were internalized by cancer cells, escaped from the lysosomes, and existed in two states: the raptured and intact liposomes. Drugs, which either are from the raptured liposomes or are released from the intact liposomes, come into play actions: **1**, dihydroartemisinin interacts with the BH3 domain of Bcl-2, thus suppressing the binding of Bcl-2 with Beclin 1, activating the class III phosphatidylinositol 3-kinase (PI3K) complex to produce phosphatidylinositol 3-phosphate (PtdIns3P) in promoting the excessive autophagy. **2**, dihydroartemisinin suppresses the binding of Bcl-2 with Bax, which allows Bax to attach onto mitochondria, to activate upstream caspase 9 and afterwards downstream caspase 3 in initiating a cascade of apoptosis via the mitochondria pathway. **3**, Epirubicin intercalates DNA strands, resulting in necrosis of cancer cells.

In vitro (Figure S3) and in vivo (Figure 5) experiments showed that dihydroartemisinin alone was moderately cytotoxic in cancer cells, while dihydroartemisinin plus epirubicin liposomes exhibited a robust cytotoxic effect. In vivo imaging also demonstrated that the liposomal formulation allowed the drugs to become significantly enriched in cancer tissues.

5. Conclusions

The present study reveals that dihydroartemisinin potentiates the efficacy of epirubicin-based treatment of heterogeneous breast cancer through the induction of autophagy and apoptosis. Dihydroartemisinin inhibits the activity of Bcl-2, which releases active Beclin 1 and Bax from their respective complexes. This results in a synergy between autophagy and apoptosis. The release of Bax activates apoptosis, leading to type I programmed death. Meanwhile, the release of Beclin 1 initiates excessive autophagy, which induces type II programmed death in cancer cells. The combinational use of dihydroartemisinin with epirubicin potentiates these effects, thereby enhancing overall cytotoxicity; namely, cancer cells can be killed by necrosis which is primarily caused by DNA damage with epirubicin, apoptosis and over-autophagy both of which are induced by dihydroartemisinin. The enhanced anticancer efficacy by liposomal formulation of dihydroartemisinin and epirubicin is evidenced in breast cancer-bearing mice. Besides, this effect may be due to the prolonged circulation of drug liposomes in the blood and the concentrated drugs in cancer tissues. Therefore, the nanostructured combinational formulation of dihydroartemisinin plus epirubicin liposomes provides a promising new strategy for the treatment of heterogeneity in breast cancer.

Supplementary Materials: The following are available online at http://www.mdpi.com/2079-4991/8/10/804/s1, Figure S1: ROS activity ratios in breast cancer MDA-MB-435S cells after treatment with varying drug formulations at 6 h, Figure S2: Morphological changes in mitochondria and nuclei of breast cancer MDA-MB-435S cells, Figure S3: Inhibitory effects to breast cancer cells, Figure S4: Body weight changes of nude mice bearing breast cancer MDA-MB-435S xenografts after treatment with varying formulations, Figure S5: White blood cells in tumor-bearing nude mice after administration of varying drug formulations, Figure S6: Real-time imaging and distribution of liposomes in nude mice bearing breast cancer MDA-MB-435S xenografts, Table S1: Characterization of liposomes, Table S2: Blood examination on tumor-bearing nude mice after administration of drug formulations.

Author Contributions: Conceptualization, Y.-J.H. and W.-L.L.; Formal analysis, Y.-J.H.; Investigation, Y.-J.H. and J.-Y.Z.; Methodology, Y.-J.H.; Project administration, W.-L.L.; Supervision, W.-L.L.; Validation, Y.-J.H., J.-Y.Z., Q.L., J.-R.X., Y.Y., L.-M.M. and J.B.; Writing: original draft, Y.-J.H.; Writing: review and editing, Q.L. and W.-L.L.

Funding: This research was funded by National Natural Science Foundation of China, grant number 81373343, and 81673367.

Acknowledgments: We thank Yong-Rui Jia and Qi-Hua He for their technical support (Peking University).

Conflicts of Interest: The authors declare no conflict of interest. The funders had no role in the design of the study; in the collection, analyses, or interpretation of data; in the writing of the manuscript, or in the decision to publish the results.

References

1. Torre, L.A.; Bray, F.; Siegel, R.L.; Ferlay, J.; Lortet-Tieulent, J.; Jemal, A. Global cancer statistics, 2012. *CA Cancer J. Clin.* **2015**, *65*, 87–108. [CrossRef] [PubMed]
2. Anderson, W.F.; Rosenberg, P.S.; Prat, A.; Perou, C.M.; Sherman, M.E. How many etiological subtypes of breast cancer: Two, three, four, or more? *J. Natl. Cancer Inst.* **2014**, *106*. [CrossRef] [PubMed]
3. Prat, A.; Pineda, E.; Adamo, B.; Galván, P.; Fernández, A.; Gaba, L.; Díez, M.; Viladot, M.; Arance, A.; Muñoz, M. Clinical implications of the intrinsic molecular subtypes of breast cancer. *Breast* **2015**, *24*, S26–S35. [CrossRef] [PubMed]
4. Rouzier, R.; Perou, C.M.; Symmans, W.F.; Ibrahim, N.; Cristofanilli, M.; Anderson, K.; Hess, K.R.; Stec, J.; Ayers, M.; Wagner, P.; et al. Breast cancer molecular subtypes respond differently to preoperative chemotherapy. *Clin. Cancer Res.* **2005**, *11*, 5678–5685. [CrossRef] [PubMed]
5. Lu, H.; Zhang, X.Y.; Wang, Y.Q.; Zheng, X.L.; Zhao, Y.; Xing, W.M.; Zhang, Q. Andrographolide sodium bisulfate-induced apoptosis and autophagy in human proximal tubular endothelial cells is a ROS-mediated pathway. *Environ. Toxicol. Pharmacol.* **2014**, *37*, 718–728. [CrossRef] [PubMed]

6. Motyl, T.; Gajkowska, B.; Zarzynska, J.; Gajewska, M.; Lamparska-Przybysz, M. Apoptosis and autophagy in mammary gland remodeling and breast cancer chemotherapy. *J. Physiol. Pharmacol.* **2006**, *57*, 17–32. [PubMed]
7. Zambrano, J.; Yeh, E.S. Autophagy and apoptotic crosstalk: Mechanism of therapeutic resistance in HER2-positive breast cancer. *Breast Cancer* **2016**, *10*, 13–23. [CrossRef] [PubMed]
8. Ravikumar, B.; Sarkar, S.; Davies, J.E.; Futter, M.; Garcia-Arencibia, M.; Green-Thompson, Z.W.; et al. Regulation of mammalian autophagy in physiology and pathophysiology. *Physiol. Rev.* **2010**, *90*, 1383–1435. [CrossRef] [PubMed]
9. Rubinsztein, D.C.; Codogno, P.; Levine, B. Autophagy modulation as a potential therapeutic target for diverse diseases. *Nat. Rev. Drug Discov.* **2012**, *11*, 709–730. [CrossRef] [PubMed]
10. Vazquez-Martin, A.; Oliveras-Ferraros, C.; Menendez, J.A. Autophagy facilitates the development of breast cancer resistance to the anti-HER2 monoclonal antibody trastuzumab. *PLoS ONE* **2009**, *4*, e6251. [CrossRef] [PubMed]
11. Yoon, J.H.; Ahn, S.G.; Lee, B.H.; Jung, S.H.; Oh, S.H. Role of autophagy in chemoresistance: Regulation of the ATM-mediated DNA-damage signaling pathway through activation of DNA-PKcs and PARP-1. *Biochem. Pharmacol.* **2012**, *83*, 747–757. [CrossRef] [PubMed]
12. Liang, X.H.; Jackson, S.; Seaman, M.; Brown, K.; Kempkes, B.; Hibshoosh, H.; Levine, B. Induction of autophagy and inhibition of tumorigenesis by beclin 1. *Nature* **1999**, *402*, 672–676. [CrossRef] [PubMed]
13. Qu, X.; Yu, J.; Bhagat, G.; Furuya, N.; Hibshoosh, H.; Troxel, A.; Rosen, J.; Eskelinen, E.L.; Mizushima, N.; Ohsumi, Y.; et al. Promotion of tumorigenesis by heterozygous disruption of the beclin 1 autophagy gene. *J. Clin. Investig.* **2003**, *112*, 1809–1820. [CrossRef] [PubMed]
14. White, E. The role for autophagy in cancer. *J. Clin. Investig.* **2015**, *125*, 42–46. [CrossRef] [PubMed]
15. Maiuri, M.C.; Le Toumelin, G.; Criollo, A.; Rain, J.C.; Gautier, F.; Juin, P.; Tasdemir, E.; Pierron, G.; Troulinaki, K.; Tavernarakis, N.; et al. Functional and physical interaction between Bcl-X(L) and a BH3-like domain in Beclin-1. *EMBO J.* **2007**, *26*, 2527–2539. [CrossRef] [PubMed]
16. Luo, S.; Garcia-Arencibia, M.; Zhao, R.; Puri, C.; Toh, P.P.C.; Sadiq, O.; Rubinsztein, D.C. Bim inhibits autophagy by recruiting Beclin 1 to microtubules. *Mol. Cell* **2012**, *47*, 359–370. [CrossRef] [PubMed]
17. Lum, J.J.; Bauer, D.E.; Kong, M.; Harris, M.H.; Li, C.; Lindsten, T.; Thompson, C.B. Growth factor regulation of autophagy and cell survival in the absence of apoptosis. *Cell* **2005**, *120*, 237–248. [CrossRef] [PubMed]
18. Tu, Y. The development of new antimalarial drugs: Qinghaosu and dihydro-qinghaosu. *Chin. Med. J.* **1999**, *112*, 976–977. [PubMed]
19. Wu, C.; Liu, J.; Pan, X.; Xian, W.; Li, B.; Peng, W.; Wang, J.; Yang, D.; Zhou, H. Design, synthesis and evaluation of the antibacterial enhancement activities of amino dihydroartemisinin derivatives. *Molecules* **2013**, *18*, 6866–6882. [CrossRef] [PubMed]
20. Flobinus, A.; Taudon, N.; Desbordes, M.; Labrosse, B.; Simon, F.; Mazeron, M.C.; Schnepf, N. Stability and antiviral activity against human cytomegalovirus of artemisinin derivatives. *J. Antimicrob. Chemother.* **2014**, *69*, 34–40. [CrossRef] [PubMed]
21. Aung, W.; Sogawa, C.; Furukawa, T.; Saga, T. Anticancer effect of dihydroartemisinin (DHA) in a pancreatic tumor model evaluated by conventional methods and optical imaging. *Anticancer Res.* **2011**, *31*, 1549–1558. [PubMed]
22. Chen, H.H.; Zhou, H.J.; Fang, X. Inhibition of human cancer cell line growth and human umbilical vein endothelial cell angiogenesis by artemisinin derivatives in vitro. *Pharmacol. Res* **2003**, *48*, 231–236. [CrossRef]
23. Jia, L.F.; Song, Q.; Zhou, C.Y.; Li, X.M.; Pi, L.H.; Ma, X.R.; Li, H.; Lu, X.; Shen, Y. Dihydroartemisinin as a putative STAT3 inhibitor, suppresses the growth of head and neck squamous cell carcinoma by targeting Jak2/STAT3 signaling. *PLoS ONE* **2016**, *11*, e0147157. [CrossRef] [PubMed]
24. Wang, S.J.; Gao, Y.; Chen, H.; Kong, R.; Jiang, H.C.; Pan, S.H.; Xue, D.B.; Bai, X.W.; Sun, B. Dihydroartemisinin inactivates NF-kB and potentiates the anti-tumor effect of gemcitabine on pancreatic cancer both in vitro and in vivo. *Cancer Lett.* **2010**, *293*, 99–108. [CrossRef] [PubMed]
25. Zhang, S.Y.; Shi, L.; Ma, H.W.; Li, H.Z.; Li, Y.R.; Lu, Y.; Wang, Q.; Li, W. Dihydroartemisinin induces apoptosis in human gastric cancer cell line BGC-823 through activation of JNK1/2 and p38 MAPK signaling pathways. *J. Recept. Signal Transduct. Res.* **2016**, *37*, 174–180. [CrossRef] [PubMed]

26. Feng, X.; Li, L.; Jiang, H.; Jiang, K.P.; Jin, Y.; Zheng, J.X. Dihydroartemisinin potentiates the anticancer effect of cisplatin via mTOR inhibition in cisplatin-resistant ovarian cancer cells: Involvement of apoptosis and autophagy. *Biochem. Biophys. Res. Commun.* **2014**, *444*, 376–381. [CrossRef] [PubMed]
27. Jia, G.; Kong, R.; Ma, Z.B.; Han, B.; Wang, Y.W.; Pan, S.H.; Li, Y.H.; Sun, B. The activation of c-Jun NH$_2$-terminal kinase is required for dihydroartemisinin-induced autophagy in pancreatic cancer cells. *J. Exp. Clin. Cancer Res.* **2014**, *33*, 8–17. [CrossRef] [PubMed]
28. Zhang, Z.S.; Wang, J.; Shen, Y.B.; Guo, C.C.; Sai, K.; Chen, F.R.; Mei, X.; Han, F.; Chen, Z.P. Dihydroartemisinin increases temozolomide efficacy in glioma cells by inducing autophagy. *Oncol. Lett.* **2015**, *10*, 379–383. [CrossRef] [PubMed]
29. Chen, K.; Shou, L.M.; Lin, F.; Duan, W.M.; Wu, M.Y.; Xie, X.; Xie, Y.F.; Li, W.; Tao, M. Artesunate induces G2/M cell cycle arrest through autophagy induction in breast cancer cells. *Anticancer Drugs* **2014**, *25*, 652–662. [CrossRef] [PubMed]
30. Woodle, M.C.; Lasic, D.D. Sterically stabilized liposomes. *Biochim. Biophys. Acta* **1992**, *1113*, 171–199. [CrossRef]
31. Maeda, H.; Tsukigawa, K.; Fang, J. A retrospective 30 years after discovery of the enhanced permeability and retention effect of solid tumors: Next-generation chemotherapeutics and photodynamic therapy–problems, solutions, and prospects. *Microcirculation* **2016**, *23*, 173–182. [CrossRef] [PubMed]
32. Zeng, F.; Ju, J.R.; Liu, L.; Xie, H.J.; Mu, L.M.; Zhao, Y.; Yan, Y.; Hu, Y.J.; Wu, J.S.; Lu, W.L. Application of functional vincristine plus dasatinib liposomes to deletion of vasculogenic mimicry channels in triple-negative breast cancer. *Oncotarget* **2015**, *6*, 36625–36642. [CrossRef] [PubMed]
33. Ju, R.J.; Zeng, F.; Liu, L.; Mu, L.M.; Xie, H.J.; Zhao, Y.; Yan, Y.; Wu, J.S.; Hu, Y.J.; Lu, W.L. Destruction of vasculogenic mimicry channels by targeting epirubicin plus celecoxib liposomes in treatment of brain glioma. *Int. J. Nanomed.* **2016**, *11*, 1131–1146.
34. Lu, W.L.; Qi, X.R.; Zhang, Q.; Li, R.Y.; Wang, G.L.; Zhang, R.J.; Wei, S.L. A pegylated liposomal platform: Pharmacokinetics, pharmacodynamics, and toxicity in mice using doxorubicin as a model drug. *J. Pharmacol. Sci.* **2004**, *95*, 381–389. [CrossRef] [PubMed]
35. Fulda, S.; Kogel, D. Cell death by autophagy: Emerging molecular mechanisms and implications for cancer therapy. *Oncogene* **2015**, *34*, 5105–5113. [CrossRef] [PubMed]
36. Kihara, A.; Kabeya, Y.; Ohsumi, Y.; Yoshimori, T. Beclin-phosphatidylinositol 3-kinase complex functions at the trans-Golgi network. *EMBO Rep.* **2001**, *2*, 330–335. [CrossRef] [PubMed]
37. He, Y.Y.; Zhao, X.D.; Subahan, N.R.; Fan, L.F.; Gao, J.; Chen, H.L. The prognostic value of autophagy-related markers beclin-1 and microtubule-associated protein light chain 3B in cancers: A systematic review and meta-analysis. *Tumour Biol.* **2014**, *35*, 7317–7326. [CrossRef] [PubMed]
38. Hassan, M.; Watari, H.; AbuAlmaaty, A.; Ohba, Y.; Sakuragi, N. Apoptosis and molecular targeting therapy in cancer. *BioMed. Res. Int.* **2014**, *2014*, 150845–150867. [CrossRef] [PubMed]
39. Elmore, S. Apoptosis: A review of programmed cell death. *Toxicol. Pathol.* **2007**, *35*, 495–516. [CrossRef] [PubMed]
40. Lim, J.Y.; Kim, D.; Kim, B.R.; Jun, J.S.; Yeom, J.S.; Park, J.S.; Seo, J.H.; Park, C.H.; Woo, H.O.; Youn, H.S.; et al. Vitamin C induces apoptosis in AGS cells via production of ROS of mitochondria. *Oncol. Lett.* **2016**, *12*, 4270–4276. [CrossRef] [PubMed]
41. Karni, R.; Jove, R.; Levitzki, A. Inhibition of pp60c-Src reduces Bcl-XL expression and reverses the transformed phenotype of cells overexpressing EGF and HER-2 receptors. *Oncogene* **1999**, *18*, 4654–4662. [CrossRef] [PubMed]
42. Cao, Y.; Klionsky, D.J. Physiological functions of Atg6/Beclin 1: A unique autophagy-related protein. *Cell Res.* **2007**, *17*, 839–849. [CrossRef] [PubMed]

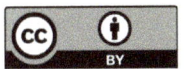

© 2018 by the authors. Licensee MDPI, Basel, Switzerland. This article is an open access article distributed under the terms and conditions of the Creative Commons Attribution (CC BY) license (http://creativecommons.org/licenses/by/4.0/).

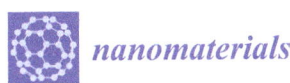

Review

Lanthanide-Doped Upconversion Nanocarriers for Drug and Gene Delivery

Gibok Lee and Yong Il Park *

School of Chemical Engineering, Chonnam National University, Gwangju 61186, Korea; 188608@jnu.ac.kr
* Correspondence: ypark@jnu.ac.kr; Tel.: +82-62-530-1886; Fax: +82-62-530-1889

Received: 4 June 2018; Accepted: 7 July 2018; Published: 9 July 2018

Abstract: Compared to traditional cancer treatments, drug/gene delivery is an advanced, safe, and efficient method. Nanoparticles are widely used as nanocarriers in a drug/gene delivery system due to their long circulation time and low multi-drug resistance. In particular, lanthanide-doped upconversion nanoparticles (UCNPs) that can emit UV and visible light by near-infrared (NIR) upconversion demonstrated more efficient and safer drug/gene delivery. Because of the low penetration depth of UV and visible light, a photoinduced reaction such as photocleavage or photoisomerization has proven restrictive. However, NIR light has high tissue penetration depth and stimulates the photoinduced reaction through UV and visible emissions from lanthanide-doped UCNPs. This review discusses the optical properties of UCNPs that are useful in bioapplications and drug/gene delivery systems using the UCNPs as a photoreaction inducer.

Keywords: upconversion nanoparticles; nanocarriers; drug delivery; gene delivery; photolysis

1. Introduction

Cancer is one of the major diseases that threatens human health worldwide. Many researchers have developed various cancer treatments such as surgery, chemotherapy, and radiotherapy. However, these methods have limitations. Because cancer lesions and normal tissue are not completely differentiated during surgery, large complex tissues are removed. Chemotherapy works on the whole body in addition to the cancerous tissues and results in low tumor-specific targeting, severe side effects, drug dependence, and multi-drug resistance (MDR) [1–4]. Radiotherapy works on a specific region with normal tissues and results in skin damage, cancer recurrence, cell mutation, dose-dependent side effects, and cardiovascular problems [5–7]. Therefore, the development of more efficient and safe methods to remove cancerous tissues is essential for improving cancer treatments. Recently, drug/gene delivery systems have been suggested as an alternative to conventional cancer treatments. In particular, nanoparticles used as drug/gene carriers are attracting attention due to advantages such as their high tumor-specific targeting with low side effects and increased loading capacity. Nanoparticles tend to accumulate in tumor lesions through the relatively leaky tumor vasculature, and this accumulation is associated with the enhanced permeability and retention (EPR) effect [8–11]. The large specific surface area of nanoparticles and mesoporous/hollow nanostructures increases the amount of drug/gene loading. To exploit these advantages, many researchers have designed nanocarriers such as liposomes [12–15], polymeric micelles [16–18], polymeric nanoparticles [19–21], carbon nanotubes [22,23], reduced graphene oxides [24–26], gold nanoparticles [27–29], magnetic nanoparticles [30–32], and lanthanide-doped upconversion nanoparticles (UCNPs) [33–38].

In this review, we discuss drug/gene delivery systems that use lanthanide-doped UCNPs. The unique and fascinating optical properties that convert near-infrared (NIR) light to visible and UV light allow UCNPs to be used as more efficient nanocarrier materials in drug/gene delivery systems. This drug/gene delivery system is based on photoinduced reactions such as photocleavage and photoisomerization. Photoinduced delivery systems enhance the efficacy of spatial and temporal control of drug/gene release and minimize normal cell death, side effects, and the tissue damage.

2. Lanthanide-Doped UCNPs

Photoinduced drug/gene delivery systems use photoreactions to control drug release and gene expression, mainly through UV light sources. However, the UV region is not only harmful to tissues and cells, but also has a disadvantage of low tissue penetration depth due to its absorption by biological substances (e.g., protein, hemoglobin, and melanin) [39,40]. Unlike UV light, NIR light exhibit the deep penetration depth due to low absorption by biological substances and minimizes photodamage to tissues and cells [39,41]. In order to use NIR light for photoinduced drug/gene delivery, an anti-Stokes shifting material that emits UV light by NIR excitation is required. Among the various materials, UCNPs have been proposed as a strong candidate. Upconversion is the process by which multiple lower energy photons are converted to higher energy photons and are emitted [42]. Various lanthanide-doped UCNPs have been extensively investigated, and ytterbium (Yb^{3+}), erbium (Er^{3+}), thulium (Tm^{3+}), and holmium (Ho^{3+}) are well-known lanthanide dopants in UCNPs (see Figure 1a) [43]. Yb^{3+} ions are usually used as a sensitizer for absorbing NIR photons, and Er^{3+}, Tm^{3+}, and Ho^{3+} ions are used as an activator to emit upconverted luminescence (i.e., visible and UV). In addition, because lanthanide ions produce long-lived luminescence emission through the forbidden 4f-4f transition between real intermediate energy states, upconversion is much more efficient than other anti-Stokes shift phenomena (e.g., two-photon absorption and second harmonic generation). Moreover, compact and inexpensive continuous wave (CW) lasers can be used as an excitation source for upconversion, while other anti-Stokes shifting materials require high power pulsed lasers [44,45]. Since energy transfer between the energy levels of lanthanide ions is possible, the choice of UCNP host material doped with lanthanide elements has a significant effect on the upconversion mechanism and its efficiency. The most widely used host material for lanthanide-mediated upconversion is sodium yttrium fluoride ($NaYF_4$) because of its relatively low phonon energy (400 cm^{-1}), which minimizes non-radiative relaxation decay [46,47]. Yb^{3+} and Er^{3+} co-doped UCNPs are primarily used as probes for in vitro and in vivo bioimaging [48–50]. The $^2H_{11/2}$, $^4S_{3/2} \to {}^4I_{15/2}$, and $^4F_{9/2} \to {}^4I_{15/2}$ transitions in trivalent Er^{3+} emit the green and red upconverted luminescence (see Figure 1b) [51]. Green emission from Yb^{3+} and Er^{3+} co-doped UCNPs shows relatively high quantum yield compared to UCNPs with other lanthanide elements [52–54]. Yb^{3+} and Tm^{3+} co-doped UCNPs are primarily used as UV sources for photoinduced reactions. The $^1I_6 \to {}^3H_6$, $^1D_2 \to {}^3H_6$, $^1D_2 \to {}^3F_4$, and $^1G_4 \to {}^3H_6$ transition in trivalent Tm^{3+} emit the UV and blue upconverted luminescence (see Figure 1b) [51]. Thus, Yb^{3+} and Tm^{3+} co-doped UCNPs can induce photocleavage and photoisomerization of photosensitive compounds for drug/gene delivery systems.

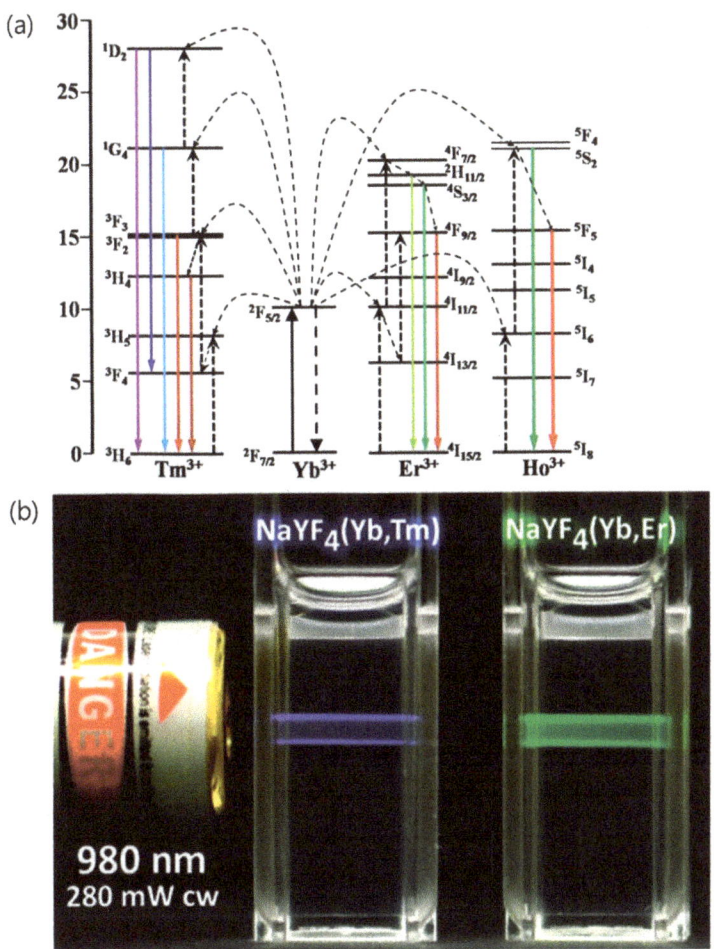

Figure 1. (a) Energy level diagrams of Tm^{3+}, Yb^{3+}, Er^{3+}, and Ho^{3+} ions, illustrating the upconversion mechanism in lanthanide-doped upconversion nanoparticles (UCNPs) [43]. (b) Photographs of upconversion emission excited by a 980 nm laser [51]. Reproduced with permission from [43]. Copyright MDPI, 2017. Reproduced with permission from [51]. Copyright IVYSPRING, 2013.

Figure 2a shows the difference in the penetration depths of UV and NIR light through pork skin placed on top of a solution containing UCNPs [55]. Figure 2b shows the penetration difference between UV and NIR lasers used to excite the fluorescein (FITC) and UCNPs, respectively. Under UV irradiation, the emission intensity from FITC decreased when the thickness of chicken breast increased, but the fluorescence signal from FITC was not observed when the thickness of chicken breast reached 6 mm. Under NIR irradiation, however, enough photons are transmitted to the UCNPs to emit green luminescence even though the thickness of the chicken is 10 mm [56]. Also, the penetration depth of NIR light for upconversion imaging was demonstrated to be 1.25 inches (3.2 cm) at the pork tissue [57]. Therefore, UCNPs can be used as effective UV sources that can cause photoinduced reactions under NIR irradiation with high penetration depth and can be used as nanocarriers for drug/gene delivery.

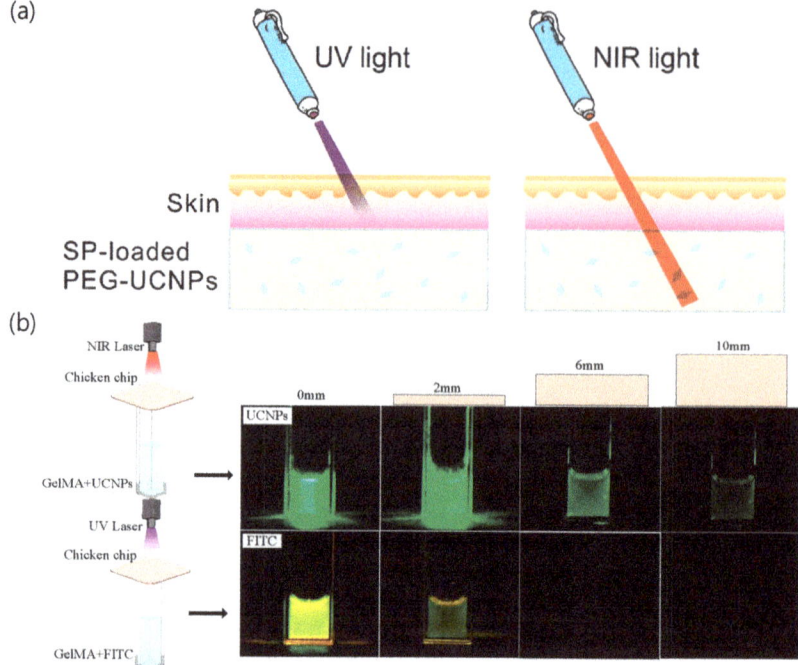

Figure 2. (a) Illustration of the penetration depths for UV and NIR light [55]. (b) Photographs of tissue penetration for NIR and UV light. Slices of chicken breast with various thicknesses (2 mm–10 mm) were placed between the laser source and the glass cuvette containing the UCNP-labeled hydrogel and fluorescein (FITC)-labeled hydrogel, respectively [56]. Reproduced with permission from [55]. Copyright The Royal Society of Chemistry, 2015. Reproduced with permission from [56]. Copyright Elsevier, 2017.

3. Drug/Gene Delivery Using Photocleavage

In drug/gene delivery, the photocleavage reaction of small molecules or polymer backbones is an attractive method to trigger drug release and gene expression. The photocleavage reaction has three methods, namely (1) the direct cleavage of the bond between the molecule and the carrier [37,58–60]; (2) a change in the charge on the carrier surface used to induce electrostatic repulsion between the molecules and the carrier [61,62]; and (3) the destruction of the carrier itself [63].

3.1. Direct Cleavage of the Bond between the Molecule and the Carrier

The photosensitive compounds are modified to bind the drug/gene to the carrier through a variety of molecular interactions, thus undergoing irreversible deformation [37,58,60,64,65]. The most commonly used photosensitive molecules are coumarinyl and o-nitrobenzyl esters. They serve as linkers that bind the drug/gene to the carriers and are broken when exposed to UV or visible light. These photoreactive molecules can also be directly destroyed by two-photon absorption of NIR light [66,67]. However, the molecules have a small two-photon absorption cross-section and slow reaction rate [68]. Thus, this photoreaction involving two-photon absorption requires a higher NIR laser power and longer reaction time than a UV (or visible) source. Due to the NIR excitation and efficient upconverted UV and visible light emission, the UCNPs can be used to induce photocleavable reactions using NIR light. When combined with the high penetration depth of NIR light, the low energy requirement of the UCNPs, which can be used with inexpensive CW lasers instead of high energy pulsed lasers, also has the advantage of increasing the delivery efficiency [69]. In 2015, He et al. reported that the UCNPs could induce photoreactive drug delivery under ultralow-intensity NIR irradiation [70]. The authors used the photocleavable reaction of the Ru complex to release the drug from the carrier (see Figure 3a). Since the absorption (~453 nm) of the Ru complex overlaps with the blue emission from the UCNPs, the upconverted light by NIR excitation induces photocleavage of the Ru complex [71]. The mesoporous silica shell of the UCNPs (UCNP@mSiO$_2$) was used as the drug carrier, and the Ru complex was attached to the pores to serve as a molecular valve. Without NIR irradiation, the release of doxorubicin from UCNP@mSiO$_2$ was not detected. When irradiated with NIR light, doxorubicin clogged with the Ru complex in the UCNP@mSiO$_2$ was released due to photocleavage of the Ru complex (see Figure 3b). Irradiation with 0.35 W cm^{-2} laser intensity was sufficient to trigger the UCNPs-assisted photoreaction and release doxorubicin. Figure 3c also shows how the drug release efficiency depends on the NIR laser output intensity. Approximately 78% of the doxorubicin was released under irradiation with 0.64 W cm^{-2} for 5 h, while ~42% of the doxorubicin was released under irradiation with 0.35 W cm^{-2} for 5 h. Direct cleavage of the photosensitive compound for the drug release is dependent on the irradiated laser power and irradiation time.

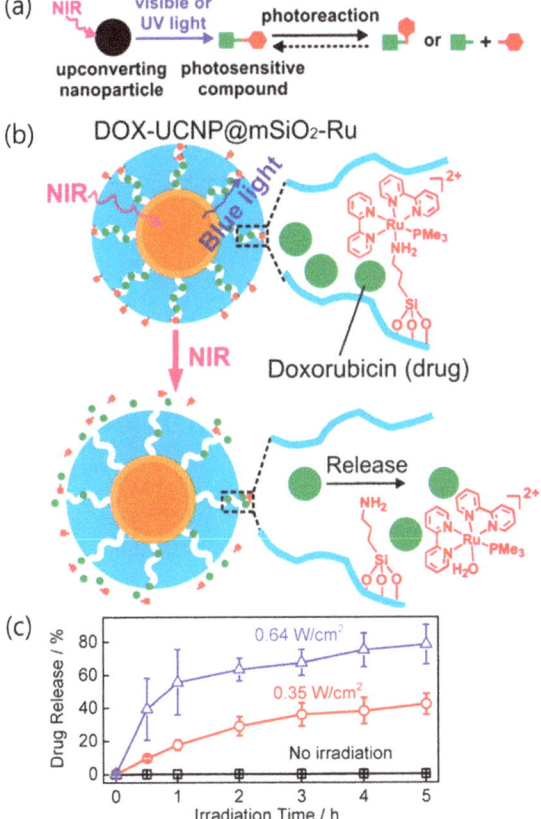

Figure 3. (a) Schematic illustration of photoreactions involving photosensitive compounds induced by UV and visible light produced by upconverted NIR radiation. (b) Under NIR irradiation, upconverted blue light triggers cleavage of the Ru complexes and drug release. (c) Doxorubicin release profiles with laser power and irradiation time. Reproduced with permission from [70]. Copyright The Royal Society of Chemistry, 2015.

3.2. Change in the Charge on the Carrier Surface To Induce Electrostatic Repulsion

The delivery of chemical drugs enables effective therapy whether the carriers internalize into a cell or not. Contrary to chemical drug delivery, the carriers containing gene expression molecules must be internalized into a cell for gene therapy [72,73]. In addition, if the payload leakage is severe, the efficacy of gene therapy is greatly reduced. Therefore, the size and surface charge of the nanocarriers are important for cellular uptake. In particular, the positively charged surface of the nanocarriers demonstrates the increased efficiency of gene loading as well as an increased binding capacity to the anionic plasma membranes. The Fan group reported NIR-induced charge-variable cationic conjugated polyelectrolyte brushes (CCPEB) that encapsulate UCNPs for promoted siRNA release and cooperative photodynamic therapy (PDT) [61]. The charge-variable cationic conjugated polyelectrolyte (CCPE) was synthesized based on the o-nitrobenzyl ester and changed the surface charge on the carrier via the photocleavage reaction (see Figure 4a). CCPE has many positively charged quaternary amine groups that act as negatively charged nucleic acid carriers. The release of o-nitrobenzyl aldehyde by NIR irradiation converts the CCPEB on the UCNPs to zwitterionic conjugated polyelectrolyte brushes (ZCPEB) and initiates siRNA release by charge repulsion (see Figure 4b). As a result, UCNP@CCPEB as an siRNA carrier promoted siRNA release (80% efficiency) at pH 5.0 under 980 nm irradiation.

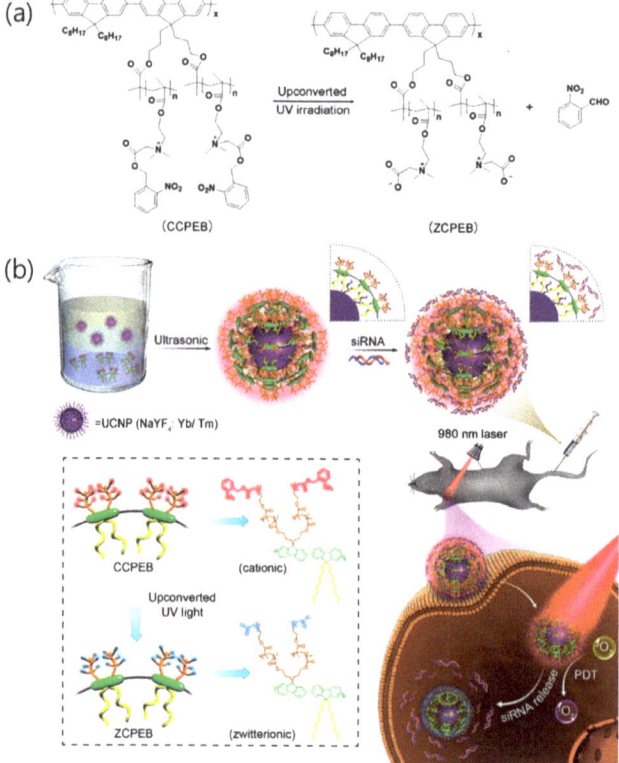

Figure 4. (**a**) Photoinduced charge-variable cationic conjugated polyelectrolyte brush (CCPEB). (**b**) Schematic representation of the NIR-induced charge-variable nanotherapeutic system (UCNP@CCPEB) for siRNA delivery and PDT. Reproduced with permission from [61]. Copyright John Wiley and Sons, 2017.

3.3. Destruction of the Carrier

The nanocomposites encapsulating the drug molecules and functionalized nanomaterials increase the payload for effective chemotherapy. This strategy has the advantage of creating multifunctional materials by adding nanomaterials with various properties to the inside of the carrier. For example, UV emission from the UCNPs can destroy the drug carrier itself. In 2011, Yan et al. reported NIR light-triggered dissociation of block copolymer (BCP) micelles containing hydrophobic drugs and UCNPs (see Figure 5a) [63]. When the UCNPs in the BCP micelle were irradiated with NIR light, the polymethacrylate block in the BCP micelle was converted to hydrophilic poly-(methacrylic acid) by photocleavage of the hydrophobic *o*-nitrobenzyl groups (see Figure 5b). This collapse of the hydrophilic-hydrophobic balance destabilizes the BCP micelles [67]. Dissociation of the BCP micelles was also confirmed using TEM analysis. Before NIR irradiation, the BCP micelles contained 4-5 UCNPs per micelle (see Figure 5c). After excitation at 980 nm, the BCP micelles completely collapsed, and the UCNPs and drugs were released from the micelles (see Figure 5d).

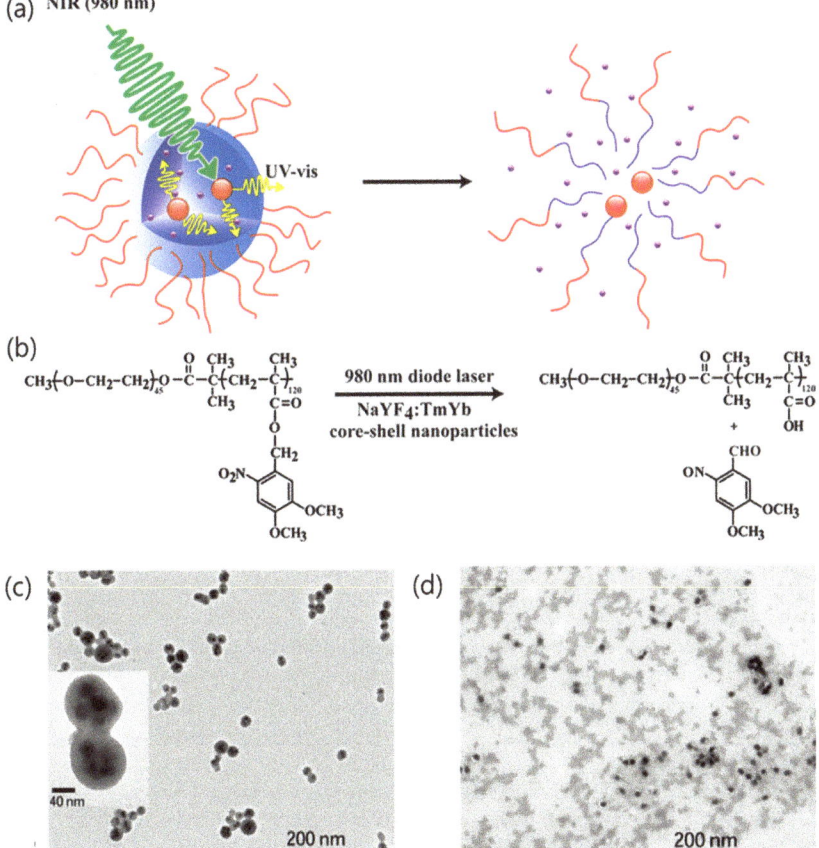

Figure 5. (a) Schematic of drug release resulting from NIR light-triggered dissociation of UCNP-loaded block copolymer (BCP) micelles. (b) Photoreaction scheme showing cleavage of the BCP backbone by NIR irradiation. (c,d) TEM images of the UCNP-loaded BCP micelles (c) before and (d) after NIR light irradiation. Reproduced with permission from [63]. Copyright American Chemical Society, 2011.

4. Drug/Gene Delivery Using Photoisomerization

Photoisomerization is a reaction in which isomers change their spatial conformation under optical irradiation [74–77]. Molecules such as azobenzene, spiropyran, and dithienylethene are mainly used, and their spatial conformation changes reversibly under UV and visible illumination [67,78]. This reaction can be used as a switch to control the drug/gene release by opening the pathway through which the drug/gene passes. In particular, azobenzene with a *trans-cis* transformation is mainly used for lanthanide-doped UCNPs [79–83]. In 2016, Yao et al. developed azobenzene-liposome/UCNPs hybrid vesicles for controlled drug delivery to overcome cancer MDR [79]. Azobenzene liposomes (Azo-Lipo) consists of 1,2-distearoyl-sn-glycero-3-phosphocholine (DSPC) phospholipids and azobenzene amphiphilic derivatives. The as-synthesized hydrophobic UCNPs ($NaGdF_4$:Yb,Tm@$NaGdF_4$) were encapsulated by DSPC phospholipids via van der Waals interaction to induce a hydrophilic surface [84]. The hydrophilic UCNPs and doxorubicin are located in the hydrophilic cavity of the vesicles along with formation of the doxorubicin-loaded Azo-Lipo/UCNPs hybrid vesicles. UV and visible light from the UCNPs enable reversible photoisomerization of the azobenzene derivatives. Continuous rotation-inversion motion by reversible *trans-cis* conversion destabilizes the lipid bilayer and releases the drug (see Figure 6a). This nanocomposite showed increased drug release efficiency with higher laser power and increased concentration of azobenzene derivatives. The release of doxorubicin reached 57 wt % in 6 h under intermittent 2.2 W cm^{-2} NIR laser irradiation, while over 90 wt % release can be reached in 6 h under intermittent 7.8 W cm^{-2} irradiation. The *trans-cis* transformation of azobenzene for drug release was also adapted to the mesopore structure on the UCNPs. In 2013, Liu et al. reported NIR-triggered anticancer drug delivery by UCNPs with an integrated azobenzene-modified mesoporous silica shell (Dox-UCNP@$mSiO_2$-azo) [80]. The back and forth wagging motion of the azobenzene groups through *trans-cis* isomerization under UV and visible illumination acts as a molecular impeller to propel the release of doxorubicin from silica mesopores (see Figure 6b). Because the azobenzene molecular impeller is activated by light emitted from the UCNPs, drug release also depends on the laser power and duration. More doxorubicin was released with higher NIR illumination intensity. Conventional mesoporous silica releases the loaded drug by diffusion, the azobenzene impeller, regulated by the NIR light, controls the drug release more precisely. The azobenzene *trans-cis* transformation property has also been studied for use in gene delivery [85–88]. In 2017, Chen et al. reported an NIR-induced UCNP-based siRNA nanocarrier that exhibited spatiotemporally controlled gene silencing [81]. The UCNPs functionalized with β-cyclodextrin (CD) form the (UCNP-(CD/Azo)-siRNA) complex with siRNA-azobenzene through a host–guest interaction. *Trans*-azobenzene derivatives have a strong host-guest interaction with CD [77,89]. Under NIR irradiation, UV emission from the UCNPs induces photoisomerization of Azo-siRNAs into the cis configuration. The isomerized cis-azobenzene derivatives exhibit polarity change and steric hindrance, which destabilizes the host–guest interaction and releases siRNA (see Figure 6c). The amount of released siRNA can be easily controlled by selecting an appropriate NIR irradiation time. About 41% and 85% of siRNA was released within 10 and 20 min under 0.75 W cm^{-2} NIR irradiation, respectively. In addition, spatial gene silencing was controlled by spatial irradiation in the cell culture dish. Cells which are half-covered by aluminum foil and irradiated with the NIR laser (0.75 W cm^{-2}, 10 min) show region-specific down-regulation of green fluorescent proteins. This controlled drug/gene delivery shows that the NIR-activated UCNPs are safer and more efficient carriers.

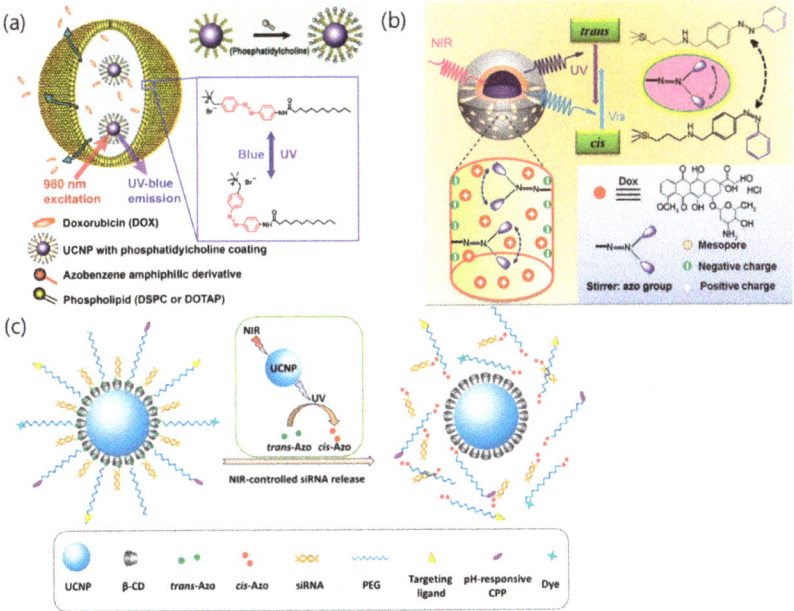

Figure 6. (a) Schematic illustration showing NIR light-triggered drug release of azobenzene-liposome/UCNPs hybrid vesicles by *trans-cis* photoisomerization [79]. (b) NIR-activated drug release from azo molecules grafted on mesopores by *trans-cis* photoisomerization [80]. (c) Illustration of NIR-triggered *trans*-to-*cis* photoisomerization of azobenzene, which subsequently leads to siRNA release from the UCNP-(CD/Azo)-siRNA [81]. Reproduced with permission from [79]. Copyright John Wiley and Sons, 2016. Reproduced with permission from [80]. Copyright John Wiley and Sons, 2013. Reproduced with permission from [81]. Copyright Elsevier, 2018.

5. Conclusions and Future Prospects

The optical properties of lanthanide-doped UCNPs, which emit UV and visible light under NIR excitation, are useful for biomedical applications such as bioimaging and drug/gene delivery. In drug/gene delivery systems, UCNPs act as a source of UV light that cleaves the chemical link between the drug/gene and the nanocarrier and induces the photoisomerization of photosensitive compounds. The photocleavage of the photosensitive compound occurs by the direct cleavage of conjugation, a change in the charge on the surface of the carrier, and the destruction of the carrier itself. The photoreaction also depends on the NIR laser output power and irradiation time, resulting in better control over drug/gene release. Photoisomerization induces conformational change of the isomer. Azobenzene derivatives have been widely used as a photoisomer. These UCNPs generate a rapid release of the drug/gene for cancer treatment. In addition, the UCNPs function as a UV source and allow spatial control of gene expression by blocking the irradiating area. Despite the development of drug/gene delivery systems using lanthanide-doped UCNPs, several problems remain. Drug/gene payload is important for effective therapy and successful gene expression. However, a constraint of the payload in nanocarriers limits the therapeutic efficacy of the drug/gene delivery system. Increasing the concentration of nanocarriers induces high toxicity in normal tissues. Thus, to overcome these limitations, further studies on drug/gene delivery systems that combine immunotherapy [90] or other therapies, such as photodynamic therapy (PDT) [91,92] or photothermal therapy (PTT) [93], have been reported. Researchers should also investigate and understand the leakage of drugs/genes from the cargo to prevent side effects. For example, Bazylińska et al. reported that the leakage of delivery cargo was prevented by encapsulating the drug and UCNPs using the double emulsion method, which forms hybrid nanocomposites [94,95]. Future research should be carried out to reduce the loss of therapeutic agents as well as the leakage of inorganic species by utilizing lanthanide-doped UCNPs as nanocarriers. In particular, dissociation of the carrier itself releases all components such as drug/gene molecules, lanthanide-doped UCNPs, and enveloping molecules. This release can interrupt metabolism and excretion behavior. Thus, future research should investigate the toxicity of the residue by long-term tracking for the biosafety of nanocomposites.

Author Contributions: G.L. and Y.I.P. outlined and mainly wrote the manuscript. All authors contributed to discussion and reviewed the manuscript.

Funding: This work was supported by the National Research Foundation of Korea (NRF) grant funded by the Korea Government (Ministry of Science, ICT & Future Planning) (No. 2016R1A4A1012224).

Conflicts of Interest: The authors declare no conflict of interest.

References

1. Chabner, B.A.; Roberts, T.G., Jr. Chemotherapy and the war on cancer. *Nat. Rev. Cancer* **2005**, *5*, 65. [CrossRef] [PubMed]
2. He, Q.; Shi, J. MSN Anti-cancer nanomedicines: Chemotherapy enhancement, overcoming of drug resistance, and metastasis inhibition. *Adv. Mater.* **2014**, *26*, 391–411. [CrossRef] [PubMed]
3. Tian, G.; Zheng, X.; Zhang, X.; Yin, W.; Yu, J.; Wang, D.; Zhang, Z.; Yang, X.; Gu, Z.; Zhao, Y. TPGS-stabilized NaYbF$_4$:Er upconversion nanoparticles for dual-modal fluorescent/CT imaging and anticancer drug delivery to overcome multi-drug resistance. *Biomaterials* **2015**, *40*, 107–116. [CrossRef] [PubMed]
4. Zhu, H.; Chen, H.; Zeng, X.; Wang, Z.; Zhang, X.; Wu, Y.; Gao, Y.; Zhang, J.; Liu, K.; Liu, R.; et al. Co-delivery of chemotherapeutic drugs with vitamin E TPGS by porous PLGA nanoparticles for enhanced chemotherapy against multi-drug resistance. *Biomaterials* **2014**, *35*, 2391–2400. [CrossRef] [PubMed]
5. Newhauser, W.D.; de Gonzalez, A.B.; Schulte, R.; Lee, C. A review of radiotherapy-induced late effects research after advanced technology treatments. *Front. Oncol.* **2016**, *6*, 13. [CrossRef] [PubMed]
6. Adams, M.J.; Lipsitz, S.R.; Colan, S.D.; Tarbell, N.J.; Treves, S.T.; Diller, L.; Greenbaum, N.; Mauch, P.; Lipshultz, S.E. Cardiovascular status in long-term survivors of hodgkin's disease treated with chest radiotherapy. *J. Clin. Oncol.* **2004**, *22*, 3139–3148. [CrossRef] [PubMed]
7. Darby, S.C.; Ewertz, M.; McGale, P.; Bennet, A.M.; Blom-Goldman, U.; Brønnum, D.; Correa, C.; Cutter, D.; Gagliardi, G.; Gigante, B.; et al. Risk of ischemic heart disease in women after radiotherapy for breast cancer. *N. Engl. J. Med.* **2013**, *368*, 987–998. [CrossRef] [PubMed]
8. Yu, M.; Zheng, J. Clearance pathways and tumor targeting of imaging nanoparticles. *ACS Nano* **2015**, *9*, 6655–6674. [CrossRef] [PubMed]
9. Albanese, A.; Tang, P.S.; Chan, W.C.W. The effect of nanoparticle size, shape, and surface chemistry on biological systems. *Annu. Rev. Biomed. Eng.* **2012**, *14*, 1–16. [CrossRef] [PubMed]
10. Maeda, H.; Nakamura, H.; Fang, J. The EPR effect for macromolecular drug delivery to solid tumors: Improvement of tumor uptake, lowering of systemic toxicity, and distinct tumor imaging in vivo. *Adv. Drug Deliv. Rev.* **2013**, *65*, 71–79. [CrossRef] [PubMed]
11. Nakamura, Y.; Mochida, A.; Choyke, P.L.; Kobayashi, H. Nanodrug delivery: Is the enhanced permeability and retention effect sufficient for curing cancer? *Bioconjug. Chem.* **2016**, *27*, 2225–2238. [CrossRef] [PubMed]
12. Torchilin, V.P. Recent advances with liposomes as pharmaceutical carriers. *Nat. Rev. Drug Discov.* **2005**, *4*, 145. [CrossRef] [PubMed]
13. Malam, Y.; Loizidou, M.; Seifalian, A.M. Liposomes and nanoparticles: Nanosized vehicles for drug delivery in cancer. *Trends Pharmacol. Sci.* **2009**, *30*, 592–599. [CrossRef] [PubMed]
14. Im, N.R.; Kim, K.M.; Young, S.J.; Park, S.N. Physical characteristics and in vitro skin permeation of elastic liposomes loaded with caffeic acid-hydroxypropyl-β-cyclodextrin. *Korean J. Chem. Eng.* **2016**, *33*, 2738–2746. [CrossRef]
15. Noh, G.Y.; Suh, J.Y.; Park, S.N. Ceramide-based nanostructured lipid carriers for transdermal delivery of isoliquiritigenin: Development, physicochemical characterization, and in vitro skin permeation studies. *Korean J. Chem. Eng.* **2017**, *34*, 400–406. [CrossRef]

16. Rapoport, N. Physical stimuli-responsive polymeric micelles for anti-cancer drug delivery. *Prog. Polym. Sci.* **2007**, *32*, 962–990. [CrossRef]
17. Kakizawa, Y.; Kataoka, K. Block copolymer micelles for delivery of gene and related compounds. *Adv. Drug Deliv. Rev.* **2002**, *54*, 203–222. [CrossRef]
18. Iyer, A.K.; Greish, K.; Seki, T.; Okazaki, S.; Fang, J.; Takeshita, K.; Maeda, H. Polymeric micelles of zinc protoporphyrin for tumor targeted delivery based on EPR effect and singlet oxygen generation. *J. Drug Target.* **2007**, *15*, 496–506. [CrossRef] [PubMed]
19. Elsabahy, M.; Wooley, K.L. Design of polymeric nanoparticles for biomedical delivery applications. *Chem. Soc. Rev.* **2012**, *41*, 2545–2561. [CrossRef] [PubMed]
20. Kumari, A.; Yadav, S.K.; Yadav, S.C. Biodegradable polymeric nanoparticles based drug delivery systems. *Colloids Surf. B* **2010**, *75*, 1–18. [CrossRef] [PubMed]
21. Zahedi, P.; Fallah-Darrehchi, M.; Nadoushan, S.A.; Aeinehvand, R.; Bagheri, L.; Najafi, M. Morphological, thermal and drug release studies of poly (methacrylic acid)-based molecularly imprinted polymer nanoparticles immobilized in electrospun poly (ε-caprolactone) nanofibers as dexamethasone delivery system. *Korean J. Chem. Eng.* **2017**, *34*, 2110–2118. [CrossRef]
22. Bianco, A.; Kostarelos, K.; Prato, M. Applications of carbon nanotubes in drug delivery. *Curr. Opin. Chem. Biol.* **2005**, *9*, 674–679. [CrossRef] [PubMed]
23. Liu, Z.; Tabakman, S.; Welsher, K.; Dai, H. Carbon nanotubes in biology and medicine: In vitro and in vivo detection, imaging and drug delivery. *Nano Res.* **2009**, *2*, 85–120. [CrossRef] [PubMed]
24. Kim, H.; Lee, D.; Kim, J.; Kim, T.-I.; Kim, W.J. Photothermally triggered cytosolic drug delivery via endosome disruption using a functionalized reduced graphene oxide. *ACS Nano* **2013**, *7*, 6735–6746. [CrossRef] [PubMed]
25. Wei, G.; Yan, M.; Dong, R.; Wang, D.; Zhou, X.; Chen, J.; Hao, J. Covalent modification of reduced graphene oxide by means of diazonium chemistry and use as a drug-delivery system. *Chem. Eur. J.* **2012**, *18*, 14708–14716. [CrossRef] [PubMed]
26. Chen, Y.-W.; Chen, P.-J.; Hu, S.-H.; Chen, I.W.; Chen, S.-Y. NIR-triggered synergic photo-chemothermal therapy delivered by reduced graphene oxide/carbon/mesoporous silica nanocookies. *Adv. Funct. Mater.* **2014**, *24*, 451–459. [CrossRef]
27. Ghosh, P.; Han, G.; De, M.; Kim, C.K.; Rotello, V.M. Gold nanoparticles in delivery applications. *Adv. Drug Deliv. Rev.* **2008**, *60*, 1307–1315. [CrossRef] [PubMed]
28. Brown, S.D.; Nativo, P.; Smith, J.-A.; Stirling, D.; Edwards, P.R.; Venugopal, B.; Flint, D.J.; Plumb, J.A.; Graham, D.; Wheate, N.J. Gold nanoparticles for the improved anticancer drug delivery of the active component of oxaliplatin. *J. Am. Chem. Soc.* **2010**, *132*, 4678–4684. [CrossRef] [PubMed]
29. Torchilin, V.P. Multifunctional, stimuli-sensitive nanoparticulate systems for drug delivery. *Nat. Rev. Drug Discov.* **2014**, *13*, 813–827. [CrossRef] [PubMed]
30. Veiseh, O.; Gunn, J.W.; Zhang, M. Design and fabrication of magnetic nanoparticles for targeted drug delivery and imaging. *Adv. Drug Deliv. Rev.* **2010**, *62*, 284–304. [CrossRef] [PubMed]
31. Sun, C.; Lee, J.S.H.; Zhang, M. Magnetic nanoparticles in MR imaging and drug delivery. *Adv. Drug Deliv. Rev.* **2008**, *60*, 1252–1265. [CrossRef] [PubMed]
32. Kazemi, S.; Sarabi, A.A.; Abdouss, M. Synthesis and characterization of magnetic molecularly imprinted polymer nanoparticles for controlled release of letrozole. *Korean J. Chem. Eng.* **2016**, *33*, 3289–3297. [CrossRef]
33. Zhao, N.; Wu, B.; Hu, X.; Xing, D. NIR-triggered high-efficient photodynamic and chemo-cascade therapy using caspase-3 responsive functionalized upconversion nanoparticles. *Biomaterials* **2017**, *141*, 40–49. [CrossRef] [PubMed]
34. Liu, J.-N.; Bu, W.; Pan, L.-M.; Zhang, S.; Chen, F.; Zhou, L.; Zhao, K.-L.; Peng, W.; Shi, J. Simultaneous nuclear imaging and intranuclear drug delivery by nuclear-targeted multifunctional upconversion nanoprobes. *Biomaterials* **2012**, *33*, 7282–7290. [CrossRef] [PubMed]
35. Liu, G.; Liu, N.; Zhou, L.; Su, Y.; Dong, C.-M. NIR-responsive polypeptide copolymer upconversion composite nanoparticles for triggered drug release and enhanced cytotoxicity. *Polym. Chem.* **2015**, *6*, 4030–4039. [CrossRef]
36. Yang, Y.; Velmurugan, B.; Liu, X.; Xing, B. NIR photoresponsive crosslinked upconverting nanocarriers toward selective intracellular drug release. *Small* **2013**, *9*, 2937–2944. [CrossRef] [PubMed]

37. Yang, Y.; Liu, F.; Liu, X.; Xing, B. NIR light controlled photorelease of siRNA and its targeted intracellular delivery based on upconversion nanoparticles. *Nanoscale* **2013**, *5*, 231–238. [CrossRef] [PubMed]
38. Lee, S.; Lin, M.; Lee, A.; Park, Y. Lanthanide-doped nanoparticles for diagnostic sensing. *Nanomaterials* **2017**, *7*, 411. [CrossRef] [PubMed]
39. Weissleder, R. A clearer vision for in vivo imaging. *Nat. Biotechnol.* **2001**, *19*, 316–317. [CrossRef] [PubMed]
40. Li, C.; Liu, J.; Alonso, S.; Li, F.; Zhang, Y. Upconversion nanoparticles for sensitive and in-depth detection of Cu^{2+} ions. *Nanoscale* **2012**, *4*, 6065–6071. [CrossRef] [PubMed]
41. Shi, J.; Wang, L.; Zhang, J.; Ma, R.; Gao, J.; Liu, Y.; Zhang, C.; Zhang, Z. A tumor-targeting near-infrared laser-triggered drug delivery system based on GO@Ag nanoparticles for chemo-photothermal therapy and X-ray imaging. *Biomaterials* **2014**, *35*, 5847–5861. [CrossRef] [PubMed]
42. Auzel, F. Upconversion and anti-Stokes processes with f and d ions in solids. *Chem. Rev.* **2004**, *104*, 139–174. [CrossRef] [PubMed]
43. Li, H.; Hao, S.; Yang, C.; Chen, G. Synthesis of multicolor core/shell $NaLuF_4:Yb^{3+}/Ln^{3+}@CaF_2$ Upconversion nanocrystals. *Nanomaterials* **2017**, *7*, 34. [CrossRef] [PubMed]
44. Bestvater, F.; Spiess, E.; Stobrawa, G.; Hacker, M.; Feurer, T.; Porwol, T.; Berchner-Pfannschmidt, U.; Wotzlaw, C.; Acker, H. Two-photon fluorescence absorption and emission spectra of dyes relevant for cell imaging. *J. Microsc.* **2002**, *208*, 108–115. [CrossRef] [PubMed]
45. Ahn, H.-Y.; Yao, S.; Wang, X.; Belfield, K.D. Near-infrared-emitting squaraine dyes with high 2PA cross-sections for multiphoton fluorescence imaging. *ACS Appl. Mater. Interfaces* **2012**, *4*, 2847–2854. [CrossRef] [PubMed]
46. Li, C.; Quan, Z.; Yang, J.; Yang, P.; Lin, J. Highly uniform and monodisperse β-$NaYF_4:Ln^{3+}$ (Ln = Eu, Tb, Yb/Er, and Yb/Tm) hexagonal microprism crystals: Hydrothermal synthesis and luminescent properties. *Inorg. Chem.* **2007**, *46*, 6329–6337. [CrossRef] [PubMed]
47. Haase, M.; Schäfer, H. Upconverting nanoparticles. *Angew. Chem. Int. Ed.* **2011**, *50*, 5808–5829. [CrossRef] [PubMed]
48. Tian, G.; Yin, W.; Jin, J.; Zhang, X.; Xing, G.; Li, S.; Gu, Z.; Zhao, Y. Engineered design of theranostic upconversion nanoparticles for tri-modal upconversion luminescence/magnetic resonance/X-ray computed tomography imaging and targeted delivery of combined anticancer drugs. *J. Mater. Chem. B* **2014**, *2*, 1379–1389. [CrossRef]
49. He, L.; Feng, L.; Cheng, L.; Liu, Y.; Li, Z.; Peng, R.; Li, Y.; Guo, L.; Liu, Z. Multilayer dual-polymer-coated upconversion nanoparticles for multimodal imaging and serum-enhanced gene delivery. *ACS Appl. Mater. Interfaces* **2013**, *5*, 10381–10388. [CrossRef] [PubMed]
50. Jo, H.L.; Song, Y.H.; Park, J.; Jo, E.-J.; Goh, Y.; Shin, K.; Kim, M.-G.; Lee, K.T. Fast and background-free three-dimensional (3D) live-cell imaging with lanthanide-doped upconverting nanoparticles. *Nanoscale* **2015**, *7*, 19397–19402. [CrossRef] [PubMed]
51. Wilhelm, S.; Hirsch, T.; Patterson, W.M.; Scheucher, E.; Mayr, T.; Wolfbeis, O.S. Multicolor upconversion nanoparticles for protein conjugation. *Theranostics* **2013**, *3*, 239–248. [CrossRef] [PubMed]
52. Boyer, J.-C.; van Veggel, F.C.J.M. Absolute quantum yield measurements of colloidal $NaYF_4:Er^{3+},Yb^{3+}$ upconverting nanoparticles. *Nanoscale* **2010**, *2*, 1417–1419. [CrossRef] [PubMed]
53. Wisser, M.D.; Fischer, S.; Maurer, P.C.; Bronstein, N.D.; Chu, S.; Alivisatos, A.P.; Salleo, A.; Dionne, J.A. Enhancing quantum yield via local symmetry distortion in lanthanide-based upconverting nanoparticles. *ACS Photonics* **2016**, *3*, 1523–1530. [CrossRef]
54. Liu, H.; Xu, C.T.; Lindgren, D.; Xie, H.; Thomas, D.; Gundlach, C.; Andersson-Engels, S. Balancing power density based quantum yield characterization of upconverting nanoparticles for arbitrary excitation intensities. *Nanoscale* **2013**, *5*, 4770–4775. [CrossRef] [PubMed]
55. Chen, W.; Chen, M.; Zang, Q.; Wang, L.; Tang, F.; Han, Y.; Yang, C.; Deng, L.; Liu, Y.-N. NIR light controlled release of caged hydrogen sulfide based on upconversion nanoparticles. *Chem. Commun.* **2015**, *51*, 9193–9196. [CrossRef] [PubMed]
56. Dong, Y.; Jin, G.; Ji, C.; He, R.; Lin, M.; Zhao, X.; Li, A.; Lu, T.J.; Xu, F. Non-invasive tracking of hydrogel degradation using upconversion nanoparticles. *Acta Biomater.* **2017**, *55*, 410–419. [CrossRef] [PubMed]

57. Chen, G.; Shen, J.; Ohulchanskyy, T.Y.; Patel, N.J.; Kutikov, A.; Li, Z.; Song, J.; Pandey, R.K.; Ågren, H.; Prasad, P.N.; et al. (α-NaYbF$_4$:Tm^{3+})/CaF$_2$ core/shell nanoparticles with efficient near-infrared to near-infrared upconversion for high-contrast deep tissue bioimaging. *ACS Nano* **2012**, *6*, 8280–8287. [CrossRef] [PubMed]
58. Michael Dcona, M.; Yu, Q.; Capobianco, J.A.; Hartman, M.C.T. Near infrared light mediated release of doxorubicin using upconversion nanoparticles. *Chem. Commun.* **2015**, *51*, 8477–8479. [CrossRef] [PubMed]
59. Chien, Y.-H.; Chou, Y.-L.; Wang, S.-W.; Hung, S.-T.; Liau, M.-C.; Chao, Y.-J.; Su, C.-H.; Yeh, C.-S. Near-infrared light photocontrolled targeting, bioimaging, and chemotherapy with caged upconversion nanoparticles in vitro and in vivo. *ACS Nano* **2013**, *7*, 8516–8528. [CrossRef] [PubMed]
60. Li, J.; Lee, W.Y.-W.; Wu, T.; Xu, J.; Zhang, K.; Hong Wong, D.S.; Li, R.; Li, G.; Bian, L. Near-infrared light-triggered release of small molecules for controlled differentiation and long-term tracking of stem cells in vivo using upconversion nanoparticles. *Biomaterials* **2016**, *110*, 1–10. [CrossRef] [PubMed]
61. Zhao, H.; Hu, W.; Ma, H.; Jiang, R.; Tang, Y.; Ji, Y.; Lu, X.; Hou, B.; Deng, W.; Huang, W.; et al. Photo-induced charge-variable conjugated polyelectrolyte brushes encapsulating upconversion nanoparticles for promoted siRNA release and collaborative photodynamic therapy under NIR light irradiation. *Adv. Funct. Mater.* **2017**, *27*, 1702592. [CrossRef]
62. Liu, C.; Zhang, Y.; Liu, M.; Chen, Z.; Lin, Y.; Li, W.; Cao, F.; Liu, Z.; Ren, J.; Qu, X. A NIR-controlled cage mimicking system for hydrophobic drug mediated cancer therapy. *Biomaterials* **2017**, *139*, 151–162. [CrossRef] [PubMed]
63. Yan, B.; Boyer, J.-C.; Branda, N.R.; Zhao, Y. Near-infrared light-triggered dissociation of block copolymer micelles using upconverting nanoparticles. *J. Am. Chem. Soc.* **2011**, *133*, 19714–19717. [CrossRef] [PubMed]
64. Wong, P.T.; Tang, S.; Cannon, J.; Chen, D.; Sun, R.; Lee, J.; Phan, J.; Tao, K.; Sun, K.; Chen, B.; et al. Photocontrolled release of doxorubicin conjugated through a thioacetal photocage in folate-targeted nanodelivery systems. *Bioconjug. Chem.* **2017**, *28*, 3016–3028. [CrossRef] [PubMed]
65. Zhang, L.; Lu, Z.; Bai, Y.; Wang, T.; Wang, Z.; Chen, J.; Ding, Y.; Yang, F.; Xiao, Z.; Ju, S.; et al. PEGylated denatured bovine serum albumin modified water-soluble inorganic nanocrystals as multifunctional drug delivery platforms. *J. Mater. Chem. B* **2013**, *1*, 1289–1295. [CrossRef]
66. Bertrand, O.; Gohy, J.-F. Photo-responsive polymers: Synthesis and applications. *Polym. Chem.* **2017**, *8*, 52–73. [CrossRef]
67. Jiang, J.; Tong, X.; Morris, D.; Zhao, Y. Toward photocontrolled release using light-dissociable block copolymer micelles. *Macromolecules* **2006**, *39*, 4633–4640. [CrossRef]
68. Aujard, I.; Benbrahim, C.; Gouget, M.; Ruel, O.; Baudin, J.-B.; Neveu, P.; Jullien, L. o-Nitrobenzyl photolabile protecting groups with red-shifted absorption: Syntheses and uncaging cross-sections for one- and two-photon excitation. *Chem. Eur. J.* **2006**, *12*, 6865–6879. [CrossRef] [PubMed]
69. Gargas, D.J.; Chan, E.M.; Ostrowski, A.D.; Aloni, S.; Altoe, M.V.P.; Barnard, E.S.; Sanii, B.; Urban, J.J.; Milliron, D.J.; Cohen, B.E.; et al. Engineering bright sub-10-nm upconverting nanocrystals for single-molecule imaging. *Nat. Nanotechnol.* **2014**, *9*, 300–305. [CrossRef] [PubMed]
70. He, S.; Krippes, K.; Ritz, S.; Chen, Z.; Best, A.; Butt, H.-J.; Mailander, V.; Wu, S. Ultralow-intensity near-infrared light induces drug delivery by upconverting nanoparticles. *Chem. Commun.* **2015**, *51*, 431–434. [CrossRef] [PubMed]
71. San Miguel, V.; Álvarez, M.; Filevich, O.; Etchenique, R.; del Campo, A. Multiphoton reactive surfaces using ruthenium(II) photocleavable cages. *Langmuir* **2012**, *28*, 1217–1221. [CrossRef] [PubMed]
72. Meng, Z.; Luan, L.; Kang, Z.; Feng, S.; Meng, Q.; Liu, K. Histidine-enriched multifunctional peptide vectors with enhanced cellular uptake and endosomal escape for gene delivery. *J. Mater. Chem. B* **2017**, *5*, 74–84. [CrossRef]
73. Park, J.S.; Park, W.; Park, S.-J.; Larson, A.C.; Kim, D.-H.; Park, K.-H. Multimodal Magnetic Nanoclusters for Gene Delivery, Directed Migration, and Tracking of Stem Cells. *Adv. Funct. Mater.* **2017**, *27*, 1700396. [CrossRef]
74. Tiberio, G.; Muccioli, L.; Berardi, R.; Zannoni, C. How does the *trans-cis* photoisomerization of azobenzene take place in organic solvents? *ChemPhysChem* **2010**, *11*, 1018–1028. [CrossRef] [PubMed]
75. Sierocki, P.; Maas, H.; Dragut, P.; Richardt, G.; Vögtle, F.; De Cola, L.; Brouwer, F.; Zink, J.I. Photoisomerization of azobenzene derivatives in nanostructured silica. *J. Phys. Chem. B* **2006**, *110*, 24390–24398. [CrossRef] [PubMed]

76. Ikeda, T.; Tsutsumi, O. Optical switching and image storage by means of azobenzene liquid-crystal films. *Science* **1995**, *268*, 1873–1875. [CrossRef] [PubMed]
77. Bandara, H.M.D.; Burdette, S.C. Photoisomerization in different classes of azobenzene. *Chem. Soc. Rev.* **2012**, *41*, 1809–1825. [CrossRef] [PubMed]
78. Huang, Y.; Dong, R.; Zhu, X.; Yan, D. Photo-responsive polymeric micelles. *Soft Matter* **2014**, *10*, 6121–6138. [CrossRef] [PubMed]
79. Yao, C.; Wang, P.; Li, X.; Hu, X.; Hou, J.; Wang, L.; Zhang, F. Near-infrared-triggered azobenzene-liposome/upconversion nanoparticle hybrid vesicles for remotely controlled drug delivery to overcome cancer multidrug resistance. *Adv. Mater.* **2016**, *28*, 9341–9348. [CrossRef] [PubMed]
80. Liu, J.; Bu, W.; Pan, L.; Shi, J. NIR-triggered anticancer drug delivery by upconverting nanoparticles with integrated azobenzene-modified mesoporous silica. *Angew. Chem. Int. Ed.* **2013**, *52*, 4375–4379. [CrossRef] [PubMed]
81. Chen, G.; Ma, B.; Xie, R.; Wang, Y.; Dou, K.; Gong, S. NIR-induced spatiotemporally controlled gene silencing by upconversion nanoparticle-based siRNA nanocarrier. *J. Control. Release* **2018**, *282*, 148–155. [CrossRef] [PubMed]
82. Hao, W.; Liu, D.; Wang, Y.; Han, X.; Xu, S.; Liu, H. Dual-stimuli responsive nanoparticles (UCNP-CD@APP) assembled by host-guest interaction for drug delivery. *Colloids Surf. A* **2018**, *537*, 446–451. [CrossRef]
83. Cui, L.; Zhang, F.; Wang, Q.; Lin, H.; Yang, C.; Zhang, T.; Tong, R.; An, N.; Qu, F. NIR light responsive core-shell nanocontainers for drug delivery. *J. Mater. Chem. B* **2015**, *3*, 7046–7054. [CrossRef]
84. Yao, C.; Wang, P.; Zhou, L.; Wang, R.; Li, X.; Zhao, D.; Zhang, F. Highly biocompatible zwitterionic phospholipids coated upconversion nanoparticles for efficient bioimaging. *Anal. Chem.* **2014**, *86*, 9749–9757. [CrossRef] [PubMed]
85. Hu, Q.-D.; Tang, G.-P.; Chu, P.K. Cyclodextrin-based host-guest supramolecular nanoparticles for delivery: From design to applications. *Acc. Chem. Res.* **2014**, *47*, 2017–2025. [CrossRef] [PubMed]
86. Mei, X.; Yang, S.; Chen, D.; Li, N.; Li, H.; Xu, Q.; Ge, J.; Lu, J. Light-triggered reversible assemblies of azobenzene-containing amphiphilic copolymer with β-cyclodextrin-modified hollow mesoporous silica nanoparticles for controlled drug release. *Chem. Commun.* **2012**, *48*, 10010–10012. [CrossRef] [PubMed]
87. Tomatsu, I.; Hashidzume, A.; Harada, A. Contrast viscosity changes upon photoirradiation for mixtures of poly(acrylic acid)-based α-cyclodextrin and azobenzene polymers. *J. Am. Chem. Soc.* **2006**, *128*, 2226–2227. [CrossRef] [PubMed]
88. Yan, H.; Teh, C.; Sreejith, S.; Zhu, L.; Kwok, A.; Fang, W.; Ma, X.; Nguyen, K.T.; Korzh, V.; Zhao, Y. Functional mesoporous silica nanoparticles for photothermal-controlled drug delivery in vivo. *Angew. Chem. Int. Ed.* **2012**, *51*, 8373–8377. [CrossRef] [PubMed]
89. Moller, N.; Hellwig, T.; Stricker, L.; Engel, S.; Fallnich, C.; Ravoo, B.J. Near-infrared photoswitching of cyclodextrin-guest complexes using lanthanide-doped LiYF$_4$ upconversion nanoparticles. *Chem. Commun.* **2017**, *53*, 240–243. [CrossRef] [PubMed]
90. Xu, J.; Xu, L.; Wang, C.; Yang, R.; Zhuang, Q.; Han, X.; Dong, Z.; Zhu, W.; Peng, R.; Liu, Z. Near-Infrared-Triggered Photodynamic Therapy with Multitasking Upconversion Nanoparticles in Combination with Checkpoint Blockade for Immunotherapy of Colorectal Cancer. *ACS Nano* **2017**, *11*, 4463–4474. [CrossRef] [PubMed]
91. Chi, Y.; Wenxing, W.; Peiyuan, W.; Mengyao, Z.; Xiaomin, L.; Fan, Z. Near-Infrared Upconversion Mesoporous Cerium Oxide Hollow Biophotocatalyst for Concurrent pH-/H$_2$O$_2$-Responsive O$_2$-Evolving Synergetic Cancer Therapy. *Adv. Mater.* **2018**, *30*, 1704833. [CrossRef]
92. Han, Y.; An, Y.; Jia, G.; Wang, X.; He, C.; Ding, Y.; Tang, Q. Theranostic micelles based on upconversion nanoparticles for dual-modality imaging and photodynamic therapy in hepatocellular carcinoma. *Nanoscale* **2018**, *10*, 6511–6523. [CrossRef] [PubMed]
93. Gulzar, A.; Xu, J.; Xu, L.; Yang, P.; He, F.; Yang, D.; An, G.; Ansari, M.B. Redox-responsive UCNPs-DPA conjugated NGO-PEG-BPEI-DOX for imaging-guided PTT and chemotherapy for cancer treatment. *Dalton Trans.* **2018**, *47*, 3921–3930. [CrossRef] [PubMed]

94. Bazylińska, U.; Wawrzyńczyk, D. Encapsulation of TOPO stabilized NaYF$_4$:Er^{3+},Yb^{3+} nanoparticles in biocompatible nanocarriers: Synthesis, optical properties and colloidal stability. *Colloids Surf. A* **2017**, *532*, 556–563. [CrossRef]
95. Bazylińska, U.; Wawrzyńczyk, D.; Kulbacka, J.; Frąckowiak, R.; Cichy, B.; Bednarkiewicz, A.; Samoć, M.; Wilk, K.A. Polymeric nanocapsules with up-converting nanocrystals cargo make ideal fluorescent bioprobes. *Sci. Rep.* **2016**, *6*, 29746. [CrossRef] [PubMed]

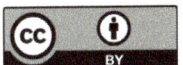

© 2018 by the authors. Licensee MDPI, Basel, Switzerland. This article is an open access article distributed under the terms and conditions of the Creative Commons Attribution (CC BY) license (http://creativecommons.org/licenses/by/4.0/).

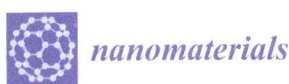

Article

Knockdown of microRNA-135b in Mammary Carcinoma by Targeted Nanodiamonds: Potentials and Pitfalls of In Vivo Applications

Romana Křivohlavá, Eva Neuhöferová, Katrine Q. Jakobsen and Veronika Benson *

Institute of Microbiology of the CAS, v.v.i., Videnska 1083, 142 20 Prague 4, Czech Republic; romule@volny.cz (R.K.); neuhoferova.eva@gmail.com (E.N.); katrineq@outlook.dk (K.Q.J.)
* Correspondence: benson@biomed.cas.cz; Tel.: +420-296-442-395

Received: 24 May 2019; Accepted: 4 June 2019; Published: 7 June 2019

Abstract: Nanodiamonds (ND) serve as RNA carriers with potential for in vivo application. ND coatings and their administration strategy significantly change their fate, toxicity, and effectivity within a multicellular system. Our goal was to develop multiple ND coating for effective RNA delivery in vivo. Our final complex (NDA135b) consisted of ND, polymer, antisense RNA, and transferrin. We aimed (i) to assess if a tumor-specific coating promotes NDA135b tumor accumulation and effective inhibition of oncogenic microRNA-135b and (ii) to outline off-targets and immune cell interactions. First, we tested NDA135b toxicity and effectivity in tumorspheres co-cultured with immune cells ex vivo. We found NDA135b to target tumor cells, but it binds also to granulocytes. Then, we followed with NDA135b intravenous and intratumoral applications in tumor-bearing animals in vivo. Application of NDA135b in vivo led to the effective knockdown of microRNA-135b in tumor tissue regardless administration. Only intravenous application resulted in NDA135b circulation in peripheral blood and urine and the decreased granularity of splenocytes. Our data show that localized intratumoral application of NDA135b represents a suitable and safe approach for in vivo application of nanodiamond-based constructs. Systemic intravenous application led to an interaction of NDA135b with bio-interface, and needs further examination regarding its safety.

Keywords: nanodiamond; targeted nanoparticles; in vivo application; cancer cell targeting; antimiR; nano-bio interaction

1. Introduction

Breast cancer is one of the most frequent women cancers worldwide and results in 13% of total cancer deaths [1]. New strategies for treatment or adjuvant therapies are needed in order to decrease its mortality. In breast cancer as well as other cancers, deregulation of microRNAs enables tumor development and promotes its progression [2–5]. In order to restore microRNA homeostasis resulting in impairment of tumor growth and its sensitization to conventional therapy, synthetic RNA is introduced into cancer cells using suitable carriers [6–9]. Such synthetic RNA can be designed to target microRNA overexpressed in tumor cells. This so-called antimiR recognizes sequence of specific microRNA and promotes its degradation.

Nanodiamonds (ND) represent rather promising material for such biomedical application [10–13]. Their capability to serve as an effective RNA carrier strongly depends on size, shape, preparation method, and on coating of the ND [10,11,13–17]. Especially suitable are the high-pressure and high-temperature (HPHT) ND possessing great biocompatibility [18]. An important feature of these ND is the presence of fluorescent centers (nitrogen-vacancy, N-V) giving them the advantage of traceability [12,14,19].

Even though the HPHT ND have been successfully used in vitro [11,13], there are only a few studies regarding their effectivity in vivo. The existing in vivo studies evaluate organ accumulation and toxicity of naked ND in *Caenorhabditis elegans* [20,21] and mice [22,23]. There is also one study reporting on red blood cells toxicity in human and rats [24]. The in vivo studies agreed the HPHT nanodiamonds were non-toxic and non-harmful even though the nanodiamonds accumulated in lungs, liver, or spleen. The potential accumulation site depends on ND size, coat, and way of administration. While targeting specific tissue such as tumor, we require negligible off-target accumulation. Here, multiple coatings preserving biocompatibility of the ND carrier but driving its cell-specific internalization is needed. Finally, yet importantly, to evaluate the suitability of the ND carriers for topical or even systemic applications, we need more specific applications in vivo showing the different effects of the particular ND-based carrier.

In this work, we focus on HPHT ND with multiple coatings consisting of tumor antigen (transferrin), polymer link (polyethylenimine 800, PEI), and sequence-specific antimiR. All of the four components possess specific function and contribute to the nanocarrier's (NDA135b) final behavior and effectivity. Our goal was to evaluate if surface coating with tumor specific antigen enables the nanodiamond-based carrier to reach the tumor in a sufficient amount to knockdown particular microRNA and to draft our first idea regarding off-targets and immune cell interactions.

We chose the model of murine breast cancer and we aimed to target oncogenic microRNA-135b that is overexpressed in the cancer cells contributing to the tumor progression and metastasis [25]. First, we successfully applied the NDA135b on cancer cells monocultures in vitro. We assumed then that in vivo, the NDA135b would encounter not only cancer cells, but also immune and endothelial cells. Therefore, we have tested and proved the effectivity of the NDA135b in a mixed co-culture of 3D mammospheres with peritoneal cavity cells, an intermediate model between in vitro and in vivo systems. Importantly, here we found, for the first time, the targeted NDA135b interact with primary granulocytes. We followed with in vivo applications of the NDA135b in a xenograft model of murine cancer and we tested the systemic effects of different ND administrations. The application directly into tumor site as well as systemic intravenous application both led to efficient knockdown of microRNA-135b in tumor tissue. Although, only the intratumoral application resulted in high accumulation of NDA135b in tumors and the NDA135b did not escape into blood. On the other hand, NDA135b applied intravenously were detectable in peripheral circulation and urine. It eventually entered the tumor in a sufficient amount to eliminate microRNA-135b but it also affected the granularity of splenocytes. We believe the intratumoral application of NDA135b represented a more suitable and safer approach for in vivo application of nanodiamond-based constructs.

2. Materials and Methods

2.1. Materials

2.1.1. Nanodiamond Complex (NDA135b) Preparation

Oxidized fluorescent nanodiamond particles (ND) were obtained from Dr. Petrakova (Faculty of Biomedical Engineering, Czech Technical University, Kladno, Czech Republic) and their preparation has been described in detail by Petrakova et al. [26]. Briefly, the nanodiamond powder (Microdiamant, Lengwil, Switzerland) was purified in a mixture of HNO_3 and H_2SO_4, washed with NaOH, HCl, and water, and freeze-dried. Purified nanodiamonds were irradiated using a 15.5 MeV proton beam, annealed at 900 °C, and air oxidized at 510 °C. Subsequently, the ND were re-purified with HNO_3 and H_2SO_4, dissolved in water (2 mg/mL), and sonicated with a probe (750 W, 30 min). Obtained suspension was filtered via polyvinylidene difluoride (PVDF) membrane with 0.2 μm pores [12]. The obtained ND possessed negative zeta-potential [13]. Before any functionalization, the nanodiamonds were sonicated in the ultrasonic bath for 30 min. Subsequently, the ND solution (1 mg/mL in deionized water) was mixed with equal amounts of PEI 800 (Sigma-Aldrich, Prague, Czech Republic; 0.9 mg/mL) and stirred overnight at room temperature. To prepare a ND complex with targeting structure-transferrin (Tf), we mixed 1 mg of ND (1 mL of water solution) with 200 µg of transferrin conjugate (Alexa Fluor 488 or Texas Red; Life Technologies, Prague, Czech Republic), incubated the mixture in room temperature for 1 h, and subsequently mixed with PEI 800 as described above. Unbound PEI and Tf were removed by centrifugation (9000× g, 60 min) and repeated dispersion of the NDs fraction in sterile deionized water in ND concentration 1 mg/mL. (Tf)-PEI-coated ND (1 mg/mL) were kept in a sonication bath, and immediately incubated for 1 h at room temperature with 270 µg of RNA.

A135b, a single-stranded short RNA (antimiR), was designed using the miRBase database (www.mirbase.org) to specifically target and inhibit microRNA-135b. The antimiR sequence was synthesized and modified by IDT (5′ UptCptAptCAUAGGAAUGAAAAGCCptAptUptA 3′, Integrated DNA Technologies; Prague, Czech republic). All the ribonucleotides were modified with 2′ O-methyl, and there were six phosphorothioate bonds (pt). Scrambled control RNA (Sc) was used in non-functional complexes (NDSc) instead of A135b. The RNA probes were purified by high-performance liquid chromatography (HPLC). The complexes of ND and RNA were freshly prepared before each experiment and sonicated in a cooled water bath before their use.

2.1.2. NDA135b Complex Characterization

Nanodiamond carriers were characterized by size, surface charge, and load of individual components. We employed dynamic light scattering (DLS) to evaluate size of the complexes. Here, we measured z-average hydrodynamic diameter at a scattering angle of 173° in 25 °C and the overall polydispersity index PdI. Surface charge of the complex estimated as a zeta potential was measured in a clear disposable zeta cells at room temperature. For the measurements and data analyses of zeta potential and DLS, we used Zetasizer Nano ZS (Malvern Instruments, Milcom, Prague, Czech Republic) and Zetasizer Software 7.11 (Malvern Instruments, Milcom, Prague, Czech Republic).

The load of transferrin (Tf) linked to nanodiamond has been determined after the subtraction of unbound Tf from the initial concentration. We used Tf conjugated with Texas Red, and the unbound Tf-Texas Red fluorescence was detected in supernatant using excitation at 595 nm and emission at 615 nm. The concentration of Tf load has been determined from a standard curve of Tf conjugate. The load of PEI was determined by subtraction of unbound PEI from the initial PEI concentration. To detect unbound PEI, we incubated 200 µL of supernatant with 500 µL of 0.150 mg/mL $CuSO_4·5H_2O$ (Sigma Aldrich, Prague, Czech Republic) and measured the absorbance at 285 nm. The PEI concentration was calculated from a standard curve of PEI. The load of nucleic acid (NA) was established by subtraction of unbound NA from its initial concentration in reaction. To obtain the unbound NA in supernatant, we pelleted the final complexes 9000× g 30 min. NA concentration was measured with a Qubit microRNA assay according to manufacturer protocol (Life Technologies, Prague, Czech Republic). Samples and standards were diluted 1:20 with reaction buffer containing dye (dye dilution 1:1000) and fluorescence was measured using excitation 488 nm and emission 540 nm. Absorbance (PEI quantitation) and fluorescence (Tf and NA quantitation) were detected with an Infinite M200 Pro plate reader (Tecan, Schoeller Instruments, Prague, Czech Republic).

2.1.3. Cell Cultures and Transfection

The 4T1 mammary carcinoma cell line were kindly provided by Dr. Jaroslav Truksa, Institute of Biotechnology, Academy of Sciences, Czech Republic. The 4T1 cells were cultured in RPMI (Sigma Aldrich, Prague, Czech republic) containing 10% (v/v) fetal bovine serum (FBS, Gibco, Thermo Fisher Scientific, Prague, Czech Republic), 44 mg/L gentamicin (Sandoz, Novartis Company, Prague, Czech Republic), 4.5 g/L glucose, and 1.1% pyruvate (both from Sigma Aldrich) in 37 °C and a humid atmosphere consisting of 5% CO_2. Cells were passaged three times a week to maintain an exponential growth phase. To obtain 2D cultures, the cells were grown on plastic Petri dishes (TPP, BioTech, Prague, Czech Republic).

Unless stated otherwise, before experimentation, cells were cultured at density 0.5×10^5 cells per well with 1 mL of media (in a 6-well plate, total volume 2 mL) overnight and then stimulated with

NDs for 48 h. The final concentration of NDs was always 25 µg/mL corresponding to 6.8 µg/mL of A135b where applicable. The control group (NC) was treated only with PBS.

In the case of 3D spheroid, we cultured 10^3 4T1 cells in a 40 µL hanging drop [27] for 10 days and then matured mammospheres were carefully transported into 6-well plate with 2% agarose covered bottoms to underwent stimulations with ND.

Control transfections of A135b without NDs were carried out using X-tremeGENE HP DNA Transfection Reagent (A135bCR, commercial reagent) according to the manufacturer protocol (Roche, Prague, Czech Republic). The ratio of X-tremeGENE HP DNA and A135b was 3:1.

2.1.4. Ex-Vivo Primary Cells Culture and Their Tracking

Cells from peritoneal cavity were obtained by lavage of peritoneal cavity with saline from 12-weeks old Balb/c female mice. The cells were collected by centrifugation and resuspended in RPMI media supplemented with 5% of sera. For cell tracking, total 5×10^6 of peritoneal cells in 3 mL of media were incubated overnight with a 6 µL of CellTracker Violet (Life Technologies, Prague, Czech Republic) in 37 °C and humid atmosphere. In the end of incubation period, the cells were washed with PBS and further used in a co-culture with 4T1 spheroids. When we used a co-culture of peritoneal cells with 4T1 cells, we combined 5×10^6 of peritoneal cells and 2.5×10^6 of 4T1 cells. The co-culture was further maintained (or stimulated) like the 2D cell culture described above.

2.1.5. Quantitative Real-Time-PCR Analysis

The miRNA was purified according to manufacturer instructions using a high pure miRNA isolation kit (Roche, Prague, Czech Republic). After elution, 4 µL of miRNA fraction (total eluted volume 100 µL) were reverse transcribed using specific primers for miR-135b (assay MI0000810) or miR-16 (assay MI0000070) and a high-capacity cDNA Archive Kit (all from Thermo Fisher Scientific, Prague, Czech Republic). PCR quantification was carried out with a TaqMan Universal PCR Master Mix and miR-specific PCR primers (Thermo Fisher Scientific, Prague, Czech Republic). MiR-16 was used as an internal control for miR quantitation. During qPCR, all samples were analyzed in triplicate using an iQ5 Real Time PCR Detection System (BioRad, Prague, Czech Republic). The obtained data were analyzed using iQ5 Optical System Software 2.1 (BioRad, Prague, Czech Republic). The expression of the miR-135b was normalized to the expression of miR-16 and fold change was calculated by the software (based on 2^{-ddct} method).

2.1.6. Lactate dehydrogenase (LDH) Assay

Lactate dehydrogenase released from damaged cells was used to evaluate direct cytotoxicity. The cells were seeded in 96-well plates (5×10^3 cells per well) in triplicates and stimulated the next day with ND complexes for 48 h. Culture media was supplemented with 1% FBS as suggested by manufacturer. A commercial lysis buffer was added to one triplicate of the control cells for the last 3 h of the experimental period (serving as an LDH assay positive control, PC). Negative control comprised from non-stimulated cells (NC).

The LDH assay was performed according to manufacturer instructions (LDH assay, Roche, Prague, Czech Republic). Briefly, when the experiment completed, a cell supernatant was collected and incubated with LDH dye for 10 min. Then, the absorbance was measured with an Infinite M200 Pro plate reader (Tecan, Schoeller Instruments, Prague, Czech Republic) using specific excitation at 490 nm and a reference excitation at 630 nm.

2.1.7. Flow Cytometry

The apoptosis of 4T1 cells was assessed using an Annexin V Dyomics/Hoechst33258 staining (Exbio Antibodies, Vestec, Czech Republic) and the assay was performed according to manufacturer's protocol. Cells positive for Annexin V and Hoechst33258 were detected by a BD LSR II flow cytometer

(BD Bioscience, Prague, Czech Republic). The settings were following: Annexin V 473/520 nm and Hoechst 405/461 nm.

The surface expression of transferrin receptor has been assessed with a transferrin (Tf) conjugated with Texas Red. One million cultured cells were incubated with 1 µL of transferrin-conjugate (1 µg/mL) for 30 min and co-stained with Hoechst 33258 for 15 min. Settings for Tf detection: Ex/Em 559/615 nm. The same settings were used to detect Texas Red in cells obtained from homogenized tissues in the end of in vivo experiments.

The percentage of positive cells for each fluorophore was analyzed by a FlowJo v9.9.4 software (BD Bioscience, Prague, Czech Republic).

2.1.8. Confocal Imaging

For confocal analysis, the 4T1 cells were plated onto 6-well glass bottom plates (10^5 cells/well) and incubated with functionalized ND for the assay-specific time points. At the end of the incubation period, cell nuclei were stained with Hoechst33342 (1 µg/mL; Invitrogen, Life Technologies, Prague, Czech Republic). In the case of spheroids, the mammospheres were transferred to a glass-bottom dish. The images were acquired with an Olympus FluoView FV1000 confocal microscope (Olympus, Prague, Czech Republic; objective 20×/NA 0.75; 40×/NA 0.95; and 60×/NA 1.35). The data were analyzed with Olympus FluoView 2.0 software (Olympus, Prague, Czech Republic). Excitation/emission parameters were as follows: Hoechst 405/461 nm; NDs 559/655–755 nm; Alexa Fluor 488 473/520 nm; Cell Tracker Violet 415/516 nm. Photo-bleaching (with a 405 nm laser) was used to distinguish a non-specific and the ND-specific signal. In order to imagine the sample depths (particularly spheroids) we performed z-stack imaging with steps of 5 µm.

2.1.9. Animal Model and In Vivo NDA135b Application

Animals' procedures followed the Czech law regarding animal protection and the Czech Academy of Sciences with number 82/2015 approved the experimental plan. To develop breast tumor, we inoculated 10^6 4T1 cells (in saline) into fads pads of six-week-old female Balb/c mice (day 1). Mice were kept under standardized conditions and the tumor development was observed carefully. We started treatment with NDA135b on day 14 when a palpable tumor with a diameter of about 0.5 cm developed. The animals were divided into several groups (3 animals per group): One control group, two groups with NDA135b administered via tail vein, and two groups with NDA135b administered directly into tumor tissue. The control group received saline intravenously. Animals administered with NDA135b received NDA135b with transferrin conjugated (i) with Alexa Fluor 488 or ii) Texas Red. The animals obtained 20 µg of ND carrying 5.4 µg of A135b per mouse for three consecutive days. One hour after the third dose, we took peripheral blood and urine from anesthetized animals, the animals were sacrificed, and different tissues were collected (liver, spleen, kidney, and tumor) for subsequent analyses of NDA135b presence (enabled by transferrin-fluorophore conjugates) and antimiR-135b effect. The in vivo experiments were repeated twice.

2.1.10. Spectrometer Measurements of NDA135b in Fluids

Blood or urine from experimental animals were diluted five times with saline and 100 µL of fluid was placed in the 96-Well optical-bottom plates (Nunc, Thermo Fisher Scientific, Brno, Czech Republic). Fluorescence of Texas Red was measured using 595/615 nm filters and Infinite M200 Pro plate reader. The amount of complexes in the experimental sample was calculated from standard curve of NDA135b samples with known concentration.

2.1.11. Whole Tissue Imaging

At the end of experimental period, the excised liver, spleen, lung, and tumor tissues were imaged with a fluorescent microscopy OV-100. The microscope setup enables to read transferrin-Alexa Fluor 488 (Tf-A; settings 473/520 nm). After visualization, the organs were homogenized, cells were separated via 70 μm filters, and used to detect transferrin–Texas Red by flow cytometry (settings described earlier).

2.1.12. Statistical Analysis

If not stated otherwise, the results are presented as means ± SD of three independent experiments. Statistically significant differences in the tested parameters were assessed using a two-tailed *t*-test with a confidence interval of 95% for paired comparison or ANOVA/post-hoc Tukey for group comparison (online tool available at http://astatsa.com/OneWay_Anova_with_TukeyHSD/). Values of $p \leq 0.05$ (*) and $p \leq 0.01$ (**) were considered to be statistically significant between the compared groups.

3. Results

In order to properly evaluate the application possibilities of NDA135b complex, we have employed different experimental systems starting with the simplest monoculture of adherent cells derived from mouse mammary tumor. Subsequently, we performed tests in advanced model such as mixed 3D co-culture imitating tumor microenvironment. Finally, we tested NDA135b in vivo, employing local as well systemic administration. Schematic composition of NDA135b and models used in this study are depicted in Figure 1.

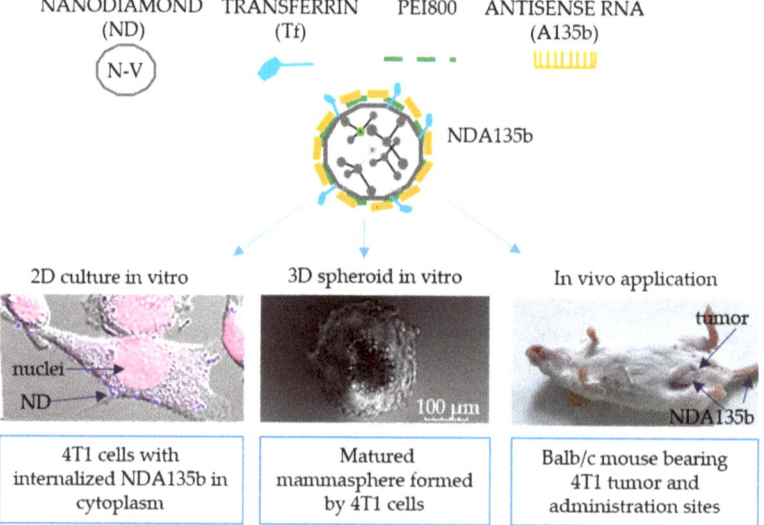

Figure 1. Composition of nanodiamond-based complex with multiple functionalization and its application onto a sequence of biological models from the easiest 2D cell culture via 3D differentiated mammospheres towards local and systemic in vivo administrations.

3.1. Characterization of the NDA135b Complex

In neutral pH, the complete NDA135b construct possessed zeta potential of −20 ± −3.42 mV, size of 353 ± 140 nm, and polydispersity index of PdI = 0.4. The PdI measured by DLS for a uniform sample equals zero and the value 0.4 represents moderate polydispersity due to transferrin–fluorophore conjugate. In comparison to the complex NDA135b, we tested plain ND and ND coated with NA but lacking Tf. The comparison is shown in Table 1.

Table 1. Basic characterization of NDA135b complex and its comparison to original nanodiamonds (ND) and similar complex ND-polyethylenimine (PEI)-RNA lacking targeting Tf-conjugate.

Sample	Zeta Potential (mV)	Average Size (nm)	PdI
NDA135b	-20 ± -3	353 ± 140	0.4
ND	-35 ± -7	73 ± 28	0.2
ND-PEI-RNA	-28 ± -4	120 ± 15	0.24

During the NDA135b preparation, we measured the amount of Transferrin, PEI, and A135b load. One milliliter of the NDA135b complex consisted of 1 mg of ND, 191 µg of transferrin conjugate, 740 µg of PEI800, and 270 µg of antimiR-135b RNA.

3.2. Effective Delivery of NDA135b into Adherent Breast Cancer Cells

Using conventional 2D culture of 4T1 mammary tumor cells enabled us to characterize the effect of antisense RNA (A135b) coated onto ND via PEI 800 without background of other cellular populations. This antisense RNA specifically targets oncogenic miR-135b overexpressed in many tumors including mammary tumor cells such as 4T1. Once A135b reaches target miR-135b in cytoplasm, it drives its degradation. Hypothetically, decreasing the level of miR-135b impairs the growth of cancer cells and eventually leads to cell death. We have used cells treated with saline and cells treated with complex NDA135b (consisting of ND, transferrin conjugated with Alexa488, PEI800, and A135b). Using confocal microscopy, we monitored internalization of the NDA135b into the vast majority of adherent 4T1 cells (Figure 2a). The complexes that were just internalized or are about to be internalized are shown in yellow (merging color from red stained ND and green stained Alexa Fluor 488) and the image has been focused on the level of cellular nuclei (in blue) to distinguish internalized complexes.

After stimulation with NDA135b, the 4T1 cells were cultured for additional two days and at the end of the incubation period, we measured amount of lactate dehydrogenase, an enzyme release from damaged cells due to increased plasma membrane permeability. Performing this assay, we added several controls such as positive control (PC) representing cells with damaged plasma membrane; cells incubated with uncoated nanodiamonds (ND), cells incubated with ND coated with scrambled control RNA instead of specific A135b (NDSc), and cells incubated with a commercial transfection reagent loaded with A135b (A135CR). We found significantly increased (p-value < 0.01) amount of lactate dehydrogenase only in cells stimulated with A135b without difference in carrier (Figure 2b).

Increased permeability of plasma membrane points towards direct toxicity but it can also occur in the very late phase of programmed cell death such as apoptosis, especially in cancer cells monoculture lacking cells phagocyting apoptotic bodies. We have further tested percentage of cells undergoing early phases of apoptosis and we found that A135b, independently on carrier, significantly increased (p-value < 0.01) the percentage of apoptotic cells (Figure 2c). However, we have also found a slightly increased rate of apoptosis in cells incubated with ND and NDSc (p-value < 0.05), suggesting that exposure of these cells to ND affects their viability up to some extent.

We observed internalization of NDA135b into cells with confocal microscopy. To prove not only delivery of A135b but also its release into cytoplasm, we performed detection of target miR-135b localized in cancer cell cytoplasm by qPCR. We observed a significant decrease (p value < 0.01) in cells incubated with A135b delivered within NDA135b or with a commercial reagent (Figure 2d). There was no decrease in miR-135b level in cells incubated with ND or NDSc, proving the specific targeting of miR-135b with antisense A135b.

Data are presented as the mean ± standard deviation; * p-value < 0.05 and ** p-value < 0.01 versus saline-treated group (NC) were calculated by ANOVA.

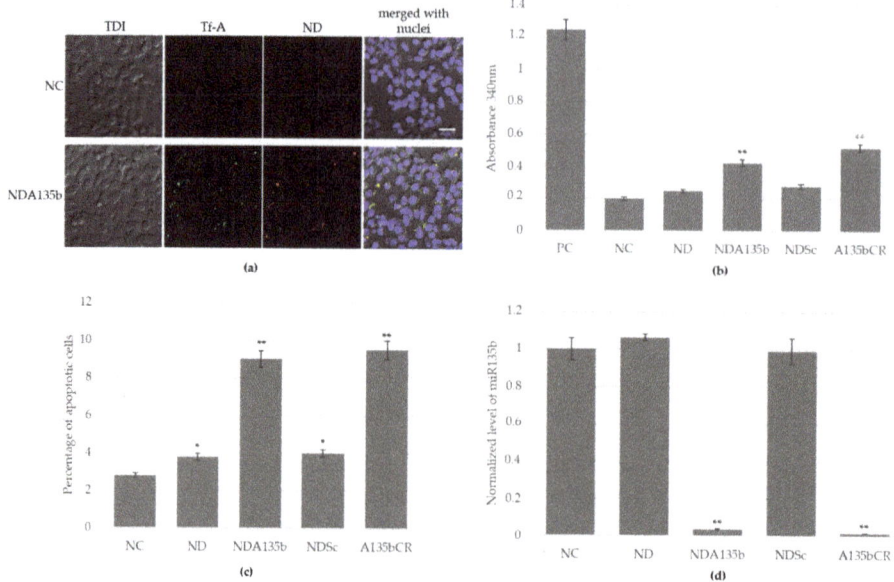

Figure 2. Internalization of functionalized nanodiamond carrier into 4T1 cells grown in 2D culture and the biological effect of antimiR-135b cargo: (**a**) Visualization of NDA135b, here decorated with transferrin conjugated to Alexa Fluor 488. Nuclei counterstained with Hoechst 33342 (blue). Fluorescence and transmission (TDI) visualized with a confocal microscopy Olympus FV1000, 40x. Scale bar is 20 µm; (**b**) release of lactate dehydrogenase indicating cell damage; (**c**) induction of apoptosis (early phase) measured with an AnnexinV assay; (**d**) detection of remaining miR-135b level in 4T1 cells after particular stimulation. Values of $p \leq 0.05$ (*) and $p \leq 0.01$ (**) were statistically significant.

3.3. Specific Internalization of NDA135b into Breast Cancer Cells Spheroids Co-Cultured with Peritoneal Lavage Cells

Adherent monocultures are great for obtaining basic characteristics of the material tested, however this setup lacks important features such as cell–cell communication and interaction and different special awareness found in in vivo conditions. To imitate the basic tumor microenvironment in vitro, we employed 3D mammospheres derived from 4T1 cells grown in conditions protecting them from the attachment to surface. The mammospheres were further co-cultured with cells obtained from peritoneal lavage of C57BL/6 mouse. The peritoneal lavage is rich in macrophages (in our samples, 45%–50% of leukocytes) that easily engulf nanoparticles and, thus, they are an important cell population to evaluate the cancer cell-targeting effectivity of transferrin adsorbed to NDA135b surface. In order to distinguish 4T1 cancer cells from peritoneal lavage cells (MF) when co-cultured, we loaded MF with cell tracking dye and it enabled us to visualize MF actively incorporating into 4T1 spheroids (Figure 3a).

To evaluate the effectivity of A135b delivered into our 3D tumor, we performed qPCR. We found that only samples incubated with A135b significantly decreased (p-value < 0.01) the level of cytoplasmic miR-135b (Figure 3b). In contrast to 4T1 cancer cells, the peritoneal lavage cells do not express miR-135b as shown in Figure A1.

4T1 cells or MF loaded with NDA135b can be also detected by flow cytometry due to transferrin conjugated with Texas Red. We used flow cytometry to quantify how many cancer cells and MF carried the NDA135b. The NDA135b was designed to carry transferrin as a targeting structure to facilitate the uptake of the particle by cancer cells expressing transferrin receptor and decrease the uptake by normal cells including phagocytes. We confirmed that in our system, most (98% ± 1.2) 4T1 cancer cells express transferrin receptor in contrast to 7% (6.6% ± 1.5) of cells present in peritoneal lavage (Figure 3c). When we checked the cells present in peritoneal lavage thoroughly, we found that 61% ± 0.5 of transferrin receptor positive cells belong to monocyte/macrophage fraction as shown in Figure 3d. Remaining populations expressed transferrin receptor from 5% to 12% of cells (8.9% ± 0.6 of erythrocytes, 12.1% ± 1.5 of lymphocytes, and 5.8% ± 0.5 of granulocytes).

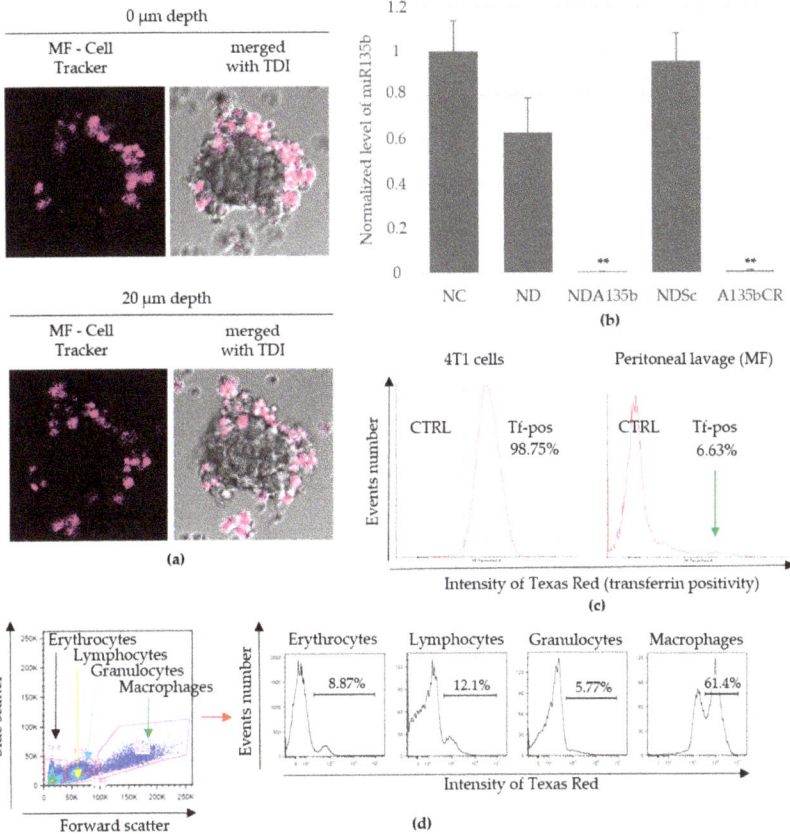

Figure 3. Targeting of 4T1 spheroids by functionalized nanodiamonds within a mixed 3D co-culture with peritoneal lavage cells imitating basic tumor microenvironment: (**a**) Determination of peritoneal lavage cells (MF, purple) integrating into matured mammosphere. Fluorescence and transmission (TDI) visualized with a confocal microscopy Olympus FV1000, 20×. Spheroid size is about 200 µm; (**b**) detection of remaining miR-135b level in mammospheres after particular stimulation. Data are presented as the mean ± standard deviation, ** p-value < 0.01 versus saline-treated group was obtained by ANOVA; (**c**) surface expression of transferrin receptor in 4T1 spheres (left) and peritoneal cells (right). CTRL stands for negative control of staining; (**d**) basic distribution of live cell sub-populations in peritoneal lavage and transferrin receptor positive cells detected within each sub-population.

In order to evaluate percentage of 4T1 cells and MF interacting with NDA135b within the tumor microenvironment, we incubated co-cultures with NDA135b and subsequently detected cells positive for transferrin. In parallel, we have incubated 4T1 spheroids and MF with ND135b separately to obtain controls of individual cell populations. While incubated alone, about 60% of 4T1 cells and about 37% of MF were positive for NDA135b (Figure 4a). The percentage of NDA135b-positive cells was calculated as positivity in both right quadrants. There is a distinct population within the MF sample (marked in right bottom quadrant) that represents about 6% of MF cells positive for NDA135b once the MF cells were incubated alone with NDA135b. This population represents live cells that carry NDA135b. We expected those cells to be macrophages present in MF population that engulfed NDA135b. Our presumption was based on the result mentioned in Figure 3d showing that in total, 4% of macrophages in our MF samples express transferrin receptor (calculated as 0.61*6.6%). To prove our hypothesis, we have gated the MF samples used for co-cultures for specific cell populations: Granulocytes, lymphocytes, and macrophages (Figure 4b). Subsequently, we tested each population for NDA135b positivity. Here, erythrocytes were not acquired due to optimal events distribution for further analyses of mixed 4T1 and MF cultures. We found that only about 30% (30% ± 1.5) of macrophages were positive for NDA135b. Surprisingly, we detected 65% of granulocytes (65% ± 3.2) and 14% (14% ± 1.7) of lymphocytes carrying NDA135b (Figure 4b).

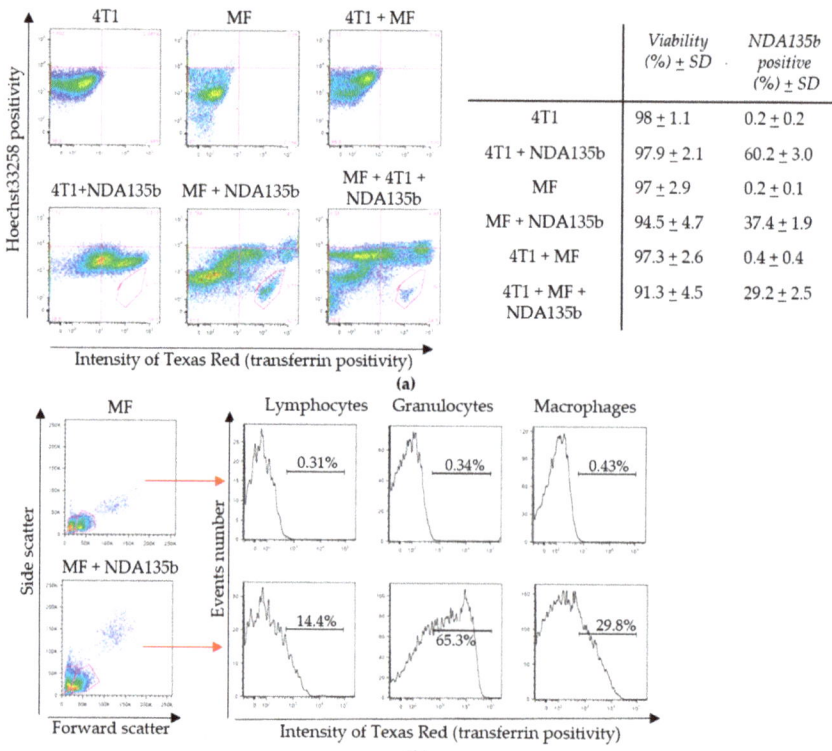

Figure 4. Targeting of 4T1 spheroids by functionalized nanodiamonds within a mixed 3D co-culture with peritoneal lavage cells (MF) imitating basic tumor microenvironment: (**a**) Uptake of targeted nanodiamond complex NDA135b by particular cells within a spheroid MF co-culture. The average percentage of positivity (and standard deviation) are listed on the right; (**b**) gating of live cells within the peritoneal lavage sample with or without stimulation by NDA135b (left) and detection of NDA135b in individual populations (right).

3.4. Local and Systemic In Vivo Application of Targeted NDA135b

Systemic administration of nanoparticles represents major challenge for most researchers. Even constructs exhibiting great effectivity in vitro might encounter difficulties such as lower stability in blood environment, decreased circulation time in blood and fast renal clearance, or unspecific internalization and accumulation in off-target tissue. All of that contributes to low effectivity of the constructs. Regarding nanodiamond particles with the average core size of 70 nm used in this study, we are aware of problematic nanoparticles clearance once administered into the blood system without good targeting and shielding structures. In this study, we employed two different types of NDA135b administration-intratumoral (i.t.) application directly into tumor mass and intravenous (i.v.) application via tail vein. Our first goal was to compare the effectivity of both approaches in order to reach the tumor cells cytoplasm and eliminate target miR-135b. We found that after three consecutive doses (1 day apart), we could detect NDA135b in tumors excised from experimental animals (Figure 5a). Here, detection of NDA135b in tumor samples was enabled by using transferrin–Alexa Fluor 488 conjugate adsorbed on the nanodiamond core. We compared tumors from animals administered with NDA135b containing Alexa Fluor 488-labeled transferrin with animals that received saline (control animals) as well as animals that received NDA135b containing transferrin without Alexa Fluor 488 label.

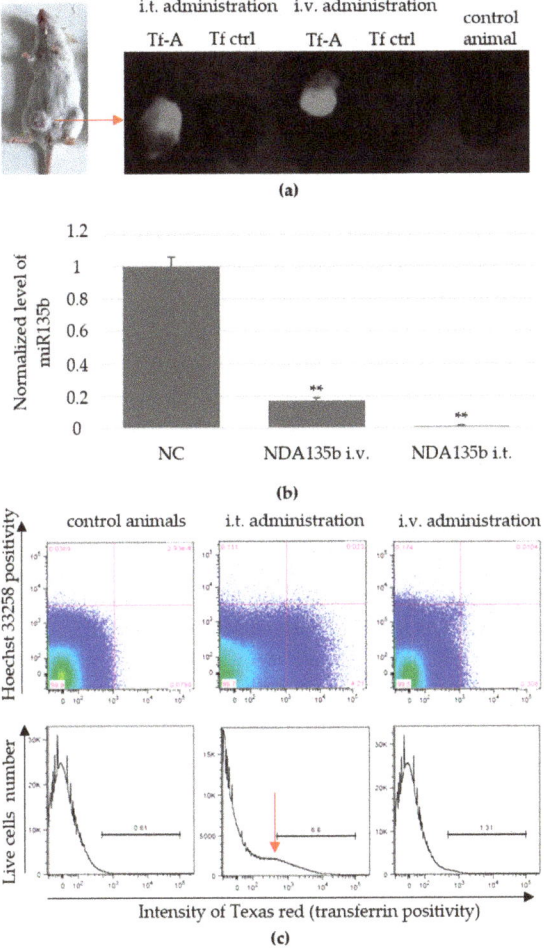

Figure 5. In vivo applications of NDA135b into breast tumor-bearing animals: (**a**) Detection of transferrin-Alexa Fluor 488 decorated NDA135b complexes (Tf-A) in tumor samples ex vivo. Tf ctrl stands for NDA135b decorated with Tf without the Alexa Fluor 488. Control animals received saline only; (**b**) detection of remaining miR-135b level in tumor after NDA135b administration. Data are presented as the mean ± standard deviation, ** p-value < 0.01 versus saline-treated group was obtained by ANOVA; (**c**) detection of NDA135b in cells obtained from excised tumors. Red arrow point to NDA135b-positive cells.

To test the presence of nanoparticles inside the tumor cells, we performed flow cytometry analysis and qPCR-based detection of target miR-135b in tumor cells after tumor homogenization. We found significantly decreased levels of miR-135b in both groups—administered intratumoral or intravenous (Figure 5b). In parallel, we performed flow cytometry analysis to evaluate the percentage of tumor cells carrying NDA135b. We found 6.54% ± 0.3 cells positive for NDA135b in samples administered intratumoral (significant, ** p-value < 0.01) as shown in Figure 5c (bottom). This positivity was rather weak in animals with intravenous administration of NDA135b (1.43 ± 0.1; ns p-value = 0.34). Here, we also did not experience a well-defined positive peak, but rather consistent slight changes in dot plot distributions (Figure 5c; top).

3.5. Accumulation of Non-Internalized NDA135b Complex in Key Tissues after In Vivo Applications

Since we found touches of NDA135b in tumors even after intravenous administration, we wondered if NDA135b circulating in peripheral blood interacted with blood elements or accumulated in tissues such as kidney, liver, or spleen. We also wondered if NDA135b administered intratumorally could escape from the tumor site and accumulate in other tissue due to its size.

In our system, transferrin also represented a targeting molecule with high affinity to 4T1 cells expressing a high amount of surface transferrin receptor (Figure 3c) and, thus, it shielded the complexes from extensive non-specific uptake. We have analyzed excised organs from the control group as well as groups administered with NDA135b by a whole-body imaging system. However, we found no signs of NDA135b presence in any of the excised tissues (Figure 6a). We also performed flow cytometry analyses of homogenized tissues and we did not detect any positive signal pointing out the presence of NDA135b in examined samples (Figure 6b). Distinguishable sub-populations such as leukocytes are marked in the liver, kidney, and spleen dot plots (yellow). We checked for any positive signal within these subpopulations and they displayed similar signal intensities like the whole tissues (Figure A2). Within spleen samples, we also checked the erythrocyte/debris population (black gate) and there was no positive signal either (Figure A3). Interestingly we found very different splenocytes granularity using side scatter parameter (Figure 6c). The granularity of splenocytes was apparently lower in animals after intravenous administration of NDA135b in contrast to control animals and animals administered with NDA135b intratumorally (Figure 6c).

The intravenous administration of NDA135b exhibited an effect on splenocytes. It would be ideal if we could prove the final effect of A135b by qPCR. However, the splenocytes, as they are not cancerous cells, do not express miR-135b (Figure A1) so we cannot use this approach. Assuming an indirect effect on splenocytes and no accumulation in spleen, liver, or kidney, we examined the presence of NDA135b in bodily fluids such as blood and urine. We also checked basic parameters of major cell populations within peripheral blood. We tested the presence of NDA135b using fluorescence spectrometer and flow cytometry. In both fluids, urine and peripheral blood, we found significantly positive (p-value < 0.01) signals in samples from animals administered with NDA135b intravenously—compared to control animals (Figure 7a). We did not detect any positivity in fluids obtained from animals administered intratumoral. We analyzed basic blood cells populations—erythrocytes, monocytes/granulocytes, and lymphocytes. Nevertheless, we did not observe any positive signal in any of the mentioned subpopulations (Figure 7b). That suggests that NDA135b was present in peripheral blood but it was not internalized by any blood cells.

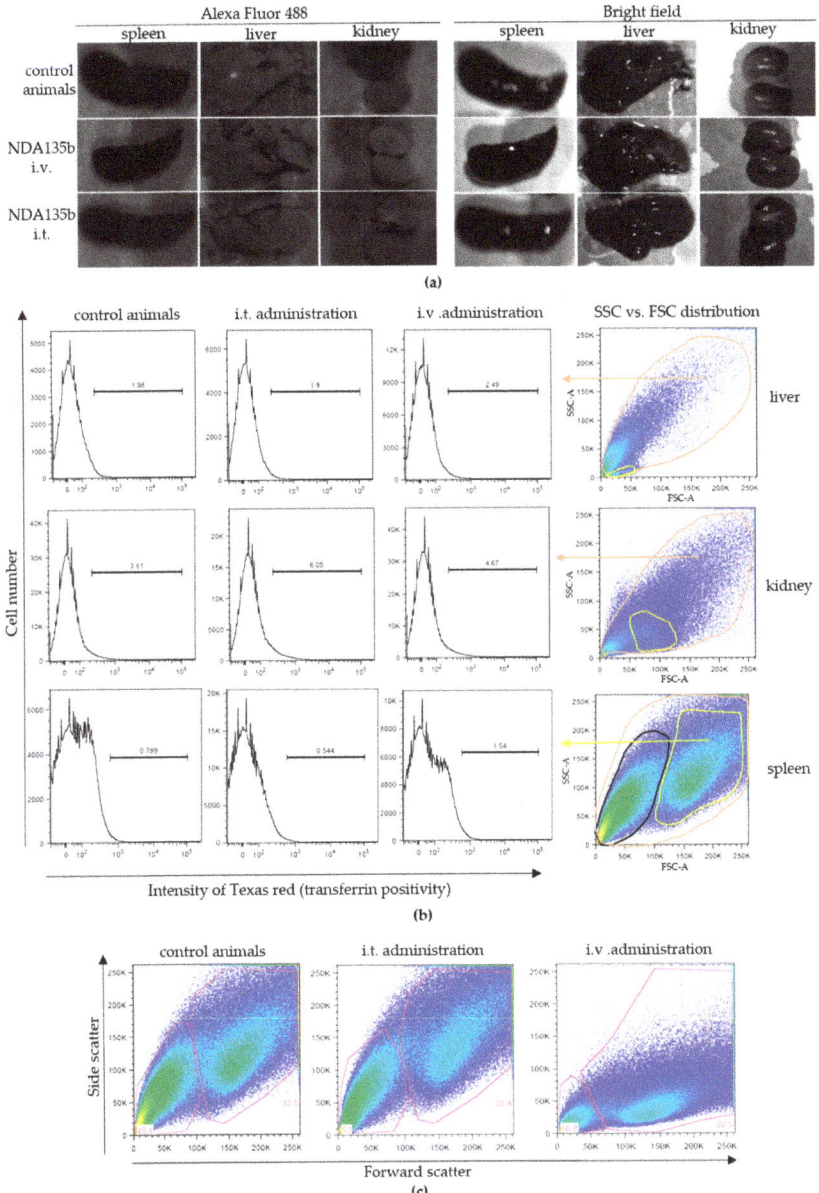

Figure 6. (a) Detection of transferrin conjugate in tissues excised from experimental animals administered with NDA135b intravenously or intratumoral: (**a**) Detection of NDA135b complexes in tissues ex vivo by microscopy. Control animals received saline only; (**b**) detection of NDA135b in excised tissues by flow cytometry. Representative dot plots and histograms are shown (exemplary gating is on the right). The histograms of liver and kidney samples consider signal from all cell-like events (orange gate). In spleen, histograms show signal in leukocytes (yellow gate in dot plots); (**c**) comparison of different splenocytes granularity after NDA135b intravenous and intratumoral applications.

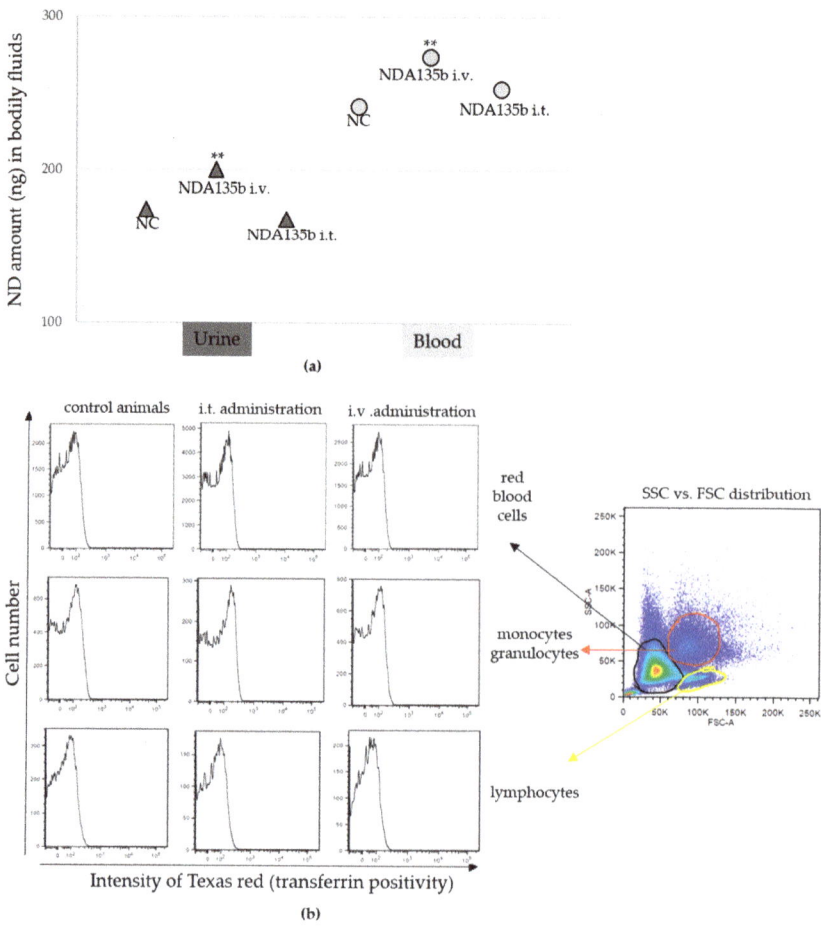

Figure 7. Detection of NDA135b decorated with transferrin-Texas red in bodily fluids obtained from tumor-bearing animals administered with ND-A135b intravenously or intratumoral: (**a**) Detection of transferrin–Texas red in acellular fraction of urine and blood. Data are presented as the mean ± standard deviation, ** p-value < 0.01 versus NC group was obtained by ANOVA; (**b**) detection of transferrin-Texas red in cellular fraction of peripheral blood. Representative dot plots and histograms are presented. The histograms show signal from different cell populations indicated in dot plot on the right side of the image (red blood cells, granulocytes/monocytes, and lymphocytes).

4. Discussion

In this report, we discuss, for the first time, the effectivity of HPHT nanodiamonds as carriers for short antisense RNAs when applied in 3D organoids as well as in vivo. Nanodiamonds prepared under HPHT possess great benefits like cyto-compatibility, cytoplasmic membrane penetration, easy surface decoration, or traceability, suggesting them for advanced biomedical use. Due to their size (in this report, an average of 70 nm), the HPHT nanodiamonds cannot be cleared from the system via renal filtration [28]. This may be a benefit since, if appropriately shielded, they can circulate in the blood stream for a longer time but on the other hand, they can accumulate in RES (reticuloendothelial system) organs. There is an abundance of particles without any specific structure that would facilitate their passage into target tissue for example tumor. Blood vessels of the majority of tumors exhibit enhanced permeability retention (EPR), supporting entrance of nanoparticles larger than 5 nm [29], so even particles without a targeting structure can reach the tumor tissue, but the efficacy is much lower [30].

Compatibility of nanomaterial with the bio-interface represents a key request every time the material is intended for any biomedical use. The compatibility evaluation primarily employs tests in vitro. So far, the only studies describing toxicity of nanodiamond particles employed detonation nanodiamonds with usual diameter 2–5 nm. Turcheniuk and Mochalin summarized that the possible cytotoxic effects reported in detonation nanodiamonds probably originated from usage of nanomaterial with a high degree of impurities [31]. Regarding HPHT nanodiamonds, all studies performed so far claimed no toxicity in vitro [32–35]. However, the surface modifications such as polyethylenimine (PEI) coating can affect the cyto-compatibility of the nanoparticle-polymer complex [36]. We support this finding as we have described it in our preceding study [13] too. The intermediate complexes consisting only of nanodiamond and PEI are not stable in colloids and tend to aggregate fast if a stabilizing component such as nucleic acid is not added immediately [13]. We suggested that large aggregates with positive total charge impair cellular membrane while adsorbing and entering the cells. In the current study, we have experienced slightly increased rate of early apoptosis (Figure 2c) in samples incubated with ND and NDSc, complexes without active A135b. The increase is rather negligible, yet statistically significant. We suspect the uptake of nanoparticles that reside in high concentration in 4T1 cell cytoplasm could interfere with the cell divisions. This hypothesis is supported by the results of direct toxicity (LDH release) shown in Figure 2b. Neither ND nor NDSc exhibited direct toxicity and significant release of LDH but the presence of those nanoparticles led, in a small percentage of cells, to apoptosis. When using NDA135b, the increase in apoptotic or dead cells was much more prominent (Figure 2b,c) due to A135b function (Figure 2d).

Unlike adherent 2D culture, the 3D tumor grown without surface attachment enables testing of nanocomplexes in an ambiance much closer to the natural situation in vivo. To imitate the tumor microenvironment and tests NDA135b specificity, we co-cultured the mammospheres with cells obtained from peritoneal cavity lavage of experimental animals. Nanodiamonds within NDA135b were decorated with transferrin in order to facilitate their uptake by tumor cells [37]. We believe it also promoted stabilization of the complexes and protected them from extensive binding of sera proteins. This hypothesis is based on recent studies that showed how adsorption of a specific protein onto ND before the exposure of ND to sera prevented formation of protein corona [38]. Decoration of ND surface with a protein such as Tf conjugated with a fluorophore increased the size of the final complex to about 300 nm and significantly increased the polydispersity index. The PdI increase might be due to uneven amount of conjugates linked to ND particle. This approach with fluorophore-labeled targeting structure is convenient for proof-of function presented in this study where we needed to control the complex location. If not necessary, we suggest using unlabeled targeting antibodies to obtain lower PdI.

The silencing of microRNA-135b in 4T1 cells by NDA135b performed in the 3D model was very effective (Figure 3b) suggesting good distribution of NDA135b in the media, which enabled its sufficient internalization into cells that are in a compact sphere not adhering and covering the bottom of the experimental dish. Flow cytometry analysis of 3D tumor spheres with intercalated cells from peritoneal lavage revealed very interesting information regarding cells carrying NDA135b. In this setup, we can benefit from existing communication between tumor and immune cells but the model is still much simpler than the situation in vivo. We expected the tumor cell will uptake most of NDA135b due to specific targeting of NDA135b with transferrin and shielding of the complex from macrophages. We believed macrophages from peritoneal lavage could up to some degree compete with tumor cells for the NDA135b since they are (in 7%) positive for transferrin receptor too. We found that the granulocytes are a major population that carries NDA135b (Figure 4). A presence of transferrin-receptor on the cell surface was ruled out by flow cytometry (Figure 3), thus, the granulocytes did carry NDA135b regardless the targeting molecule. So far, mostly monocyte/macrophage cells were studied regarding transportation of internalized nanoparticles within multicellular organism [39]. Now, we found granulocytes play an important role too and the future research regarding nanoparticle interaction should consider deeper study of this cell population. To our knowledge, there is only one report describing interaction of nanodiamonds with granulocytes specifically with neutrophils in air pouches of lungs [40].

Detailed reports describing the effect of HPHT nanodiamond particles on the immune system in vivo or complex organ toxicity are rare. So far, the non-targeted ND particles applied in vivo exhibited neither direct toxicity nor inflammatory and stress responses [23,24]. If nanodiamonds accumulated, predominantly in lungs, liver, or spleen, there were no symptoms of abnormalities [20,22]. Also, mice injected with ND did not show any weight-loss or other clinical signs of toxicity even after exposure for four weeks [22]. On the other hand, ND coated with hemagglutinin significantly enhanced the immunostimulatory effect of hemagglutinin in mice—however, it was more likely because of increased stability and concentration of the hemagglutinin than presence of nanodiamond carrier [41]. Modified ND in hydrosol applied intravenously into rabbits showed a short-term increase in serum bilirubin (sign of erythrocyte lysis) and other changes associated with the sequestering of the nanodiamonds in the liver [42].

As mentioned earlier specific coating and targeting of nanoparticles significantly effects their fate and final accumulation site [30]. Since we applied, in vivo, a newly developed construct (combination of RNA, protein, and polymer coating), we performed basic compatibility tests to assess particles' fate and their interactions with biological structures. We wondered if localized application would trigger any side effects because of possible NDA135b leakage from tumor into peripheral blood system. Using intratumoral as well as intravenous application of NDA135b targeted with transferrin led to accumulation of NDA135b in the excised tumor mass (Figure 5a) and significant downregulation of cytoplasmic microRNA-135b. It shows that even the NDA135b circulating in blood after intravenous application effectively reached tumor cells. Once we isolated tumor cells in order to perform flow cytometry and quantitative estimate, we yielded a significantly different amount of NDA135b-positive cells concerning the type of administration. In samples after intratumoral application, we found a well-defined peak pointing out cells positive for NDA135b (Figure 5c). In samples after intravenous application, we did not see any specific peak but we still experienced some shift in cells' positivity as shown in histograms (Figure 5c, top). We are aware the lower amount of cells positive for NDA135b in samples after intravenous application reflected the way of administration. However, the whole tumor (after intravenous application) exhibited quite strong fluorescence but the isolated tumor cells were insignificantly positive for NDA135b. We believe that after intratumoral application, NDA135b resided in the tumor site for a longer time, increasing its chance to be internalized. After intravenous administration, we assume that some circulating NDA135b reached the tumor and were internalized by tumor cells, but the amount of internalized complexes was too low to detect it. In addition, the non-internalized NDA135b within tumor mass were washed away during tumor cells isolation.

The lower amount of positive tumor cells after intravenous application suggested persisting of NDA135b in blood or its off-target accumulation. Our data show that NDA135b did not significantly accumulate in liver, kidney, or spleen, suggesting the coating prevented ND accumulation in those key tissues. In animals, after intravenous application of NDA135b, we found positivity in urine. Since the core particle is about 70 nm big, it is not possible that the fully coated complex would pass via renal filtration into urine [28]. There is a small chance that when the NDA135b entered blood cells, transferrin–fluorophore conjugate separated from the ND core and left the body via renal clearance. For example, dextrans conjugated with Texas Red are renal clearable [43].

Interestingly, analyzing splenocytes obtained from homogenized spleen samples, we found a remarkable shift in their granularity after intravenous application of NDA135b (Figure 6c). We suggested an indirect effect since we did not detect any presence of NDA135b in excised spleen tissues or different splenocytes populations. Assuming an indirect effect on splenocytes, we examined basic blood cells populations—erythrocytes, monocytes/granulocytes, and lymphocytes within peripheral blood. We expected to find positive signal in monocytes/granulocytes that could potentially interact with or internalize NDA135b. We found NDA135b-positive blood samples after intravenous application but we did not observe any positive signal in any of the cellular subpopulations (Figure 7). The data suggest that NDA135b was present in peripheral blood, it was not carried by any blood cells, but it interacted with a blood element to affect granularity of spleen tissue.

Within multicellular organism, an inflammatory reaction is a response to infection but also to non-infectious agents. Recently, Li et al. [44] described non-infectious inflammation after intraperitoneal application of hydrocarbon oil. This inflammation recruited neutrophils, dendritic cells, and macrophages into spleen based on elevated levels of interleukin-6 and tumor necrosis factor—alpha (TNF—α). Intravenous application of NDA135b could induce non-infections inflammation too. This hypothesis is supported by Munoz et al. [40]. The authors proposed that small (10 nm) naked or PEG-coated ND damage plasma membrane and trigger instability of lysosomal compartment and formation of neutrophil extracellular traps. It initialized inflammatory response comprising synthesis of pro-inflammatory cytokines. Larger particles (100 nm) seemed inert [40]. Our data (Figure A4) and other authors' [22–24] reports reinforce the relative inertness regarding cytokine production too.

Comparing the two different in vivo administrations, the localized intratumoral application was effective in order to knockdown target microRNA-135b and exhibited no leakage of NDA135b into bodily fluids or other tissues. The intravenous application was effective in order to knockdown target microRNA-135b. It was accompanied with circulation of NDA135b in blood and it affected splenocytes parameters. According to our data, the intratumoral application represents a much safer mean of NDA135b application with much less side effects. We believe that localized and targeted application is the most effective and the safest approach regarding any biomedical use of non-degradable inorganic carriers with diameter exceeding limits for renal clearance. Keeping this approach in mind, we still can benefit from extraordinary characteristics of nanodiamond particles even though they are non-biodegradable. Thus nanodiamond-based complexes that are stabilized and decorated with nucleic acids and/or peptides are prospective in topical treatments of skin disorder such as chronic wound-healing, dermatitis, or skin tumors. Next to the therapeutic function (nucleic acid) performed only in particular cells (antibody), the nanodiamond core keeps its luminescence and with a suitable optical system, we could track the process of construct diffusion within the treated tissue. Using intravenous application of coated ND carriers requires further detailed analysis of cell interaction triggering changes in organ (spleen) characteristics. Since the immune response is dependent on carrier size as well as on way of administration [40], each ND carrier has to be evaluated with regard to its anticipated use. Importantly, our findings contribute to the understanding of ND carriers' fate and trafficking in vivo. It has revealed new interesting interactions between ND carrier and biological interface as well as future challenges regarding signal transport and response mechanisms within in vivo systems.

Author Contributions: Conceptualization, V.B.; investigation, R.K., E.N., K.Q.J., and V.B.; methodology, R.K., E.N., and V.B.; resources, V.B.; writing—original draft, R.K., E.N., and V.B.; writing—review and editing, V.B.

Funding: This research was funded by the Ministry of Health of the Czech Republic, grant number 15-33094A.

Acknowledgments: The HPHT ND were kindly provided by Vladimira Petráková (Czech Technical University). The authors thank to the Core of Cytometry and Microscopy, Institute of Microbiology CAS for support during flow cytometry and microscopy measurements.

Conflicts of Interest: The authors declare no conflict of interest. The funders had no role in the design of the study; in the collection, analyses, or interpretation of data; in the writing of the manuscript, or in the decision to publish the results.

Appendix A

Comparison of miR135b levels in cell fraction of peritoneal lavage (MF), splenocytes (SPL), and mammary tumor (4T1) obtained from homogenized tissues ex vivo. Samples were obtained from tumor (derived from 4T1) bearing animals. Peritoneal cells and splenocytes exhibited minimal level of miR135b in contrast to the tumor tissue.

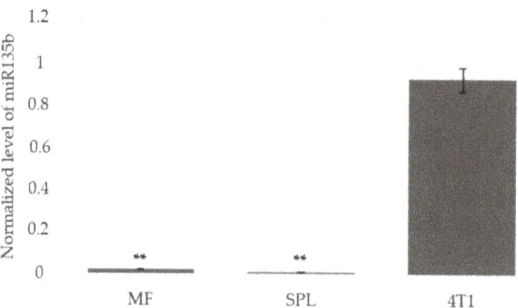

Figure A1. Expression of miR135b in different tissues. MF stands for peritoneal cells, SPL stands for splenocytes, and 4T1 represents tumor cells with high expression of miR-135b. Data are presented as the mean ± standard deviation, ** p-value < 0.01 versus 4T1 group was obtained by ANOVA.

Appendix B

Flow cytometry analyses of NDA135b signal presence in leukocytes obtained from homogenized liver and kidney after different administration of NDA135b complex can reveal uptake of NDA135b from blood and its accumulation in this cell fraction. Measuring the signal intensity within the whole organ homogenate could cover up the potential positivity in leukocyte population so we took a closer look by gating out distinguishable populations. Regarding spleen, the NDA135b could accumulate within the debris fraction so we checked that portion of spleen homogenate too. Detection was enabled by administration of NDA135b containing transferrin conjugated with Texas Red. Control animals received saline. The data complement analyses mentioned in Figure 5.

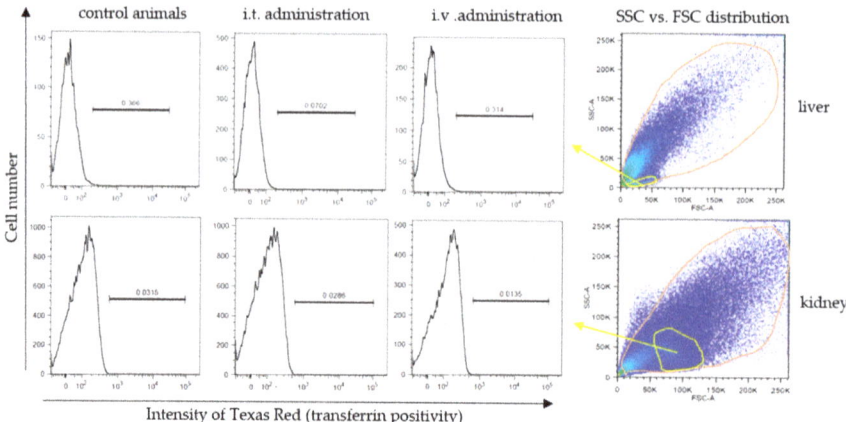

Figure A2. Texas Red signal in leukocytes obtained from homogenized liver and kidney after NDA135b administration.

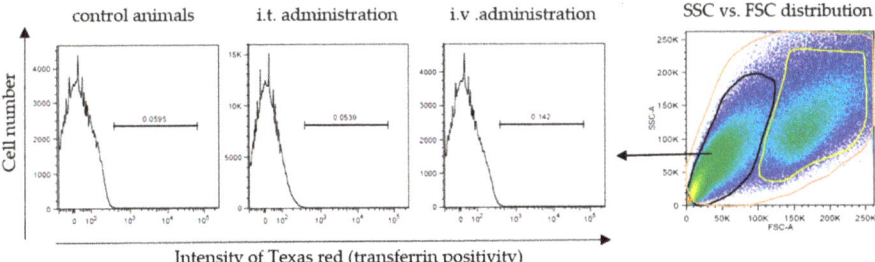

Figure A3. Texas Red signal in debris/erythrocytes fraction of unfiltered spleen samples from animals administered with NDA135b.

Appendix C

Flow cytometry analyses of cytokine secretion in response to NDA135b administrations. Basic cytokines IFN—γ, TNF—α, and IL—6 were analyzed in blood of experimental animals (1 h after 3rd dose) using Cytometric Bead Array (BD Biosciences). Here we followed manufacturer protocol. Briefly, whole blood was diluted five times, mixed with specific beads, and incubated for 3 h. After that, samples were washed with PBS, and beads were analyzed with flow cytometry. APC fluorophore determines bead/cytokine type and PE fluorophore represents cytokine positivity. The levels of all three cytokines were equal in all tested samples.

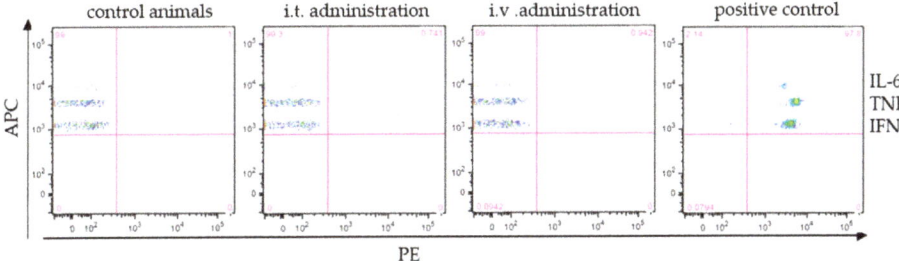

Figure A4. Levels of secreted cytokines (IL—6, IFN—γ, and TNF—α) in peripheral blood of control animals, animals who received NDA135b intratumorally, and animals who received NDA135b intravenously. Positive control stands for mixture of 625 pg/mL of each of the three cytokines (test standards). Representative images are shown.

References

1. Bray, F.; Ferlay, J.; Soerjomataram, I.; Siegel, R.L.; Torre, L.A.; Jemal, A. Global cancer statistics 2018: GLOBOCAN estimates of incidence and mortality worldwide for 36 cancers in 185 countries. *CA Cancer J. Clin.* **2018**, *68*, 394–424. [CrossRef] [PubMed]
2. Bandrés, E.; Cubedo, E.; Agirre, X.; Malumbres, R.; Zárate, R.; Ramirez, N.; Abajo, A.; Navarro, A.; Moreno, I.; Monzó, M.; et al. Identification by Real-time PCR of 13 mature microRNAs differentially expressed in colorectal cancer and non-tumoral tissues. *Mol. Cancer* **2006**, *5*, 29–39. [CrossRef] [PubMed]
3. Tong, A.W.; Fulgham, P.; Jay, C.; Chen, P.; Khalil, I.; Liu, S.; Senzer, N.; Eklund, A.C.; Han, J.; Nemunaitis, J. MicroRNA profile analysis of human prostate cancers. *Cancer Gene Ther.* **2009**, *16*, 206–216. [CrossRef] [PubMed]
4. Lowery, A.J.; Miller, N.; Devaney, A.; McNeill, R.E.; Davoren, P.A.; Lemetre, C.; Benes, V.; Schmidt, S.; Blake, J.; Ball, G.; et al. MicroRNA signatures predict oestrogen receptor, progesterone receptor and HER2/neu receptor status in breast cancer. *Breast Cancer Res.* **2009**, *11*, R27. [CrossRef] [PubMed]
5. Lin, S.L.; Chang, D.C.; Ying, S.Y. Isolation and identification of gene-specific microRNAs. *Methods Mol. Biol.* **2013**, *936*, 271–278. [PubMed]

6. Hayward, S.L.; Francis, D.M.; Kholmatov, P.; Kidambi, S. Targeted Delivery of MicroRNA125a-5p by Engineered Lipid Nanoparticles for the Treatment of HER2 Positive Metastatic Breast Cancer. *J. Biomed. Nanotechnol.* **2016**, *12*, 554–568. [CrossRef] [PubMed]
7. Tyagi, N.; Arora, S.; Deshmukh, S.K.; Singh, S.; Marimuthu, S.; Singh, A.P. Exploiting Nanotechnology for the Development of MicroRNA-Based Cancer Therapeutics. *J. Biomed. Nanotechnol.* **2016**, *12*, 28–42. [CrossRef] [PubMed]
8. Wang, S.; Zhang, J.; Wang, Y.; Chen, M. Hyaluronic acid-coated PEI-PLGA nanoparticles mediated co-delivery of doxorubicin and miR-542-3p for triple negative breast cancer therapy. *Nanomedicine* **2016**, *12*, 411–420. [CrossRef] [PubMed]
9. Zhong, S.; Chen, X.; Wang, D.; Zhang, X.; Shen, H.; Yang, S.; Lv, M.; Tang, J.; Zhao, J. MicroRNA expression profiles of drug-resistance breast cancer cells and their exosomes. *Oncotarget* **2016**, *7*, 19601–19609. [CrossRef]
10. Faklaris, O.; Joshi, V.; Irinopoulou, T.; Tauc, P.; Sennour, M.; Girard, H.; Gesset, C.; Arnault, J.C.; Thorel, A.; Boudou, J.P.; et al. Photoluminescent diamond nanoparticles for cell labeling: Study of the uptake mechanism in mammalian cells. *ACS Nano* **2009**, *3*, 3955–3962. [CrossRef]
11. Alhaddad, A.; Durieu, C.; Dantelle, G.; Le Cam, E.; Malvy, C.; Treussart, F.; Bertrand, J.R. Influence of the internalization pathway on the efficacy of siRNA delivery by cationic fluorescent nanodiamonds in the Ewing sarcoma cell model. *PLoS ONE* **2012**, *7*, e52207. [CrossRef] [PubMed]
12. Petrakova, V.; Benson, V.; Buncek, M.; Fiserova, A.; Ledvina, M.; Stursa, J.; Cigler, P.; Nesladek, M. Imaging of transfection and intracellular release of intact, non-labeled DNA using fluorescent nanodiamonds. *Nanoscale* **2016**, *8*, 12002–12012. [CrossRef] [PubMed]
13. Lukowski, S.; Neuhoferova, E.; Kinderman, M.; Krivohlava, R.; Mineva, A.; Petrakova, V.; Benson, V. Fluorescent Nanodiamonds are Efficient, Easy-to-Use Cyto-Compatible Vehicles for Monitored Delivery of Non-Coding Regulatory RNAs. *J. Biomed. Nanotechnol.* **2018**, *14*, 946–958. [CrossRef] [PubMed]
14. Chang, Y.R.; Lee, H.Y.; Chen, K.; Chang, C.C.; Tsai, D.S.; Fu, C.C.; Lim, T.S.; Tzeng, Y.K.; Fang, C.Y.; Han, C.C.; et al. Mass production and dynamic imaging of fluorescent nanodiamonds. *Nat. Nanotechnol.* **2008**, *3*, 284–288. [CrossRef] [PubMed]
15. Zhang, X.Q.; Chen, M.; Lam, R.; Xu, X.; Osawa, E.; Ho, D. Polymer-functionalized nanodiamond platforms as vehicles for gene delivery. *ACS Nano* **2009**, *3*, 2609–2616. [CrossRef] [PubMed]
16. Ho, D.; Wang, C.H.; Chow, E.K. Nanodiamonds: The intersection of nanotechnology, drug development, and personalized medicine. *Sci. Adv.* **2015**, *1*, e1500439. [CrossRef] [PubMed]
17. Zheng, T.; Perona Martínez, F.; Storm, I.M.; Rombouts, W.; Sprakel, J.; Schirhagl, R.; de Vries, R. Recombinant Protein Polymers for Colloidal Stabilization and Improvement of Cellular Uptake of Diamond Nanosensors. *Anal. Chem.* **2017**, *89*, 12812–12820. [CrossRef] [PubMed]
18. Chipaux, M.; van der Laan, K.J.; Hemelaar, S.R.; Hasani, M.; Zheng, T.; Schirhagl, R. Nanodiamonds and Their Applications in Cells. *Small* **2018**, *14*, e1704263. [CrossRef] [PubMed]
19. Hsiao, W.W.; Hui, Y.Y.; Tsai, P.C.; Chang, H.C. Fluorescent Nanodiamond: A Versatile Tool for Long-Term Cell Tracking, Super-Resolution Imaging, and Nanoscale Temperature Sensing. *Acc. Chem. Res.* **2016**, *49*, 400–407. [CrossRef] [PubMed]
20. Mohan, N.; Chen, C.S.; Hsieh, H.H.; Wu, Y.C.; Chang, H.C. In vivo imaging and toxicity assessments of fluorescent nanodiamonds in Caenorhabditis elegans. *Nano Lett.* **2010**, *10*, 3692–3699. [CrossRef]
21. Van der Laan, K.; Hasani, M.; Zheng, T.; Schirhagl, R. Nanodiamonds for In Vivo Applications. *Small* **2018**, *14*, e1703838. [CrossRef] [PubMed]
22. Yuan, Y.; Chen, Y.; Liu, J.H.; Wang, H.; Liu, Y. Biodistribution and fate of nanodiamonds in vivo. *Diam. Relat. Mater.* **2009**, *18*, 95–100. [CrossRef]
23. Vaijayanthimala, V.; Cheng, P.Y.; Yeh, S.H.; Liu, K.K.; Hsiao, C.H.; Chao, J.I.; Chang, H.C. The long-term stability and biocompatibility of fluorescent nanodiamond as an in vivo contrast agent. *Biomaterials* **2012**, *33*, 7794–7802. [CrossRef] [PubMed]
24. Tsai, L.W.; Lin, Y.C.; Perevedentseva, E.; Lugovtsov, A.; Priezzhev, A.; Cheng, C.L. Nanodiamonds for Medical Applications: Interaction with Blood in Vitro and in Vivo. *Int. J. Mol. Sci.* **2016**, *17*, 1111. [CrossRef] [PubMed]
25. Hua, K.; Jin, J.; Zhao, J.; Song, J.; Song, H.; Li, D.; Maskey, N.; Zhao, B.; Wu, C.; Xu, H.; et al. miR-135b, upregulated in breast cancer, promotes cell growth and disrupts the cell cycle by regulating LATS2. *Int. J. Oncol.* **2016**, *48*, 1791–2423. [CrossRef] [PubMed]

26. Petrakova, V.; Rehor, I.; Stursa, J.; Ledvina, M.; Nesladek, M.; Cigler, P. Charge-sensitive fluorescent nanosensors created from nanodiamonds. *Nanoscale* **2015**, *7*, 12307–12311. [CrossRef]
27. Upreti, M.; Jamshidi-Parsian, A.; Koonce, N.A.; Webber, J.S.; Sharma, S.K.; Asea, A.A.; Mader, M.J.; Griffin, R.J. Tumor-Endothelial Cell Three-dimensional Spheroids: New Aspects to Enhance Radiation and Drug Therapeutics. *Transl. Oncol.* **2011**, *4*, 365–376. [CrossRef]
28. Longmire, M.; Choyke, P.L.; Kobayashi, H. Clearance properties of nano-sized particles and molecules as imaging agents: Considerations and caveats. *Nanomed. Lond.* **2008**, *3*, 703–717. [CrossRef]
29. Fang, J.; Nakamura, H.; Maeda, H. The EPR effect: Unique features of tumor blood vessels for drug delivery, factors involved, and limitations and augmentation of the effect. *Adv. Drug Deliv. Rev.* **2011**, *63*, 136–151. [CrossRef]
30. Yu, M.; Zheng, J. Clearance Pathways and Tumor Targeting of Imaging Nanoparticles. *ACS Nano* **2015**, *9*, 6655–6674. [CrossRef]
31. Turcheniuk, K.; Mochalin, V.N. Biomedical applications of nanodiamond (Review). *Nanotechnology* **2017**, *28*, 252001. [CrossRef]
32. Yu, S.J.; Kang, M.W.; Chang, H.C.; Chen, K.M.; Yu, Y.C. Bright fluorescent nanodiamonds: No photobleaching and low cytotoxicity. *J. Am. Chem. Soc.* **2005**, *127*, 17604–17605. [CrossRef]
33. Liu, K.K.; Cheng, C.L.; Chang, C.C.; Chao, J.I. Biocompatible and detectable carboxylated nanodiamond on human cell. *Nanotechnology* **2007**, *18*, 325102. [CrossRef]
34. Blaber, S.P.; Hill, C.J.; Webster, R.A.; Say, J.M.; Brown, L.J.; Wang, S.C.; Vesey, G.; Herbert, B.R. Effect of labeling with iron oxide particles or nanodiamonds on the functionality of adipose-derived mesenchymal stem cells. *PLoS ONE* **2013**, *8*, e52997. [CrossRef]
35. Hsu, T.C.; Liu, K.K.; Chang, H.C.; Hwang, E.; Chao, J.I. Labeling of neuronal differentiation and neuron cells with biocompatible fluorescent nanodiamonds. *Sci. Rep.* **2014**, *4*, 5004–5015. [CrossRef]
36. Feng, Q.; Liu, Y.; Huang, J.; Chen, K.; Xiao, K. Uptake, distribution, clearance, and toxicity of iron oxide nanoparticles with different sizes and coatings. *Sci. Rep.* **2018**, *8*, 2082–2095. [CrossRef]
37. Daniels, T.R.; Bernabeu, E.; Rodríguez, J.A.; Patel, S.; Kozman, M.; Chiappetta, D.A.; Holler, E.; Ljubimova, J.Y.; Helguera, G.; Penichet, M.L. The transferrin receptor and the targeted delivery of therapeutic agents against cancer. *Biochim. Biophys. Acta* **2012**, *1820*, 291–317. [CrossRef]
38. Hemelaar, S.R.; Nagl, A.; Bigot, F.; Rodríguez-García, M.M.; de Vries, M.P.; Chipaux, M.; Schirhagl, R. The interaction of fluorescent nanodiamond probes with cellular media. *Mikrochim. Acta* **2017**, *184*, 1001–1009. [CrossRef]
39. Yuan, Y.; Wang, X.; Jia, G. Pulmonary toxicity and translocation of nanodiamond in mice. *Diam. Relat. Mater.* **2010**, *19*, 291–300. [CrossRef]
40. Muñoz, L.E.; Bilyy, R.; Biermann, M.H.; Kienhöfer, D.; Maueröder, C.; Hahn, J.; Brauner, J.M.; Weidner, D.; Chen, J.; Scharin-Mehlmann, M.; et al. Nanoparticles size-dependently initiate self-limiting NETosis-driven inflammation. *Proc. Natl. Acad. Sci. USA* **2016**, *113*, 5856–5865. [CrossRef]
41. Pham, N.B.; Ho, T.T.; Nguyen, G.T.; Le, T.T.; Le, N.T.; Chang, H.C.; Pham, M.D.; Conrad, U.; Chu, H.H. Nanodiamond enhances immune responses in mice against recombinant HA/H7N9 protein. *J. Nanobiotechnol.* **2017**, *15*, 69–81. [CrossRef]
42. Puzyr, A.P.; Baron, A.V.; Purtov, K.V.; Bortnikov, E.V.; Skobelev, N.N.; Mogilnaya, O.A.; Bondar, V.S. Nanodiamonds with novel properties: A biological study. *Diam. Relat. Mater.* **2007**, *16*, 2124–2128. [CrossRef]
43. Wang, E.; Sandoval, R.M.; Campos, S.B.; Molitoris, B.A. Rapid diagnosis and quantification of acute kidney injury using fluorescent ratio-metric determination of glomerular filtration rate in the rat. *Am. J. Physiol. Renal Physiol.* **2010**, *299*, 1048–1055. [CrossRef]
44. Li, Y.; Wu, J.; Xu, L.; Wu, Q.; Wan, Z.; Li, L.; Yu, H.; Li, X.; Li, K.; Zhang, Q.; et al. Regulation of Leukocyte Recruitment to the Spleen and Peritoneal Cavity during Pristane-Induced Inflammation. *J. Immunol. Res.* **2017**, *2017*, 9891348. [CrossRef]

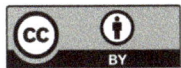

© 2019 by the authors. Licensee MDPI, Basel, Switzerland. This article is an open access article distributed under the terms and conditions of the Creative Commons Attribution (CC BY) license (http://creativecommons.org/licenses/by/4.0/).

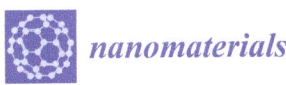

Article

Elaboration of *Trans*-Resveratrol Derivative-Loaded Superparamagnetic Iron Oxide Nanoparticles for Glioma Treatment

Fadoua Sallem [1], Rihab Haji [2], Dominique Vervandier-Fasseur [2], Thomas Nury [3], Lionel Maurizi [1], Julien Boudon [1], Gérard Lizard [3] and Nadine Millot [1,*]

[1] Laboratoire Interdisciplinaire Carnot de Bourgogne (ICB), UMR 6303 CNRS/Université Bourgogne Franche-Comté, 21000 Dijon, France; fadouasallem@gmail.com (F.S.); lionelmaurizi@gmail.com (L.M.); julien.boudon@u-bourgogne.fr (J.B.)
[2] Institut de Chimie Moléculaire de l'Université de Bourgogne (ICMUB), UMR 6302 CNRS/Université Bourgogne Franche-Comté, 21000 Dijon, France; hajirihab22@yahoo.com (R.H.); dominique.vervandier-fasseur@u-bourgogne.fr (D.V.-F.)
[3] Laboratoire Bio-PeroxIL, EA7270, Université de Bourgogne Franche-Comté/Inserm, 21000 Dijon, France; thomas.nury@u-bourgogne.fr (T.N.); gerard.lizard@u-bourgogne.fr (G.L.)
* Correspondence: nadine.millot@u-bourgogne.fr

Received: 9 January 2019; Accepted: 15 February 2019; Published: 18 February 2019

Abstract: In this work, new nanohybrids based on superparamagnetic iron oxide nanoparticles (SPIONs) were elaborated and discussed for the first time as nanovectors of a derivative molecule of trans-resveratrol (RSV), a natural antioxidant molecule, which can be useful for brain disease treatment. The derivative molecule was chemically synthesized (4′-hydroxy-4-(3-aminopropoxy) trans-stilbene: HAPtS) and then grafted onto SPIONs surface using an organosilane coupling agent, which is 3-chloropropyltriethoxysilane (CPTES) and based on nucleophilic substitution reactions. The amount of HAPtS loaded onto SPIONs surface was estimated by thermogravimetric analysis (TGA) and X-ray photoelectron spectroscopy (XPS) analyses at 116 µMol·g^{-1} SPIONs. The synthesized HAPtS molecule, as well as the associated nanohybrids, were fully characterized by transmission electron microscopy (TEM), XPS, TGA, infrared (IR) and UV-visible spectroscopies, dynamic light scattering (DLS), and zeta potential measurements. The in vitro biological assessment of the synthesized nanohybrid's efficiency was carried out on C6 glioma cells and showed that the nanovector SPIONs-CPTES-HAPtS do not affect the mitochondrial metabolism (MTT test), but damage the plasma membrane (FDA test), which could contribute to limiting the proliferation of cancerous cells (clonogenic test) at a HAPtS concentration of 50 µM. These nanoparticles have a potential cytotoxic effect that could be used to eliminate cancer cells.

Keywords: iron oxide superparamagnetic nanoparticles; *trans*-resveratrol derivative; drug delivery; glioma

---

1. Introduction

Trans-resveratrol, or 3,4′,5-trihydroxy-trans-stilbene (RSV) (Figure 1A), is a polyphenolic compound that belongs to the stilbene family. It is widespread in the plant kingdom and found especially in peanuts, grapes, and accordingly, in wine [1,2]. The discovery of RSV in red wine and interest in its ability to prevent cardiovascular diseases was the starting point of this molecule [3]. Since then, numerous in vitro and in vivo studies in animals have shown various biological properties of RSV, such as antioxidant [4], anti-microbial [5], anti-inflammatory [6], estrogenomimetic effects, anti-cancer [7], and chemopreventive activities [8]. Indeed, thanks to its potent antioxidant power, it has proven its effectiveness against skin, breast, lung, prostate, and pancreas cancers [9].

As oxidative damage has been considered the main cause of many neurodegenerative diseases, including Alzheimer's disease (AD), Parkinson's disease (PD), and stroke [10,11], RSV has extensively been studied as a therapeutic molecule for these kinds of diseases based on its antioxidant properties [12]. In fact, the neuroprotective effects of RSV against oxidative stress was proved by R. Alyssa et al. [13]. Moreover, a study by Wang et al. showed that RSV can cross the blood brain barrier (BBB) and protect against cerebral ischemic injury [14]. RSV was also shown to inhibit the formation of amyloid-beta (Aβ) aggregation characterizing Alzheimer's disease (AD), and to reduce its secretion in numerous cell lines [12]. It was also suggested that RSV reduces neurodegeneration in the hippocampus and prevents learning deficits [15].

Currently, the use of RSV in humans remains limited due to its photosensitivity, easy oxidation [16], and low biodisponibility [1]. In addition, pharmacokinetic evaluations of free RSV have reported a very short half-life (30–45 min) and a rapid metabolism in rats [17]. Therefore, large doses of this polyphenol would be necessary to be effective in humans, which is limited by its low water solubility [18]. In order to overcome those limits, RSV has been encapsulated in order to favor its biological activity and increase its half-life [18]. Thus, many encapsulation methods have been used for this purpose, such as microemulsion [19,20], liposomes [21–24], and biopolymers [25,26]. Recent studies have focused on the association of RSV to nanoparticles. Indeed, Wang et al. modified liposomes encapsulating RSV with iron oxide nanoparticles for targeted PD treatment application [27]. RSV was also conjugated to silver and gold nanoparticles in order to enhance their antibacterial efficacy [28,29], or was used as an anticancer delivery system [30]. To the best of our knowledge, RSV has never been linked covalently to iron oxide nanoparticles. Therefore, the latter strategy has been chosen and herein we aim at delivering a RSV derivative, the molecules of which were grafted to the surface of superparamagnetic iron oxide nanoparticles (SPIONs), for further studies in neurodegenerative disease or glioma treatment.

SPIONs are considered as one of the most developed nanoparticles for various biomedical applications thanks to their small size, high magnetic moment, high surface to volume ratio, and biocompatibility [31]. They have been used for magnetic resonance imaging (MRI) as a contrast agent [32,33], cell labeling, tissue repair, gene and drug delivery, hyperthermia [34], and nano-sensors [35]. One of the most promising biomedical applications of SPIONs is drug delivery, thanks to the magnetic response of the iron oxide allowing magnetic targeting, which makes the retention of nanoparticles in the target tissue longer [36]. The most challenging targets for SPIONs are in the brain because of the presence of the BBB, a natural boundary between the neural tissue and the blood circulation, which limits the entrance of most drugs intended for the central nervous system (CNS). Many kinds of nanoparticles, polymeric and inorganic, have been studied for drug delivery across the BBB, however, the advantage of using inorganic nanoparticles (silica, gold, SPIONs, etc.) is the facility in modulating them in terms of shape, size, and surface modification [37]. The surface modification of nanoparticles increases their ability to cross this barrier. Indeed, unlike bare SPIONs, it has been reported that ligand-coated SPIONs or BBB disruption (BBB-targeting peptides, curcumin, polyethylene glycol (PEG)/chitosan, etc.) make them capable of crossing the BBB because they facilitate SPIONs uptake by the endothelial cells via specific receptors [38]. Moreover, the magnetic targeting of SPIONs not only enhances their penetration in brain cells, as has been proved by Chertok et al. on glioma cells [39,40], but also can transiently increase the BBB permeability following from magnetic heating (hyperthermia), as was proved by Tabatabaei et al. for rat brains [41]. The percentage of SPIONs that reach the CNS via the bloodstream has varied from 17 to 30% according to rodent studies [42].

Herein, we studied the surface modification of SPIONs with a derivative molecule of RSV, used as a therapeutic molecule, for further application in neurodegenerative diseases. This molecule has the same stilbene core as RSV—4'-hydroxy-4-(3-aminopropoxy) trans-stilbene, hereafter referred to as HAPtS (Figure 1)—and it was exclusively synthesized for this purpose. The anti-tumor and anti-microbial activities of compounds structurally close to HAPtS have been proven in previous studies [5,43]. The feature of this phenolic stilbene is an organic alkyl chain with a terminal functional group (primary amine) capable of linking to SPION's surface, as shown in Figure 1.

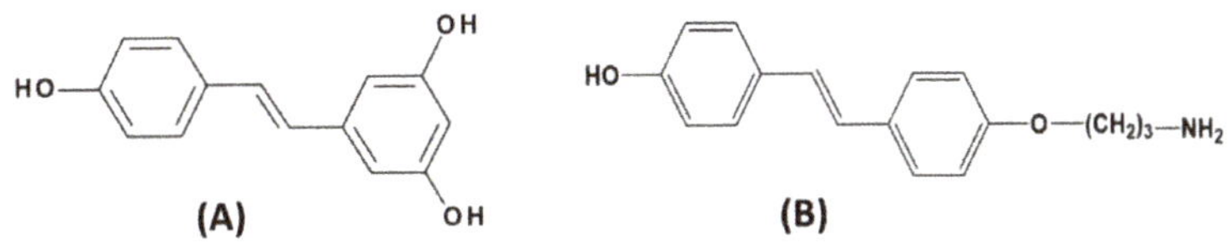

Figure 1. Chemical structure of (**A**) the natural trans-resveratrol molecule (RSV) and (**B**) the trans-resveratrol derivative molecule: 4'-hydroxy-4-(3-aminopropoxy) trans-stilbene (HAPtS).

2. Materials and Methods

2.1. Chemicals and Reagents

Iron (III) chloride hexahydrate ($FeCl_3.6H_2O$, 97%), and iron (II) chloride tetrahydrate ($FeCl_2.4H_2O$, 98%) were purchased from Alfa Aesar (Haverhill, MA, USA). Sodium hydroxide (NaOH, $\geq$97%), ammonium hydroxide solution (NH_4OH, 28%), hydrochloric acid (HCl, 37%), nitric acid (HNO_3, 69%), 3-chloropropyltriethoxysilane (CPTES, 95%), dimethylsulfoxide (DMSO, $\geq$99.7%), crystal violet, 2,2'-azobis (2-amidinopropane) dihydrochloride (AAPH), fluorescein sodium salt, N,N-diisopropylethylamine, ReagentPlus®(DIEA, $\geq$99%), 3-(4,5-dimethylthiazol-2-yl)-2,5-diphenyl tetrazolium bromide (MTT, 98%), 7β-hydroxycholesterol (7β-OHC), and Trolox (97%) were purchased from Sigma-Aldrich (St. Louis, MO, USA). Absolute ethanol (EtOH, $\geq$99.8%) was purchased from Fluka (Seelze, Germany). Phosphate buffer saline (PBS) 1× solution was purchased from Fisher Chemicals (Fair Lown, NJ, USA). Dulbecco's modified Eagle medium (DMEM), trypan blue, fetal bovine serum (FBS), and antibiotic (Penicillin, Streptomycin) were purchased from Dominique Dutscher and Pan Biotech (Brumath, France). Ultrafiltration membranes (regenerated cellulose 100 kDa) were acquired from Merck Millipore (Darmstadt, Germany).

2.2. Characterization Techniques

An X-Ray diffraction (XRD) pattern of bare SPIONs was obtained using a Bruker D8 Advance diffractometer (Billerica, MA, USA). Cu K$\alpha_{1,2}$ radiations ($\lambda\alpha_1$ = 1.540598 Å and $\lambda\alpha_2$ = 1.544426 Å) were applied. Scans were measured over a 2θ range of 10–80°. A step of 0.026° and a scan speed of 52 s per angle unit were set. The data analysis was carried out with Topas®software (Billerica, MA, USA). The Le Bail method was used to obtain lattice parameters and mean crystallite size.

The morphology of synthesized nanoparticles (NPs) were observed by Transmission electron microscopy (TEM, Tokyo, Japan) using a JEOL JEM 2100F microscope operating at 200 kV (point-to-point resolution of 0.19 nm). The samples were prepared by evaporating a diluted suspension of SPIONs in deionized (DI) water on a carbon-coated copper grid. About 150 nanoparticles were counted in order to estimate their average size (imageJ software, 1.52a, NIH, MD, USA).

X-ray photoelectron spectroscopy (XPS) measurements were collected with a PHI 5000 Versaprobe instrument (ULVAC-PHI, Osaka, Japan) using an Al Kα monochromatic radiation (EKα(Al) = 1486.7 eV with a 200 μM diameter spot size)). Powders were pressed on an indium sheet. Data were analyzed with CasaXPS processing and ULVAC-PHI MultiPak software (ver. 9.0.1, Osaka, Japan) for quantitative analysis. Neutralization was used to minimize charge effects. C1s peak at 284.5 eV was used as reference. Shirley background was subtracted, and Gauss (70%)–Lorentz (30%) profiles were used. Full width at half maximum (FWHM) were fixed between 1.4 and 1.6 eV for O 1s, 1.6–1.7 eV for C 1s, and 1.7–1.8 eV for N 1s.

Specific surface area measurement (S_{BET}) was carried out using a Micromeritics Tristar II apparatus. Samples were outgassed in situ at 100 °C under a pressure of $ca.\approx$30 μbar. The measurements were performed at liquid N_2 temperature using N_2 as the adsorbing gas. The BET method was used in the calculation of surface area value from the isotherm of nitrogen adsorption. The mean apparent particle diameter was determined from surface area.

Zeta potentials were measured with a Malvern ZetasizerNano ZSP instrument (Worcestershire, UK) supplied by a DTS Nano V7.11 software (Worcestershire, UK). The suspensions of SPIONs were prepared in 10^{-2} M NaCl aqueous solutions. The pH of the suspension was adjusted from 3 to 11 by addition of HCl (0.1 M) or NaOH (0.1 M and 0.01 M) solutions. Hydrodynamic diameters were determined by Dynamic Light Scattering (DLS, Malvern, Worcestershire, UK) curves, which are derived from the number distribution calculation on the same instrument. Measurements were carried out three times at 25.0 °C, immediately after homogenization by ultrasound bath for 5 min, and using refractive index 2.42 for Fe_3O_4 and 1.33 for water (viscosity 0.8872 cP).

The weight losses of bare and grafted SPIONs were studied by thermogravimetric analyses (TGA) with a TA Instruments Discovery TGA (Newcastle, UK) under an air flow rate of 25 mL min^{-1}. The analyses were done using the following thermal program: ramp 1 of 20 °C.min^{-1} from 25 °C to 100 °C, isotherm at 100 °C for 30 min (to remove the remaining moisture), and ramp 2 of 5 °C min^{-1} from 100 °C to 700 °C. TGA weight losses were considered only from the second ramps.

Fourier transform infrared (FTIR) measurements were recorded on a Bruker IFS 28 (Billerica, MA, USA) using OPUS version 3.1 in the wavenumber range of 4000–400 cm^{-1}, with a resolution of 4 cm^{-1} and a total of 50 scans per measurement. Pellets were made of 0.5 mg sample mixed in 199.5 mg of dried KBr.

UV-visible spectroscopy (UV-vis) measurements were carried out using a Shimadzu UV-2550 UV-Vis spectrophotometer (Tokyo, Japan). All spectra were measured in the range of 220-800 nm and recorded at 23 °C using UV cuvettes of 1 cm path length.

2.3. Synthesis of 4'-Hydroxy-4-(3-aminopropoxy) Trans-Stilbene (HAPtS) Molecule

The 4'-hydroxy-4-(3-aminopropoxy)*trans*-stilbene (HAPtS) was synthesized by a Wittig reaction from 4-acetoxybenzyltriphenylphosphonium and N-3-(4-carbaldehydephenoxy)propylphtalimide. The Wittig reaction was carried out in phase transfer conditions [44] to give 4-acetoxy-4'-N-(3-O-propylphtalimide) *trans*-stilbene. The protective groups of latter molecule were removed to afford HAPtS. A detailed description, scheme, and NMR data of each reaction step of HAPtS synthesis are given in the Supplementary Materials (SM1).

2.4. Synthesis of Bare and Modified Nanoparticles

2.4.1. Synthesis of Bare SPIONs

Bare superparamagnetic iron oxide nanoparticles (SPIONs) were synthesized following a simple co-precipitation protocol. Briefly, a stoichiometric mixture of $FeCl_2 \cdot 4H_2O$ (12.72 g) solution and $FeCl_3 \cdot 6H_2O$ (34.58 g) solution was prepared in 1.5 L of deionized (DI) water in the molar ratio Fe^{2+}:Fe^{3+} = 1:2 at 25 °C. After the total dissolution of salts, 120 mL of ammonium hydroxide (28%) was added quickly to the solution and the SPIONs were precipitated immediately. The solution was kept under magnetic stirring for 2–3 minutes and then washed thoroughly with deionized (DI) water, using a magnetic separation, until the solution reached pH 8. The pH of the suspension was adjusted to pH 3 with HNO_3 solution (0.1 M). The obtained suspension was dialyzed for 76 h against pH 3 HNO_3 solution. After that, the suspension was centrifuged at 20,000 g for 15 min and only the supernatant was kept as a homogeneous and stable suspension. The final SPION concentration of 9.2 mg·mL^{-1} of nanoparticles was used for further surface modifications. A small amount of the obtained suspension was freeze-dried for characterization.

2.4.2. Synthesis of 3-Chlorporyltriethoxysilane-Modified SPIONs: SPIONs-CPTES

A total of 50 mg of as prepared SPIONs were dispersed in a mixture of EtOH and DI water, with a volume ratio 3:1. 600 µL of CPTES, which was added to the suspension and the pH was then adjusted to 4 with NaOH solution (0.1 M). The suspension was kept under magnetic stirring at 360 rpm for 24 h at 25 °C.

The purification of the grafted SPIONs from the unreacted CPTES was realized using an ultrafiltration device through an ultrafiltration membrane (regenerated cellulose, 30 kDa). The purification was carried on until the conductivity of the filtrate reached that of DI water (0.5 μS·cm^{-1}).

2.4.3. Synthesis of 4'-hydroxy-4-(3-aminopropoxy)-trans-stilbene-Modified SPIONs: SPIONs-CPTES-HAPtS

A total of 7.5 mg of CPTES-modified SPIONs (SPIONs-CPTES) were dispersed in anhydrous DMSO and 80 μL of DIEA (organic base), and 1.9 mg of HAPtS was added in excess to the SPIONs suspension (molar ratio HAPtS/grafted CPTES is 7:0.4). The suspension was kept under magnetic stirring (360 rpm) for 24 h at 25 °C. The purification was carried out by a magnetic decantation with DMSO and then DI water. The purification efficiency was controlled by UV-visible spectrometry (of the washing water).

After each synthesis step, a small amount of the SPIONs in suspension was freeze dried for 48 h to perform the suitable characterizations, and the rest of the samples were kept in suspension to avoid nanoparticles agglomeration during the drying step and to keep a good dispersion of SPIONs in water. Figure 2 summarizes the surface modification steps of bare SPIONs.

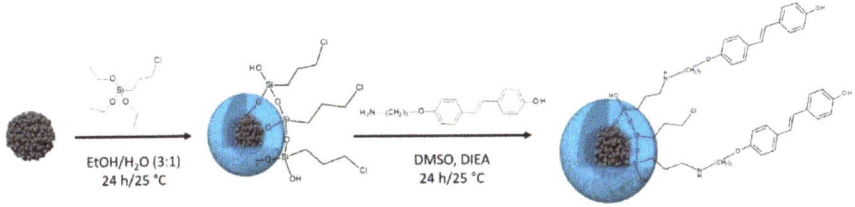

Figure 2. Schematic representation of the *trans*-resveratol derivative-modified SPIONs (SPIONs-CPTES-HAPtS) nanohybrid synthesis.

2.5. Biological Assays

2.5.1. Antioxidant Test: the Oxygen Radical Absorbance Capacity (ORAC) Assay

The antioxidant capacity of HAPtS was evaluated by the ORAC test, which measures the ability of a molecule to prevent or delay the oxidation of a fluorescent molecule (in this case fluorescein) in the presence of a free radical-generating (oxidizing) molecule, which is AAPH. The experiment was carried out according to the literature [6,45]. Briefly, the reaction was carried in a 96-well black plate, in 75 mM phosphate buffer (pH 7.4), and the final reaction mixture was 200 μL; 20μL of antioxidant (Trolox for calibration curves, HAPtS or RSV) molecules and 120 μL of fluorescein solution (final concentration of 50 nM) were added in the 96 wells of the microplate. The mixtures were incubated for 15 min at 37 °C, and 20 μL of AAPH solution (40 mM, final concentration) was added rapidly using the automate (Tecan machine). The fluorescence was recorded every minute for 80 min. The microplate was automatically shaken prior each reading.

The calibration curve was carried out using five calibration solutions of Trolox (1–50 μM, final concentration) and a blank of only fluorescein and AAPH was also used. All the reaction mixtures were prepared in triplicate. The obtained curves (fluorescence versus time) were normalized and the ORAC values (AUC) were calculated from the area under the fluorescence decay curve according to the following formula:

$$\text{AUC} = 1 + \sum_{i=1}^{i=80} f_i / f_0$$

where f_0: fluorescence read at 0 min and f_i: fluorescence read at i min.

The relative AUC values (expressed in equivalent Trolox) are determined as following:

$$AUC_{relative} = \frac{(AUC)_{sample}}{(AUC)_{Trolox}} \times \frac{[Trolox]}{[sample]}$$

2.5.2. Cell Culture

The C6 rat glioma cells were cultured at 25,000 cells.cm^{-2}, in 6-well or 96-well plates, in Dulbecco's modified Eagle medium (DMEM) with 10% heat inactivated fetal bovine serum FBS and 1% antibiotic (Penicillin, Streptomycin), as described by Nury et al. [46]. The cells were incubated at 37 °C in a humidified atmosphere containing 5% CO_2 and passaged twice a week. At each passage, cells were trypsinized with a 0.05% trypsin–0.02% ethylenediaminetetraacetic acid (EDTA) solution (Pan Biotech).

2.5.3. Clonogenic Survival Assay

Cell clonogenic survival assay is an in vitro cell survival assay based on the ability of a single cell to grow into a colony following insult with physical or chemical agents [47]. After cell incubation for 24 h with a density of 25,000 cells cm^{-2}, cells were exposed to the following compounds: RSV (50 µM), HAPtS (50 µM), grafted SPION (SPIONs-CPTES-HAPtS (determined volume of nanohybrids suspension which corresponds to 50 µM of grafted HAPtS)), SPIONs-CPTES, bare SPIONs, positive control (cells treated with a toxic molecule, 7β-hydroxycholesterol (7β-OHC), 100 µM). Data were compared to untreated cells. It is important to note that the masse of SPIONs-CPTES sample corresponds to that included in the sample SPIONs-CPTES-HAPtS and it is the same for bare SPIONs. At the end of treatment in 6-well plates, cells were trypsinized, counted on a Malassez hemocytometer using trypan blue dye (v:v), and 1000 cells were cultured in a 100 mm diameter Petri dish containing 10 mL of culture medium for 8 days. After 8 days of culture, the cells were stained with crystal violet solution to visualize the cell colonies (the culture medium was changed twice a week).

2.5.4. Cytotoxicity: MTT Assay

MTT (3-(4-,5-dimethylthiazol-2-yl)-2,5-diphenyltetrazolium bromide) assay was used to evaluate the effects of molecules and nanoparticles on cell viability and was carried out as described by Lizard et al. [48]. Cell viability was assessed as a function of the mitochondrial activity. Cells were seeded in 96-well plates at an initial seeding density of 25,000 cells·cm^{-2}, and incubated for 24 h at 37 °C, 5% CO_2. After exposure to RSV (0.5–50 µM), HAPtS (0.5–50 µM), bare SPIONs (50–500 µg·mL^{-1} of SPIONs), SPIONs-CPTES (50-500 µg·mL^{-1} of SPIONs), SPIONs-CPTES- HAPtS (50–500 µg·mL^{-1} of SPIONs), and 7β-OHC (100 µM) for 24 h, cells were incubated with MTT (0.05 mg·mL^{-1}) for 3 h in the dark. The formazan crystals formed were solubilized using 200 µL DMSO and absorbance was read at 570 nm with a microplate reader (Tecan, France).

2.5.5. Cytotoxicity: FDA (Fluorescein Diacetate) Assay

The FDA assay stains cells fluorescently green when they have intact cell membrane esterase activity. All non-FDA-fluorescent cells are considered dead [49]. Cells were seeded in 96-well plates at an initial seeding density of 25,000 cells/cm^{-2}, and incubated for 24 h at 37 °C, 5% CO_2. After exposure to RSV (0.5–50 µM), HAPtS (0.5–50 µM), bare SPIONs (50–500 µg·mL^{-1} of SPIONs), SPIONs-CPTES (50–500 µg·mL^{-1} of SPIONs), SPIONs-CPTES- HAPtS (50–500 µg·mL^{-1} of SPIONs), and 7β-OHC (100 µM) for 24 h, cells were washed twice with 200 µL PBS and then treated with 150 µL of FDA solution (50 µM) for 5 min at 37 °C. FDA solution was then removed and 150 µL of lysis buffer (aqueous solution with 10% (v/v) SDS and 0.079% (m/v) Tris HCl) was added. The 96-well plate was kept under magnetic stirring for 3 min and the fluorescence was read (λ_{exc} = 485 nm, λ_{em} = 528 nm) with a microplate reader (Tecan).

3. Results and Discussion

3.1. Characterization of the New RSV Derivative Molecule: HAPtS

Figure 3A shows the FTIR spectrum of the as-synthesized RSV derivative molecule. It proves the presence of most of the characteristic bands of the stilbene derivative—the stretching vibration bands of NH$_2$ and OH groups are situated at 3400 and 3290 cm^{-1}, respectively, and those of -CH$_2$ (νCH$_2$) are at 2951 and 2880 cm^{-1}. The stretching vibration band of ν C-O-C, ν C-O-H, and ν C-N bonds is illustrated by an intense wide band at 1250 cm^{-1}, as well as by two less intense and finer bands around 1030 and 1070 cm^{-1}. The vibration bands of C=C bonds in the aromatic and inter-aromatic rings are observed at 1560 cm^{-1} and 1600 cm^{-1}, respectively. Moreover, the bending vibration band of C-H in aromatic rings (δ C-H) is observed at 830 cm^{-1} [50]. All these bands are in common with those observed in the commercial RSV molecule and are consistent with the data in literature [51].

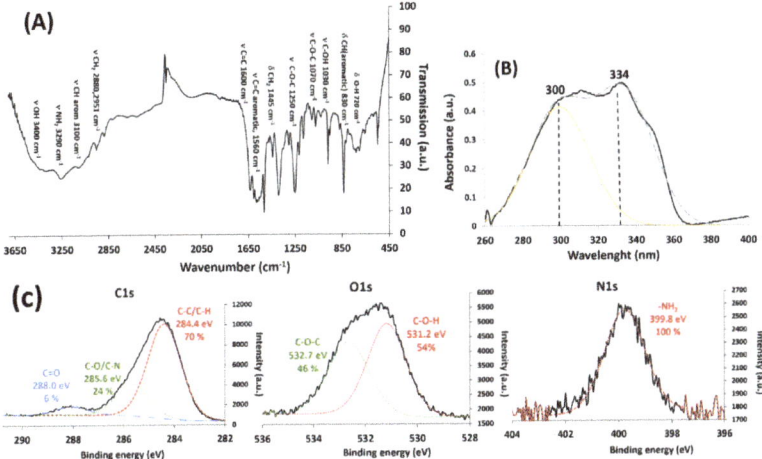

Figure 3. (**A**) Fourier-transform infrared (FTIR) spectrum, (**B**) UV-visible spectrum, and (**C**) fitted X-ray photoelectron spectroscopy (XPS) spectra of C1s, O1s, and N1s peaks of the synthesized RSV derivative molecule (HAPtS).

The fitted UV-Visible spectrum (fityk software) of HAPtS in DMSO, shown in Figure 3B, proves the presence of a broad band with two contributions centered at 300 and 334 nm, which are characteristic of the trans isomer of resveratrol molecule [52]. The second absorbance peak at 334 nm indicates the deprotonated form of resveratrol according to the study by Manuel et al. [53]. This form of stilbene derivative is justified by the use of potassium hydroxide (KOH) during the synthesis and the extraction process of HAPtS molecules (see Supplementary Materials SM1).

XPS analysis shows the experimental and the calculated elemental analysis of the synthesized stilbene derivative (Table 1). The presence of a small amount of silicon and calcium in the final product is due to the purification step, in which a chromatography on silica gel column was used. In order to better understand the type of chemical bonds in HAPtS molecule, a fitting of C1s, O1s, and N1s XPS spectra was carried out.

Table 1. Experimental and calculated XPS elemental analysis of HAPtS.

Element (%)	C1s	O1s	N1s	Si2p	Ca2p	C/N
Calculated	85.0	10.0	5.0	-	-	17
Experimental	81.1	14.3	3.4	0.4	0.8	23

Figure 3C shows three components in C1s XPS peak, which can be assigned to three types of carbons: C=O, C-O/C-N, and C-C/C-H, situated, respectively, at 288.0, 285.6, and 284.4 eV binding energies. However, according to the chemical structure of HAPtS (Figure 1), only two types of carbon should exist, which are C-C/C-H and C-O/C-N. This suggests that the presence of carbonyl groups (-C=O) could be attributed to the presence of calcium carbonate compounds, as the calcium exists as an impurity in the final product, and since K_2CO_3 is used along the synthesis (see SM1). This result explains the difference in the C/N ratio between the calculated and the experimental structure Table 1. On the other hand, Table 2 shows a similarity between the calculated or theoretical and the experimental percentages of the carbon, oxygen, and nitrogen chemical bonds, obtained from the fitting of XPS spectra in Figure 3C. Additionally, NMR data show the presence of the characteristic peak of HAPtS (SM1).

FTIR, UV-vis XPS, and NMR results suggest that the molecule synthesized is the sought stilbene derivative molecule—HAPtS.

Table 2. Comparison between the calculated and the experimental proportion of the chemical bonds obtained from the fitting of C1s, O1s, and N1s XPS peaks.

Element	C1s			O1s		N1s
Chemical bonds	C-C/C-H	C-O/C-N	C=O	H-O-C	C-O-C	$-NH_2$
Calculated (%)	76.5	23.5	-	50.0	50.0	100.0
Experimental (%)	70.0	24.0	6.0	54.0	46.0	100.0

Figure 4 gives the antioxidant capacity of RSV and HAPtS molecules, estimated by ORAC test and expressed in Trolox equivalent. The result indicates that the HAPtS has almost the same ORAC value as the RSV molecule, with 1.1 ± 0.1 and 0.9 ± 0.2 Trolox equivalent, respectively. This proves that the antioxidant capacity of HAPtS remains despite the chemical change and the presence of an alkyl chain.

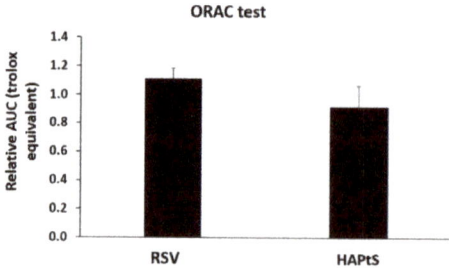

Figure 4. Antioxidant capacity measurement of *trans*-resveratrol (RSV) and chemically synthesized molecules (HAPtS).

3.2. Elaboration of HAPtS Nanocarrier Based on Superparamagnetic Iron Oxide Nanoparticles (SPIONs)

The crystallinity of the synthesized powder of bare SPIONs was checked by the XRD pattern, shown in Figure S1 (in Supplementary Materials), which corresponds to the spinel crystallographic phase of either magnetite (Fe_3O_4) or maghemite (γ-Fe_2O_3) with a crystallite size of 10.1 ± 0.1 nm. The lattice parameter, determined from XRD pattern, is 8.368 ± 0.001 Å and the diffracting planes are (220), (311), (400), (511), and (440). The interatomic distances observed on the selected area diffraction pattern of Fe_3O_4 are in agreement with the spinel structure (ICDD: 19-0629) [54]. The lattice parameter suggests that the powder is slightly oxidized ($Fe_{3(1-\delta)}O_4$ crystallites, with δ the deviation from oxygen stoichiometry and a small presence of γ-Fe_2O_3 on the surface) [55,56].

The specific surface area (S_{BET}) of bare SPIONs is 114.0 ± 0.5 $m^2 \cdot g^{-1}$. The calculated crystallite size from S_{BET} value is 10.1 ± 0.2 nm, which is in a good agreement with the XRD result. Moreover, the counting of hundreds of SPION nanoparticles from TEM images (Figure 5) gives an average size of 9.0 ± 2.0 nm, illustrating the two previous methods of crystallite size measurement (S_{BET} and XRD).

Figure 5 shows the evolution in the size of bare and functionalized SPIONs, assessed by dynamic light scattering (DLS) and TEM images. Unlike the latter that do not show a significant increase in the size of SPIONs after grafting, DLS measurements prove considerable changes in the hydrodynamic size (d_H) of the functionalized SPIONs. Indeed, the statistic measurement of nanoparticle size using TEM images shows an average size of about 9 nm for bare and grafted SPIONs (Table 3), however, Figure 5B,C suggests also the presence of an organic shell around the iron oxide inorganic core. The organic shell is considered for size measurements by DLS, but it cannot be the main reason for the increase of the d_H. Indeed, the particle size as measured by DLS is generally higher than the size of nanoparticles observed via TEM because it takes into account not only the hydration layer surrounding the nanoparticles but also the aggregated nanoparticles. This explains the size of bare SPIONs of 21 ± 8 nm and the increase in the hydrodynamic size after CPTES and HAPtS grafting to 26 ± 7 nm and 92 ± 20 nm, respectively (Figure 5D, Table 3).

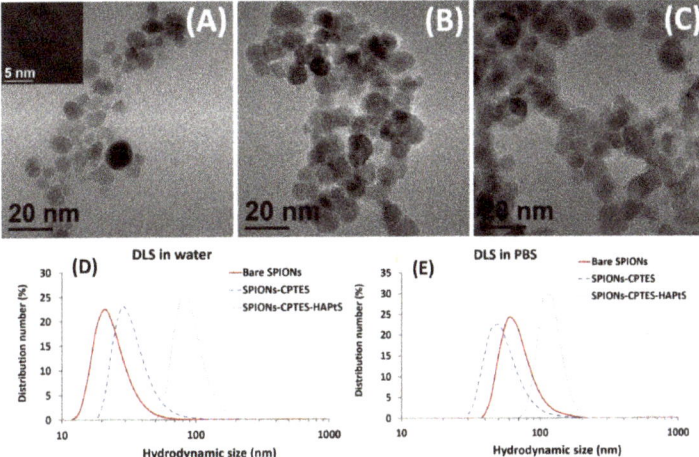

Figure 5. Transmission electron microscopy (TEM) images of (**A**) bare superparamagnetic iron nanoparticles (SPIONs) (inset: high resolution (HR)-TEM image of one nanoparticle), (**B**) SPIONs-CPTES, and (**C**) SPIONs-CPTES-HAPtS and dynamic light scattering (DLS) curves of bare and functionalized SPIONs in (**D**) water (10^{-2} NaCl) and (**E**) phosphate buffer solution (PBS) 0.1× (pH 7.4).

On the other side, the hydrodynamic size of bare SPIONs in water (pH 5) is different from that measured in PBS medium (60 ± 9 nm), since the pH of the latter is close to the isoelectric point (IEP) of bare SPIONs (Figure 6), which makes nanoparticles aggregate rapidly. The aggregation of bare SPIONs in PBS medium is also proved by the increase of the polydispersion index (PDI) from 0.157 to 0.489.

Table 3. Physico-chemical characteristics of bare and modified SPIONs.

Parameter		Bare SPIONs	SPIONs-CPTES	SPIONs-CPTES-HAPtS
	Isoelectric point	8.3	5.9	8.2
Hydrodynamic size in water	dH (number) (nm)	21 ± 8	26 ± 7	92 ± 20
	PDI	0.157 ± 0.004	0.189 ± 0.003	0.329 ± 0.026
	Z-average (nm)	67 ± 1	96 ± 5	145 ± 10
Hydrodynamic size in PBS 0.1×	dH (number) (nm)	60 ± 9	50 ± 8	118 ± 25
	PDI	0.489 ± 0.016	0.230 ± 0.004	0.410 ± 0.012
	Z-average (nm)	299 ± 16	135 ± 12	220 ± 8
	TEM measured diameter (nm)	9.0 ± 2.0	8.7 ± 1.5	9.6 ± 1.6

Figure 5E suggests that SPIONs-CPTES is the most stable sample in PBS medium, with the smallest hydrodynamic size (50 ± 8 nm), compared to SPIONs-CPTES-HAPtS sample (118 ± 25 nm). Moreover, Figure S2 in the Supplementary Information (SI) illustrates the improvement in the colloidal stability between the bare and functionalized SPIONs in PBS medium (pH 7.4) after 24 h. In fact, functionalized SPIONs remain in suspension with good colloidal stability compared to the poor stability of bare SPIONs, which completely settled. Nanoparticle aggregation of bare SPIONs are not observed in Figure 5E, since DLS measurements were carried out immediately after homogenization. We can conclude from the previous results that the increase of the hydrodynamic size in water (pH 5, 10^{-2} M NaCl) after the sequential grafting is explained by the increase of the hydration layer around the nanoparticles, but also due to nanoparticle aggregation, explained by the increase of interaction between nanohybrids. This interaction seems to increase after the grafting of the hydrophobic molecule, which is HAPtS through the pi-stacking bonds between the aromatic rings that could be intra and inter-nanoparticles during or after the surface modification of SPIONs. On the other side, when the medium changes, in particular the pH (7.4) and the ionic strength (PBS, 0.1×), the dH of all samples increases continuously, compared to dH in water. We notice also that the negatively charge nanoparticles as SPIONs-CPTES (Figure 6) have better colloidal stability in PBS medium than the positively charged samples (Bare SPIONs and SPIONs-CPTES-HAPtS). This result shows that the colloidal stability of the samples is also governed by the electrostatic interactions. On one side, the Debye length decreases with the increasing ionic strength, which favors the decrease of the particle repulsion, and thus the agglomeration. On the other side, when the pH of the medium increases, it becomes close to IEP of bare and SPIONs-CPTES-HAPtS, which explains also the increase of dH of these two samples. However, the aggregation phenomenon in SPIONs-CPTES-HAPtS is reduced compared to bare SPIONs due to the presence of two organic layers (CPTES and HAPtS). These two molecules bring steric repulsion that limit the interactions to pH 7.4. Otherwise, these results suggest that the surface modification of nanoparticles participate to stabilize the nanoparticles.

In order to better understand the evolution of the colloidal stability of the synthesized nanohybrids in biological medium, the hydrodynamic size of all samples was followed up in PBS medium (0.1×, pH7.4), with addition of bovine serum albumin as a function of the time at 37 °C. The results presented in Figure S3 show that bare SPIONs and SPIONs-CPTES-HAPtS have almost a constant dH during the time, approximately 125 nm and 65 nm, respectively, however, dH of SPIONs-CPTES decreases from 290 nm to about 200 nm. We notice that contrarily to PBS medium only, the addition of BSA has contributed to stabilizing bare SPIONs at physiological pH and decreases the dH of bare and HAPtS-modified SPIONs. However, BSA addition increases the dH of CPTES-modified SPIONs compared to PBS only. This result shows that the dispersion medium composition is very important in the control of the colloidal stability of nanoparticles, which was also proved in our previous work for titanate nanotubes [57]. The poor stability of SPIONs-CPTES sample can be explained by the interaction between BSA and the latter sample due to the presence of proteins containing free amine groups, which could interact with the free chloride in CPTES molecule.

Zeta potential measurements provide information about the surface modification of SPIONs following a molecule grafting, as well as about their colloidal stability. Figure 6 shows the evolution in the zeta potential curves as a function of pH for the synthesized nanohybrids. It illustrates a decrease in the zeta potential from about 40 mV to 20 mV, at the lowest imposed pH of about 3, and in the isoelectric point (IEP) from 8.2 to 5.9 after CPTES grafting. Although the organic chain in CPTES should not change the IEP of grafted SPIONs because it is considered as a neutral organofunctional silane, the decrease in the global surface charge may be due to the presence of silanol groups (Si-OH) on SPIONs surface, as is the case in silica nanoparticles, which exhibit a low IEP (below pH 3) [58]. After HAPtS grafting, the zeta potential as well as the IEP increase to about +30 and 8.3 mV, respectively, at the lowest imposed pH of about 3. Such a considerable shift is due to the presence of protonated amine group (pk_a between 9 and 10) in the trans-resveratrol derivative molecule, which leads to a positive surface charge on SPIONs' surface [58].

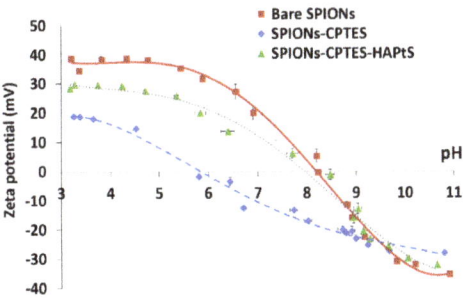

Figure 6. Zeta potential measurements of bare and functionalized SPIONs (10^{-2} M NaCl).

The synthesized nanohybrids were analyzed by infrared spectroscopy, where only the interesting part of the spectra are shown in Figure 7A, while the whole spectra are shown in Figure S4. The IR spectra illustrate the grafting of CPTES by the presence of its characteristic vibration bands, which are mainly the broad stretching vibration band of siloxane bonds (ν Si-O-Si) in the range between 1045 and 1000 cm^{-1} and the bending vibration band of Si-OH at 880 cm^{-1} [50,59]. Indeed, the vibration of Si-O-Si bond formation is due to the hydrolysis condensation mechanism of oligosiloxane containing Si-OH bonds [60]. In addition, the immobilization of HAPtS on SPION's surface is illustrated in Figure 7B by the presence of the stretching vibration band of the aromatic rings (ν C=C at 1560 and 1515 cm^{-1} and δ CH at 1308 cm^{-1}) and C-O bonds (ν C-O at 1250 and 1070 cm^{-1}). The stretching vibration bands of the alkyl chain (-CH$_2$-CH$_2$-) are also observed at 2960-2930 cm^{-1}.

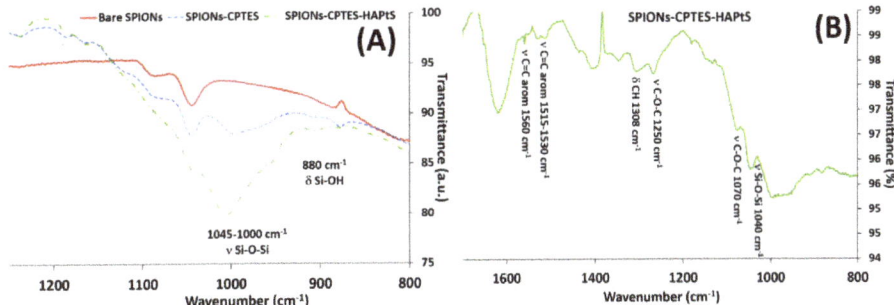

Figure 7. Infrared spectra of (**A**) bare SPIONs, SPIONs-CPTES, and SPIONs-CPTES-HAPtS (spectra range from 1250 to 800 cm^{-1}), and (**B**) SPIONs-CPTES-HAPtS (from 1700 to 800 cm^{-1}).

The elemental analysis by XPS shows the evolution in the surface chemistry of SPIONs depending on the kind of the grafted molecule (Table 4). Indeed, the CPTES grafting is proved by the appearance of new elements, which are silicon (5.3%) and chlorine (2.2%), besides the increase of the carbon proportion from 3% for bare SPIONs to 15% for SPIONs-CPTES sample. The amount of carbon continues to increase following the surface modification of SPIONs-CPTES with HAPtS to 21.6%. However, the decrease in Cl/Si ratio from 0.4 to 0.2 after HAPtS immobilization proves the reaction between CPTES and the stilbene derivative through a nucleophile substitution occurred between nitrogen and chlorine. This result corroborates the re-appearance of nitrogen in the SPIONs-CPTES-HAPtS sample (Table 4). On the other hand, the atomic percentages of iron and silicon decrease continuously after each grafting step, which can be explained by a partial hiding of the inorganic core by the organic shell on the surface.

Table 4. XPS elemental analysis of bare and functionalized SPIONs (atomic percentage).

Element (%)	C1s	O1s	Fe2p	N1s	Si2p	Cl2p	Cl/Si
Bare SPIONs	3.0	57.5	38.4	1.1	-	-	-
Element SPIONs/Fe	0.08	1.50	1.00	0.03			
SPIONs-CPTES	15.2	49.1	28.2	-	5.3	2.2	0.4
Element SPIONs-CPTES/Fe	0.54	1.74	1.00	-	0.19	0.07	-
SPIONs-CPTES-HAPtS	21.6	48.0	24.7	0.4	4.2	1.1	0.2
Element SPIONs-CPTES-HAPtS/Fe	0.87	1.94	1.00	0.02	0.17	0.04	-

In order to better investigate the change occurring in the chemical bonds on SPIONs surface, C1s and O1s XPS peaks are fitted, as is shown in Figure 8. It should be noted that the carbon present in bare SPIONs comes from the adventitious carbon contamination. C1s XPS peak of SPIONs-CPTES shows two components that correspond to two types of carbon bonds in this sample, which are C-C/C-H at 284.5 eV (77%), assigned to the organic alkyl chain, and C-Cl bond at 286.2 eV (23%). The high binding energy of C-Cl component can be explained by the high electronegativity of chlorine compared to hydrogen. It should be noted that it is not possible, in our case, to see the Si-C bond that must be overlapped by C-C/C-H peak. However, the experimental ratio of the percentage of Si-C bond (23%) regarding the total carbon bond is similar to the theoretical one (25%) (Figure 8). The C1s XPS peak for SPIONs-CPTES-HAPtS shows a decrease in the ratio between both contributions located at 286.0 eV and 284.5 eV (18%/80%), compared to that obtained for SPIONs-CPTES sample (23%/77%), which can be explained by the high amount of C-C/C-H bonds in HAPtS molecules.

The oxygen O1s XPS peak of bare SPIONs (Figure 8) shows the presence of two components—one is located at 530.1 eV and is attributed to the oxygen of the inorganic core (Fe-O-Fe), and the second at 531.7 eV corresponds to the surface oxygen bond Fe-OH [54]. After the first grafting step of the organosilane, a third component appears at high binding energy (532.5 eV) in the O1s peak of the SPIONs-CPTES sample. This component could be assigned to the Si-O-Si bonds of the oligosiloxane generated onto SPIONs surface. Moreover, the increase in O-H bond from 11% to 15% (Figure 8) can be also explained by the presence of silanol bonds (Si-O-H) in addition to those of Fe-OH. These results agree with the previous infrared analysis (Figure 7A). The percentage of O-H contribution increases continuously after the HAPtS grafting (19%), since in addition to Si-OH and Fe-OH bonds, there are C-OH bonds belonging to the RSV derivative. On the other hand, there is a decrease in the amount of Si-O bonds in SPIONs-CPTES-HAPtS to 3% instead of 7% in SPIONs-CPTES due to the presence of a thick organic shell that hides the inorganic core. The existence of N1s peak for SPIONs-CPTES-HAPtS, shown in Figure S5, proves the presence of HAPtS in this sample at a position almost similar to that of free HAPtS molecules (399.6 eV). It should be noted that the nitrogen present in bare SPIONs comes from the washing process in which HNO_3 solution is used.

The quantification of the immobilized trans-resveratrol derivatives (HAPtS) on SPIONs' surface is carried out using thermogravimetric and XPS analyses. Indeed, the TGA curve of bare SPIONs reveals the weight loss of physisorbed water at low temperatures (100–200 °C) and chemisorbed water at high temperatures (200–700 °C) (Figure 9). The weight loss of functionalized SPIONs comes not only from physi- and chemisorbed waters, but also from the loss of the organic layers on SPIONs' surface. This is also observed through the derivative curves of TG analysis (DTG), presented in Figure S6, which shows an increase in the DTG signal and the appearance of an additional peak after each grafting step. The grafting rate of SPIONs is expressed in molecule·nm^{-2} of SPIONs or μMol of grafted molecule·g^{-1} SPIONs (the calculation details are given in Supplementary Materials (SM2)). The weight loss of CPTES corresponds to the difference between the bare SPIONs and the SPIONs-CPTES sample, which is 2.6%, and the grafting rate is estimated at 1.8 CPTES/nm^2 (Table 5). However, on the subsequent functionalization step, the estimation of the grafting rate of HAPtS becomes more difficult, since two different molecules are present on SPIONs' surface (free CPTES and CPTES-HAPtS). Indeed, during the HAPtS grafting, 50% chlorine reacts with HAPtS, according to

XPS data (Table 4), and since chlorine represents about 46% of the molecular weight of the degraded molecules during the heating process (M(Cl) = 35.5 g·mol^{-1} and M((-CH$_2$-)$_3$) = 42 g·mol^{-1}), the real weight loss corresponding to the last grafting can be estimated at 3.6% (2.4 + (2.6 × 0.46)) instead of 2.4%.

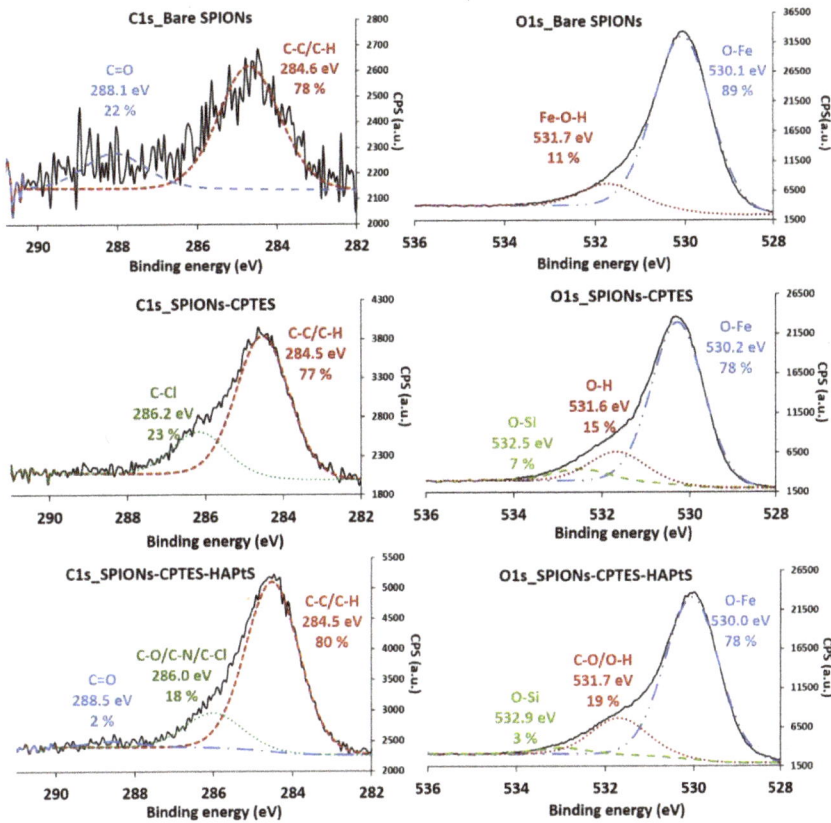

Figure 8. XPS spectra of C1s and O1s of bare SPIONs, SPIONs-CPTES, and SPIONs-CPTES-HAPtS samples.

Table 5. Thermogravimetric data and calculation of the number of molecules on SPIONs' surface.

Samples	Weight Loss (%)	Degraded Molecule during Heating		Compounds on SPIONs Surface	
		Chemical Formula	Molecular Weight (g·mol^{-1})	molecule·nm^{-2}	µmol·g^{-1} SPIONs
Bare SPIONs	3.5	H$_2$O	18	10.3 (OH)	1944 (OH)
SPIONs-CPTES	2.6	-(CH$_2$)$_3$-Cl	78	1.8 (CPTES)	340 (CPTES)
SPIONs-CPTES- HAPtS	3.6	-(CH$_2$)$_3$-NH-C$_{17}$H$_{17}$O$_2$	310	0.6 (HAPtS)	116 (HAPtS)

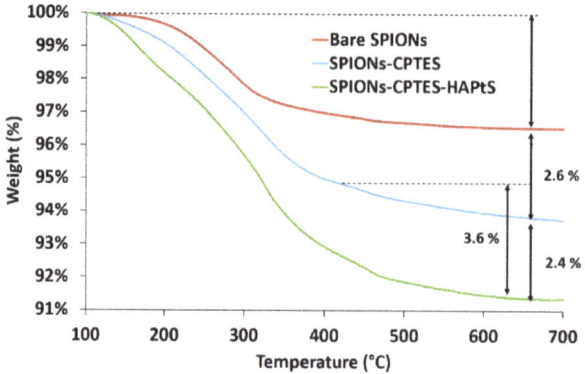

Figure 9. Thermogravimetric analysis (TGA) curves of bare and grafted SPIONs under air (100–700 °C).

3.3. Assessment of Nanohybrids Biological Efficiency

3.3.1. Cytotoxicity Assessment

The nanoparticles' cytotoxicity was studied by MTT and FDA tests in order to assess the effect of nanoparticles on the viability of C6 rat glioma cells. Indeed, the FDA test is a test for estimation of viable cells, where the fluorescein diacetate (FDA) passes through cell membranes and is then hydrolyzed by intracellular esterases (in living cells) to produce fluorescein, which is accumulated inside cells and exhibits green fluorescence [31]. This test assesses the cells viability through the cellular membrane injuries or damages. This test was carried out for RSV (50 µM), HAPtS (50 µM in RSV equivalent), bare, and grafted SPIONs (SPIONs-CPTES and SPIONs-CPTES-HAPtS) compared to the untreated cells (Ctrl), and the 7β-hydroxycholesterol (7β-OHC, 100 µM) was used as a positive control of toxicity.

The results of the FDA test suggest that the surface modified SPIONs (SPIONs-CPTES and SPIONs-CPTES-HAPtS) have a different effect on the cells membrane. Indeed, Figure 10A shows that no significant damage in the cellular membrane is observed for bare SPIONs, free RSV, and HAPtS molecules. However, a decrease in the fluorescence signal of cells treated with SPIONs-CPTES and SPIONs-CPTES-HAPtS is observed compared to the untreated cells, which supposes that these nanoparticles could damage the plasma membrane. This result does not exclude the interference of nanoparticles with this kind of assay, as it is known for the colorimetric and fluorimetric tests. Indeed, Arenda et al. [61] reported that the aggregation of nanoparticles has an effect on the quenching of the fluorescein's fluorescence. In order to illustrate this kind of interference, a fluorescence measurement was carried out for fluorescein with and without the presence of bare SPIONs (60 µg·mL^{-1}) (Figure S7). The result shows the decrease of the fluorescence signal to half immediately after the SPIONs addition, which illustrates the capacity of nanoparticles in the quenching of FITC fluorescence. As the interaction of cells–nanoparticles depends on the latter's surface chemistry, it is difficult to estimate the interference of the nanoparticles via this method. On the other hand, the MTT test evaluates the cells viability through assessing their metabolic activity (metabolically active mitochondria). Figure 10B shows that the quantity of cells remains almost the same for all studied samples. This suggests that the nanoparticles do not affect the mitochondrial activity. We should notice that the cell's viability of 120%, observed for SPIONs-CPTES, could be explained by nanoparticle interference [62]. To conclude, the obtained results with FDA and MTT tests suggest a negative impact of the SPIONs-CPTES-HAPtS on the plasma membrane without any effect on the mitochondrial activity. This does not allow any clear conclusion regarding the effect of nanoparticles on cell viability, which led to performing the clonogenic test.

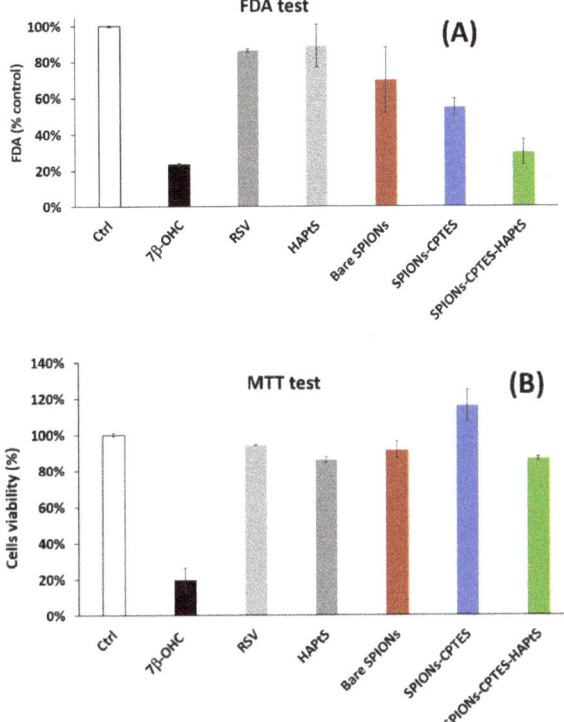

Figure 10. Cytotoxicity tests ((**A**) FDA and (**B**) MTT) for control (Ctrl; untreated cells), positive cytotoxic control (7β-OHC, 100 μM), RSV (50 μM), HAPtS (50 μM in RSV equivalent), bare SPIONs (the same amount as in SPIONs-CPTES-HAPtS), SPIONs-CPTES (the same amount as in SPIONs-CPTES-HAPtS), and SPIONs-CPTES-HAPtS (amount equivalent to 50 μM HAPtS). Incubation time of cells with molecules or nanoparticles was 24 h and cells are C6 rat glioma cells.

3.3.2. Clonogenic Assay

The clonogenic test evaluates the capacity of molecule/mixtures of molecules/nanoparticles to avoid the proliferation of cancerous cells after incubation for 24 h. This test permits assessment of the proliferation capacity of potentially viable cells (based on cells counting using trypan blue) after exposure to nanoparticles [28]. It was carried out on C6 rat glioma cells. The obtained results, shown in Figure 11, prove that RSV and HAPtS molecules have almost the same effect in reducing cell proliferation at a concentration of 50 μM, since they reduce the number and the size of colonies compared to control (untreated cells). On the other hand, bare SPIONs (500 μg·mL^{-1}) do not show any significant anti-clonogenic effect, since a similar number of colonies is formed with almost the same size. However, cells treated with functionalized SPIONs lose their capacity of proliferation (colonies formation), which is illustrated by the small number of the developed colonies for SPIONs-CPTES and SPIONs-CPTES-HAPtS samples. The slight cytotoxic effect observed in this work, with FDA and clonogenic tests for SPIONs-CPTES, has been also observed in the study of Bollu et al. for CPTES-modified mesoporous silica nanoparticles [63]. This result could be explained by the presence of the chlorinated organic carbon chain in the CPTES molecule [64]. We can consider that the cytotoxic effect linked to the CPTES molecule in the SPIONs-CPTES-HAPtS sample is neglected, since the amount of chlorine is reduced to the half (according to XPS analysis) and HAPtS is the main molecule that is in direct contact with the cells. The number of C6 cell colonies is expressed as anti-clonogenic activity and the results are shown in Figure S8 (control value is set to 0%). The anti-clonogenic activity of SPIONs-CPTES-HAPtS is higher than that obtained for free RSV and HAPtS, which proves the HAPtS molecule has the best efficiency in limiting the proliferation of cancerous C6 cells when it is associated with SPIONs at the same concentration.

The results obtained with clonogenic assay could be correlated with FDA results showing a possible damage of the cellular membrane caused by SPIONs-CPTES and SPIONs-CPTES-HAPtS nanoparticles, as is shown in Figure 10, which could be the main cause of the cell's incapacity to replicate. These preliminary results could be explained by the fact that SPIONs could: (i) favor the deregulation of localized signaling pathways at the level of plasma membrane involved in the life-death balance of the cells; (ii) contribute to better internalization of HAPtS inside the cell through endocytic vesicles [62,65]; (iii) increase the half-life of HAPtS in the cell by delaying its catabolism. These different points could contribute, at least in part, to the anti-proliferative and cytotoxic activity of HAPtS.

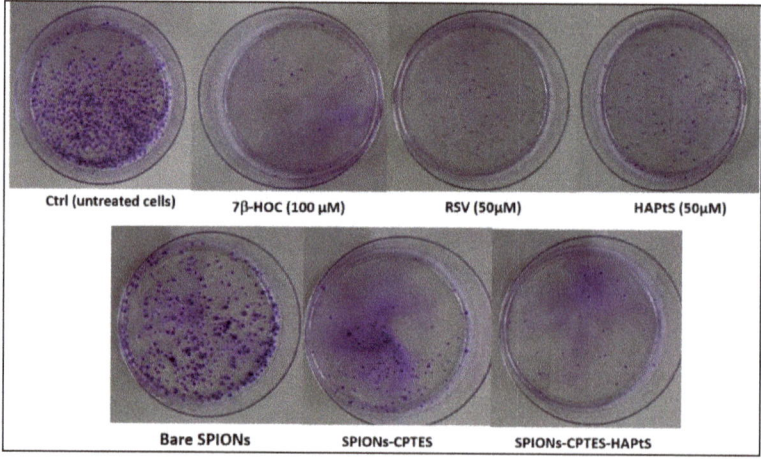

Figure 11. Pictures of Petri dishes of C6 cells at the end of the clonogenic assay (24 h of incubation with nanoparticles or molecules and 8 days of culture). Ctrl (untreated cells), positive cytotoxic control (7β-OHC, 100 µM), RSV (50 µM), HAPtS (50 µM in RSV equivalent), bare SPIONs (the same amount as in SPIONs-CPTES-HAPtS), SPIONs-CPTES (the same amount as in SPIONs-CPTES-HAPtS), and SPIONs-CPTES-HAPtS (amount equivalent to 50 µM HAPtS).

4. Conclusions

In this work, new nanohybrid materials based on superparamagnetic iron oxide nanoparticles have been elaborated to deliver a derivative of the RSV molecule, a natural compound known for its antioxidant activity, in order to elaborate new nanovectors for brain disease treatment. This molecule, HAPtS, was exclusively synthesized to be adapted for grafting onto SPIONs through an alkyl chain ending with a functional amine group. The evaluation of the antioxidant potential of this molecule by the ORAC test showed a similar antioxidant capacity to that obtained for RSV. The surface modification of SPIONs with HAPtS was carried out using the organosilane CPTES as a coupling agent and happened via a nucleophilic substitution reaction to yield 116 µMol of HAPtS per g of SPIONs, an amount estimated by thermogravimetric analysis. The elaborated nanohybrids were fully characterized by DLS and TEM images that show the evolution of the nanohybrids size and colloidal stability after the sequential grafting. The immobilized molecules grafted onto SPION's surface were also analyzed using zeta potential measurement, IR spectra, and XPS analysis, which permits illustration of the evolution of the surface chemistry of SPIONs and confirms the presence of an organic shell. The biological efficiency of elaborated nanoparticles was assessed by MTT, FDA, and clonogenic tests. The results show that SPIONs-CPTES-HAPtS damage the plasma membrane of C6 rat glioma cells; this side effect could subsequently limit the cell proliferation of C6 cells, making SPIONs-HAPtS potential candidates for targeted cancer treatment, including the glioma.

Supplementary Materials: The following are available online at http://www.mdpi.com/2079-4991/9/2/287/s1, Figure S1: XRD pattern of bare SPIONs (λ = 1.540598 Å). Figure S2: Photo showing the difference in the colloidal stability between bare SPIONs, SPIONs-CPTES, and SPIONs-HAPtS samples in PBS medium after 24 h (pH 7.4, 100 µg/mL of nanoparticles concentration). Figure S3: Hydrodynamic size vs. time of bare SPIONs, SPIONs-CPTES, and SPIONs-CPTES-HAPtS in PBS medium with bovine serum albumin (BSA, 40 g/L) at 37 °C. Figure S4: IR spectra of bare and functionalized SPIONs. Figure S5: XPS spectrum of N1s peak for SPIONs-HAPtS sample. Figure S6. Derivative of TGA curves of bare SPIONs, SPIONs-CPTES, and SPIONs-CPTES-HAPtS. Figure S7: Excitation and emission spectra of fluorescein with and without the presence of bare SPIONs showing the fluorescence quenching effect of SPIONs at the concentration 60 µg·mL^{-1} in PBS 0.1×. Figure S8: Anti-clonogenic activity (expressed in %, control value is set to 0%) on C6 cells after 24 h of incubation with nanoparticles or molecules and 8 days of culture. Ctrl, untreated cells, positive cytotoxic control (7β-OHC, 100 µM), RSV (50 µM), HAPtS (50 µM), bare SPIONs (the same amount as in SPIONs-CPTES-HAPtS), SPIONs-CPTES (the same amount as in SPIONs-CPTES-HAPtS), and SPIONs-CPTES-HAPtS (amount equivalent to 50 µM HAPtS).

Author Contributions: Conceptualization and methodology, F.S., D.V.-F., G.L., and N.M.; investigation, J.B., L.M., and F.S.; writing—original draft preparation, F.S.; writing—review and editing, N.M., J.B., L.M., and G.L.; supervision and project administration, N.M.; chemical organic synthesis, R.H. and D.V.-F.; biological experiments, F.S. and T.N.; biological data analysis, F.S. and G.L.

Funding: This research was funded by the French Government through the CNRS, the "Université de Bourgogne" and the "Conseil Régional de Bourgogne" through the 3MIM integrated project ("Marquage de Molécules par les Métaux pour l'Imagerie Médicale"). This work is also part of the projects "Pharmacoimagerie et agents théranostiques" and "Nano2bio", both funded by the "Université de Bourgogne" and the "Conseil Régional de Bourgogne" through the "Plan d'Actions Régional pour l'Innovation (PARI") and the European Union through the PO FEDER-FSE Bourgogne 2014/2020 programs.

Acknowledgments: The authors would like to thank Olivier Heintz for XPS analysis, Rémi Chassagnon for TEM images, Christine Goze for fluorescence measurements, and Nicolas Geoffroy for XRD pattern.

Conflicts of Interest: The authors declare no conflict of interest.

References

1. Wenzel, E.; Somoza, V. Metabolism and bioavailability of trans-resveratrol. *Mol. Nutr. Food Res.* **2005**, *49*, 472–481. [CrossRef] [PubMed]
2. Siemann, E.; Creasy, L. Concentration of the phytoalexin resveratrol in wine. *Am. J. Enol. Vitic.* **1992**, *43*, 49–52.
3. Frankel, E.; German, J.; Kinsella, J.; Parks, E.; Kanner, J. Inhibition of oxidation of human low-density lipoprotein by phenolic substances in red wine. *Lancet* **1993**, *341*, 454–457. [CrossRef]
4. Stivala, L.A.; Savio, M.; Carafoli, F.; Perucca, P.; Bianchi, L.; Maga, G.; Forti, L.; Pagnoni, U.M.; Albini, A.; Prosperi, E. Specific structural determinants are responsible for the antioxidant activity and the cell cycle effects of resveratrol. *J. Boil. Chem.* **2001**, *276*, 22586–22594. [CrossRef] [PubMed]
5. Chalal, M.; Klinguer, A.; Echairi, A.; Meunier, P.; Vervandier-Fasseur, D.; Adrian, M. Antimicrobial activity of resveratrol analogues. *Molecules* **2014**, *19*, 7679–7688. [CrossRef] [PubMed]
6. Tili, E.; Michaille, J.-J.; Adair, B.; Alder, H.; Limagne, E.; Taccioli, C.; Ferracin, M.; Delmas, D.; Latruffe, N.; Croce, C.M. Resveratrol decreases the levels of miR−155 by upregulating miR-663, a microRNA targeting JunB and JunD. *Carcinogenesis* **2010**, *31*, 1561–1566. [CrossRef] [PubMed]
7. Aggarwal, B.B.; Bhardwaj, A.; Aggarwal, R.S.; Seeram, N.P.; Shishodia, S.; Takada, Y. Role of resveratrol in prevention and therapy of cancer: Preclinical and clinical studies. *Anticancer Res.* **2004**, *24*, 2783–2840. [PubMed]
8. Holmes-McNary, M.; Baldwin, A.S. Chemopreventive properties of trans-resveratrol are associated with inhibition of activation of the IκB kinase. *Cancer Res.* **2000**, *60*, 3477–3483. [PubMed]
9. Athar, M.; Back, J.H.; Tang, X.; Kim, K.H.; Kopelovich, L.; Bickers, D.R.; Kim, A.L. Resveratrol: A review of preclinical studies for human cancer prevention. *Toxicol. Appl. Pharmacol.* **2007**, *224*, 274–283. [CrossRef] [PubMed]
10. Perez-Campo, R.; López-Torres, M.; Cadenas, S.; Rojas, C.; Barja, G. The rate of free radical production as a determinant of the rate of aging: Evidence from the comparative approach. *J. Comp. Physiol. B* **1998**, *168*, 149–158. [CrossRef] [PubMed]

11. Beckman, K.B.; Ames, B.N. The Free Radical Theory of Aging Matures. *Physiol. Rev.* **1998**, *78*, 547–581. [CrossRef] [PubMed]
12. Sun, A.Y.; Wang, Q.; Simonyi, A.; Sun, G.Y. Resveratrol as a Therapeutic Agent for Neurodegenerative Diseases. *Mol. Neurobiol.* **2010**, *41*, 375–383. [CrossRef] [PubMed]
13. Ranney, A.; Petro, M.S. Resveratrol protects spatial learning in middle-aged C57BL/6 mice from effects of ethanol. *Behav. Pharmacol.* **2009**, *20*, 330–336. [CrossRef] [PubMed]
14. Wang, Q.; Xu, J.; Rottinghaus, G.E.; Simonyi, A.; Lubahn, D.; Sun, G.Y.; Sun, A.Y. Resveratrol protects against global cerebral ischemic injury in gerbils. *Brain Res.* **2002**, *958*, 439–447. [CrossRef]
15. Kim, D.; Nguyen, M.D.; Dobbin, M.M.; Fischer, A.; Sananbenesi, F.; Rodgers, J.T.; Delalle, I.; Baur, J.A.; Sui, G.; Armour, S.M.; et al. SIRT1 deacetylase protects against neurodegeneration in models for Alzheimer's disease and amyotrophic lateral sclerosis. *EMBO J.* **2007**, *26*, 3169–3179. [CrossRef] [PubMed]
16. Kuhnle, G.; Spencer, J.P.; Chowrimootoo, G.; Schroeter, H.; Debnam, E.S.; Srai, S.K.S.; Rice-Evans, C.; Hahn, U. Resveratrol is absorbed in the small intestine as resveratrol glucuronide. *Biochem. Biophys. Res. Commun.* **2000**, *272*, 212–217. [CrossRef] [PubMed]
17. Bertelli, A.; Giovannini, L.; Stradi, R.; Urien, S.; Tillement, J.; Bertelli, A. Kinetics of trans-and cis-resveratrol (3,4′,5-trihydroxystilbene) after red wine oral administration in rats. *Int. J. Clin. Pharmacol. Res.* **1996**, *16*, 77–81. [PubMed]
18. Summerlin, N.; Soo, E.; Thakur, S.; Qu, Z.; Jambhrunkar, S.; Popat, A. Resveratrol nanoformulations: Challenges and opportunities. *Int. J. Pharm.* **2015**, *479*, 282–290. [CrossRef] [PubMed]
19. Spigno, G.; Donsì, F.; Amendola, D.; Sessa, M.; Ferrari, G.; De Faveri, D.M. Nanoencapsulation systems to improve solubility and antioxidant efficiency of a grape marc extract into hazelnut paste. *J. Food Eng.* **2013**, *114*, 207–214. [CrossRef]
20. Lee, C.-W.; Yen, F.-L.; Huang, H.-W.; Wu, T.-H.; Ko, H.-H.; Tzeng, W.-S.; Lin, C.-C. Resveratrol nanoparticle system improves dissolution properties and enhances the hepatoprotective effect of resveratrol through antioxidant and anti-inflammatory pathways. *J. Agric. Food Chem.* **2012**, *60*, 4662–4671. [CrossRef] [PubMed]
21. Isailović, B.D.; Kostić, I.T.; Zvonar, A.; Đorđević, V.B.; Gašperlin, M.; Nedović, V.A.; Bugarski, B.M. Resveratrol loaded liposomes produced by different techniques. *Innov. Food Sci. Emerg. Technol.* **2013**, *19*, 181–189. [CrossRef]
22. Blond, J.; Denis, M.; Bezard, J. Antioxidant action of resveratrol in lipid peroxidation. *Sci. Aliment. (France)* **1995**, *15*, 347–358.
23. Pando, D.; Gutiérrez, G.; Coca, J.; Pazos, C. Preparation and characterization of niosomes containing resveratrol. *J. Food Eng.* **2013**, *117*, 227–234. [CrossRef]
24. Pando, D.; Caddeo, C.; Manconi, M.; Fadda, A.M.; Pazos, C. Nanodesign of olein vesicles for the topical delivery of the antioxidant resveratrol. *J. Pharm. Pharmacol.* **2013**, *65*, 1158–1167. [CrossRef] [PubMed]
25. Peng, H.; Xiong, H.; Li, J.; Xie, M.; Liu, Y.; Bai, C.; Chen, L. Vanillin cross-linked chitosan microspheres for controlled release of resveratrol. *Food Chem.* **2010**, *121*, 23–28. [CrossRef]
26. Kim, S.; Ng, W.K.; Dong, Y.; Das, S.; Tan, R.B. Preparation and physicochemical characterization of trans-resveratrol nanoparticles by temperature-controlled antisolvent precipitation. *J. Food Eng.* **2012**, *108*, 37–42. [CrossRef]
27. Wang, M.; Li, L.; Zhang, X.; Liu, Y.; Zhu, R.; Liu, L.; Fang, Y.; Gao, Z.; Gao, D. Magnetic Resveratrol Liposomes as a New Theranostic Platform for Magnetic Resonance Imaging Guided Parkinson's Disease Targeting Therapy. *ACS Sustain. Chem. Eng.* **2018**, *6*, 17124–17133. [CrossRef]
28. Shukla, S.P.; Roy, M.; Mukherjee, P.; Das, L.; Neogy, S.; Srivastava, D.; Adhikari, S. Size Selective Green Synthesis of Silver and Gold Nanoparticles: Enhanced Antibacterial Efficacy of Resveratrol Capped Silver Sol. *J. Nanosci. Nanotechnol.* **2016**, *16*, 2453–2463. [CrossRef] [PubMed]
29. Park, S.; Cha, S.-H.; Cho, I.; Park, S.; Park, Y.; Cho, S.; Park, Y. Antibacterial nanocarriers of resveratrol with gold and silver nanoparticles. *Mater. Sci. Eng. C* **2016**, *58*, 1160–1169. [CrossRef] [PubMed]
30. Ganesh Kumar, C.; Poornachandra, Y.; Mamidyala, S.K. Green synthesis of bacterial gold nanoparticles conjugated to resveratrol as delivery vehicles. *Colloids Surf. B Biointerfaces* **2014**, *123*, 311–317. [CrossRef] [PubMed]
31. Laurent, S.; Forge, D.; Port, M.; Roch, A.; Robic, C.; Vander Elst, L.; Muller, R.N. Magnetic Iron Oxide Nanoparticles: Synthesis, Stabilization, Vectorization, Physicochemical Characterizations, and Biological Applications. *Chem. Rev.* **2008**, *108*, 2064–2110. [CrossRef] [PubMed]

32. Canet, E.; Revel, D.; Forrat, R.; Baldy-Porcher, C.; de Lorgeril, M.; Sebbag, L.; Vallee, J.-P.; Didier, D.; Amiel, M. Superparamagnetic iron oxide particles and positive enhancement for myocardial perfusion studies assessed by subsecond T1-weighted MRI. *Magn. Reson. Imaging* **1993**, *11*, 1139–1145. [CrossRef]
33. Thomas, G.; Demoisson, F.; Chassagnon, R.; Popova, E.; Millot, N. One-step continuous synthesis of functionalized magnetite nanoflowers. *Nanotechnology* **2016**, *27*, 135604. [CrossRef] [PubMed]
34. Gupta, A.K.; Gupta, M. Synthesis and surface engineering of iron oxide nanoparticles for biomedical applications. *Biomaterials* **2005**, *26*, 3995–4021. [CrossRef] [PubMed]
35. Perez, J.M.; Josephson, L.; Weissleder, R. Use of Magnetic Nanoparticles as Nanosensors to Probe for Molecular Interactions. *ChemBioChem* **2004**, *5*, 261–264. [CrossRef] [PubMed]
36. Arruebo, M.; Fernández-Pacheco, R.; Ibarra, M.R.; Santamaría, J. Magnetic nanoparticles for drug delivery. *Nano Today* **2007**, *2*, 22–32. [CrossRef]
37. Saraiva, C.; Praça, C.; Ferreira, R.; Santos, T.; Ferreira, L.; Bernardino, L. Nanoparticle-mediated brain drug delivery: Overcoming blood–brain barrier to treat neurodegenerative diseases. *J. Control. Release* **2016**, *235*, 34–47. [CrossRef] [PubMed]
38. Champagne, P.-O.; Westwick, H.; Bouthillier, A.; Sawan, M. Colloidal stability of superparamagnetic iron oxide nanoparticles in the central nervous system: A review. *Nanomedicine* **2018**, *13*, 1385–1400. [CrossRef] [PubMed]
39. Chertok, B.; Moffat, B.A.; David, A.E.; Yu, F.; Bergemann, C.; Ross, B.D.; Yang, V.C. Iron oxide nanoparticles as a drug delivery vehicle for MRI monitored magnetic targeting of brain tumors. *Biomaterials* **2008**, *29*, 487–496. [CrossRef] [PubMed]
40. Chertok, B.; David, A.E.; Yang, V.C. Polyethyleneimine-modified iron oxide nanoparticles for brain tumor drug delivery using magnetic targeting and intra-carotid administration. *Biomaterials* **2010**, *31*, 6317–6324. [CrossRef] [PubMed]
41. Tabatabaei, S.N.; Girouard, H.; Carret, A.-S.; Martel, S. Remote control of the permeability of the blood–brain barrier by magnetic heating of nanoparticles: A proof of concept for brain drug delivery. *J. Control. Release* **2015**, *206*, 49–57. [CrossRef] [PubMed]
42. Dan, M.; Cochran, D.B.; Yokel, R.A.; Dziubla, T.D. Binding, Transcytosis and Biodistribution of Anti-PECAM–1 Iron Oxide Nanoparticles for Brain-Targeted Delivery. *PLoS ONE* **2013**, *8*, e81051. [CrossRef] [PubMed]
43. Chalal, M.; Delmas, D.; Meunier, P.; Latruffe, N.; Vervandier-Fasseur, D. Inhibition of cancer derived cell lines proliferation by synthesized hydroxylated stilbenes and new ferrocenyl-stilbene analogs. Comparison with resveratrol. *Molecules* **2014**, *19*, 7850–7868. [CrossRef] [PubMed]
44. Daubresse, N.; Francesch, C.; Rolando, C. Phase transfer Wittig reaction with 1,3-dioxolan-2-yl-methyltriphenyl phosphonium salts: An efficient method for vinylogation of aromatic aldehydes. *Tetrahedron* **1998**, *54*, 10761–10770. [CrossRef]
45. Sabale, S.; Kandesar, P.; Jadhav, V.; Komorek, R.; Motkuri, R.K.; Yu, X.-Y. Recent developments in the synthesis, properties, and biomedical applications of core/shell superparamagnetic iron oxide nanoparticles with gold. *Biomater. Sci.* **2017**, *5*, 2212–2225. [CrossRef] [PubMed]
46. Nury, T.; Zarrouk, A.; Ragot, K.; Debbabi, M.; Riedinger, J.-M.; Vejux, A.; Aubourg, P.; Lizard, G. 7-Ketocholesterol is increased in the plasma of X-ALD patients and induces peroxisomal modifications in microglial cells: Potential roles of 7-ketocholesterol in the pathophysiology of X-ALD. *J. Steroid Biochem. Mol. Boil.* **2017**, *169*, 123–136. [CrossRef] [PubMed]
47. Franken, N.A.P.; Rodermond, H.M.; Stap, J.; Haveman, J.; van Bree, C. Clonogenic assay of cells in vitro. *Nat. Protoc.* **2006**, *1*, 2315. [CrossRef] [PubMed]
48. Lizard, G.; Gueldry, S.; Deckert, V.; Gambert, P.; Lagrost, L. Evaluation of the cytotoxic effects of some oxysterols and of cholesterol on endothelial cell growth: Methodological aspects. *Pathol. Biol. (Paris)* **1997**, *45*, 281–290. [PubMed]
49. Garvey, M.; Moriceau, B.; Passow, U. Applicability of the FDA assay to determine the viability of marine phytoplankton under different environmental conditions. *Mar. Ecol. Prog. Ser.* **2007**, *352*, 17–26. [CrossRef]
50. Socrates, G. *Infrared and Raman Characteristic Group Frequencies: Tables and Charts*; John Wiley & Sons: Chichester, UK, 2004.
51. Zhou, Z.; Li, W.; Sun, W.-J.; Lu, T.; Tong, H.H.; Sun, C.C.; Zheng, Y. Resveratrol cocrystals with enhanced solubility and tabletability. *Int. J. Pharm.* **2016**, *509*, 391–399. [CrossRef] [PubMed]

52. Trela, B.C.; Waterhouse, A.L. Resveratrol: Isomeric Molar Absorptivities and Stability. *J. Agric. Food Chem.* **1996**, *44*, 1253–1257. [CrossRef]
53. López-Nicolás, J.M.; García-Carmona, F. Aggregation state and p K a values of (E)-resveratrol as determined by fluorescence spectroscopy and UV– visible absorption. *J. Agric. Food Chem.* **2008**, *56*, 7600–7605. [CrossRef] [PubMed]
54. Thomas, G.; Demoisson, F.; Boudon, J.; Millot, N. Efficient functionalization of magnetite nanoparticles with phosphonate using a one-step continuous hydrothermal process. *Dalton Trans.* **2016**, *45*, 10821–10829. [CrossRef] [PubMed]
55. Guigue-Millot, N.; Champion, Y.; Hÿtch, M.J.; Bernard, F.; Bégin-Colin, S.; Perriat, P. Chemical Heterogeneities in Nanometric Titanomagnetites Prepared by Soft Chemistry and Studied Ex Situ: Evidence for Fe-Segregation and Oxidation Kinetics. *J. Phys. Chem. B* **2001**, *105*, 7125–7132. [CrossRef]
56. Perriat, P.; Fries, E.; Millot, N.; Domenichini, B. XPS and EELS investigations of chemical homogeneity in nanometer scaled Ti-ferrites obtained by soft chemistry. *Solid State Ion.* **1999**, *117*, 175–184. [CrossRef]
57. Sallem, F.; Boudon, J.; Heintz, O.; Séverin, I.; Megriche, A.; Millot, N. Synthesis and characterization of chitosan-coated titanate nanotubes: Towards a new safe nanocarrier. *Dalton Trans.* **2017**, *46*, 15386–15398. [CrossRef] [PubMed]
58. Jesionowski, T.; Ciesielczyk, F.; Krysztafkiewicz, A. Influence of selected alkoxysilanes on dispersive properties and surface chemistry of spherical silica precipitated in emulsion media. *Mater. Chem. Phys.* **2010**, *119*, 65–74. [CrossRef]
59. Ishida, H.; Koenig, J.L. Fourier transform infrared spectroscopic study of the structure of silane coupling agent on E-glass fiber. *J. Colloid Interface Sci.* **1978**, *64*, 565–576. [CrossRef]
60. Chuang, W.; Geng-sheng, J.; Lei, P.; Bao-lin, Z.; Ke-zhi, L.; Jun-long, W. Influences of surface modification of nano-silica by silane coupling agents on the thermal and frictional properties of cyanate ester resin. *Results Phys.* **2018**, *9*, 886–896. [CrossRef]
61. Aranda, A.; Sequedo, L.; Tolosa, L.; Quintas, G.; Burello, E.; Castell, J.V.; Gombau, L. Dichloro-dihydro-fluorescein diacetate (DCFH-DA) assay: A quantitative method for oxidative stress assessment of nanoparticle-treated cells. *Toxicol. Vitro* **2013**, *27*, 954–963. [CrossRef] [PubMed]
62. Maurizi, L.; Papa, A.-L.; Dumont, L.; Bouyer, F.; Walker, P.; Vandroux, D.; Millot, N. Influence of surface charge and polymer coating on internalization and biodistribution of polyethylene glycol-modified iron oxide nanoparticles. *J. Biomed. Nanotechnol.* **2015**, *11*, 126–136. [CrossRef] [PubMed]
63. Bollu, V.S.; Barui, A.K.; Mondal, S.K.; Prashar, S.; Fajardo, M.; Briones, D.; Rodríguez-Diéguez, A.; Patra, C.R.; Gómez-Ruiz, S. Curcumin-loaded silica-based mesoporous materials: Synthesis, characterization and cytotoxic properties against cancer cells. *Mater. Sci. Eng. C* **2016**, *63*, 393–410. [CrossRef] [PubMed]
64. Geerlings, P.; Tafazoli, M.; Kirsch-Volders, M.; Baeten, A. In vitro mutagenicity and genotoxicity study of a number of short-chain chlorinated hydrocarbons using the micronudeus test and the alkaline single cell gel electrophoresis technique (Comet assay) in human lymphocytes: A structure–activity relationship (QSAR) analysis of the genotoxic and cytotoxic potential. *Mutagenesis* **1998**, *13*, 115–126. [CrossRef]
65. Sruthi, S.; Maurizi, L.; Nury, T.; Sallem, F.; Boudon, J.; Riedinger, J.M.; Millot, N.; Bouyer, F.; Lizard, G. Cellular interactions of functionalized superparamagnetic iron oxide nanoparticles on oligodendrocytes without detrimental side effects: Cell death induction, oxidative stress and inflammation. *Colloids Surf. B Biointerfaces* **2018**, *170*, 454–462. [CrossRef] [PubMed]

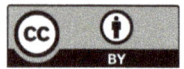

© 2019 by the authors. Licensee MDPI, Basel, Switzerland. This article is an open access article distributed under the terms and conditions of the Creative Commons Attribution (CC BY) license (http://creativecommons.org/licenses/by/4.0/).

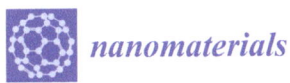

Article

Magnetic Alginate/Chitosan Nanoparticles for Targeted Delivery of Curcumin into Human Breast Cancer Cells

Wenxing Song [1,2], Xing Su [3], David Alexander Gregory [1], Wei Li [4], Zhiqiang Cai [2] and Xiubo Zhao [1,2,*]

1. Department of Chemical and Biological Engineering, University of Sheffield, Sheffield S1 3JD, UK; wsong4@sheffield.ac.uk (W.S.); d.a.gregory@sheffield.ac.uk (D.A.G.)
2. School of Pharmaceutical Engineering and Life Science, Changzhou University, Changzhou 213164, China; zhqcai@cczu.edu.cn
3. Department of Materials Science and Engineering, University of Sheffield, Sheffield S1 3JD, UK; whitesnowleopard@126.com
4. Department of Electronic and Electrical Engineering, University of Sheffield, Sheffield S3 7HQ, UK; WLi27@sheffield.ac.uk
* Correspondence: xiubo.zhao@sheffield.ac.uk; Tel.: +44-114-222-8256

Received: 27 September 2018; Accepted: 2 November 2018; Published: 5 November 2018

Abstract: Curcumin is a promising anti-cancer drug, but its applications in cancer therapy are limited, due to its poor solubility, short half-life and low bioavailability. In this study, curcumin loaded magnetic alginate/chitosan nanoparticles were fabricated to improve the bioavailability, uptake efficiency and cytotoxicity of curcumin to Human Caucasian Breast Adenocarcinoma cells (MDA-MB-231). Alginate and chitosan were deposited on Fe_3O_4 magnetic nanoparticles based on their electrostatic properties. The nanoparticle size ranged from 120–200 nm, within the optimum range for drug delivery. Controllable and sustained release of curcumin was obtained by altering the number of chitosan and alginate layers on the nanoparticles. Confocal fluorescence microscopy results showed that targeted delivery of curcumin with the aid of a magnetic field was achieved. The fluorescence-activated cell sorting (FACS) assay indicated that MDA-MB-231 cells treated with curcumin loaded nanoparticles had a 3–6 fold uptake efficiency to those treated with free curcumin. The 3-(4,5-Dimethylthiazol-2-yl)-2,5-Diphenyltetrazolium Bromide (MTT) assay indicated that the curcumin loaded nanoparticles exhibited significantly higher cytotoxicity towards MDA-MB-231 cells than HDF cells. The sustained release profiles, enhanced uptake efficiency and cytotoxicity to cancer cells, as well as directed targeting make MACPs promising candidates for cancer therapy.

Keywords: alginate; chitosan; layer-by-layer; magnetic nanoparticles; drug delivery; cancer; curcumin

1. Introduction

Curcumin (CUR) is a yellow, hydrophobic, polyphenolic compound of turmeric that is extracted from the rhizomes of *Curcuma longa*, which are widely cultivated in Asian countries, such as India and China, and have been historically used as a spice [1]. CUR is generally recognised as safe (GRAS) by the Food and Drug Administration (FDA) [1], and has been widely used in medicine due to its anti-oxidant [2–4], anti-inflammatory [5–7], wound-healing [8,9] and anti-bacterial [10,11] properties. Recent research has demonstrated that CUR has the ability to inhibit carcinogenesis in various cell lines, including breast, colon and gastric cancer cells, which has resulted in an increased interest as a promising anticancer drug [12–15]. However, CUR exhibits poor solubility in aqueous solutions, limiting its applications for cancer therapy [16–18].

It has been reported that after an oral administration of 2 g/kg of CUR in humans an extremely low serum concentration (0.006 ± 0.005 µg/mL) of CUR was observed after 1 h [19]. As a result, the bioavailability and anti-cancer efficiency of CUR is limited by its low solubility [16–18]. In order to improve the bioavailability, various nanocarriers have been used, including lipid-based nanoparticles [20–24], polymer nanoparticles [17,25–30] and inorganic nanoparticles [31]. The main advantages of the CUR loaded nanocarriers are their small size and large surface area, which enable them to pass through the cell membranes with an enhanced uptake efficiency [1,29]. Research has increasingly focused on the fabrication of biopolymer nanoparticles for CUR delivery, due to advantages of low cytotoxicity, excellent biocompatibility and biodegradability [29]. Two of the most commonly used biopolymers in medical applications are alginate and chitosan (CHI). Alginate is an anionic polysaccharide composed of (1–4)-linked β-D-mannuronate (M) and α-L-guluronate (G) residues, while CHI is a cationic polysaccharide composed of N-acetyl-β-D-glucosamine and β-D-glucosamine [32] and is positively charged below neutral pH, due to the protonation of amino groups [33]. Moreover, alginate based nanoparticles can be fabricated by simple processes, such as Ca^{2+}, cross-linking or altering of pH [34]. CHI based nanoparticles can be prepared by via polyanion of tripolyphosphate (TPP) without introducing harsh cross-linking agents or organic solvents [35]. Electrostatic interactions between positive CHI chains and negative drugs, such as CUR, enable the retention of the drug in CHI based nanoparticles providing a prolonged drug release profile [36]. These advantages of alginate and CHI make them promising candidates as nanocarriers for drug delivery [37]. Various alginate or CHI based nanoparticles have been developed for the delivery of CUR [30,38–41].

Targeted delivery by magnetic nanoparticles (MNPs) has been reported as a promising strategy for cancer therapy with the advantages ranging from visualisation of the targeting process, rapid targeting and accumulation of drug carriers at the tumour sites via magnetic forces. The MNPs can be heated in a magnetic field to promote the drug release [42]. MNPs have been reported to have very low toxicity within the human body [43]. Their small size and large surface area make them suitable for polyelectrolyte layer-by-layer deposition. The incorporation of MNPs has shown the targeted delivery of drugs to tumour sites with the help of external magnetic fields [42]. For example, Mancarella et al. [44] developed layer-by-layer functionalized nanoparticles by coating MNPs with positively charged Poly-L-lysine and negatively charged Dextran. The layer-by-layer coating enabled a high loading efficiency of CUR into the particles, and the MNP cores promoted the uptake of CUR into SKOV-3 cells. In another example Pavlov et al. [45] prepared luciferase enzyme and plasmid DNA loaded particles with alternative layers of poly-L-arginine hydrochloride and dextran sulphate sodium salt. MNPs were incorporated into the particles and the resulting MNPs improved the delivery of enzymes and plasmids into 293T cells. In addition, MNPs could be efficiently navigated to cells with a magnet below the targeted tissue culture wells [45].

Exploiting the electrostatic properties of alginate and CHI, a layer-by-layer coating method can be employed to prepare multilayer alginate/CHI polyelectrolyte nanoparticles, allowing desired surface features to be engineered for specific applications [46]. By altering the number of layers deposited, it is possible to encapsulate a high payload of drugs and control the drug release rate [47–50]. In this paper, magnetic alginate/CHI layer-by-layer nanoparticles (MACPs) were fabricated for the delivery of CUR into MDA-MB-231 breast cancer cells and HDF cells.

2. Materials and Methods

2.1. Materials

Curcumin (C8069) was purchased from LKT Laboratories (Cambridge, UK). Paraformaldehyde (sc-253236A) was purchased from Chem Cruz® (Dallas, TX, USA). $Ca(OH)_2$ (21181) was purchased from Honeywell Fluka™ (Bucharest, Romania). Sodium alginate (W201502), Na_2HPO_4 (S7907), NaH_2PO_4 (S8282), ammonium hydroxide (221228), and DMSO (Dimethyl sulfoxide, D5879) were purchased from SIGMA-ALDRICH (Gillingham, UK). RPMI (Roswell Park Memorial Institute) 1640 Medium (BE 12-167F), PBS (Dulbecco's Phosphate Buffered Saline, BE17-512F), Penicillin 5000 U/ml-Streptomycin 5000 U/mL (DE17-603E), L-Glutamine (17-605F) were purchased from Lonza® (Manchester, UK). Chitosan (349051000), Iron (II) chloride tetrahydrate (44939), Iron (III) chloride hexahydrate (44944), $NaHCO_3$ (A17005), Alexa Fluor® 568 phalloidin (A12380), MTT (3-(4,5-Dimethylthiazol-2-yl)-2,5-Diphenyltetrazolium Bromide, M6494) assay, FBS (Fetal Bovine Serum, 10500064) and DAPI (4′,6-Diamidino-2-phenylindole dihydrochloride, D1306) were purchased from Thermo Fisher Scientific (Waltham, MA, USA). MDA-MB-231 cells (Human Caucasian Breast Adenocarcinoma cells) were purchased from ECACC (Salisbury, UK). Neonatal foreskin HDFs (Human Dermal Fibroblasts) were obtained from the Sheffield RNAi Screening Facility (Sheffield, UK).

2.2. Preparation of Nanoparticles

2.2.1. Preparation of Fe_3O_4 Magnetic Nanoparticles

Fe_3O_4 MNPs were prepared by co-precipitation as previously described in Song et al. [27]. 4 g Iron (III) chloride hexahydrate and 4.5 g Iron (II) chloride tetrahydrate were each dissolved in 150 mL deionized (DI) water and degassed with nitrogen for 30 min to remove any dissolved oxygen. The solutions were then mixed in a 500 mL round-bottom flask and 15 mL of ammonium hydroxide was added under vigorous stirring under a nitrogen atmosphere at room temperature. The solution was then vigorously stirred for 2 h and the synthesised MNPs were collected with strong Neodymium magnets and washed several times with DI water until neutral pH. Finally, the magnetic nanoparticles were dried over night at room temperature and stored for future usage.

2.2.2. Preparation of Magnetic Alginate Nanoparticles

Magnetic alginate nanoparticles (MAPs) were prepared based on the procedure described by Liu et al. [51] Briefly, 20 mL of ethanol and 10 mL of DI water was mixed into a beaker and 0.25 g of MNPs were suspended in the prepared mixture. Next, 40 mL of sodium alginate (SA) solution (20 mg/mL) was added into the beaker, upon which the mixture was sonicated for 10 min to allow full homogenous dispersion of MNPs in the suspension. The resulting suspension was vigorously stirred for 30 min at room temperature. Subsequently, 128 mL of $Ca(OH)_2$ solution (0.74 mg/mL) was added into the suspension and stirred for 1 h before 16 mL of $NaHCO_3$ solution (10 mg/mL) was added. The suspension was then stirred for a further 12 h at room temperature and the resulting MAPs were collected with strong Neodymium magnets, washing thoroughly with ethanol and water to remove any excess salts. Finally, purified MAPs were re-suspended in DI water before being used for the layer-by-layer coating process.

2.2.3. Preparation of Magnetic Alginate/Chitosan Layer-by-Layer Nanoparticles

The preparation of magnetic alginate/chitosan layer-by-layer nanoparticles (MACPs) was based on the layer-by-layer self-assembly of SA and CHI on MAPs. Chitosan solution (10 mg/mL) was prepared in 1% (v/v) acetic acid aqueous solution. The first layer was deposited by adding 1 g of MAPs into 100 mL of the chitosan solution under vigorous stirring for 20 min at room temperature. The resulting MA/CHI particles were collected with a Neodymium magnet and the excess CHI was removed by washing the particles several times with DI water. The next SA layer was deposited by adding the previously prepared particles into 100 mL of SA solution (10 mg/mL) under vigorous stirring for 20 min thus forming MA/CHI/SA particles. For each layer the previously described purification process was used. Particles with more layers were fabricated by alternatively coating positively charged CHI and negatively charged SA on MACPs until the desired number of layers was reached.

2.3. Curcumin Loaded Magnetic Alginate/Chitosan Layer-by-Layer Nanoparticles

20 mL of CUR solution (7.5 mg/mL in DMSO) was added into 30 mL of DI water to prepare the CUR mixture (3 mg/mL). Then 30 mg of MACPs were added into 20 mL of the CUR mixture and stirred for 24 h. The resulting CUR loaded magnetic alginate/chitosan layer-by-layer nanoparticles (CMACPs) were collected with a Neodymium magnet and washed three times with DI water. The supernatants were collected and analysed with a UV-Vis spectrometry (JENWAY 6715, Bibby Scientific, Stone, UK) to determine the concentration of residual CUR. The CMACPs were dispersed in 5 mL of DI water and the concentration of these particles was determined by weighing dried particles from 1 mL solution. Encapsulation and loading efficiencies were determined by Equation (1), where $EE\%$ is the Encapsulation Efficiency, mP_{CUR} is the amount of CUR encapsulated in particles, and m_{intCUR} is the amount of CUR initially added. In Equation (2), $LE\%$ is the Loading Efficiency and N_P is the total amount of CUR loaded particles:

$$EE\%_{(w/w\%)} = \frac{mP_{CUR}}{m_{intCUR}} \times 100\%, \tag{1}$$

$$LE\%_{(w/w\%)} = \frac{mP_{CUR}}{N_P} \times 100\%. \tag{2}$$

2.4. Release of CUR from CMACPs

5 mg of CMACPs were suspended in 5 mL PBS buffer (pH 7.4) in vials and incubated at 37 °C under constant agitation (200 rpm). The particles were collected with strong Neodymium magnets at pre-determined time points and the supernatants were carefully removed before re-dispersing the particles in 5 mL fresh PBS. The CUR concentrations of the supernatants were analysed using UV-Vis-spectrometry and the percentage of cumulative CUR release was plotted as a function of incubation time.

2.5. Particle Characterisation

2.5.1. Nanoparticle Tracking and Zeta Potential Analysis

MACPs and CMACPs were dispersed in sodium phosphate solution (10 mM, pH 7) and injected into the scattering cell of an NTA (Nanoparticle Tracking Analysis, Nanosight LM10, Malvern, UK) where their motion was analysed and average size was calculated. The zeta potential measurement of particles was carried out by a Dynamic Light Scattering analyser (DLS, NanoBrook 90 plus Pals Particle size Analyzer, Brookhaven Instrument, Holtsville, NY, USA). Particles were washed several times and dispersed in DI water (pH 6.5–7.5) or 10 mM sodium phosphate buffer (pH 7) prior to zeta potential measurements.

2.5.2. Fourier Transform Infrared Spectroscopy

Fourier transform infrared spectroscopy (FTIR) analysis was conducted with a Spectrum 100 spectrophotometer (PerkinElmer, Waltham, MA, USA). Particles were washed three times with DI water and dried in an oven at 60 °C for 24 h before being placed on the diamond attenuated total reflectance (ATR) accessory and compressed. The wavenumber region was set from 4000 to 600 cm^{-1} with a resolution of 1 cm^{-1}. The spectral processing was conducted with IRPal 10 software.

2.5.3. Atomic Force Microscopy Analysis

The aggregation size and morphology of particles was characterised using Atomic Force Microscopy (AFM, Dimension Icon with ScanAsyst, Bruker Corporation, Billerica, MA, USA). Particle suspensions were dropped on mica substrates and air dried before being placed on the sample stage. AFM measurements were conducted using ScanAsyst mode and SCANASYST-AIR tips (spring constant: 0.4 N/m, length: 115 μm, width: 25 μm, resonant frequency: 70 kHz) and data were analysed with NanoScope Analysis 1.5 software.

2.5.4. Transmission Electron Microscopy Analysis

MACPs or CMACPs were dispersed in DI water and dropped onto copper TEM (transmission electron microscope) grids and incubated at room temperature for 30 s. Excess solution on the grids was then removed with filter paper, by gently dapping the edge and allowing excess liquid to be absorbed prior to TEM imaging (Tecnai G2 Spirit, FEI, Hillsboro, OR, USA). An acceleration voltage of 80 kV was used and images were recorded using a Gatan Orius SC1000B bottom mounted digital camera and analysed in Gatan Digital Micrograph software (version 3.9.1).

2.6. Cellular Uptake Assays

CUR medium solutions were prepared by adding CUR dissolved in DMSO (50 mg/mL) dropwise into media to obtain different final CUR concentrations (0.5, 1.5, 5, 15, 30 μg/mL). CMACPs were dispersed in media to reach the final CUR concentrations equivalent to those of CUR medium solutions. MDA-MB-231 and HDF cells were seeded onto 6 well plates at a density of 3×10^5 cells per well and incubated overnight at 37 °C and 5% CO_2. Then the media were replaced with 2 mL CUR or CMACPs medium solutions and incubated for a further 24 h. After this, the cells were harvested with trypsin and washed twice with PBS to remove any free CUR or CMACPs. The resulting cells were collected and analysed with an BD™ LSR II flow cytometer (BD Biosciences, USA) to investigate the cells CUR uptake.

2.7. Magnetically Targeted Delivery Assay

MDA-MB-231 cells were seeded in glass bottom dishes (Nunc™, diameter 35 mm, Thermo Fisher Scientific, Loughborough, UK) at a density of 3×10^5 cells per dish and incubated overnight to allow attachment. Free CUR and CMACPs were added into cell cultures to reach a final CUR concentration of 5 μg/mL and incubated for 4 h. Magnetically targeted delivery was conducted by initially placing a Neodymium magnet under the dish for the first 15 min during incubation. Cells were then washed twice with PBS buffer and fixed with 4% paraformaldehyde. The fixed cells were stained with Alexa Fluor 568 Phalloidin and DAPI for 1 h. Confocal fluorescence images of cellular uptake of CUR were taken with an Inverted Zeiss LSM 510 NLO microscope (Zeiss, Oberkochen, Germany) and analysed with LSM Image Browser software version 4.2.0.121.

2.8. In Vitro Cytotoxicity Assay

The cytotoxicity of free CUR, MACPs, and CMACPs against MDA-MB-231 and HDF cells was investigated using the MTT assay. MDA-MB-231 or HDF cells were seeded into 96-well plates at a density of 5×10^3 cells per well and incubated overnight at 37 °C and 5% CO_2. The media were then removed and replaced with CUR medium solution, MACPs or CMACPs dispersions (CUR content in the particles is equivalent to the dosage of free CUR) to reach the final CUR concentrations of 0.5, 1.5, 5, 15, 30 μg/mL. After 48 h of incubation, 50 μL of 3 mg/mL MTT was added to each well and incubated at 37 °C for 3 h followed by removing the supernatants and adding 200 μL DMSO. A plate reader (FLUOstar galaxy, BMG LABTECH, Ortenberg, Germany) was used to measure the absorbance of each well, including control wells, containing only cells and medium at 570 nm. The relative cell viability was determined by comparing the absorbance with control wells.

3. Results and Discussion

3.1. Characterisation of Magnetic Alginate/Chitosan Layer-by-Layer Nanoparticles and Curcumin Loaded Magnetic Alginate/Chitosan Nanoparticles

3.1.1. Zeta Potential, Size and FTIR Spectra

As shown in Scheme 1, magnetic alginate particles (MAPs) were prepared via the self-assembly of alginate on the surface of MNPs in Ca^{2+} solution (Stage 1). Following this the formation of MACPs (Stage 2) was achieved by coating MAPs with CHI. Stage 3: Particles with 1 layer of SA and CHI were then coated with SA again. Stage 2 and 3 were then repeated consecutively for the desired number of layers.

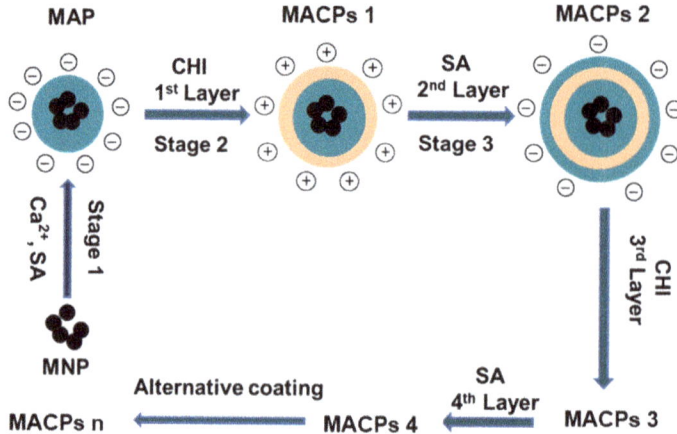

Scheme 1. Schematic illustration for the preparation of MAPs and MACPs. MAPs were fabricated by coating cross-linked alginate on MNPs using Ca^{2+} as the cross-linker. MACPs were prepared by alternatively depositing CHI and sodium alginate (SA) on MAPs based on the electrostatic interaction between the two biopolymers. The alternative coating was repeated until MACPs with desired number of layers were obtained (Stage 2 and 3). MACPs 1, 2, 3, 4 and n represent CMACPs that possess 1, 2, 3, 4 and n layers of polymers coated on MNPs respectively.

MAPs and MACPs with different number of layers were dispersed in DI water (pH was adjusted to 7 using HCl and NaOH) or sodium phosphate solution (pH 7) and their zeta potential was analysed using DLS. As shown in Figure 1a, the zeta potential of MAPs in water was −21.4 mV which was similar to the results of Ca^{2+} crosslinked alginate particles reported in previous literature [52,53]. The zeta potential of free SA in water has been reported as −50 mV [54]. The reason for the increased zeta potential of MAPs is due to crosslinking with Ca^{2+}. The carboxyl groups contribute to the anionic charge of the alginate polymer [55]. Upon gelation, the negatively charged carboxyl groups from the G blocks in the alginate chains interact with Ca^{2+} ions and form an 'egg-box'-like structure, reducing the density of free carboxyl groups, as well as the anionic charges [55]. Therefore, an increase of zeta potential was observed for MAPs. After deposition of the first layer (CHI), the zeta potential of the particles became positive (+19.2 mV) followed by a reduction to −44.8 mV after the negatively charged alginate polymer was coated as the second layer. Positive charges ranging from +12.1 to +19.2 mV were observed when CHI was coated as the outermost layer and negative charges ranging from −43 to −48.5 mV were associated with alginate coatings as the outermost layer. An oscillation of zeta potential was observed with the alternative deposition of SA and CHI, indicating the successful coating of the two polymers.

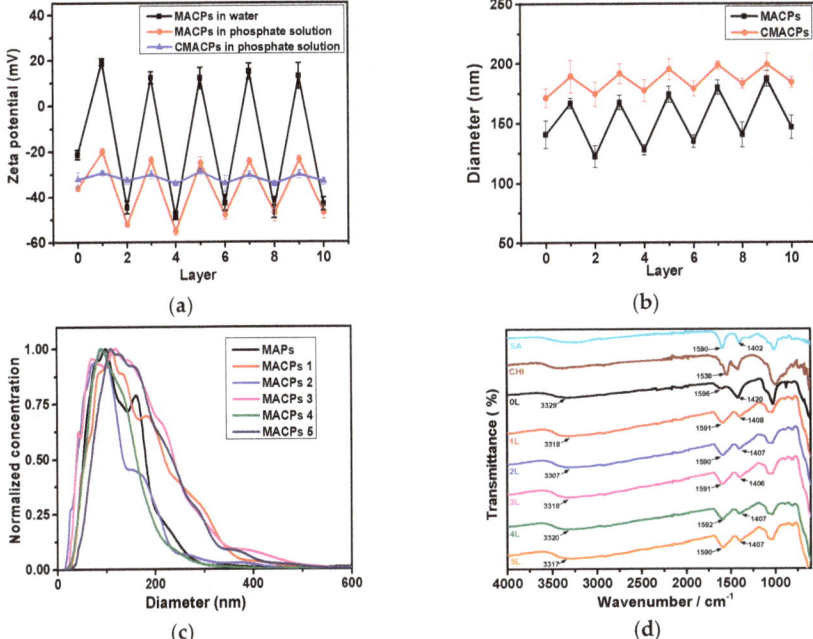

Figure 1. Zeta potential (**a**) and average diameter (**b**) of MACPs and CMACPs as a function of the number of coated layers. Zeta potential of particles was analysed in water (pH 7) and phosphate solution (10 mM, pH 7). Particle size was analysed in phosphate solution. Oscillations of zeta potential and average diameter were observed with the alternate coating of SA and CHI; (**c**) Size distribution of MAPs and MACPs with 1–5 layers of coated polymers; (**d**) FTIR spectra of MAPs and MACPs with the number of deposited polymer layers from 1 to 5. The results are shown in mean ± SD, n ≥ 3.

The zeta potential of particles in sodium phosphate solution (10 mM) is also shown in Figure 1a and exhibited a similar oscillation behaviour between coatings. However, negative surface charges were observed for MACPs (layer number: 1, 3, 5, 7, 9) with CHI outermost layer. This phenomenon is due to the adsorption of the phosphate anions onto the surface of the chitosan polymers. Phosphates contain small multivalent anions and therefore tend to interact or complex with cationic amino groups on CHI surfaces via electrostatic interactions [35]. Therefore, the phosphate anions adsorbed onto CHI layers increased the overall negative charge of the particles. Similar phenomena have been reported previously: For example, Swain et al. [56] analysed the zeta potential of CHI in both 1 and 10 mM NaCl and found that the zeta potential value decreased as the ionic strength of NaCl increased. The authors suggested the reduced surface charge was attributed to the adsorption of anions onto the surface of CHI polymers [56]. Further to this, Acevedo et al. [57] analysed the zeta potential of CHI (5 mg/mL) in water and NaCl solution (0.2 M) and reported zeta potential values of +72 mV in water and +33 mV in NaCl. It was suggested that this reduced absolute zeta potential value was governed by a compression of the electrical double layer, due to the electrostatic interactions with Cl^- in the solvent [57]. As shown in Figure 1a, the zeta potential of MACPs with alginate as the outermost layer in phosphate solution exhibited similar values as they were in water, which is in agreement with previously reported data [54]. On the other hand, MAPs exhibited a more negative zeta potential values in phosphate solution (−36 mV) compared to water (−21.4 mV). This is due to reaction between Ca^{2+} and phosphate ions to form insoluble calcium phosphate, which leads to the loss of Ca^{2+} and the increased density of free carboxyl groups thus resulting in an overall increased negative charge. The zeta potential behaviour of drug carriers can be utilised to control the drug loading and release processes. For example, cationic drug carriers, such as CHI nanoparticles, can be used to improve the loading of anionic drug molecules and prolong their release time based on electrostatic interactions between positive CHI and negative drug molecules [36]. In the case of MACPs, different numbers of polymer layers with different zeta potentials can potentially be used to improve drug loading.

The average diameter of MACPs was analysed by NTA, as shown in Figure 1b, where the diameter of MACPs was found to be 141 nm which increased to 167 nm after the first CHI layer coating. The size of particles increased gradually per bi-layer of SA/CHI and reached 187 nm for 9 layers. Size differences were observed depending on the outermost polymer of MACPs. For example, the average diameter of MACPs decreased from 167 (3 layers) to 128 nm (4 layers) and then increased to 174 nm after the deposition of CHI as the fifth polymer layer. This leaves a mean size difference of ~40 nm between CHI and SA. In addition, the size distribution of MAPs and MACPs (with 1–5 layers of coated polymers) is shown in Figure 1c. Broader size distributions were observed for particles with CHI as the outermost layer (MACPs 1, 3 and 5) compared to particles with alginate as the outermost layer (MAPs and MACPs 2 and 4). These results illustrate that particles with CHI outermost layers are larger and less condensed than particles with alginate as the outermost layer. This is most likely due to the different surface charges of the particles. For MACPs with CHI as the outermost layer, the zeta potential ranged from −20 to −25.1 mV in phosphate buffer solutions, while the zeta potential for alginate as the outermost layer ranged from −47 to −55.2 mV. Particles with absolute zeta potential values higher than 30 mV can be considered stable in solution [58]. Therefore, MACPs with alginate outermost layers were very stable in solution, due to their sufficient surface charges. On the other hand, particles with CHI as the outermost layer were less stable and more likely to aggregate in aqueous solutions forming larger particles.

The zeta potential of CMACPs in sodium phosphate solution at pH 7 is shown in Figure 1a. A significant change in surface charge was observed for particles after CUR loading. The zeta potential of free CUR sodium phosphate solution was −31.1 mV. In contrast, the zeta potentials of MAPs and MACPs with the outermost layer of alginate (layer number: 0, 2, 4, 6, 8, 10) was within the range from −36 to −55.5 mV (Figure 1a) while the zeta potentials of the particles with CHI outermost layer (layer number: 1, 3, 5, 7, 9) were around −20 mV. After CUR loading, the zeta potentials of CMACPs were found between −28.7 and −34.2 mV suggesting CUR was encapsulated in or adsorbed onto the particles, reducing the difference of the zeta potentials between MACPs with alginate and CHI outermost layers. Increased particle sizes (between 172–199 nm) were observed for CMACPs (Figure 1b) compared to MACPs (122–187 nm), which can be attributed to the loading of CUR. For CMACPs with the same outermost polymer (SA or CHI), the average diameter of particles increased as the number of layers increased, due to the fact that larger polymer matrixes encapsulate more CUR molecules. Larger particle size was observed for CMACPs with the outermost polymer being CHI for the same reason as described above. The resulting particle sizes are optimal for drug delivery applications [59]. The chemical compositions and interactions between different polymer layers were analysed by FTIR, as shown in Figure 1d. For SA, the peaks at 1590 cm^{-1} and 1402 cm^{-1} were characteristic for the asymmetric stretching and symmetric stretching of -COOH groups respectively [60,61]. In MAPs and MACPs with the number of layers (1, 2, 3, 4 and 5), these two peaks moved towards higher wavenumbers, indicating the formation of Ca^{2+}-alginate ionic cross-linking [62]. This is because of the changes in charge density, atomic radius and atomic weight of the cations [62,63]. For CHI, the peak at 1538 cm^{-1} was characteristic of -NH$_2$ bonds [64]. The presence of CHI in the MACPs was also confirmed by comparing the curves of MAPs (0 L) and MACPs (1–5 L). The broad characteristic adsorption at 3329 cm^{-1} for -OH groups in MAPs shifted to a lower frequency for MACPs (1–5 L), demonstrating the superposition of amine N-H stretching in chitosan and -OH groups of alginate and chitosan [64,65]. The peak at 1596 cm^{-1} in MAPs became broader, and moved to a lower frequency for MACPs, which can be attributed to the overlapped -NH$_2$ stretching from chitosan and -COOH stretching from alginate [66]. These results confirmed that CHI and alginate chains were successfully incorporated into the MACPs.

3.1.2. Morphology Characterisation

The size distribution and morphology of MAPs and MACPs were also analysed by AFM and TEM (Figure 2). As shown in Figure 2a, the particles exhibited heights of 50 nm with bottom diameters around 140 nm, which is due to (1) The tip-sample convolution effect, leading to the lateral broadening of surface protrusions [67]; and (2) The aggregation of small MAPs, flattened on mica substrates, leading to the expanded bottom diameter. MACPs (Figure 2b,d,f) with CHI as the outermost layer showed larger bottom diameters than those (Figure 2c,e) with SA as the outermost layer, suggesting larger aggregation occurred for particles with CHI as the outermost layer. This is also due to the fact that the mica surface is negatively charged, therefore particles with positive net charges attach tightly and become more fat and flat. This result is consistent with the data obtained from NTA, confirming that MACPs with CHI as the outermost layer are loosely packed due to their lower net surface charges. Particles with alginate as the outermost layer are negatively charged and expected to be less attached therefore are more roundly shaped. Cross section AFM images indicated that MAPs (Figure 2a) possess rough topography, which were attributed to the aggregation of small solid MAPs. After alternate coating with SA and CHI, the resultant MACPs (Figure 2b–f) exhibited more spherical shapes and smooth surfaces, which further confirmed the successful coating of both polymers. For MACPs, inter-digitation among the adjacent CHI/SA layers were constructed due to the existence of surface charges. Therefore, after the removal of excess polymers, stable films were formed by soft polymers of CHI and SA leading to the smooth surface of MACPs.

Characterisation of MAPs and MACPs via TEM revealed magnetic cores (dark areas) surrounded by polymer shells, which were the chitosan and alginate layers, as shown in Figure 2. The inset in Figure 2i. is an enlarged section of the image clearly showing magnetic core particles and the surrounding CHI/SA layers. It can be observed from Figure 2 that particle aggregates were formed on the TEM grids. This is most likely due to the aggregation of particles during the drying process. In solutions, the magnetic core-shall particles are stabilized by the charged polymer layers (chitosan and alginate) and the aggregation degree of particles is related to the balance between the repulsive electrostatic interactions and the attractive interactions. During the drying process, the concentration of particles increased, which will increase the probability of particle collisions and enhance the attractive interactions, leading to promoted aggregation of particles.

AFM was also used to investigate the morphology of CMACPs. As shown in Figure 3a, the bottom diameter of CUR loaded MAPs was ~150 nm and increased layer by layer, reaching a maximum of ~200 nm for 9 layers (Figure 3f), which is in agreement with the size tendency analysed by NTA, as shown in Figure 1b. However, rougher surface morphology was observed for CMACPs compared to MACPs, as shown in Figure 2. CUR is known as a highly hydrophobic drug [68–70] and the loading of CUR into MACPs increased the hydrophobicity of the particles. This meant that the particles rapidly dehydrated during AFM analysis and exhibited rough surfaces, indicating the successful loading of CUR into MACPs.

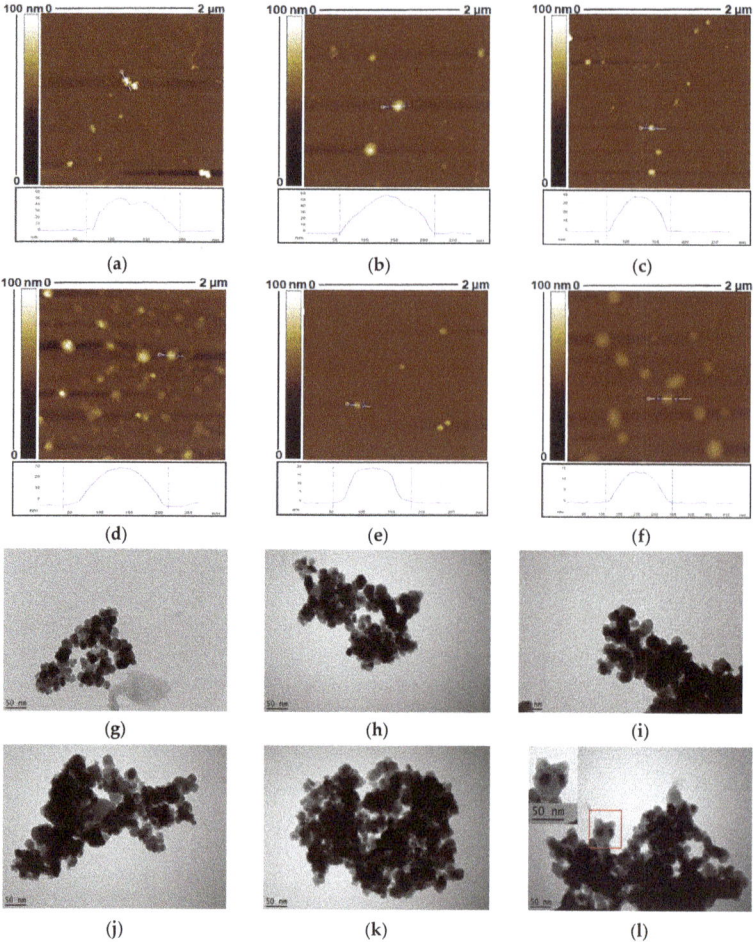

Figure 2. Atomic force microscopy (AFM) and transmission electron microscope (TEM) images of MAPs (**a**,**g**) and MACPs with the layer number of 1 (**b**,**h**), 4 (**c**,**i**), 5 (**d**,**j**), 8 (**e**,**k**) and 9 (**f**,**l**). Smaller particles were observed for MACPs with SA as the outermost layer.

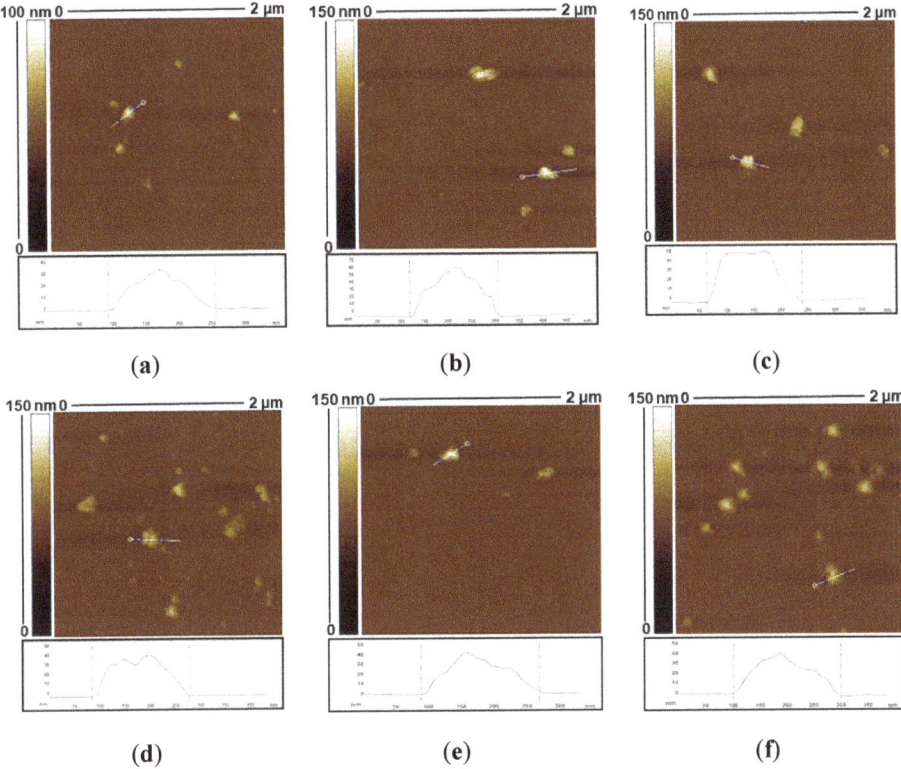

Figure 3. AFM images of Curcumin (CUR)-loaded MAPs (**a**) and CUR loaded MACPs (CMACPs) with the layer number of 1 (**b**), 4 (**c**), 5 (**d**), 8 (**e**) and 9 (**f**).

3.2. Loading and Release of Curcumin

CUR loaded MACPs were prepared by dispersing MACPs in CUR water/DMSO solution and incubated under stirring for 24 h. The addition of DMSO increases CUR solubility and its permeability into MACPs. The volume ratio of water:DMSO was 3:2, resulting in a homogeneous CUR solution (3 mg/mL) without sedimentation during the 24 h of incubation [71]. Figure 4a clearly demonstrates that the resultant CMACPs can be collected with a Neodymium magnet while CUR itself in the bulk solution was not affected by the magnetic field. Therefore, MACPs can be potentially used for targeted delivery of CUR via external magnetic fields.

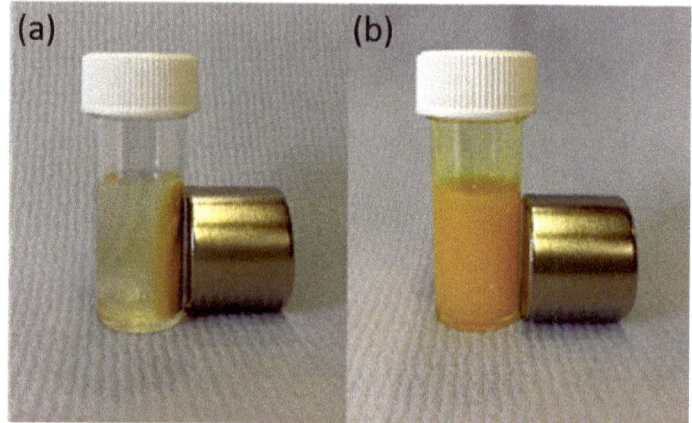

Figure 4. CMACPs were prepared by suspending MACPs in CUR water/DMSO solution and incubating for 24 h under stirring. The resulting CMACPs can be rapidly collected by a Neodymium magnet (pull force 25 Kg, 25.4 mm diameter × 30 mm thick) within 1 min (**a**). The free CUR in solution on the other hand was not affected by the magnetic force (**b**).

Encapsulation efficiency results reveal that 49.2% of CUR was loaded into CMAPs and the encapsulation efficiency increased to 67.5% with increasing number of layers of CHI and SA (see Figure 5a). For particles with the same type of polymer (CHI or SA) on the outermost surface an increased trend of encapsulation efficiency was observed with increasing layer number. However, as illustrated in Figure 5a, a higher encapsulation efficiency of CUR was observed for CMACPs with CHI as the outermost layer (layer number: 1, 3, 5, 7 and 9) compared to SA as the outermost layer (layer number: 2, 4, 6, 8, 10). The most feasible explanation for this is the different surface charges between the particle outermost layers. As illustrated in Figure 1a, CHI layers exhibited positive surface charges in water while SA layers exhibited negative surface charges. Therefore, the negatively charged CUR molecules are adsorbed on the surface of the CHI layer more readily, facilitating a more efficient and faster encapsulation into polymer matrix. On the other hand, SA layer was negatively charged in water, and thus CUR molecules were less readily to interact with the particle surface, due to the electrostatic repulsion. Moreover, larger amount of CUR molecules were expected on the surface of CHI layer, which also led to a higher encapsulation efficiency. The same hypothesis can be used to explain the loading efficiency of CMAPs and CMACPs. As shown in Figure 5b, a higher loading efficiency of CUR was observed for MACPs with CHI as the outermost layer to those with SA as the outermost layer. Higher loading efficiencies from 54.8% to 64.9% were achieved for CMAPs and CMACPs compared to many previously reported CUR loaded CHI and alginate based particles [25,28,38] with loading efficiencies from 2.7% to 48%, suggesting CMAPs and CMACPs possess great potential loading CUR into nanoparticles for drug delivery applications.

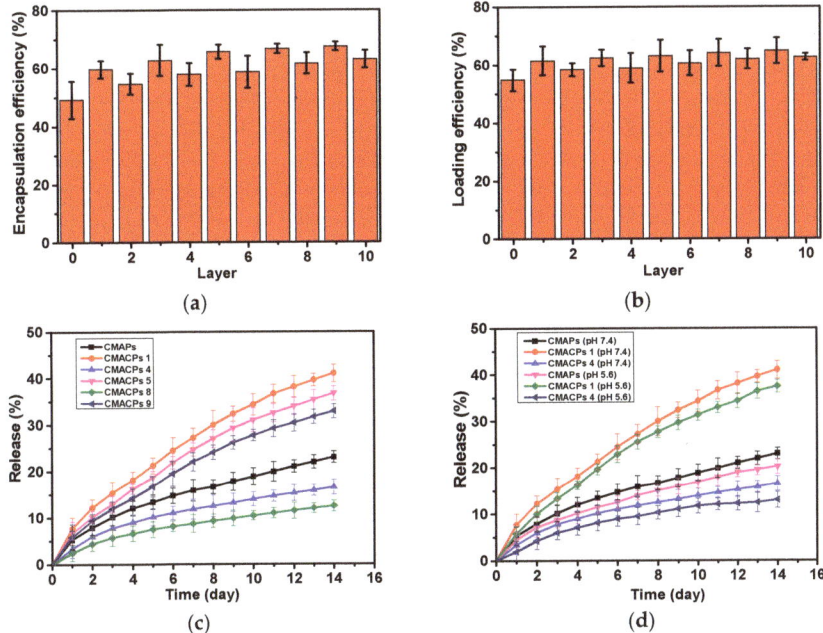

Figure 5. The drug loading and release profiles of the CMAPs and CMACPs are affected by the type of outermost polymers and the number of layers. Encapsulation efficiency of CMAPs and CMACPs (**a**). Curcumin loading efficiency into CMAPs and CMACPs (**b**). Curcumin release profile of CMAPs and CMACPs with different layers (1, 4, 5, 8, 9) of deposited polymers (**c**). Curcumin release profile of CMAPs and CMACPs (layer number: 1 and 4) in PBS buffer at pH 7.4 and pH 5.6 (**d**). The results are shown in mean ± SD, n = 3.

In order to investigate the release profile of CMAPs and CMACPs, 5 mg of particles were dispersed in 5 mL PBS buffer at pH 7.4 and incubated at 37 °C under shaking (200 rpm) at predetermined time intervals. The particles were collected with strong Neodymium magnets and the CUR concentration in supernatants were analysed to obtain the accumulative CUR release profiles. As shown in Figure 5c, for all particles, CUR was released more rapidly within the first two days and then released slower, but at more sustained rates in PBS for up to 2 weeks. The faster release in the first two days is most likely due to the loss of weakly adsorbed CUR molecules on the surface of the particles or in the polymer matrix close to particle surfaces. The sustained CUR release after the first two days was then dependent on the diffusion of CUR molecules through the polymer matrixes into the bulk PBS solution, thus exhibiting a slower and more sustained release pattern. No significant burst release was observed during the whole release process [26,72]. CMACPs with CHI as the outermost layer exhibited a faster release rate of CUR than CMAPs and CMACPs with SA as the outermost layer (CMACPs 4 and 8). As mentioned previously in Section 3.3.1, CHI is positively charged in water, but negatively in phosphate solution, due to the adsorption of negative phosphate ions [35], therefore more negatively charged CUR molecules are adsorbed onto the CHI layer surface when these particles were dispersed in CUR water/DMSO solution than on alginate, as illustrated in Figure 5a,b. When CMACPs with layer numbers of 1, 5 and 9 were dispersed in PBS, CUR molecules were released from the particle surface, due to CUR and phosphate ions competing for free amino groups on the CHI chains, this in turn facilitates the loss of CUR molecules from the inner layers to the surface via a concentration gradient driven diffusion. Thus, faster CUR release rates were observed for CMACPs with layer numbers of 1, 5 and 9. On the other hand, CMAPs and CMACPs with layer numbers of 4 and 8, where alginate was deposited as the outermost layer, showed similar negative surface charges in water and phosphate solutions, less CUR molecules were adsorbed during the loading process and thus the drug release rate was not promoted in phosphate solutions. For particles with the same type of polymer, reduced release rates were observed as the number of layers increased (release rate: CMACPs 1 > CMACPs 5 > CMACPs 9, CMAPs > CMACPs 4 > CMACPs 8). By increasing the number of polymer layers it was more difficult for the innermost CUR to permeate out. This is in agreement with previously reported data [47–49], where Chai et al. [47] fabricated doxorubicin loaded poly (lactic-co-glycolic acid) nanoparticles and layer-by-layer coated the particles with CHI and alginate. After comparing the drug release rates of uncoated and polymer coated particles, the authors found that with the CHI/SA coating the initial drug burst release was reduced from 55.1% to 5.8% and the overall drug release rate was also reduced. In another example Haidar et al. [48] prepared bovine serum albumin loaded liposomes and layer-by-layer coated them with CHI/SA. The polymer coated liposomes showed a reduced albumin release rate to the uncoated ones. Further to this Zhou et al. [49] developed polyethyleneimine coated PLGA nanoparticles and reported that the drug release rate reduced with increasing layers.

In order to investigate the drug release profile of CMAPs and CMACPs at different pH, CMAPs, CMACPs with 1 and 4 layers were dispersed in PBS with pH 7.4 and pH 5.6. As illustrated in Figure 5d, the release pattern of CUR from particles at pH 5.6 was similar to those at pH 7.4, but slightly slower. In 14 days, about 23%, 41% and 17% of CUR were released from CMAPs, CMACPs 1 and CMACPs 4 at pH 7.4 respectively, while about 20%, 37% and 13% of CUR were released at pH 5.6. The data are in agreement with previously published work by Martins et al. [41] who investigated the release profiles of CUR from N-trimethyl chitosan/alginate complexes at pH 7.4 and pH 1.2 and reported that 80% of CUR was released at pH 7.4 within the first hour while only 22% of CUR was released at pH 1.2. The pH dependent release pattern can be attributed to the altered surface charge and hydrophobicity of polymers at different pH values.

3.3. Cellular Uptake Assays

3.3.1. CUR Uptake Assay by Flow Cytometry

To investigate the cellular uptake kinetics of CMAPs and CMACPs, MDA-MB-231 breast cancer cells and HDF cells were incubated with free CUR and particles containing equivalent amounts of CUR for 24 h. Except for skin cancers, breast cancer is most commonly diagnosed among US women and the second leading cause of cancer death among women [73]. Therefore, MDA-MB-231 breast cancer cells were selected as a cancer model and HDF cells were selected as a non-cancer model to investigate the uptake effect of the drug loaded particles.

The cells were analysed by flow cytometry to determine the cellular uptake of CUR by different cells. As shown in Figure 6a, it is evident that the percentage of MDA-MB-231 cells taking up CUR was dose dependent. Significant higher uptake efficiency was observed for MDA-MB-231 cells treated with CMAPs and CMACPs than those treated with free CUR, indicating that the nanoparticles facilitate the CUR uptake. This is in agreement with previously reported data [1,17,74–76]. Here, at a CUR concentration of 1.5 μg/mL, an uptake efficiency of 31.2%, 39.6% and 24.2% was observed for MDA-MB-231 cells treated with CMAPs, CMACPs 1 and 4 respectively, which is 3–6 fold higher than the uptake efficiency of cells treated with free CUR. The increased CUR uptake of CMAPs can be attributed to the fact that the CUR loaded nanoparticles were more easily taken up by cells via endocytosis, due to their smaller size (172–199 nm), while highly hydrophobic CUR was insoluble in aqueous solutions forming larger aggregates, which are more difficult to be internalised by cells [75,77]. The order of uptake efficiency of free CUR and CUR loaded particles was CMACPs 1 > CMAPs >CMACPs 4 > free CUR. Particles with CHI as the outermost layer exhibited the highest uptake efficiency (39.6%). This result is in agreement with work by Zhou et al. [46], who compared the uptake efficiency of CHI/alginate coated poly (lactide-co-glycolide) nanoparticles and observed the uptake efficiency of particles with CHI as the outermost layer was the highest. The promoted CUR uptake by the CHI surface is because of the protonated amino groups, which interact with the negatively charged cell surfaces and promote the accumulation of CMACPs 1 onto the surface of MDA-MB-231 cells. Figure 6b shows the CUR uptake efficiency for HDF cells after being treated with free CUR and CUR loaded particles. HDF cells exhibited a similar uptake pattern, but an overall much lower CUR uptake efficiency compared to MDA-MB-231 cells, suggesting CMAPs and CMACPs target cancer cells rather than normal cells. This is in agreement with many previously published reports [28,78–80] as cancer cells possess a higher metabolic activity than normal cells and their surfaces overexpress various receptors that in turn increase the available binding sites promoting a higher uptake efficiency of particles and drugs [81–83].

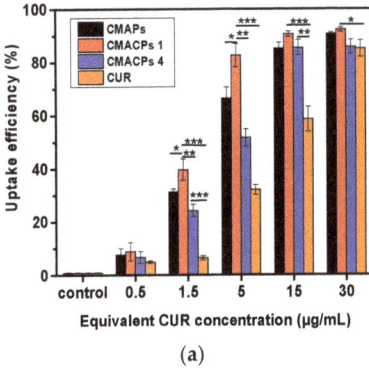
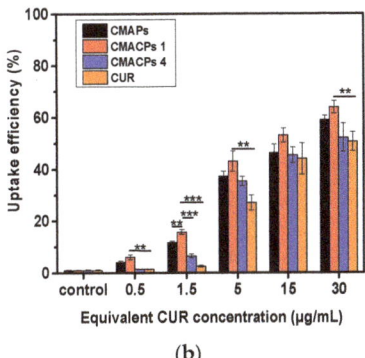

(a) (b)

Figure 6. Cellular uptake analysis of CUR in MDA-MB-231 cells (**a**) and HDF cells (**b**) after incubation with CMAPs, CMACPs 1 and 4 and free CUR for 24 h. The CUR uptake was analysed by flow cytometry. The dosages of CUR in particles were equivalent to the amounts of free CUR used. CMACPs 1 and 4 represent CMACPs that possess 1 and 4 layers of polymers coated on MNPs respectively. The results are shown in mean ± SD, n = 3. The statistical significance is expressed as *** $p < 0.001$, ** $p < 0.01$, * $p < 0.05$.

3.3.2. Magnetically Targeted Delivery Assay

To investigate the potential of CMAPs and CMACPs for magnetically targeted delivery of CUR, free CUR, CMAPs and CMACPs were incubated with MDA-MB-231 cells in glass bottom dishes. A Neodymium magnet was placed under the target area of the dish to allow for the accumulation of magnetic nanoparticles within the selected area. Taking advantage of the auto-fluorescent property of CUR, the confocal fluorescence images show the cellular uptake of CUR in and out of the target (magnet-affected) areas. The overall fluorescent intensity of MDA-MB-231 cells within the target areas that were treated with free CUR (Figure 7a) was lower than cells treated with CUR loaded nanoparticles (Figure 7c,e,g), suggesting CMAPs and CMACPs have enhanced the uptake of CUR. This result is consistent with the uptake efficiency shown in Figure 6. No obvious difference in fluorescent intensities was observed between Figures 7a and 7b, showing that the free CUR uptake is not affected by the presence of magnetic forces. In contrast, cells treated with CMAPs (Figure 7c), CMACPs 1 (Figure 7e) and CMACPs 4 (Figure 7g) within the magnet-affected area showed significant increase of fluorescent intensity compared to the cells treated with same particles, but outside of the target (magnet-affected) areas (Figure 7d,f,h). The enhanced CUR uptake in the target areas was attributed to the accumulation of CUR loaded magnetic nanoparticles to the target areas driven by the magnetic force. On the other hand, the local concentration of CUR loaded magnetic particles outside the target areas was significantly lower, thus showing much lower fluorescent intensities. This result clearly shows that CMAPs and CMACPs have the potential for targeted drug delivery.

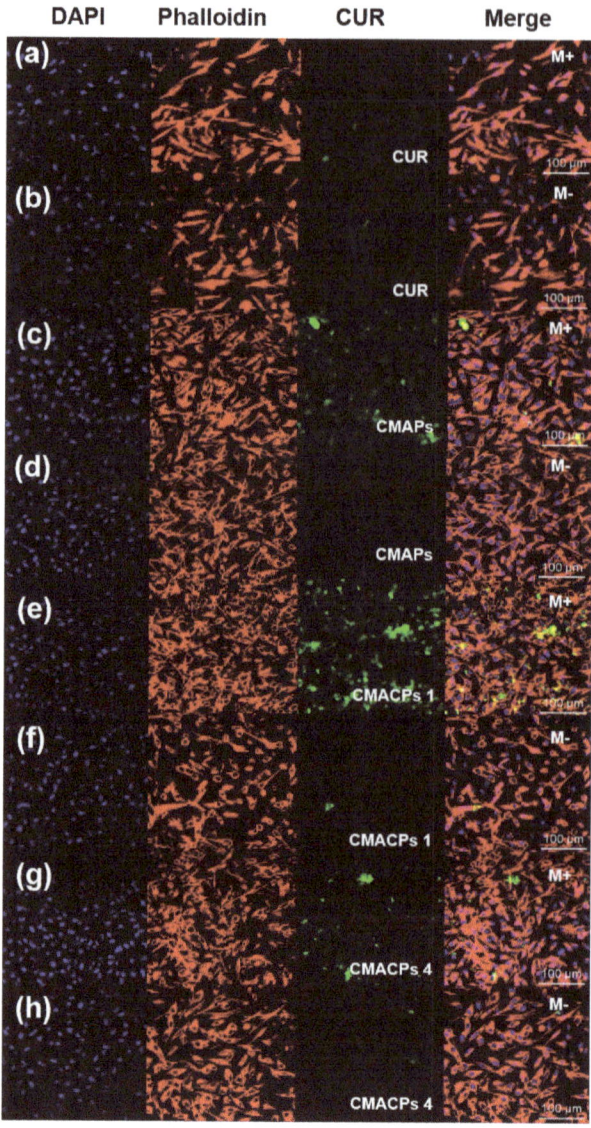

Figure 7. Confocal fluorescence microscopy images of MDA-MB-231 cells incubated with free CUR (**a,b**), CMAPs (**c,d**), CMACPs 1 (**e,f**) and CMACPs 4 (**g,h**). CMACPs 1 and 4 represent CMACPs that possess 1 and 4 layers of polymers coated on MNPs respectively. CUR loaded particles contained equivalent amount of drug as free CUR (5 μg/mL). Cell nucleus and cytoskeleton were stained with DAPI (blue) and Alexa Fluor 568 Phalloidin (red). M+ denotes the images taken within the magnet affected area and M- denotes the images taken outside of the magnet-affected target area.

3.4. In Vitro Cytotoxicity Assay

In order to investigate the cytotoxicity of CMACPs towards cancer and normal cells, MDA-MB-231 breast cancer cells and HDF cells were incubated with free CUR, CMACPs 1, CMACPs 4 and blank MACPs for 48 h. The in vitro MTT assay results are shown in Figure 8. It can be observed in Figure 8a,b that both free CUR and CMACPs exhibited increased cytotoxicity towards MDA-MB-231 cells with increasing CUR concentration, which was in agreement with previously reported data that CUR possesses dose dependent cytotoxicity towards cancer cells [1,17,74–76]. Both CMACPs 1 and 4 showed enhanced cytotoxicity towards MDA-MB-231 cells compared to free CUR, which can be attributed to an enhanced uptake of CMACPs. As discussed in Section 3.3.1, the uptake efficiency of MDA-MB-231 cells treated with CMACPs was 3–6-fold greater than those treated with free CUR. It is expected that the sustained release of CUR from internalised CMACPs maintained a high CUR concentration within the MDA-MB-231 cells, thus leading to lower viability of cells. CMACPs 1 were observed to exhibit higher cytotoxicity towards MDA-MB-231 cells than CMACPs 4, which was due to a higher CUR release rate (Figure 5c) and uptake efficiency (Figure 6a). As shown in Figure 8c,d, the viability of HDF cells after treatment with free CUR and CMACPs was reduced at higher CUR concentrations (>15 µg/mL), but a high viability was observed in contrast to MDA-MB-231 cancer cells at CUR concentrations below 15 µg/mL. One of the major accepted theories is that cancer cells possess lower glutathione levels than normal cells, due to their reprogrammed metabolic pathways [29]. Depletion of glutathione, which is important for the sensitivity of cells to CUR can lead to the enhancement of CUR sensitivity of cancer cells [29,78,84]. In addition, most cancer cells, but not normal cells, express constitutively active NF-KB that mediates their survival. CUR can suppress NF-κB regulated gene products, thus suppressing the proliferation of cancer cells [78,85]. High viabilities were observed for both MDA-MB-231 cells and HDF cells after they were treated with blank MACPs, demonstrating that MACPs are non-toxic towards these cells.

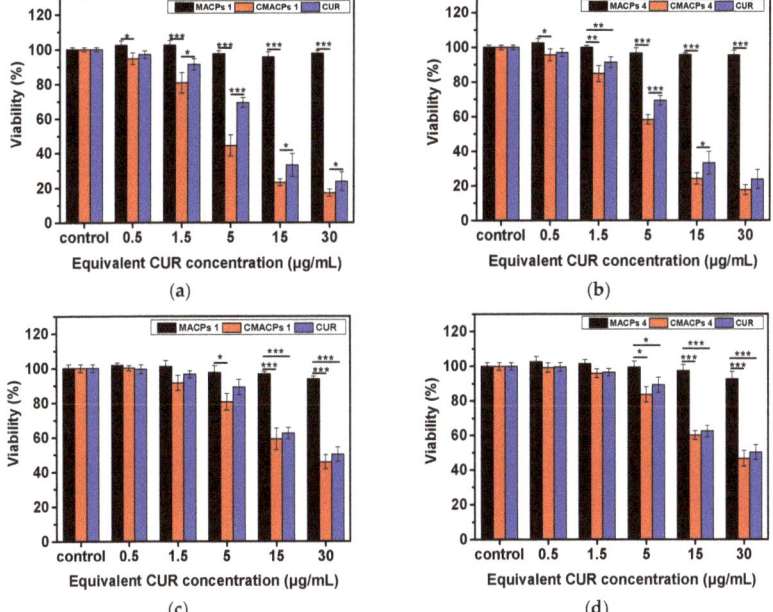

Figure 8. The in vitro MTT assay suggested CMACPs exhibited significantly higher cytotoxicity towards MDA-MB-231 breast cancer cells than to HDF cells. MDA-MB-231 cells (**a**,**b**) and HDF cells (**c**,**d**) were treated with free CUR, CMACPs 1, CMACPs 4 and blank MACPs 1, MACPs 4 for 48 h. CMACPs 1 and 4 (or MACPs 1 and 4) represent CMACPs (or MACPs) that possess 1 and 4 layers of polymers, respectively. The amounts of CUR in CUR loaded nanoparticles were equivalent to the amounts of free CUR (0.5–30 µg/mL), respectively. The results are shown in mean ± SD, n ≥ 3. The statistical significance is expressed as *** $p < 0.001$, ** $p < 0.01$, * $p < 0.05$.

4. Conclusions

MACPs were prepared by a layer-by-layer coating of CHI and SA onto the surface of Fe_3O_4 nanoparticles. The successful coating of CHI and SA was confirmed by the zeta potential and FTIR spectral measurements of the particles. Incorporation of CUR was confirmed by a change in surface charge and morphology of CMACPs, while the mean diameter of CMACPs was lower than 200 nm and within the optimum size range for drug delivery applications. In vitro drug release profiles illustrated the sustained release of CUR from CMACPs and indicated that it was possible to control the release rate by altering the outermost polymer (CHI or SA), as well as by changing the number of layers. More biopolymer layers resulted in a slower CUR drug release profile, where CHI as the outermost layer showed a faster CUR release. Confocal fluorescence microscopic images confirmed the successful internalisation of CUR into MDA-MB-231 breast cancer cells and indicated that rapid and targeted delivery of CUR could be achieved in the presence of an external magnetic field. FACS analysis indicated the CMACPs mediated uptake of CUR by MDA-MB-231 cells was 3–6 fold greater than that of free CUR. MDA-MB-231 cancer cells showed a significantly higher uptake efficiency of CUR than that of HDF normal cells after being treated with CMACPs. The MTT assay indicated that CMACPs exhibited a significantly higher cytotoxicity towards MDA-MB-231 cancer cells than towards HDF cells. In summary, the sustained release profiles, enhanced uptake efficiency and strong cytotoxicity to cancer cells, as well as the potential for targeted delivery make MACPs a promising candidate for anti-cancer drug delivery.

Author Contributions: Conceptualisation, X.Z. and W.S.; Methodology, experiments and data analysis, W.S., X.S., and W.L.; manuscript Preparation, W.S., D.A.G., Z.C., and X.Z. All authors read and approved the manuscript.

Funding: The authors would like to thank EPSRC (EP/N007174/1 and EP/N023579/1), Royal Society (RG160662) and Jiangsu specially-appointed professor program for support.

Acknowledgments: The authors thank Qingyou Xia from state key laboratory of silkworm genome biology, Southwest University, China for providing silk cocoons.

Conflicts of Interest: The authors declare no conflicts of interest.

Abbreviations

CUR, curcumin; CHI, chitosan; MNPs, magnetic nanoparticles; MAPs, Magnetic alginate nanoparticles; MACPs, magnetic alginate/CHI layer-by-layer nanoparticles; CMACPs, Curcumin loaded magnetic alginate/chitosan layer-by-layer nanoparticles; CMACPs 1 and 4, Curcumin loaded magnetic alginate/chitosan layer-by-layer nanoparticles with 1 and 4 layers of CHI/SA coating; HDF, Human Dermal Fibroblasts.

References

1. Yallapu, M.M.; Jaggi, M.; Chauhan, S.C. Curcumin nanomedicine: A road to cancer therapeutics. *Curr. Pharm. Des.* **2013**, *19*, 1994–2010. [CrossRef] [PubMed]
2. Masuda, T.; Hidaka, K.; Shinohara, A.; Maekawa, T.; Takeda, Y.; Yamaguchi, H. Chemical studies on antioxidant mechanism of curcuminoid: Analysis of radical reaction products from curcumin and Linoleate. *J. Agric. Food Chem.* **1999**, *47*, 71–77. [CrossRef] [PubMed]
3. Ruby, A.; Kuttan, G.; Babu, K.D.; Rajasekharan, K.; Kuttan, R. Anti-tumour and antioxidant activity of natural curcuminoids. *Cancer Lett.* **1995**, *94*, 79–83. [CrossRef]
4. Ak, T.; Gulcin, I. Antioxidant and radical scavenging properties of curcumin. *Chem. Biol. Interact.* **2008**, *174*, 27–37. [CrossRef] [PubMed]
5. Brouet, I.; Ohshima, H. Curcumin, an anti-tumor promoter and anti-inflammatory agent, inhibits induction of nitric oxide synthase in activated macrophages. *Biochem. Biophys. Res. Commun.* **1995**, *206*, 533–540. [CrossRef] [PubMed]
6. Kawamori, T.; Lubet, R.; Steele, V.E.; Kelloff, G.J.; Kaskey, R.B.; Rao, C.V.; Reddy, B.S. Chemopreventive effect of curcumin, a naturally occurring anti-inflammatory agent, during the promotion/progression stages of colon cancer. *Cancer Res.* **1999**, *59*, 597–601. [PubMed]

7. Aggarwal, B.B.; Harikumar, K.B. Potential therapeutic effects of curcumin, the anti-inflammatory agent, against neurodegenerative, cardiovascular, pulmonary, metabolic, autoimmune and neoplastic diseases. *Int. J. Biochem. Cell Biol.* **2009**, *41*, 40–59. [CrossRef] [PubMed]
8. Sidhu, G.S.; Singh, A.K.; Thaloor, D.; Banaudha, K.K.; Patnaik, G.K.; Srimal, R.C.; Maheshwari, R.K. Enhancement of wound healing by curcumin in animals. *Wound Repair Regen.* **1998**, *6*, 167–177. [CrossRef] [PubMed]
9. Panchatcharam, M.; Miriyala, S.; Gayathri, V.S.; Suguna, L. Curcumin improves wound healing by modulating collagen and decreasing reactive oxygen species. *Mol. Cell. Biochem.* **2006**, *290*, 87–96. [CrossRef] [PubMed]
10. Negi, P.; Jayaprakasha, G.; Jagan Mohan Rao, L.; Sakariah, K. Antibacterial activity of turmeric oil: A byproduct from curcumin manufacture. *J. Agric. Food Chem.* **1999**, *47*, 4297–4300. [CrossRef] [PubMed]
11. Mun, S.H.; Joung, D.K.; Kim, Y.S.; Kang, O.H.; Kim, S.B.; Seo, Y.S.; Kim, Y.C.; Lee, D.S.; Shin, D.W.; Kweon, K.T.; et al. Synergistic antibacterial effect of curcumin against methicillin-resistant Staphylococcus aureus. *Phytomedicine* **2013**, *20*, 714–718. [CrossRef] [PubMed]
12. Rezaee, R.; Momtazi, A.A.; Monemi, A.; Sahebkar, A. Curcumin: A potentially powerful tool to reverse cisplatin-induced toxicity. *Pharmacol. Res.* **2016**, *117*, 218–227. [CrossRef] [PubMed]
13. Wilken, R.; Veena, M.S.; Wang, M.B.; Srivatsan, E.S. Curcumin: A review of anti-cancer properties and therapeutic activity in head and neck squamous cell carcinoma. *Mol. Cancer* **2011**, *10*, 12. [CrossRef] [PubMed]
14. Aggarwal, B.B.; Kumar, A.; Bharti, A.C. Anticancer potential of curcumin: Preclinical and clinical studies. *Anticancer Res.* **2003**, *23*, 363–398. [PubMed]
15. Li, M.; Zhang, Z.; Hill, D.L.; Wang, H.; Zhang, R. Curcumin, a dietary component, has anticancer, chemosensitization, and radiosensitization effects by down-regulating the MDM2 oncogene through the PI3K/mTOR/ETS2 pathway. *Cancer Res.* **2007**, *67*, 1988–1996. [CrossRef] [PubMed]
16. Tapal, A.; Tiku, P.K. Complexation of curcumin with soy protein isolate and its implications on solubility and stability of curcumin. *Food Chem.* **2012**, *130*, 960–965. [CrossRef]
17. Liu, J.; Xu, L.; Liu, C.; Zhang, D.; Wang, S.; Deng, Z.; Lou, W.; Xu, H.; Bai, Q.; Ma, J. Preparation and characterization of cationic curcumin nanoparticles for improvement of cellular uptake. *Carbohydr. Polym.* **2012**, *90*, 16–22. [CrossRef] [PubMed]
18. Sahu, A.; Bora, U.; Kasoju, N.; Goswami, P. Synthesis of novel biodegradable and self-assembling methoxy poly (ethylene glycol)–palmitate nanocarrier for curcumin delivery to cancer cells. *Acta Biomater.* **2008**, *4*, 1752–1761. [CrossRef] [PubMed]
19. Shoba, G.; Joy, D.; Joseph, T.; Majeed, M.; Rajendran, R.; Srinivas, P. Influence of piperine on the pharmacokinetics of curcumin in animals and human volunteers. *Planta Med.* **1998**, *64*, 353–356. [CrossRef] [PubMed]
20. Liu, A.; Lou, H.; Zhao, L.; Fan, P. Validated LC/MS/MS assay for curcumin and tetrahydrocurcumin in rat plasma and application to pharmacokinetic study of phospholipid complex of curcumin. *J. Pharm. Biomed. Anal.* **2006**, *40*, 720–727. [CrossRef] [PubMed]
21. Tiyaboonchai, W.; Tungpradit, W.; Plianbangchang, P. Formulation and characterization of curcuminoids loaded solid lipid nanoparticles. *Int. J. Pharm.* **2007**, *337*, 299–306. [CrossRef] [PubMed]
22. Li, L.; Braiteh, F.S.; Kurzrock, R. Liposome-encapsulated curcumin: In vitro and in vivo effects on proliferation, apoptosis, signaling, and angiogenesis. *J. Clin. Oncol.* **2005**, *104*, 1322–1331. [CrossRef] [PubMed]
23. Hajj Ali, H.; Michaux, F.; Ntsama, B.; Sandrine, I.; Durand, P.; Jasniewski, J.; Linder, M. Shea butter solid nanoparticles for curcumin encapsulation: Influence of nanoparticles size on drug loading. *Eur. J. Lipid Sci. Technol.* **2016**, *118*, 1168–1178. [CrossRef]
24. Wang, T.; Ma, X.; Lei, Y.; Luo, Y. Solid lipid nanoparticles coated with cross-linked polymeric double layer for oral delivery of curcumin. *Colloid Surf. B Biointerfaces* **2016**, *148*, 1–11. [CrossRef] [PubMed]
25. Zhang, J.; Tang, Q.; Xu, X.; Li, N. Development and evaluation of a novel phytosome-loaded chitosan microsphere system for curcumin delivery. *Int. J. Pharm.* **2013**, *448*, 168–174. [CrossRef] [PubMed]
26. Xie, M.-B.; Li, Y.; Zhao, Z.; Chen, A.-Z.; Li, J.-S.; Hu, J.-Y.; Li, G.; Li, Z. Solubility enhancement of curcumin via supercritical CO_2 based silk fibroin carrier. *J. Supercrit. Fluids* **2015**, *103*, 1–9. [CrossRef]

27. Song, W.; Muthana, M.; Mukherjee, J.; Falconer, R.J.; Biggs, C.A.; Zhao, X. Magnetic-silk core-shell nanoparticles as potential carriers for targeted delivery of curcumin into human breast cancer cells. *ACS Biomater. Sci. Eng.* **2017**, *3*, 1027–1038. [CrossRef]
28. Anitha, A.; Maya, S.; Deepa, N.; Chennazhi, K.; Nair, S.; Tamura, H.; Jayakumar, R. Efficient water soluble O-carboxymethyl chitosan nanocarrier for the delivery of curcumin to cancer cells. *Carbohydr. Polym.* **2011**, *83*, 452–461. [CrossRef]
29. Montalbán, M.G.; Coburn, J.M.; Lozano-Pérez, A.A.; Cenis, J.L.; Víllora, G.; Kaplan, D.L. Production of curcumin-loaded silk fibroin nanoparticles for cancer therapy. *Nanomaterials* **2018**, *8*, 126. [CrossRef] [PubMed]
30. Chuah, L.H.; Billa, N.; Roberts, C.J.; Burley, J.C.; Manickam, S. Curcumin-containing chitosan nanoparticles as a potential mucoadhesive delivery system to the colon. *Pharm. Dev. Technol.* **2013**, *18*, 591–599. [CrossRef] [PubMed]
31. Bhandari, R.; Gupta, P.; Dziubla, T.; Hilt, J.Z. Single step synthesis, characterization and applications of curcumin functionalized iron oxide magnetic nanoparticles. *Mater. Sci. Eng. C* **2016**, *67*, 59–64. [CrossRef] [PubMed]
32. Lee, K.Y.; Mooney, D.J. Alginate: Properties and biomedical applications. *Prog. Polym. Sci.* **2012**, *37*, 106–126. [CrossRef] [PubMed]
33. Agnihotri, S.A.; Mallikarjuna, N.N.; Aminabhavi, T.M. Recent advances on chitosan-based micro-and nanoparticles in drug delivery. *J. Control. Release* **2004**, *100*, 5–28. [CrossRef] [PubMed]
34. Ching, S.H.; Bansal, N.; Bhandari, B. Alginate gel particles–A review of production techniques and physical properties. *Crit. Rev. Food Sci. Nutr.* **2017**, *57*, 1133–1152. [CrossRef] [PubMed]
35. Rampino, A.; Borgogna, M.; Blasi, P.; Bellich, B.; Cesàro, A. Chitosan nanoparticles: Preparation, size evolution and stability. *Int. J. Pharm.* **2013**, *455*, 219–228. [CrossRef] [PubMed]
36. Bernkop-Schnürch, A.; Dünnhaupt, S. Chitosan-based drug delivery systems. *Eur. J. Pharm. Biopharm.* **2012**, *81*, 463–469. [CrossRef] [PubMed]
37. Bhunchu, S.; Rojsitthisak, P. Biopolymeric alginate-chitosan nanoparticles as drug delivery carriers for cancer therapy. *Die Pharmazie-An Int. J. Pharm. Sci.* **2014**, *69*, 563–570. [CrossRef]
38. Anitha, A.; Deepagan, V.; Rani, V.D.; Menon, D.; Nair, S.; Jayakumar, R. Preparation, characterization, in vitro drug release and biological studies of curcumin loaded dextran sulphate–chitosan nanoparticles. *Carbohydr. Polym.* **2011**, *84*, 1158–1164. [CrossRef]
39. Ahmadi, F.; Ghasemi-Kasman, M.; Ghasemi, S.; Tabari, M.G.; Pourbagher, R.; Kazemi, S.; Alinejad-Mir, A. Induction of apoptosis in hela cancer cells by an ultrasonic-mediated synthesis of curcumin-loaded chitosan–alginate–sTPP nanoparticles. *Int. J. Nanomed.* **2017**, *12*, 8545–8556. [CrossRef] [PubMed]
40. Maghsoudi, A.; Yazdian, F.; Shahmoradi, S.; Ghaderi, L.; Hemati, M.; Amoabediny, G. Curcumin-loaded polysaccharide nanoparticles: Optimization and anticariogenic activity against Streptococcus mutans. *Mater. Sci. Eng. C* **2017**, *75*, 1259–1267. [CrossRef] [PubMed]
41. Martins, A.F.; Bueno, P.V.; Almeida, E.A.; Rodrigues, F.H.; Rubira, A.F.; Muniz, E.C. Characterization of N-trimethyl chitosan/alginate complexes and curcumin release. *Int. J. Biol. Macromol.* **2013**, *57*, 174–184. [CrossRef] [PubMed]
42. Arruebo, M.; Fernández-Pacheco, R.; Ibarra, M.R.; Santamaría, J. Magnetic nanoparticles for drug delivery. *Nano Today* **2007**, *2*, 22–32. [CrossRef]
43. Iannone, A.; Magin, R.; Walczak, T.; Federico, M.; Swartz, H.; Tomasi, A.; Vannini, V. Blood clearance of dextran magnetite particles determined by a noninvasive in vivo ESR method. *Magn. Reson. Med.* **1991**, *22*, 435–442. [CrossRef] [PubMed]
44. Mancarella, S.; Greco, V.; Baldassarre, F.; Vergara, D.; Maffia, M.; Leporatti, S. Polymer-coated magnetic nanoparticles for curcumin delivery to cancer cells. *Macromol. Biosci.* **2015**, *15*, 1365–1374. [CrossRef] [PubMed]
45. Pavlov, A.M.; Gabriel, S.A.; Sukhorukov, G.B.; Gould, D.J. Improved and targeted delivery of bioactive molecules to cells with magnetic layer-by-layer assembled microcapsules. *Nanoscale* **2015**, *7*, 9686–9693. [CrossRef] [PubMed]
46. Zhou, J.; Romero, G.; Rojas, E.; Ma, L.; Moya, S.; Gao, C. Layer by layer chitosan/alginate coatings on poly (lactide-co-glycolide) nanoparticles for antifouling protection and Folic acid binding to achieve selective cell targeting. *J. Colloid Interface Sci.* **2010**, *345*, 241–247. [CrossRef] [PubMed]

47. Chai, F.; Sun, L.; He, X.; Li, J.; Liu, Y.; Xiong, F.; Ge, L.; Webster, T.J.; Zheng, C. Doxorubicin-loaded poly (lactic-co-glycolic acid) nanoparticles coated with chitosan/alginate by layer by layer technology for antitumor applications. *Int. J. Nanomed.* **2017**, *12*, 1791. [CrossRef] [PubMed]
48. Haidar, Z.S.; Hamdy, R.C.; Tabrizian, M. Protein release kinetics for core–shell hybrid nanoparticles based on the layer-by-layer assembly of alginate and chitosan on liposomes. *Biomaterials* **2008**, *29*, 1207–1215. [CrossRef] [PubMed]
49. Zhou, J.; Moya, S.; Ma, L.; Gao, C.; Shen, J. Polyelectrolyte coated PLGA nanoparticles: Templation and release behavior. *Macromol. Biosci.* **2009**, *9*, 326–335. [CrossRef] [PubMed]
50. Becker, A.L.; Johnston, A.P.; Caruso, F. Layer-by-layer-assembled capsules and films for therapeutic delivery. *Small* **2010**, *6*. [CrossRef] [PubMed]
51. Liu, X.; Chen, X.; Li, Y.; Wang, X.; Peng, X.; Zhu, W. Preparation of superparamagnetic Fe3O4@ alginate/chitosan nanospheres for Candida rugosa lipase immobilization and utilization of layer-by-layer assembly to enhance the stability of immobilized lipase. *ACS Appl. Mater. Interfaces* **2012**, *4*, 5169–5178. [CrossRef] [PubMed]
52. Ching, S.H.; Bhandari, B.; Webb, R.; Bansal, N. Visualizing the interaction between sodium caseinate and calcium alginate microgel particles. *Food Hydrocoll.* **2015**, *43*, 165–171. [CrossRef]
53. Dos Santos Silva, M.; Cocenza, D.S.; Grillo, R.; de Melo, N.F.S.; Tonello, P.S.; de Oliveira, L.C.; Cassimiro, D.L.; Rosa, A.H.; Fraceto, L.F. Paraquat-loaded alginate/chitosan nanoparticles: preparation, characterization and soil sorption studies. *J. Hazard. Mater.* **2011**, *190*, 366–374. [CrossRef] [PubMed]
54. Maldonado, L.; Kokini, J. An optimal window for the fabrication of Edible Polyelectrolyte Complex Nanotubes (EPCNs) from bovine serum albumin (BSA) and sodium alginate. *Food Hydrocoll.* **2018**, *77*, 336–346. [CrossRef]
55. Donati, I.; Paoletti, S. Material properties of alginates. In *Alginates: Biology and Applications*; Springer: Berlin/Heidelberg, Germany, 2009; pp. 1–53.
56. Swain, S.; Dey, R.; Islam, M.; Patel, R.; Jha, U.; Patnaik, T.; Airoldi, C. Removal of fluoride from aqueous solution using aluminum-impregnated chitosan biopolymer. *Sep. Sci. Technol.* **2009**, *44*, 2096–2116. [CrossRef]
57. Acevedo-Fani, A.; Salvia-Trujillo, L.; Soliva-Fortuny, R.; Martín-Belloso, O. Layer-by-layer assembly of food-grade alginate/chitosan nanolaminates: Formation and physicochemical characterization. *Food Biophys.* **2017**, *12*, 299–308. [CrossRef]
58. Rivera, M.C.; Pinheiro, A.C.; Bourbon, A.I.; Cerqueira, M.A.; Vicente, A.A. Hollow chitosan/alginate nanocapsules for bioactive compound delivery. *Int. J. Biol. Macromol.* **2015**, *79*, 95–102. [CrossRef] [PubMed]
59. Wasan, K.M. *Role of Lipid Excipients in Modifying Oral and Parenteral Drug Delivery: Basic Principles and Biological Examples*; John Wiley & Sons: Hoboken, NJ, USA, 2007.
60. Qiu, H.; Qiu, Z.; Wang, J.; Zhang, R.; Zheng, F. Enhanced swelling and methylene blue adsorption of polyacrylamide-based superabsorbents using alginate modified montmorillonite. *J. Appl. Polym. Sci.* **2014**, *131*. [CrossRef]
61. Kevadiya, B.D.; Joshi, G.V.; Patel, H.A.; Ingole, P.G.; Mody, H.M.; Bajaj, H.C. Montmorillonite-alginate nanocomposites as a drug delivery system: Intercalation and in vitro release of vitamin B1 and vitamin B6. *J. Biomater. Appl.* **2010**, *25*, 161–177. [CrossRef] [PubMed]
62. Sartori, C.; Finch, D.S.; Ralph, B.; Gilding, K. Determination of the cation content of alginate thin films by FTIR spectroscopy. *Polymer* **1997**, *38*, 43–51. [CrossRef]
63. Daemi, H.; Barikani, M. Synthesis and characterization of calcium alginate nanoparticles, sodium homopolymannuronate salt and its calcium nanoparticles. *Sci. Iran.* **2012**, *19*, 2023–2028. [CrossRef]
64. Zeng, M.; Feng, Z.; Huang, Y.; Liu, J.; Ren, J.; Xu, Q.; Fan, L. Chemical structure and remarkably enhanced mechanical properties of chitosan-graft-poly (acrylic acid)/polyacrylamide double-network hydrogels. *Polym. Bull.* **2017**, *74*, 55–74. [CrossRef]
65. Su, X.; Mahalingam, S.; Edirisinghe, M.; Chen, B. Highly stretchable and highly resilient polymer–clay nanocomposite hydrogels with low hysteresis. *ACS Appl. Mater. Interfaces* **2017**, *9*, 22223–22234. [CrossRef] [PubMed]
66. Lawrie, G.; Keen, I.; Drew, B.; Chandler-Temple, A.; Rintoul, L.; Fredericks, P.; Grøndahl, L. Interactions between alginate and chitosan biopolymers characterized using FTIR and XPS. *Biomacromolecules* **2007**, *8*, 2533–2541. [CrossRef] [PubMed]

67. Shen, J.; Zhang, D.; Zhang, F.-H.; Gan, Y. AFM tip-sample convolution effects for cylinder protrusions. *Appl. Surf. Sci.* **2017**, *422*, 482–491. [CrossRef]
68. Aditya, N.; Aditya, S.; Yang, H.; Kim, H.W.; Park, S.O.; Ko, S. Co-delivery of hydrophobic curcumin and hydrophilic catechin by a water-in-oil-in-water double emulsion. *Food Chem.* **2015**, *173*, 7–13. [CrossRef] [PubMed]
69. Altunbas, A.; Lee, S.J.; Rajasekaran, S.A.; Schneider, J.P.; Pochan, D.J. Encapsulation of curcumin in self-assembling peptide hydrogels as injectable drug delivery vehicles. *Biomaterials* **2011**, *32*, 5906–5914. [CrossRef] [PubMed]
70. Yang, F.; Lim, G.P.; Begum, A.N.; Ubeda, O.J.; Simmons, M.R.; Ambegaokar, S.S.; Chen, P.P.; Kayed, R.; Glabe, C.G.; Frautschy, S.A. Curcumin inhibits formation of amyloid β oligomers and fibrils, binds plaques, and reduces amyloid in vivo. *J. Biol. Chem.* **2005**, *280*, 5892–5901. [CrossRef] [PubMed]
71. Manju, S.; Sreenivasan, K. Conjugation of curcumin onto hyaluronic acid enhances its aqueous solubility and stability. *J. Colloid Interface Sci.* **2011**, *359*, 318–325. [CrossRef] [PubMed]
72. Cui, J.; Yu, B.; Zhao, Y.; Zhu, W.; Li, H.; Lou, H.; Zhai, G. Enhancement of oral absorption of curcumin by self-microemulsifying drug delivery systems. *Int. J. Pharm.* **2009**, *371*, 148–155. [CrossRef] [PubMed]
73. DeSantis, C.E.; Fedewa, S.A.; Goding Sauer, A.; Kramer, J.L.; Smith, R.A.; Jemal, A. Breast cancer statistics, 2015: Convergence of incidence rates between black and white women. *CA A Cancer J. Clin.* **2016**, *66*, 31–42. [CrossRef] [PubMed]
74. Mohanty, C.; Acharya, S.; Mohanty, A.K.; Dilnawaz, F.; Sahoo, S.K. Curcumin-encapsulated MePEG/PCL diblock copolymeric micelles: A novel controlled delivery vehicle for cancer therapy. *Nanomedicine* **2010**, *5*, 433–449. [CrossRef] [PubMed]
75. Zaman, M.S.; Chauhan, N.; Yallapu, M.M.; Gara, R.K.; Maher, D.M.; Kumari, S.; Sikander, M.; Khan, S.; Zafar, N.; Jaggi, M. Curcumin nanoformulation for cervical cancer treatment. *Sci. Rep.* **2016**, *6*, 20051. [CrossRef] [PubMed]
76. Mohan Yallapu, M.; Ray Dobberpuhl, M.; Michele Maher, D.; Jaggi, M.; Chand Chauhan, S. Design of curcumin loaded cellulose nanoparticles for prostate cancer. *Curr. Drug Metab.* **2012**, *13*, 120–128. [CrossRef]
77. Jagannathan, R.; Abraham, P.M.; Poddar, P. Temperature-dependent spectroscopic evidences of curcumin in aqueous medium: A mechanistic study of its solubility and stability. *J. Phys. Chem. B* **2012**, *116*, 14533–14540. [CrossRef] [PubMed]
78. Mangalathillam, S.; Rejinold, N.S.; Nair, A.; Lakshmanan, V.-K.; Nair, S.V.; Jayakumar, R. Curcumin loaded chitin nanogels for skin cancer treatment via the transdermal route. *Nanoscale* **2012**, *4*, 239–250. [CrossRef] [PubMed]
79. Rejinold, N.S.; Sreerekha, P.; Chennazhi, K.; Nair, S.; Jayakumar, R. Biocompatible, biodegradable and thermo-sensitive chitosan-g-poly (N-isopropylacrylamide) nanocarrier for curcumin drug delivery. *Int. J. Biol. Macromol.* **2011**, *49*, 161–172. [CrossRef] [PubMed]
80. Kunwar, A.; Barik, A.; Mishra, B.; Rathinasamy, K.; Pandey, R.; Priyadarsini, K. Quantitative cellular uptake, localization and cytotoxicity of curcumin in normal and tumor cells. *Biochim. Biophys. Acta (BBA)-Gen. Subj.* **2008**, *1780*, 673–679. [CrossRef] [PubMed]
81. Chaves, N.L.; Estrela-Lopis, I.; Böttner, J.; Lopes, C.A.; Guido, B.C.; de Sousa, A.R.; Báo, S.N. Exploring cellular uptake of iron oxide nanoparticles associated with rhodium citrate in breast cancer cells. *Int. J. Nanomed.* **2017**, *12*, 5511–5523. [CrossRef] [PubMed]
82. Kettler, K.; Veltman, K.; van de Meent, D.; van Wezel, A.; Hendriks, A.J. Cellular uptake of nanoparticles as determined by particle properties, experimental conditions, and cell type. *Environ. Toxicol. Chem.* **2014**, *33*, 481–492. [CrossRef] [PubMed]
83. Kohler, N.; Sun, C.; Wang, J.; Zhang, M. Methotrexate-modified superparamagnetic nanoparticles and their intracellular uptake into human cancer cells. *Langmuir* **2005**, *21*, 8858–8864. [CrossRef] [PubMed]

84. Syng-ai, C.; Kumari, A.L.; Khar, A. Effect of curcumin on normal and tumor cells: Role of glutathione and bcl-2. *Mol. Cancer Ther.* **2004**, *3*, 1101–1108. [PubMed]
85. Shishodia, S.; Amin, H.M.; Lai, R.; Aggarwal, B.B. Curcumin (diferuloylmethane) inhibits constitutive NF-κB activation, induces G1/S arrest, suppresses proliferation, and induces apoptosis in mantle cell lymphoma. *Biochem. Pharmacol.* **2005**, *70*, 700–713. [CrossRef] [PubMed]

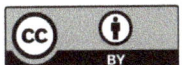

© 2018 by the authors. Licensee MDPI, Basel, Switzerland. This article is an open access article distributed under the terms and conditions of the Creative Commons Attribution (CC BY) license (http://creativecommons.org/licenses/by/4.0/).

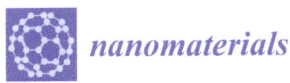

Article

Polydopamine Modified Superparamagnetic Iron Oxide Nanoparticles as Multifunctional Nanocarrier for Targeted Prostate Cancer Treatment

Nimisha Singh [1], Fadoua Sallem [2], Celine Mirjolet [3], Thomas Nury [4], Suban Kumar Sahoo [1], Nadine Millot [2,*] and Rajender Kumar [1,*]

1. Department of Applied Chemistry, Sardar Vallabhbhai National Institute of Technology, 395007 Surat, India; nimisha.singh01@gmail.com (N.S.); sks@chem.svnit.ac.in (S.K.S.)
2. Laboratoire Interdisciplinaire Carnot de Bourgogne (ICB), UMR 6303 CNRS/Université Bourgogne Franche-Comté, 21 000 Dijon, France; fadouasallem@gmail.com
3. Radiotherapy Department, Centre Georges-François Leclerc, 21 000 Dijon, France; CMirjolet@cgfl.fr
4. Laboratoire Bio-PeroxIL, Université Bourgogne Franche-Comté/Inserm, 21 000 Dijon, France; thomas.nury@u-bourgogne.fr
* Correspondence: nmillot@u-bourgogne.fr (N.M.); rajenderkumar@chem.svnit.ac.in (R.K.)

Received: 11 December 2018; Accepted: 12 January 2019; Published: 22 January 2019

Abstract: Polydopamine (pDA)-modified iron oxide core-shell nanoparticles (IONPs) are developed and designed as nanovectors of drugs. Reactive quinone of pDA enhances the binding efficiency of various biomolecules for targeted delivery. Glutathione disulfide (GSSG), an abundant thiol species in the cytoplasm, was immobilized on the pDA-IONP surface. It serves as a cellular trigger to release the drug from the nanoparticles providing an efficient platform for the drug delivery system. Additionally, GSSG on the surface was further modified to form S-nitrosoglutathione that can act as nitric oxide (NO) donors. These NPs were fully characterized using a transmission electronic microscopy (TEM), thermogravimetric analysis (TGA), dynamic light scattering (DLS), zeta potential, X-ray photoelectron spectroscopy (XPS), Fourier transform infrared (FTIR) and UV-vis spectroscopies. Doxorubicin (DOX) and docetaxel (DTX) are two anticancer drugs, which were loaded onto nanoparticles with respective loading efficiencies of 243 and 223 µmol/g of IONPs, calculated using TGA measurements. DOX release study, using UV-vis spectroscopy, showed a pH responsive behavior, making the elaborated nanocarrier a potential drug delivery system. (3-(4,5-dimethylthiazol-2-yl)-5-(3-carboxymethoxyphenyl)-2-(4-sulfophenyl) -2H-tetrazolium (MTS) and apoptosis assays were performed on PC3 cell lines to evaluate the efficiency of the developed nanocarriers. These nanoparticles thus can prove their worth in cancer treatment on account of their easy access to the site and release of drug in response to changes to internal parameters such as pH, chemicals, etc.

Keywords: core-shell nanoparticles; biocompatible; drug delivery; anticancer

1. Introduction

Multifunctional nanohybrid systems offer several advantages for integrating functional nanocomponents into one entity to manifest different roles in cancer therapeutics. They provide an ideal platform to construct the nanostructure material that can be tuned to the required physical and chemical properties. Although new chemotherapeutic molecules have been continuously developed to treat cancer, medical advancement has failed to control the serious side effects caused by such compounds [1]. Thus, to address these issues and have a targeted anticancer treatment, efficient drug delivery carrier is required. Nano drug delivery carrier shows the potential of carrying the anticancer drug to the targeted site and delivering it according to the required pharmacology activity. Consequently, core shell nanoparticles have emerged as a promising nanocarrier for targeting tumor cells [2].

Uniform core shell nanoparticles systems, having a magnetic core with a functional shell, have been widely explored in protein separation, targeted drug delivery, magnetic resonance imaging, etc. [3–5]. Polydopamine (pDA) coated iron oxide nanoparticles (IONPs) are such a class of nanohybrids that have been developed with considerable interest as a multifunctional platform, thanks to their unique biocompatibility, enhanced magnetic resonance (MR) contrast and facile surface modification [6]. pDA is the polymerized structure of dopamine (DA) monomer that undergoes self-polymerization at alkaline pH giving both catechol and amine functional groups on the surface [7]. During the polymerization step, it results in the formation of a conformal and continuous coating layer on any substrate material via strong binding affinity of catechol functional groups. Moreover, this shell thickness can be potentially monitored by varying the reaction condition and the amount of DA in the medium [8].

Recent years have witnessed an exponential growth in research concerning advance functionalization and application of pDA-based nanohybrids in medical fields [9]. Thus, we chose pDA-coated IONPs for immobilizing glutathione disulfide (GSSG), which can serve as an efficient nanocarrier to carry doxorubicin (DOX) and docetaxel (DTX) for prostate cancer treatment. pDA is known to carry highly functional groups on the surface that allows the immobilization of biomolecules via Michael addition [9]. Immobilizing biomolecules on the pDA surface can increase the efficacy of drug release in the system [10].

It was reported that nanocarriers bearing reducible disulfide bonds can be easily cleaved with GSSG by thiol/disulfide exchange [11]. Glutathione in living cells exists in a redox equilibrium state between the disulfide (GSSG, oxidized form) and sulfhydryl (GSH, reduced form) where the change in the concentration of glutathione level marks the change in the oxidative stress caused by the tumor cells. Thus, the triggered release largely depends on the redox potential controlled by the oxidation and the reduction of glutathione (GSH/GSSG) [12] and, therefore, can attain the intracellular delivery of loaded drug [13], DNA [14], and siRNA for cancer therapeutics [15]. Thus, biocompatible nanohybrids with disulfide/thiol groups are of great interest in improving the drug delivery system.

Our objective is focused on immobilizing GSSG on pDA-IONPs to serve as a dual purpose towards prostate cancer treatment. Since GSH plays an important role in determining various cellular processes, it has also been reported that it can be a determining factor for the sensitivity of some tumors to several chemotherapeutic agents [16]. It may also turn out to be a successful biomarker for selecting tumors potentially responsive to chemotherapeutic regimens.

Thus, firstly, we chose GSSG to reduce its disulfide bond in order to have thiol groups on IONP's surface. These free thiol groups can serve as nitric oxide (NO) donors in the system by forming S-nitrosothiols (SNOs). SNOs possess the same physiological functions as NO, which include neurotransmission, hormone secretion and vasodilation in living bodies [17,18]. Additionally, NO has also emerged as antimicrobial agent [19] and has a tumoricidal factor [20] that makes it a promising pharmaceutical agent. Secondly, reduced GSSG (GSH) can carry DOX or DTX drugs for targeted prostate cancer cell treatment. While DOX has been widely used in the treatment of hematological and solid tumor malignancies, DTX is popularly used in the treatment of prostate cancers. Thus, in the present work we explored DOX activity in treating prostate cancer along with DTX. The details of the objective can be better understood with Scheme 1.

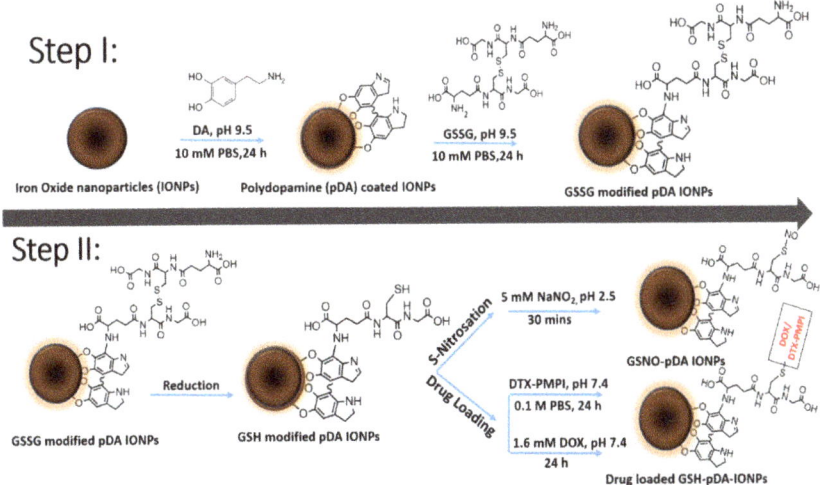

Scheme 1. Schematic representation showing the sequential synthesis of Step I: GSSG functionalized pDA-coated IONPs; and Step II: GSSG reduced to GSH-modified pDA-IONPs followed by S-nitrosation and loading of anticancer drugs (DOX and DTX).

2. Materials and Methods

Doxorubicin HCl (DOX), dopamine (DA), dithiothreitol (DTT), sodium hydroxide (NaOH, ≥97%), hydrochloric acid (HCl, 37%), nitric acid (HNO_3, 69%), Elman's reagent 5-dithiobis[2 nitrobenzoicacid] (DTNB) and ammonium hydroxide (NH_4OH, 28%) were obtained from Sigma Aldrich (St. Louis, MO, USA). p-maleimidophenyl isocyanate (PMPI) was purchased from Thermo Scientific (Fair Lown, NJ, USA). Iron (II) chloride tetrahydrate ($FeCl_2·4H_2O$, 98%) and iron (III) chloride hexahydrate ($FeCl_3·6H_2O$, 97%) were purchased from Alfa Aesar (Karlsruhe, Germany). Docetaxel (DTX) was purchased from BIOTREND Chemikalien GmbH (Cologne, Germany). PBS 1× solution (Fisher Bioreagents, Fair Lown, NJ, USA), and dimethyl sulfoxide (DMSO, ≥99.7%) (Acroseal) were also purchased from Fisher Chemicals (Leicestershire, UK). Annexin V-FITC (fluorescein isothiocyanate) detection kit with PI (propidium iodide) staining for cell apoptosis was obtained from BD biosciences (Franklin Lakes, NJ, USA). Borate buffered saline was prepared from boric acid (99.8%). Acetate buffer was prepared from sodium acetate and acetic acid. The ultrafiltration stirred cell (Model 8400, 400 mL) and membranes (ref. #PLHK07610, regenerated cellulose 100 kDa) were acquired from Merck Millipore (Darmstadt, Germany). All other chemicals were used of analytical grade and without further purification.

2.1. Characterization Techniques

The size and the morphology of the nanoparticles were analyzed using a JEOL JEM-2100 LaB6 transmission electronic microscope (TEM, Tokyo, Japan) with an acceleration voltage of 200 kV and equipped with a high tilt pole-piece achieving a point-to point resolution of 0.25 nm. The samples were prepared by evaporating a diluted suspension of NPs in deionized water on a carbon-coated copper grid. The average size of nanoparticles was determined by counting individual IONPs on each sample (150 nanoparticles).

The chemical composition of the NPs' surface, involved during the process of nanohybrid synthesis, was investigated with X-ray photoelectron spectroscopy (XPS) using PHI 5000 Versaprobe apparatus (ULVAC-PHI, Osaka, Japan) with a monochromatic Al Kα1 X-ray source (energy of 1486.7 eV with a 200 μm spot size, accelerating voltage of 12 kV, and power of 200 W). The applied pass energy

(PE) was 180 eV for the spectra and 50 eV for windows. Powders were pressed on an indium sheet. Data were analyzed using CasaXPS software for processing the peaks. Neutralization was used to minimize charge effects and the carbon C1s peak at 284.5 eV was used as the reference. A Shirley background was subtracted and Gauss (70%)–Lorentz (30%) profiles were used. Full width at half maximum (FWHM) was fixed between 1.5 and 1.9 eV. ULVAC-PHI MultiPak software (ver. 9.0.1, Osaka, Japan) was employed for quantitative analysis.

To confirm the functionalization of pDA and the immobilization of GSSG over the IONPs, a Bruker Vertex 70v (Billerica, MA, USA) using OPUS version 3.1 was used to obtain Fourier transform infrared (FT-IR) spectra using the KBr method with the wavenumber range of 400–4000 cm^{-1}, resolution of 4 cm^{-1} and a total of 30 scans per measurement.

UV-visible spectroscopic measurements were carried out to study the absorbance of the as prepared nanoparticles and drug release kinetics using a Shimadzu UV-2550 UV-Vis spectrophotometer (Tokyo, Japan). All the spectra were measured in the range of 220–800 nm and recorded at room temperature using quartz cuvette of 1 cm path length.

Drug kinetics were also analyzed using fluorescence spectroscopy using a Cary Eclipse fluorescent spectrophotometer (Santa Clara, CA, USA) in the emission range of 380–700 nm. The selected excitation and emission slits were 5 and 10 nm, respectively.

Hydrodynamic diameter and zeta potential measurements were carried out using Malvern Nano ZS instrument (Worcestershire, UK) supplied by DTS Nano V7.11 software (Worcestershire, UK). The Smoluchowski equation was used for zetametry measurements. For each measurement, powders were dispersed in 12 mL of NaCl aqueous solution (10^{-2} M). pH titrations were performed using HCl (0.1 M), NaOH (0.1 M) or NaOH (0.01 M) aqueous solutions. Standard deviations were calculated from three measurements performed on the same sample. Samples were analyzed using a backscattering angle (173°). The refractive index of Fe_3O_4 NPs is 2.42 and the absorption is equal to 0.029. Hydrodynamic diameters in this paper refer to the Z-average, which is the intensity weighted mean diameter derived from the cumulants analysis. Hydrodynamic diameter was determined by dynamic light scattering (DLS, Malvern, Worcestershire, UK) curves, which were derived from a number distribution calculation process.

The diffraction data were collected at room temperature, using a D8 Advance X-ray diffractometer (Vantack detector) (Billerica, MA, USA), in the 2θ range 10–100°. The Cu $K_{\alpha 1,2}$ radiations ($\lambda_{\alpha 1}$ = 1.540598 Å and $\lambda_{\alpha 2}$ = 1.544426 Å) were applied. The data analysis was carried out with Topas® software (Billerica, MA, USA). Le Bail method was used to obtain lattice parameters and mean crystallite size. The phase identification was established by comparison of the diffraction patterns to the ICDD: The International Centre for Diffraction Data Powder Diffraction File Reference.

Powders were analyzed using a Discovery TGA-TA instrument (Newcastle, UK) with a gas (nitrogen:oxygen 80:20) flow rate of 25 mL min^{-1}. The applied thermal program was as following: ramp 1 of 20 °C.min^{-1} from 25 to 100 °C; isotherm at 100 °C for 30 min (to remove the remaining moisture) and ramp 2 of 5 °C.min^{-1} from 100 to 800 °C.

Magnetic susceptibility measurements were performed on a Bartington MS3 magneto-susceptometer (Witney, England) at 300 K. A MS2G mono frequency sensor at 1.3 kHz from Bartington (Oxford, England) was used for around 1 mL cells operated at 1.3 kHz.

2.2. Preparation of Coated Iron Oxide Nanoparticles

2.2.1. Synthesis of Bare IONPs

Iron oxide nanoparticles (Fe_3O_4, IONPs) were prepared by a facile chemical co-precipitation method [21] where $FeCl_3·6H_2O$ (34.6 g) and $FeCl_2·4H_2O$ (12.7 g), in the molar ratio of 2:1, were dissolved in 1.5 L of water. Then, Fe_3O_4 nanoparticles were precipitated quickly by adding ammonia (120 mL, 28%) in the solution at 22 °C. The obtained black suspension was stirred for 2–3 min. The obtained black precipitate was then magnetically decanted and washed thoroughly with deionized

(DI) water until the solution reached pH 8. The precipitate was then kept in nitric acid solution (1 mM, pH 3) and dialyzed against nitric acid solution (10 mM) for 48 h. Dialyzed nanoparticles were then centrifuged for 15 min at 20,000 G with deceleration to obtain stable IONPs. The supernatant was then used for further characterizations and surface modification.

2.2.2. Synthesis of Polydopamine-modified IONPs: pDA-IONPs

A quantity of 100 mg of Fe_3O_4 (10 mg mL^{-1}) was dispersed under continuous stirring in 25 mL of 10 mM DA solution (PBS, 10 mM, pH 9.0) for 24 h at 22 °C. After, polydopamine-modified nanoparticles (pDA-IONPs) were magnetically decanted, washed thoroughly 5 times with ultrapure water using ultrafiltration to remove the non-reacted DA (ensured using UV), and further dispersed in water.

2.2.3. Preparation of GSSG-modified Nanoparticles

GSSG-modified nanoparticles were prepared using 20 mg of pDA-IONPs, which were dispersed in 1 mg mL^{-1} GSSG solution (10 mM PBS, pH 9.4) for 24 h under continuous magnetic agitation (700 rpm) at 22 °C. The GSSG-modified nanoparticles (GSSG-pDA-IONPs) were magnetically separated using magnetic syringe [22], washed with PBS buffer and checked with DTT to ensure the complete removal of unreacted GSSG. DTT reduces the unreacted disulfide, giving a yellow color solution indicating the presence of disulfide group. The resultant nanoparticles were then washed and re-dispersed in PBS.

The above nanoparticles were then reduced to glutathione to get free –SH. Briefly, GSSG modified nanoparticles (800 µL of the suspension) were first mixed with Tris buffer (0.2 M, pH 9), after which, DTT (0.01 M) was added and the reduction of disulfide was allowed to proceed for 1 h at 22 °C. To ensure the reduction, DTNB (0.01 M) in acetate buffer (0.2 M, pH 5) was reacted with the sample and the absorbance was measured at 408 nm.

S-nitrosation was then performed using $NaNO_2$ (0.4 mM). The reaction took place when GSH-pDA-IONPs were successively added in $NaNO_2$ solution at 37 °C and pH 2.5 for 30 min in the dark. UV-vis spectra were recorded to see the formation of S-nitrosation and the resultant nanoparticles were finally washed with PBS buffer and re-dispersed in PBS.

2.3. Drug Loading

For the incorporation of doxorubicin (DOX), the DOX solution (600 µL, 1 mg mL^{-1}) was added dropwise with stirring to an aqueous dispersion of GSH-pDA-IONPs (3 mg of particles in 5 mL of water) at 22 °C. Stirring was continued for 24 h to allow the partitioning of the drug into the nanoparticles. The absorbance of the supernatant was measured to determine the loading efficiency of the nanoparticles before and after the reaction. The obtained nanoparticles were then washed with deionized water (DI), magnetically separated using magnetic syringe and resuspended in DI water for further studies. Quantification and release kinetics of loaded drug were performed using UV-vis spectroscopy and TGA.

For the incorporation of docetaxel (DTX), DTX was first activated using PMPI, where prior to loading, DTX was initially dispersed in DMSO and mixed with PMPI (1:4 molar ratio) in borate buffer saline solution (0.1 M, pH 8.5) for 24 h at 22 °C [23]. The resultant solution was then dialyzed against water to eliminate unreacted PMPI. DTX-PMPI was then analyzed using nuclear magnetic resonance NMR and infrared spectroscopy (FTIR), and loaded on GSH-pDA-IONPs in a reaction medium of PBS (0.1 M, pH 7.4) for 24 h at 22 °C. The developed nanoparticles were then magnetically washed, separated and freeze dried for further characterizations.

2.4. Release Profile

After purification of DOX-loaded nanoparticles, the dialysis tube filled with DOX-loaded nanoparticles suspension was transferred to a beaker containing 25 mL of phosphate buffer (10 mM) to study the drug release at 37 °C with continuous stirring at 100 rpm. To quantify the drug release, 2 mL of samples were analyzed at different time interval. The amount of released DOX was analyzed with a spectrophotometer at 485 nm. The release was studied in 3 different pH (3.5, 5.4 and 7.4) where it was adjusted with HCl and NaOH. The experiments were performed in triplicate for all samples.

2.5. In Vitro Assays

Cytotoxicity was measured on PC-3 cell lines. The cells, at a concentration of 3000 cells/well, were seeded in 96-well plates and incubated at 37 °C in 190 µL of drug-free culture medium (DMEM) with 10% of fetal bovine serum for 24 h before treatment (when cells were at around 20% confluence). The cytotoxicity assays were performed using the following compounds: free drug (DOX or DTX), GSH-pDA-IONPs, and drug loaded GSH-pDA IONPs. Tumor cells were incubated (10 µL of drug on 190 µL of culture medium) with a range of equivalent drug concentrations. After 48 h incubation, cell viability was evaluated using MTS (3-(4,5-dimethylthiazol-2-yl)-5-(3-carboxymethoxyphenyl)-2-(4-sulfophenyl)-2H-tetrazolium) assay (Promega Corporation, Madison, WI, USA) according to Mirjolet et al. [24]. Experiments were performed 6 times and the results were calculated as the mean of the measurements.

2.6. Analysis of Cell Proliferation by Flow Cytometry

Flow cytometry was used to analyze cells' proliferation after their incubation with a DOX-loaded sample, by estimating the proportion of cells in apoptosis. After 24 h of incubation in 6-well plates, PC-3 cells were exposed to GSH-pDA-IONPs and DOX-GSH-pDA-IONPs for 24 h plus a negative control well. After the treatment, a double staining with annexin V-FITC and propidium iodide (PI) was performed with an FITC annexin V apoptosis detection kit obtained from Thermo Scientific (Fair Lown, NJ, USA). The cells were washed twice in PBS without Ca^{2+} and Mg^{2+}, trypsinized with 1 mL of trypsine solution 1× and then centrifuged for 5 min at 300 g. After 2 washes with cold PBS, 1 mL of annexin V binding buffer (1×), 10 µL of annexin V-FITC and 10 µL of PI staining solutions were added to each sample. Finally, cells were incubated for 15 min at 37 °C. Cell suspensions were analyzed with a Galaxy flow cytometer (Partec, Görlitz, Germany). Red fluorescence of PI was collected through a 590-nm long-pass filter and green fluorescence was collected through a 520-nm band-pass filter. For each sample, about 10,000 cells were analyzed and the data were treated with FlowJo (Tree Star Inc., Ashland, OR, USA) software.

3. Results

The morphology and the size of the synthesized nanoparticles were analyzed using TEM, XRD and DLS measurements as shown in Figure 1, where the size of bare IONPs is calculated to be 9.0 ± 4.0 nm from TEM measurements and 10.1 ± 0.1 nm from XRD (Figure S1). The lattice parameter determined from XRD is 8.368 ± 0.001 Å. The diffracting planes (222), (311), (422) and (511) and the interatomic distances observed on the selected area diffraction pattern of Fe_3O_4 (Figures S1 and S2) are in good agreement with the spinel structure (ICDD: 19-0629) [25]. This lattice parameter suggests that the powder is slightly oxidized (Fe_3O_4 crystallites and a small presence of γ-Fe_2O_3 on the surface) [26,27]. Additionally, with DLS measurements, the hydrodynamic diameter of IONPs at pH 5.0–6.0, is observed to be 33 ± 5 nm (PDI = 0.38 ± 0.07). The TEM image of the polydopamine coated IONPs (Figure 1B) reveals the presence of a homogeneous layer of pDA on the surface with a thickness of about 2 nm, calculated using ImageJ software. It is also observed that even with pDA coating, the crystalline nature of IONPs is retained (inset Figure 1B and Figure S2).

The hydrodynamic diameter, obtained from DLS measurements, is 164 ± 8 nm (PDI = 0.66 ± 0.01) in the case of pDA-IONPs, which is larger than that of bare IONPs. Indeed, pDA form an organic shell with reactive functional groups, which increases the interaction between IONPs and forms small aggregates. This large size can be due to the swelling effect of the polymer when coated over IONPs [28]. During the polymerization step of dopamine, it tends to produce oligomers having from four to eight 5,6-dihydroxyindole units which are assembled in an orderly manner via π stacking to form nanoaggregates [29]. This results in the formation of continuous film on the surface that can be seen in the TEM image (Figure 1B).

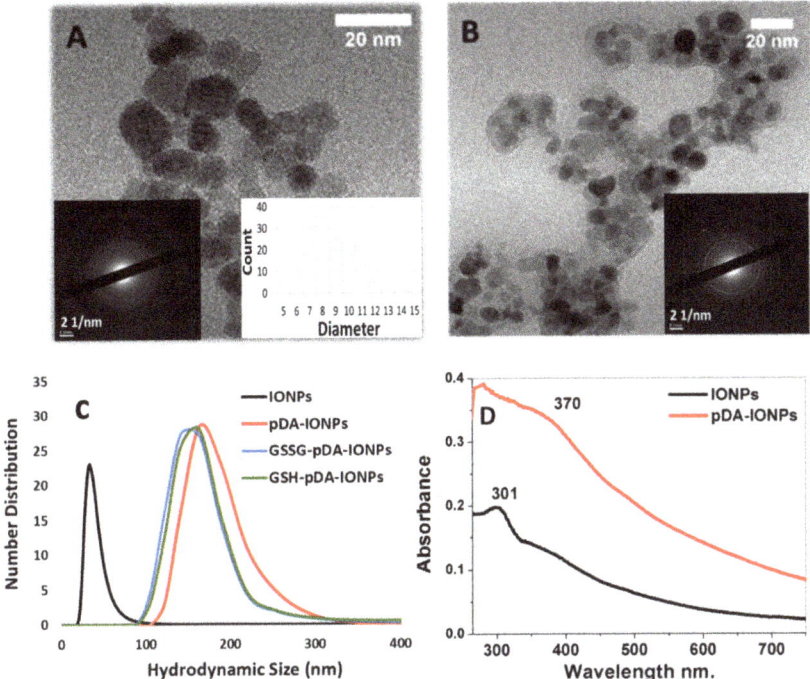

Figure 1. Transmission electronic microscope (TEM) images of (**A**) bare IONPs; and (**B**) pDA-coated IONPs (inset selected area (electron) diffraction (SAED) patterns and size distribution); (**C**) Dynamic light scattering (DLS) measurements showing the hydrodynamic diameter at pH = 5.0–6.0 and in 10^{-2} M NaCl; and (**D**) UV-vis spectra of the synthesized nanoparticles.

UV-vis absorbance spectra are recorded to understand the polymerization step of DA on the surface of IONPs. In Figure 1D, the pDA-IONPs show an absorbance band at 370 nm, which is the characteristic of polymerized layer of quinone, the intermediate molecule of pDA, onto the IONP surface [21]. On the other hand, the characteristic absorbance band of IONPs is observed at 301 nm as shown in Figure 1D.

Since our objective is to have thiol groups on the surface for a wide range of applicability of the developed nanoparticles in the field of medicine, upon binding of GSSG to pDA-IONPs, similar hydrodynamic size (141 ± 2 nm, PDI = 0.68 ± 0.15) is observed. After the reduction of GSSG to GSH, the DLS measurements indicate the same hydrodynamic size as the previous step (140 ± 2 nm, polydispersity index (PDI) = 0.33 ± 0.03). This result shows that reduction step does not affect the hydrodynamic size of coated IONPs.

It has been reported that physicochemical properties such as shape, size and surface charge mark an important role in the cellular uptake of nanoparticles [30]. Indeed, nanoparticles with a negative surface charge show greater cellular uptake due to their high interaction with cells or organs such as the liver [31]. Thus, zeta potential measurements were used to explore the surface charge of coated IONPs. The zeta potential of the synthesized nanoparticles with and without the surface modification with pDA and GSSG as a function of pH is measured as shown in Figure 2. The hydroxyl groups (Fe–OH) on the surface of bare IONPs are responsible for their surface charge. Indeed, in basic condition, it results in negative values of zeta potential due to the formation of Fe–O$^-$ and positive values in acidic conditions due to the formation of Fe-OH$_2^+$ [32]. The isoelectric point (IEP) of bare IONPs is measured to be 8.2 which decreases to 6.4, 4.7 and 4.5 upon functionalization with pDA, GSSG and GSH respectively. This shift in the IEP from 8.2 for bare IONPs to 4.5 for GSH-pDA-IONPs suggests the successful immobilization of GSH molecules onto the surface of IONPs [33]. Moreover, the decrease in the zeta potential values, after pDA and GSH grafting, proves the presence of an organic shell which hides a part of the surface charge of IONPs [34]. Also, at physiological pH, the colloidal stability of the synthesized nanoparticles, on the successive molecules' conjugation, is improved as shown in Figure S3, thanks to the increase in the absolute value of zeta potential and the steric hindrance of the organic molecules, thereby making them suitable nanocarriers for drug loading.

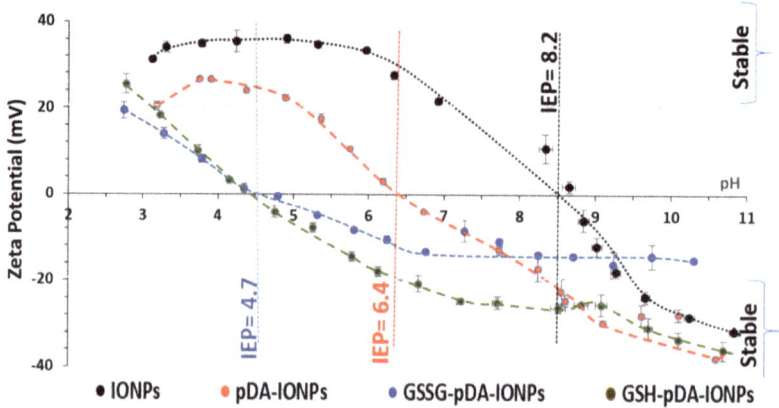

Figure 2. Zeta potential vs pH curves showing the isoelectric point of differently functionalized nanoparticles in 10^{-2} M NaCl.

The magnetic nature was also analyzed as a calibration curve shown in Figure S4, supporting information (SI) showing the magnetic susceptibility of the prepared IONPs increases with increase in the concentration of nanoparticles used.

Chemical and thermal properties of pDA- and GSSG-functionalized IONPs are further characterized using FTIR, XPS and TGA measurements. The presence of pDA layer is confirmed from IR stretching frequencies at 1611, 1460 and 1270 cm^{-1}, which correspond to the vibration bands of aromatic rings of pDA (Figure 3A) [21]. Naked IONPs exhibit the magnetite characteristic Fe–O stretching band at 580 cm^{-1}, which remains constant even after the formation of a pDA layer on the surface. FTIR spectrum of GSSG-modified pDA-IONPs gives an additional strong stretching band of C=O at 1690 cm^{-1}, attributed to the carboxylic group of GSSG, which remains after the reduction of GSSG into GSH (Figure 3B). Furthermore, a broad stretching band of primary amine is observed on GSSG modification at 3300 cm^{-1}, which is shifted to 3400 cm^{-1} on the reduction step of GSSG to GSH. This shift may be explained by the intramolecular hydrogen bonding between NH$_2$ and carboxylic oxygen. The GSH modified nanoparticles show a slightly quenched fluorescence emission when compared to only pDA-IONPs (Figure 3C), measured at the same concentration, which supports the immobilization step of glutathione onto pDA-IONPs. Indeed, pDA nanoparticles are known to show an inherent fluorescence property [35]. Since pDA possesses reactive quinone and amine groups, it can actively bind to the GSSG molecule and consequently GSH serves as an excellent fluorescent quencher. Thus, GSSG-pDA shows the potential to quench fluorescence via plausible electron-electron transfer energy process [36].

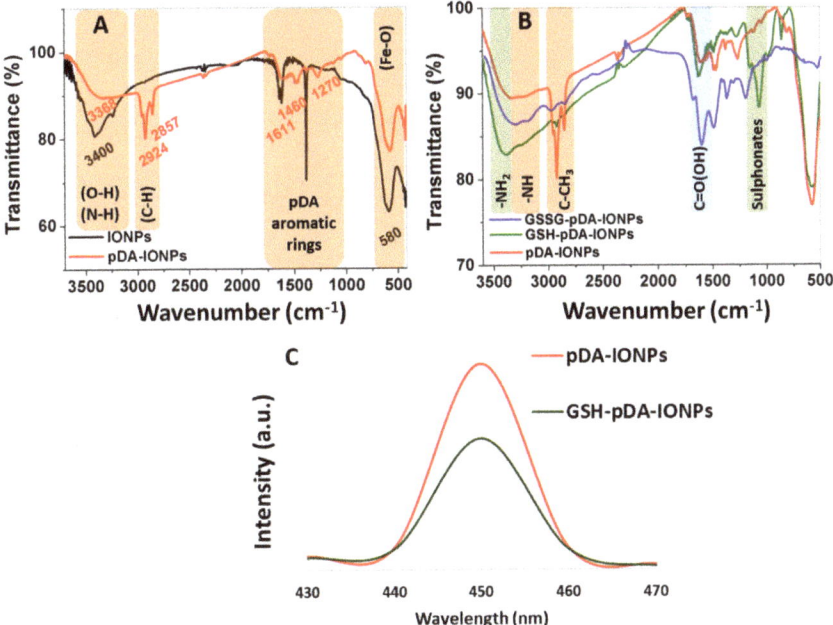

Figure 3. (**A**,**B**) Fourier transform infrared (FTIR) spectra showing the successful conjugation of pDA and GSSG molecules on IONPs; and (**C**) fluorescence spectra of pDA-IONPs and GSH-pDA-IONPs with $\lambda_{excitation}$ = 400 nm, $\lambda_{emission}$ = 450 nm.

X-ray photoelectron spectroscopy is a highly surface sensitive technique and provides accurate information about surface properties [37,38]. The XPS survey scans of IONPs, pDA-IONPs and GSSG-pDA-IONPs are shown in Figure 4. The elemental composition, calculated from XPS (Table 1), explains that after pDA coating, the atomic percentages of carbon and nitrogen increase drastically from 3.0% to 41.8% and from 1.1% to 4.5%, respectively, which confirms the presence of a pDA shell, where Fe atomic percentage decreases. Indeed, as the XPS is a surface analysis technique (about 5 nm of depth) and the thickness of organic shell increases progressively after each grafting, the inorganic core becomes more and more covered and not easily accessible. On immobilizing GSSG onto pDA-IONPS, the atomic percentage of carbon (C) further increases to 51.1% and a similar trend is observed for nitrogen. This is also observed on analyzing the survey spectra shown in Figure 4A, where the intensity of carbon and nitrogen increase on reacting IONPs with pDA and GSSG.

To understand the nature of the chemical bonds of Fe and O in bare IONPs, decomposition of XPS spectra was realized. On fitting Fe 2p spectrum, it is split into $2p_{1/2}$ and $2p_{3/2}$ due to spin orbit j-j coupling as shown in Figure 4B [39]. In addition to the two major peaks (Fe $2p_{3/2}$ at 710.7 eV and Fe $2p_{1/2}$ at 724.3 eV), two satellite peaks are also observed, which are Fe(II) $2p_{3/2}$ satellite peak at 719.1 eV and Fe(III) $2p_{1/2}$ satellite peak at 732.7 eV (Figure 4B). The oxidation state of iron species present in the sample may be evaluated thanks to these data. Indeed, the binding energy difference between Fe $2p_{3/2}$ and its satellite peaks is related to the oxidation state of the iron cations; this difference is close to 6 eV for Fe^{2+} and 8 eV for Fe^{3+}. In our case, this difference is equal to 8.4 eV for bare IONPs [40]. Thus, XPS shows that the surface of bare IONPs is oxidized with the presence of mainly Fe^{3+}. The other contributions, respectively located at 712.6 and 726.2 eV, could not be attributed to Fe^{2+} contribution, because they should be located at lower energies (about 709 eV) [41]. However, they may be assigned to Fe–O–OH [42]. Similarly, the XPS spectrum of oxygen in bare IONPs shows two peaks at 530.2 eV and 531.6 eV, which are attributed to the binding energies of Fe–O–Fe and Fe–OH bonds as shown in Figure 4C [43].

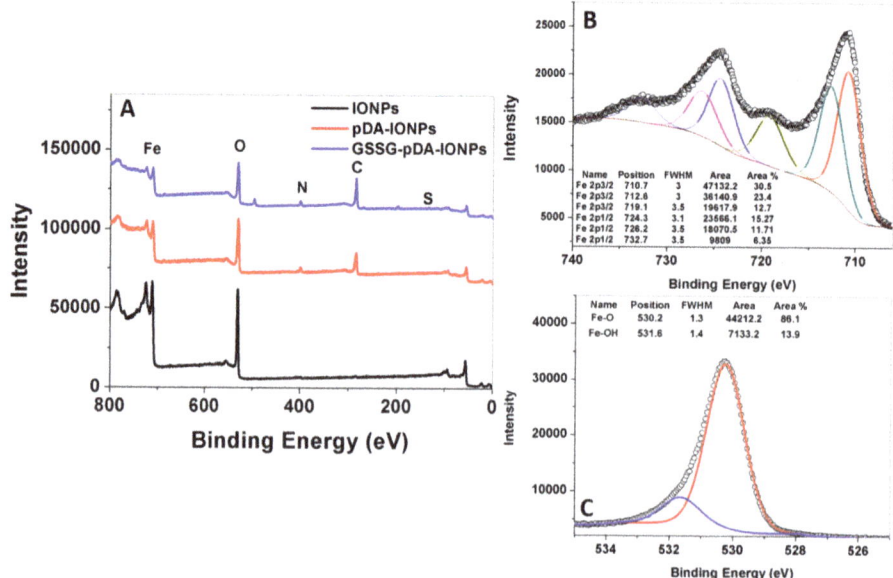

Figure 4. (**A**) X-ray photoelectron spectroscopy (XPS) survey spectra of the prepared nanoparticles with the fitted peaks of (**B**) Fe (2p); and (**C**) oxygen (1s) of bare IONPs.

Table 1. XPS elemental analysis (atomic percentage) of the prepared nanoparticles.

Samples	Fe	O	C	N	S	N/C	Fe/O	Fe/C
IONPs	38	57	3	1	–	0.3	0.7	13
pDA-IONPs	16	37	42	5	–	0.1	0.4	0.4
GSSG-pDA-IONPs	9	28	59	3	0.1	0.1	0.3	0.2

XPS peak fittings, performed for pDA-IONPs and GSSG-pDA-IONPs, describe the chemical interaction between the grafted molecules as shown in Figure 5. The C 1s peak region is fitted into three components for pDA-IONPs and GSSG-pDA-IONPs (Figure 5A,B). pDA shell on IONPs shows two dominant peaks attributed to C–C/C–H at 284.8 eV and C–N/C–O at 286.2 eV of the dopamine polymerized structure and one weak peak attributed to C=O at 288.4 eV that corresponds to the possible tautomers of pDA [44].

The incorporation of GSSG into the pDA shell reveals a slight shift in the peak position of C–N/C–O and O–C=O bonds to 285.8 and 288.1 eV, respectively, which suggests the immobilization of GSSG by introducing additional amine and carboxyl functional groups on pDA shell. To ensure the immobilization of GSSG, N (1s) peaks of the functionalized nanoparticles (Figure 5C,D) are fitted into two peaks at 398.4 eV for =N–R and at 400.1 eV for R–NH–R that correspond to the tertiary/aromatic and the secondary amines of dopamine intermediate structures [45,46]. The GSSG immobilization displays an additional peak corresponding to –NH$_2$ at 402.1 eV, which is attributed to the free amine groups of glutathione structure [44]. Further, the XPS survey scan of GSSG-pDA-IONPs (Figure 4A) shows the presence of sulfur which confirms the immobilization of GSSG onto pDA-IONPs.

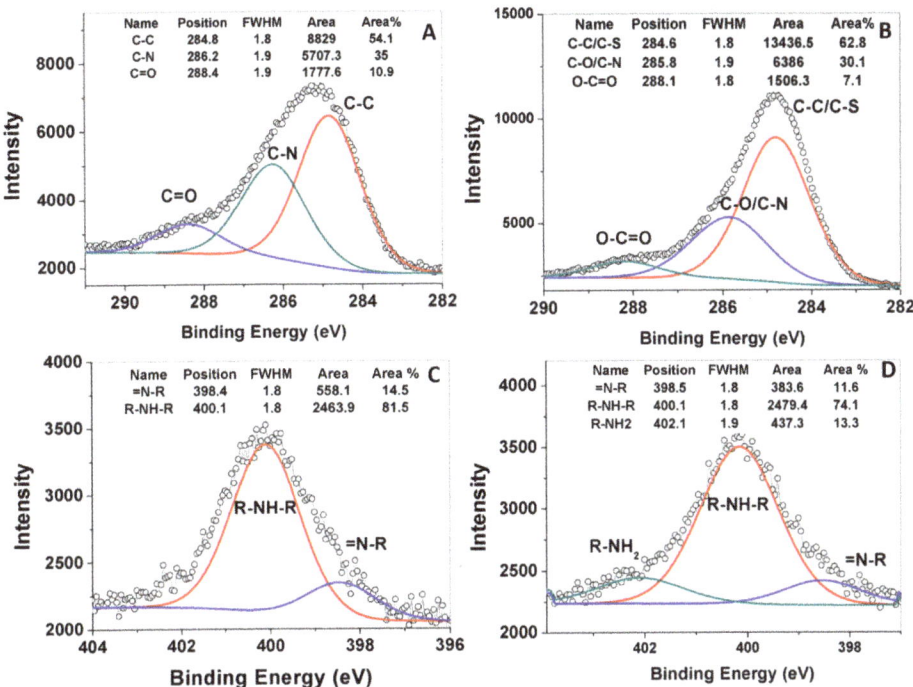

Figure 5. Fitted spectra of C (1s) for (**A**) pDA-IONPs; (**B**) GSSG functionalized pDA-IONPs; and of N (1s) for (**C**) pDA-IONPs; (**D**) GSSG functionalized pDA-IONPs.

3.1. Reduction and S-nitrosation of GSSG-pDA-IONPs

To serve as a dual modality to treat the cancer cells, GSSG-pDA-IONPs were first reduced to GSH using Elman's reagent and then S-nitrosated using sodium nitrite. UV-visible spectra of reduced nanoparticles (Figure 6A), show a sharp shift in the absorbance peak from 325 to 408 nm on successive addition of GSSG-pDA-IONPs into 5,5-dithiobis-[2-nitrobenzoicacid] (DTNB) which confirms the presence of –SH in GSH-pDA-IONPs. Indeed, DTNB shows its characteristic absorbance band at 325 nm. When it reacts with the free sulfhydryl group in the reaction mixture, it gives a mixed disulfide or TNB (2-nitro-5-thiobenzoic acid), characterized by the absorbance band at 408 nm, which is in good agreement with the FTIR spectra (Figure 6C). The biological effect of S-nitrosothiol is attributed to the NO release from the breaking of the S–N bond to act as NO donor under physiological conditions. NO formation has the potential to influence the chemotherapy and contribute significantly to cancer biology [47]. Thus, with successive addition of GSH-pDA-IONPs in sodium nitrite solution, the formation of S-nitrosothiols is observed through the appearance of a broad and weak band at 320 nm (Figure 6B), which is in conformity with the weak absorbance shown by S-nitrosothiols [48].

The FTIR spectrum of GSNO-pDA-IONPs in Figure 6C shows the NO vibration band at ~1500 cm^{-1} which confirms the presence of S–NO in GSNO-pDA-IONPs. It is also shown that the broad band of GSH-pDA-IONPs, observed due to intramolecular hydrogen bonds, disappears on the formation of the S–NO bond, giving rise to the N–H bending band at 3440 cm^{-1} and suggesting the successful formation of S-nitrosothiols.

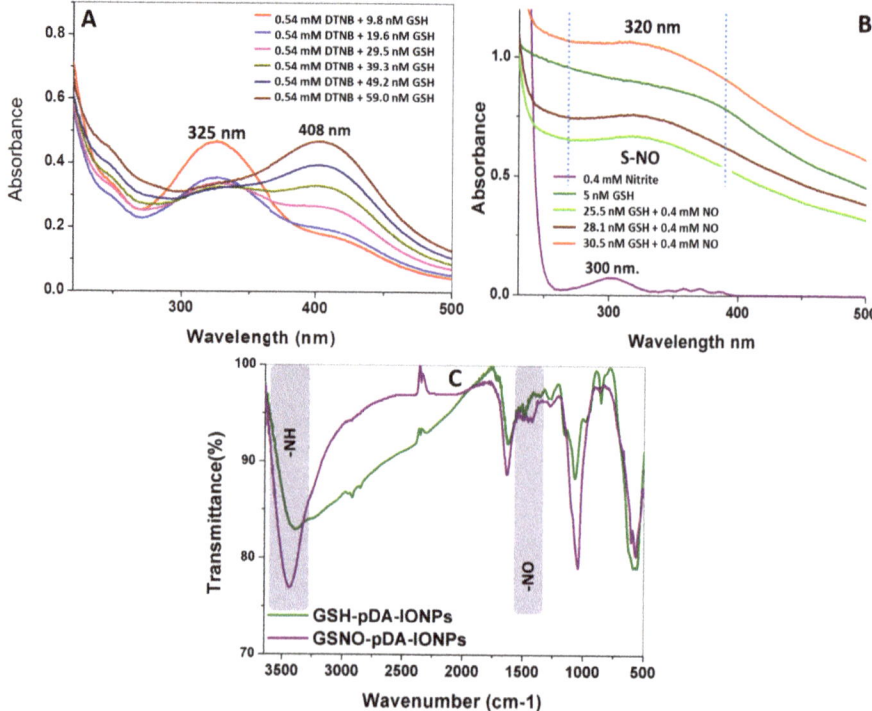

Figure 6. UV-visible spectra showing (**A**) the reduction of GSSG into GSH-pDA-IONPs; (**B**) S-nitrosation of GSH-pDA-IONPs; and (**C**) FTIR spectra of GSNO-pDA-IONPs and GSH-pDA-IONPs.

3.2. In-Vitro Drug Loading and Release Kinetics

DTX was first modified with PMPI prior to its loading and was characterized using FTIR and NMR (Figures S5 and S6). The hydroxyl group of DTX reacts with PMPI isocyanate and induces the disappearance of the isocyanate bond (Figure S5) and the formation of –CN, –NH and –CONH bonds, which are assigned respectively to 1310, 1520 and 1640 cm^{-1} vibration bands. This confirms the covalent bonding of DTX-PMPI, which was then loaded on GSH-pDA-IONPs. DOX- and DTX-loaded nanoparticles were further analyzed using DLS size measurement to ensure the stability of the nanocarrier in the biological medium (RPMI (Roswell Park Memorial Institute medium) and Albumin) at 37 °C where DTX-modified nanoparticles show an enhanced colloidal stability as compared to DOX-loaded nanoparticles (Figure S7).The PDI values of the nanocarrier dispersed in water were also measured where DOX-loaded nanoparticles had a value of 0.71 ± 0.24 and DTX-loaded 0.61 ± 0.10.

To evaluate the efficiency of the nanocarriers, it is very important to evaluate the drug loading efficiency of the designed drug delivery system. Since DOX is responsive in UV-vis spectroscopy due to its inherent chromophore, DOX loading and release kinetics were measured using both UV and TG analyses while quantification of loaded DTX was determined using TGA only. A comparative chart (Table S1, SI) shows the loading percentages of DOX and DTX analyzed using UV-vis spectroscopy and the High-performance liquid chromatography (HPLC) method, and observed in the literature.

The surface loading efficiency of DOX, on the developed nanocarrier, is estimated to be 78% for 24 h of loading reaction (Figure 7A) using UV-vis absorbance measurement at 490 nm, which is the characteristic absorbance band of DOX molecule. The drug loading efficiency was calculated as given in Equation (1) [49].

$$\% \text{ EE} = \frac{\text{Concentration (Drug added} - \text{Free unentrapped Drug)}}{\text{Concentration of Drug Added}} \times 100 \qquad (1)$$

Drug release studies were carried out at three different pH (3.5, 5.4 and 7.4) with respect to the pH value of the endocytic compartment, which is lower than that of the normal physiological pH. Figure 7B shows that the release behavior of DOX from the GSH-pDA-IONPs is pH responsive because of the greater solubility of DOX in acid medium (low pH) [50]. This explanation is in good agreement with the results obtained from the zeta potential curves when measured at different pH (Figure 7C). Indeed, in acid medium, greater solubility and increased hydrophilicity of DOX is obtained due to the protonation of its –NH$_2$ functional group [51]. The rate of DOX release is higher at low pH (3.5), but when the pH of the release medium increases to 5.4 and 7.4, the rate of the drug release decreases and the maximum release is observed during the initial 6 h as shown in Figure 7B.

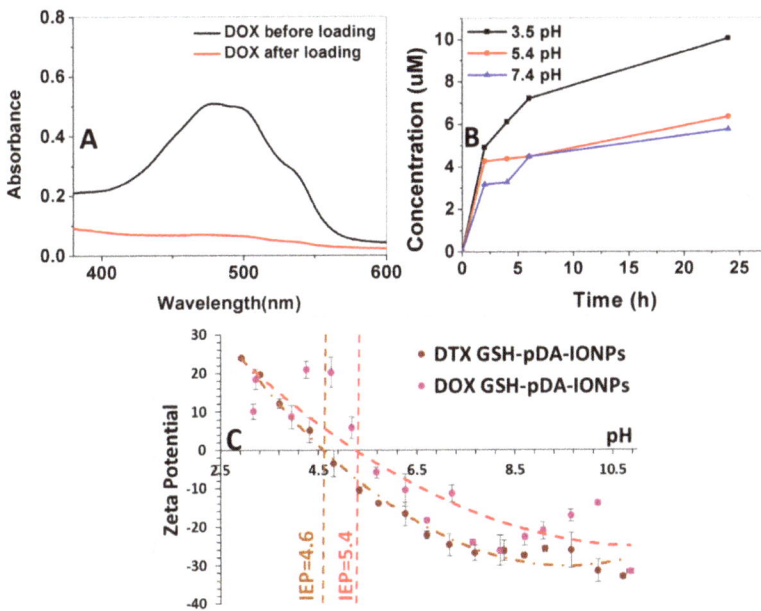

Figure 7. UV-vis absorbance spectra showing (**A**) doxorubicin loading on GSH-pDA-IONPs; (**B**) doxorubicin release at different pH in PBS (10 mM); and (**C**) zeta potential vs. pH curves of DOX- and DTX-drug loaded nanoparticles.

Conclusively, moving from pH 7.4 to pH 3.5, the amount of released DOX has doubled. This could be due to the positively charged amine group and its effect on the drug's solubility which depends on its protonation degrees [52]. Moreover, it has also been reported that at low pH condition, the ionization of the DOX molecule enhances its solubility which leads to an increased diffusion ability, preventing all non-bonding interactions with the polymeric layer of pDA [53]. On comparing the release profile at all pH, two stages of drug release are observed defining the DOX interaction: the first is between 0 and 2 h, where the drug release is fast and can be attributed to the adsorbed drug. The second stage is between 2 and 24 h, where the drug release is slow and could be attributed to the covalently linked drug. As the low pH favors the protonation of the DOX molecule, so the maximum drug release is observed at pH 3.5.

Thus, 78% of DOX loading can result in generating enough concentration of drug within a short span of time, thereby providing a great potential in developing an excellent nanocarrier and a positive approach towards an improved targeted cancer therapy.

TGA measurements (under air flow; nitrogen:oxygen 80:20), on the other hand, support quantifying the drug and immobilization steps. They indicate a weight loss of 6.1% (Figure 8) for bare IONPs, which later helps in the quantification of the organic coating. This weight loss, in the range of 100 to 800 °C, is due to the desorption of the physically adsorbed water and the dehydroxylation of hydroxyl groups on the surface. On heating pDA-IONPs, the weight loss increases to 22%, suggesting the degradation of the polymeric pDA coating on the surface. When GSH is immobilized on pDA-IONPs, the weight loss further increases to 25%, which corresponds to 97.6 µmol of GSH/g of IONPs. The amount of the loaded drug on GSH-pDA-IONPs is also calculated using TGA where 13.2% of weight loss is obtained for DOX and 18.0% for DTX. Drug-loading efficiency is then estimated to be 243 µmol/g for doxorubicin (DOX) and 223 µmol/g for docetaxel (DTX). The details of the analysis are presented in Table 2.

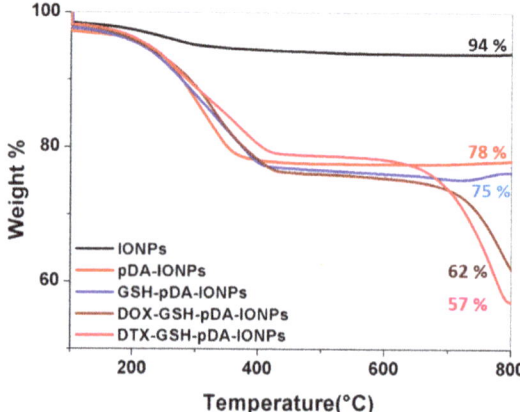

Figure 8. Thermogravimetric analysis (TGA) curves showing the sequential grafting of different organic molecules on the surface of IONPs.

Table 2. Detailed analysis of the weight loss of synthesized nanoparticles and quantification of the grafted molecules.

Samples	Weight Loss %	Amount of Organic Content %	Amount of DOX/DTX Loaded (µmol g^{-1} of IONPs)
IONPs	6	0.0	–
pDA-IONPs	22	16	–
GSH-pDA-IONPs	25	19	–
DOX-GSH-pDA-IONPs	38	32	243
DTX-GSH-pDA-IONPs	43	37	223

3.3. Cytotoxicity Assay

In vitro cytotoxicity activity of DOX was assessed using MTS assay against PC3 cell lines where cells were exposed to the DOX-loaded nanoparticles for 48 h. The results obtained were preliminary but effective to explore the applicability of drug-loaded nanoparticles. Elevated dose studies were done with respect to the concentration of DOX as shown in Figure 9. The IC50 (the half maximal inhibitory concentration) value for DOX was reported to be 334.4–836.1 nM for 48 h [54,55]. On the other hand, our calculated IC50 value for the free drug is observed at 1,200 nM, which is increased to 3,400 nM when loaded on GSH-pDA-IONPs. It is also observed that the free drug is more toxic than the drug-loaded nanoparticles for maximum concentration. Indeed, the percentage of cell survival is 17.2 ± 4.3% for free DOX, while DOX-loaded nanoparticles show cell survival of 37.1 ± 9.5% in the studied range of concentration. This difference could be explained by the different behavior of the free and loaded DOX inside the cells [56,57]. DOX shows antiproliferative activity against many tumor cells and has the potential to permeate through the cell membrane very easily thanks to its hydrophobic nature. Unfortunately, DOX alone can also affect the growth of other healthy cells, leading to many side effects. These ultimately result in the depletion of the immune system and the human body becomes more prone to microbial infection, fatigue and, thus, the healing time decreases significantly [58]. Nanocarriers thus come into the role that can be used to target the cancer cells, thereby reducing the side effect of using a drug alone.

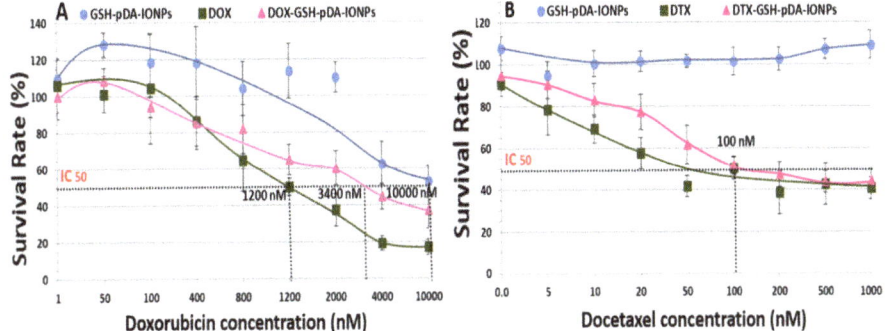

Figure 9. MTS ((3-(4,5-dimethylthiazol-2-yl)-5-(3-carboxymethoxyphenyl)-2-(4-sulfophenyl)-2H-tetrazolium)) assay showing the average percent of cell survival against various concentration of (**A**) DOX; and (**B**) DTX drug on PC3 cell lines when incubated for 48 h. (Standard deviations were calculated with six measurements).

When MTS assay is performed with the DTX drug, the reported IC50 value is 11 nM [59]. However, in our case, the IC50 value of the loaded DTX drug increases to 100 nM due to the chemical modification of the molecule. This value is lower than that obtained by Loiseau et al. for DTX-modified titanate nanotubes where the obtained IC50 value was 390 nM [23]. Also, the percentage of surviving cells at a higher concentration is 43.9 ± 5.7% for DTX-loaded nanoparticles and 40.5 ± 5.2% for free DTX, as shown in Figure 9B. This suggests that it can be used as effective nanocarrier.

The targeting specificity of the developed nanoparticles were further quantified using flow cytometry by an Annexin V-FITC detection kit with PI staining. Necrosis and apoptosis are measured as shown in Figure 10.

At an equivalent drug concentration where the concentration of only GSH-pDA-IONPs in the nanohybrid is in the range of 0.01 to 5.3 µg mL^{-1}, it is observed that DOX-loaded nanoparticles reveal a slightly lower antitumor activity compared to free DOX. This may be due to the interaction mechanism of DOX-GSH-pDA-IONPs as it is observed in MTS and confocal studies (Figure S8) [60]. However, in this test, PC-3 cells were exposed to DOX for 24 h, whereas MTS assay cells were exposed for 48 h. On further analyzing the nature of cell apoptosis, it is observed that DOX-loaded nanoparticles show 24.9% of early apoptotic (Annexin positive / PI negative) for only 24 h of exposure compared to 16.7% for free drug nanoparticles (GSH-pDA-IONPs). These results suggest that even a small concentration is able to induce cell apoptosis, which confirms the antiproliferative effect of DOX-loaded nanoparticles.

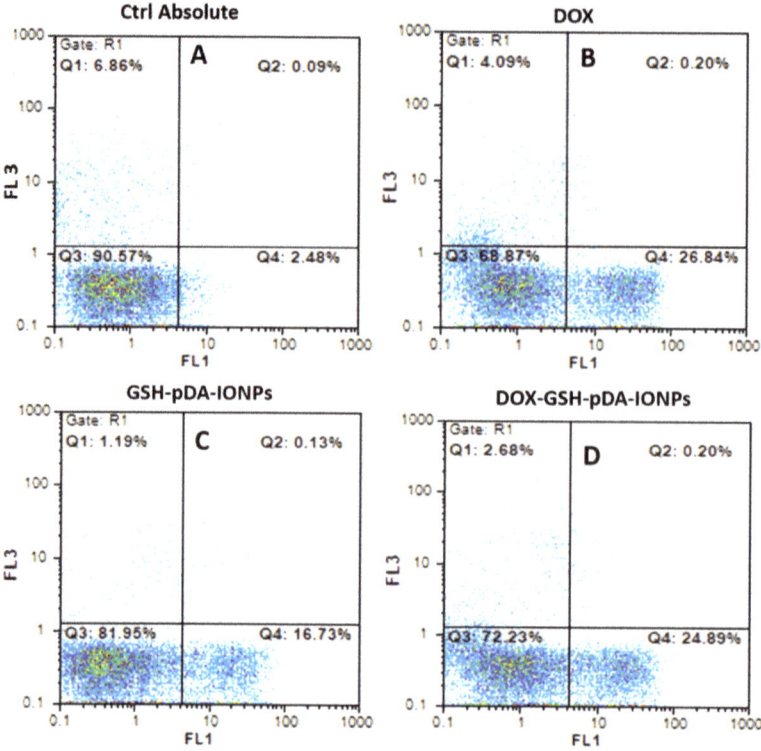

Figure 10. Representative dot plot of Annexin V-FITC/PI ((fluorescein isothiocyanate) detection kit with PI (propidium iodide) staining of PC3 (prostate cancer) cells incubated for 24 h A. Without any sample B. with DOX, C. GSH-pDA-IONPs and D. DOX-GSH-pDA-IONPs (flow cytometry: x axis (Fluorescence 1, FL1) Annexin V-FITC and y axis (FL3) propidium iodide). The Q1 quadrant represents unviable cells (PI positive and annexin negative). The Q2 quadrant represents cells that are in late apoptosis or necrosis (both annexin and PI positive). The Q3 quadrant represents viable cells (both annexin-FITC and PI negative). The Q4 quadrant represents cells in early apoptosis (annexin positive and PI negative).

4. Conclusions

In this work, we attempted to develop nanocarriers based on IONPs to treat prostate cancer. IONPs were first coated with a biocompatible polymer, pDA, which provides an anchor for further functionalization. Then, glutathione was successfully grafted onto pDA-IONPs in order to increase the efficacy of the developed nanocarrier thanks to its intrinsic biological properties. Before going to the biological assays, the developed nanocarriers were fully characterized using different techniques (TEM, XPS, XRD, TGA, FTIR, UV-vis, DLS and zeta potential measurements) to ensure the successive coating and immobilization of pDA and GSSG onto the IONPs' surface. Two therapeutic molecules were studied in this work: DOX and DTX. These two anticancer drugs have been widely used in the treatment of cancer but they have several side effects when used alone. Thus, to overcome these limitations, we developed nanocarriers that can decrease these side effects. This was preliminarily proved with MTS and apoptosis studies, performed on PC3 cell lines. Drug release studies were also carried out with DOX-loaded nanoparticles to explore the interaction behavior of drugs in physiological and cancerous cell environments (imitated by an acid medium). Subsequently, the GSSG grafted onto pDA-IONPs was reduced to obtain free thiols on the surface, which provides an additional advantage to the nanocarrier by forming S-nitrosothiols. This could also be used as a NO donor agent and, thus, proves its worth in cancer treatments.

Supplementary Materials: The following are available online at http://www.mdpi.com/2079-4991/9/2/138/s1, Figure S1: XRD pattern of the bare IONPs (λ = 1.540598 Å), Figure S2: SAED patterns obtained via TEM analyses of A. bare IONPs and B. pDA-IONPs, Figure S3: Suspension images of (A). pDA-IONPs and (B). GSSG-pDA-IONPs after 24 h in PBS (10 mM, pH 7.4), Figure S4: Calibration curve showing the magnetic susceptibility vs. concentration of bare IONPs. Measurements were carried out in deionized water at pH 5.0–6.0, Figure S5: FTIR spectrum of the prepared DTX-PMPI, Figure S6: 1H-NMR predicted spectrum of DTX-PMPI, Figure S7: DLS size measurements to check the colloidal stability of the developed nanoparticles drug loaded FDG (GSH-pDA-SPIONs) in biological media (RPMI and albumin in NaCl) at 37 °C, Figure S8: Confocal images of PC3 cell lines with A. no treatment, B. only DOX and C. DOX loaded nanoparticles; Table S1: Comparative chart showing the drug loading efficiencies of doxorubicin and docetaxel, calculated using different method.

Author Contributions: Conceptualization and methodology, N.S., and F.S.; writing—original draft preparation by N.S. writing—review and editing was done by N.M., F.S., R.K. and S.K.S. Under the supervision of N.M. and R.K. Biological experiments were performed by T.N. and C.M.

Funding: This research was funded by the French Government through the CNRS, the "Université de Bourgogne" and the "Conseil Régional de Bourgogne" through the 3MIM integrated project ("Marquage de Molécules par les Métaux pour l'Imagerie Médicale"). This work is also part of the project "Pharmacoimagerie et agents théranostiques", funded by the "Université de Bourgogne" and the "Conseil Régional de Bourgogne" through the "Plan d'Actions Régional pour l'Innovation (PARI)" and the European Union through the PO FEDER-FSE Bourgogne 2014/2020 programs. We would also like to acknowledge DST (YSS/2015/001184) for financial grant in India.

Acknowledgments: The authors would like to thank Julien Boudon and Lionel Maurizi for their help in some experiments, Olivier Heintz for XPS analysis, Rémi Chassagnon for TEM images, Nicolas Geoffroy for XRD pattern, Christine Goze for fluorescence measurements, Véronique Morgand, Christine Arnould, and Gérard Lizard for in vitro investigations.

Conflicts of Interest: The authors declare no conflict of interest.

References

1. Soppimath, K.S.; Liu, L.-H.; Seow, W.Y.; Liu, S.-Q.; Powel, R.; Chan, P.; Yang, Y.Y. Multifunctional Core/Shell Nanoparticles Self-Assembled from pH-Induced Thermosensitive Polymers for Targeted Intracellular Anticancer Drug Delivery. *Adv. Funct. Mater.* **2007**, *17*, 355–362. [CrossRef]
2. Liu, F.; Eisenberg, A. Preparation and pH Triggered Inversion of Vesicles from Poly(acrylic Acid)-block-Polystyrene-block-Poly(4-vinyl Pyridine). *J. Am. Chem. Soc.* **2003**, *125*, 15059–15064. [CrossRef] [PubMed]
3. Liu, J.; Qiao, S.Z.; Hu, Q.H.; Lu, G.Q. Magnetic nanocomposites with mesoporous structures: Synthesis and applications. *Small* **2011**, *7*, 425–443. [CrossRef] [PubMed]
4. Lu, A.H.; Salabas, E.L.; Schuth, F. Magnetic nanoparticles: Synthesis, protection, functionalization, and application. *Angew. Chem. Int. Ed.* **2007**, *46*, 1222–1244. [CrossRef] [PubMed]
5. Polshettiwar, V.; Luque, R.; Fihri, A.; Zhu, H.; Bouhrara, M.; Basset, J.M. Magnetically recoverable nanocatalysts. *Chem. Rev.* **2011**, *111*, 3036–3075. [CrossRef] [PubMed]
6. Lee, D.-E.; Koo, H.; Sun, I.-C.; Ryu, J.H.; Kim, K.; Kwon, I.C. Multifunctional nanoparticles for multimodal imaging and theragnosis. *Chem. Soc. Rev.* **2012**, *41*, 2656–2672. [CrossRef] [PubMed]
7. Lee, H.; Dellatore, S.M.; Miller, W.M.; Messersmith, P.B. Mussel-inspired surface chemistry for multifunctional coatings. *Science* **2007**, *318*, 426–430. [CrossRef] [PubMed]
8. Liu, N.; Wu, H.; McDowell, M.T.; Yao, Y.; Wang, C.; Cui, Y. A yolk-shell design for stabilized and scalable li-ion battery alloy anodes. *Nano Lett.* **2012**, *12*, 3315–3321. [CrossRef]
9. Batul, R.; Tamanna, T.; Khaliq, A.; Yu, A. Recent progress in the biomedical applications of polydopamine nanostructures. *Biomater. Sci.* **2017**, *5*, 1204–1229. [CrossRef]
10. Cui, J.; Yan, Y.; Such, G.K.; Liang, K.; Ochs, C.J.; Postma, A.; Caruso, F. Immobilization and intracellular delivery of an anticancer drug using mussel-inspired polydopamine capsules. *Biomacromolecules* **2012**, *13*, 2225–2228. [CrossRef]
11. Yi, M.C.; Khosla, C. Thiol–Disulfide exchange reactions in the mammalian extracellular environment. *Annu. Rev. Chem. Biomol. Eng.* **2016**, *7*, 197–222. [CrossRef] [PubMed]

12. Zhang, Z.; Jiao, Y.; Wang, Y.; Zhang, S. Core-shell self-assembly triggered via a thiol-disulfide exchange reaction for reduced glutathione detection and single cells monitoring. *Sci. Rep.* **2016**, *6*, 29872. [CrossRef] [PubMed]
13. Ghaz-Jahanian, M.A.; Abbaspour-Aghdam, F.; Anarjan, N.; Berenjian, A.; Jafarizadeh-Malmiri, H. Application of chitosan-based nanocarriers in tumor-targeted drug delivery. *Mol. Biotechnol.* **2015**, *57*, 201–218. [CrossRef] [PubMed]
14. Chuang, C.C.; Chang, C.W. Complexation of bioreducible cationic polymers with gold nanoparticles for improving stability in serum and application on nonviral gene delivery. *ACS Appl. Mater. Interfaces* **2015**, *7*, 7724–7731. [CrossRef] [PubMed]
15. Israel, L.L.; Lellouche, E.; Ostrovsky, S.; Yarmiayev, V.; Bechor, M.; Michaeli, S.; Lellouche, J.P. Acute in vivo toxicity mitigation of PEI-coated maghemite nanoparticles using controlled oxidation and surface modifications toward siRNA delivery. *ACS Appl. Mater. Interfaces* **2015**, *7*, 15240–15255. [CrossRef] [PubMed]
16. Traverso, N.; Ricciarelli, R.; Nitti, M.; Marengo, B.; Furfaro, A.L.; Pronzato, M.A.; Marinari, U.M.; Domenicotti, C. Role of glutathione in cancer progression and chemoresistance. *Oxid. Med. Cell. Longev.* **2013**, *2013*, 972913. [CrossRef] [PubMed]
17. Ignarro, L.J. Nitric oxide: A unique endogenous signaling molecule in vascular biology. *Biosci. Rep.* **1999**, *19*, 51–71. [CrossRef]
18. Furchgott, R.F. Endothelium-derived relaxing factor: Discovery, early studies, and identification as nitric oxide. *Biosci. Rep.* **1999**, *19*, 235–251. [CrossRef]
19. Carlsson, S.; Weitzberg, E.; Wiklund, P.; Lundberg, J.O. Intravesical nitric oxide delivery for prevention of catheter-associated urinary tract infections. *Antimicrob. Agents Chemother.* **2005**, *49*, 2352–2355. [CrossRef]
20. Thomsen, L.L.; Miles, D.W.; Happerfield, L.; Bobrow, L.G.; Knowles, R.G.; Moncada, S. Nitric oxide synthase activity in human breast cancer. *Br. J. Cancer* **1995**, *72*, 41–44. [CrossRef]
21. Martin, M.; Salazar, P.; Villalonga, R.; Campuzano, S.; Pingarron, J.M.; Gonzalez-Mora, J.L. Preparation of core-shell Fe_3O_4@poly(dopamine) magnetic nanoparticles for biosensor construction. *J. Mater. Chem. B* **2014**, *2*, 739–746. [CrossRef]
22. Kläser, K.; Graeser, M.; Steinhagen, D.; Luedtke-Buzug, K. Construction of a device for magnetic separation of superparamagnetic iron oxide nanoparticles. *Curr. Dir. Biomed. Eng.* **2015**, *1*, 306–309. [CrossRef]
23. Loiseau, A.; Boudon, J.; Mirjolet, C.; Crehange, G.; Millot, N. Taxane-Grafted Metal-Oxide Nanoparticles as a New Theranostic Tool against Cancer: The Promising Example of Docetaxel-Functionalized Titanate Nanotubes on Prostate Tumors. *Adv. Healthc. Mater.* **2017**, *6*, 1700245. [CrossRef] [PubMed]
24. Mirjolet, J.; Barberi-Heyob, M.; Merlin, J.; Marchal, S.; Etienne, M.; Milano, G.; Bey, P. Thymidylate synthase expression and activity: Relation to S-phase parameters and 5-fluorouracil sensitivity. *Br. J. Cancer* **1998**, *78*, 62. [CrossRef] [PubMed]
25. Thomas, G.; Demoisson, F.; Boudon, J.; Millot, N. Efficient functionalization of magnetite nanoparticles with phosphonate using a one-step continuous hydrothermal process. *Dalton Trans.* **2016**, *45*, 10821–10829. [CrossRef] [PubMed]
26. Millot, N.; Aymes, D.; Bernard, F.; Niepce, J.C.; Traverse, A.; Bourée, F.; Cheng, B.L.; Perriat, P. Particle Size Dependency of Ternary Diagrams at the Nanometer Scale: Evidence of TiO_2 Clusters in Fe-Based Spinels. *J. Phys. Chem. B* **2003**, *107*, 5740–5750. [CrossRef]
27. Guigue-Millot, N.; Champion, Y.; Hÿtch, M.J.; Bernard, F.; Bégin-Colin, S.; Perriat, P. Chemical Heterogeneities in Nanometric Titanomagnetites Prepared by Soft Chemistry and Studied Ex Situ: Evidence for Fe-Segregation and Oxidation Kinetics. *J. Phys. Chem. B* **2003**, *107*, 5740–5750. [CrossRef]
28. Ju, K.-Y.; Lee, Y.; Lee, S.; Park, S.B.; Lee, J.-K. Bioinspired polymerization of dopamine to generate melanin-like nanoparticles having an excellent free-radical-scavenging property. *Biomacromolecules* **2011**, *12*, 625–632. [CrossRef]
29. Jiang, J.; Zhu, L.; Zhu, L.; Zhu, B.; Xu, Y. Surface Characteristics of a Self-Polymerized Dopamine Coating Deposited on Hydrophobic Polymer Films. *Langmuir* **2011**, *27*, 14180–14187. [CrossRef]
30. Honary, S.; Zahir, F. Effect of zeta potential on the properties of nano-drug delivery systems-a review (Part 2). *Trop. J. Pharm. Res.* **2013**, *12*, 265–273.
31. Maurizi, L.; Papa, A.-L.; Dumont, L.; Bouyer, F.; Walker, P.; Vandroux, D.; Millot, N. Influence of surface charge and polymer coating on internalization and biodistribution of polyethylene glycol-modified iron oxide nanoparticles. *J. Biomed. Nanotechnol.* **2015**, *11*, 126–136. [CrossRef] [PubMed]

32. Yu, S.; Chow, G.M. Carboxyl group (-CO2H) functionalized ferrimagnetic iron oxide nanoparticles for potential bio-applications. *J. Mater. Chem.* **2004**, *14*, 2781–2786. [CrossRef]
33. Losic, D.; Yu, Y.; Aw, M.S.; Simovic, S.; Thierry, B.; Addai-Mensah, J. Surface functionalisation of diatoms with dopamine modified iron-oxide nanoparticles: Toward magnetically guided drug microcarriers with biologically derived morphologies. *Chem. Commun.* **2010**, *46*, 6323–6325. [CrossRef] [PubMed]
34. Sallem, F.; Boudon, J.; Heintz, O.; Séverin, I.; Megriche, A.; Millot, N. Synthesis and characterization of chitosan-coated titanate nanotubes: Towards a new safe nanocarrier. *Dalton Trans.* **2017**, *46*, 15386–15398. [CrossRef] [PubMed]
35. Zhang, D.; Wu, M.; Zeng, Y.; Wu, L.; Wang, Q.; Han, X.; Liu, X.; Liu, J. Chlorin e6 Conjugated Poly(dopamine) Nanospheres as PDT/PTT Dual-Modal Therapeutic Agents for Enhanced Cancer Therapy. *ACS Appl. Mater. Interfaces* **2015**, *7*, 8176–8187. [CrossRef] [PubMed]
36. Chen, D.; Zhao, L.; Hu, W. Protein immobilization and fluorescence quenching on polydopamine thin films. *J. Colloid Interface Sci.* **2016**, *477*, 123–130. [CrossRef]
37. Pauleau, Y. *Materials Surface Processing by Directed Energy Techniques*; Elsevier: Amsterdam, The Netherlands, 2006.
38. Perriat, P.; Fries, E.; Millot, N.; Domenichini, B. XPS and EELS investigations of chemical homogeneity in nanometer scaled Ti-ferrites obtained by soft chemistry. *Solid State Ion.* **1999**, *117*, 175–184. [CrossRef]
39. Petran, A.; Radu, T.; Nan, A.; Olteanu, D.; Filip, A.; Clichici, S.; Baldea, I.; Suciu, M.; Turcu, R. Synthesis, characterization, and cytotoxicity evaluation of high-magnetization multifunctional nanoclusters. *J. Nanopart. Res.* **2017**, *19*, 10. [CrossRef]
40. Thomas, G.; Demoisson, F.; Chassagnon, R.; Popova, E.; Millot, N. One-step continuous synthesis of functionalized magnetite nanoflowers. *Nanotechnology* **2016**, *27*, 135604. [CrossRef]
41. Yamashita, T.; Hayes, P. Analysis of XPS spectra of Fe^{2+} and Fe^{3+} ions in oxide materials. *Appl. Surf. Sci.* **2008**, *254*, 2441–2449. [CrossRef]
42. Barr, T.L. An ESCA study of the termination of the passivation of elemental metals. *J. Phys. Chem.* **1978**, *82*, 1801–1810. [CrossRef]
43. Martine, M.; Varsha, K.; Christian, R. XPS study of Fe(II)—Fe(III) (oxy)hydroxycarbonate green rust compounds. *Surf. Interface Anal.* **2008**, *40*, 323–328.
44. Zangmeister, R.A.; Morris, T.A.; Tarlov, M.J. Characterization of Polydopamine Thin Films Deposited at Short Times by Autoxidation of Dopamine. *Langmuir* **2013**, *29*, 8619–8628. [CrossRef] [PubMed]
45. Clark, M.B.; Gardella, J.A.; Schultz, T.M.; Patil, D.G.; Salvati, L. Solid-state analysis of eumelanin biopolymers by electron spectroscopy for chemical analysis. *Anal. Chem.* **1990**, *62*, 949–956. [CrossRef]
46. Bernsmann, F.; Ponche, A.; Ringwald, C.; Hemmerlé, J.; Raya, J.; Bechinger, B.; Voegel, J.-C.; Schaaf, P.; Ball, V. Characterization of Dopamine−Melanin Growth on Silicon Oxide. *J. Phys. Chem. C* **2009**, *113*, 8234–8242. [CrossRef]
47. Sinha, B.K.; Bhattacharjee, S.; Chatterjee, S.; Jiang, J.; Motten, A.G.; Kumar, A.; Espey, M.G.; Mason, R.P. Role of Nitric Oxide in the Chemistry and Anticancer Activity of Etoposide (VP-16,213). *Chem. Res. Toxicol.* **2013**, *26*, 379–387. [CrossRef] [PubMed]
48. Diers, A.R.; Keszler, A.; Hogg, N. Detection of S-nitrosothiols. *Biochim. Biophys. Acta* **2014**, *1840*, 892–900. [CrossRef]
49. Awotwe-Otoo, D.; Zidan, A.S.; Rahman, Z.; Habib, M.J. Evaluation of Anticancer Drug-Loaded Nanoparticle Characteristics by Nondestructive Methodologies. *AAPS PharmSciTech* **2012**, *13*, 611–622. [CrossRef]
50. Wang, J.; Chen, J.-S.; Zong, J.-Y.; Zhao, D.; Li, F.; Zhuo, R.-X.; Cheng, S.-X. Calcium Carbonate/Carboxymethyl Chitosan Hybrid Microspheres and Nanospheres for Drug Delivery. *J. Phys. Chem. C* **2010**, *114*, 18940–18945. [CrossRef]
51. Wu, S.; Zhao, X.; Li, Y.; Du, Q.; Sun, J.; Wang, Y.; Wang, X.; Xia, Y.; Wang, Z.; Xia, L. Adsorption properties of doxorubicin hydrochloride onto graphene oxide: Equilibrium, kinetic and thermodynamic studies. *Materials* **2013**, *6*, 2026–2042. [CrossRef]
52. Di Martino, A.; Kucharczyk, P.; Capakova, Z.; Humpolicek, P.; Sedlarik, V. Chitosan-based nanocomplexes for simultaneous loading, burst reduction and controlled release of doxorubicin and 5-fluorouracil. *Int. J. Biol. Macromol.* **2017**, *102*, 613–624. [CrossRef] [PubMed]
53. Johnson, R.P.; Jeong, Y.I.; John, J.V.; Chung, C.-W.; Kang, D.H.; Selvaraj, M.; Suh, H.; Kim, I. Dual stimuli-responsive poly (N-isopropylacrylamide)-b-poly (L-histidine) chimeric materials for the controlled delivery of doxorubicin into liver carcinoma. *Biomacromolecules* **2013**, *14*, 1434–1443. [CrossRef] [PubMed]

54. Tanaka, M.; Rosser, C.J.; Grossman, H.B. PTEN gene therapy induces growth inhibition and increases efficacy of chemotherapy in prostate cancer. *Cancer Detect. Prev.* **2005**, *29*, 170–174. [CrossRef] [PubMed]
55. Salim, E.I.; Farara, K.; Maria, D. Antitumoral and antioxidant potential of Egyptian propolis against the PC3 prostate cancer cell line. *Asian Pac. J. Cancer Prev.* **2015**, *16*, 7641–7651. [CrossRef] [PubMed]
56. Speelmans, G.; Staffhorst, R.W.H.M.; Steenbergen, H.G.; de Kruijff, B. Transport of the anti-cancer drug doxorubicin across cytoplasmic membranes and membranes composed of phospholipids derived from Escherichia coli occurs via a similar mechanism. *Biochim. Biophys. Acta Biomembr.* **1996**, *1284*, 240–246. [CrossRef]
57. Nizamov, T.R.; Garanina, A.S.; Grebennikov, I.S.; Zhironkina, O.A.; Strelkova, O.S.; Alieva, I.B.; Kireev, I.I.; Abakumov, M.A.; Savchenko, A.G.; Majouga, A.G. Effect of Iron Oxide Nanoparticle Shape on Doxorubicin Drug Delivery Toward LNCaP and PC-3 Cell Lines. *BioNanoScience* **2018**, *8*, 394–406. [CrossRef]
58. Tacar, O.; Sriamornsak, P.; Dass, C.R. Doxorubicin: An update on anticancer molecular action, toxicity and novel drug delivery systems. *J. Pharm. Pharmacol.* **2013**, *65*, 157–170. [CrossRef]
59. Ernsting, M.J.; Murakami, M.; Undzys, E.; Aman, A.; Press, B.; Li, S.-D. A docetaxel-carboxymethylcellulose nanoparticle outperforms the approved taxane nanoformulation, Abraxane, in mouse tumor models with significant control of metastases. *J. Control. Release* **2012**, *162*, 575–581. [CrossRef]
60. Li, M.; Song, W.; Tang, Z.; Lv, S.; Lin, L.; Sun, H.; Li, Q.; Yang, Y.; Hong, H.; Chen, X. Nanoscaled poly (L-glutamic acid)/doxorubicin-amphiphile complex as pH-responsive drug delivery system for effective treatment of nonsmall cell lung cancer. *ACS Appl. Mater. Interfaces* **2013**, *5*, 1781–1792. [CrossRef]

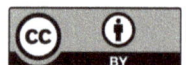

© 2019 by the authors. Licensee MDPI, Basel, Switzerland. This article is an open access article distributed under the terms and conditions of the Creative Commons Attribution (CC BY) license (http://creativecommons.org/licenses/by/4.0/).

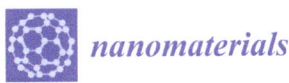

Article

Coating Dependent In Vitro Biocompatibility of New Fe-Si Nanoparticles

Mihaela Balas [1],*, Florian Dumitrache [2], Madalina Andreea Badea [1], Claudiu Fleaca [2], Anca Badoi [2], Eugenia Tanasa [3] and Anca Dinischiotu [1]

1. Department of Biochemistry and Molecular Biology, University of Bucharest, 91–95 Splaiul Independenței, 050095 Bucharest, sector 5, Romania; badea_andreea08@yahoo.com (M.A.B.); ancadinischiotu@yahoo.com (A.D.)
2. National Institute for Lasers, Plasma and Radiation Physics (NILPRP), Atomistilor 409, 077125 Magurele, Romania; dumitracheflorian@yahoo.com (F.D.); claudiufleaca@yahoo.com (C.F.); anca.badoi@inflpr.ro (A.B.)
3. Department of Oxide Materials and Nanomaterials, Faculty of Applied Chemistry and Materials Science, University Politehnica of Bucharest, Gh. Polizu 1-7, 11061 Bucharest, sector 1, Romania; eugenia.vasile27@gmail.com
* Correspondence: radu_mihaella@yahoo.com or mihaela.radu@bio.unibuc.ro; Tel./Fax: +40-21-3181575 (ext. 103)

Received: 24 May 2018; Accepted: 2 July 2018; Published: 5 July 2018

Abstract: Magnetic nanoparticles offer multiple utilization possibilities in biomedicine. In this context, the interaction with cellular structures and their biological effects need to be understood and controlled for clinical safety. New magnetic nanoparticles containing metallic/carbidic iron and elemental silicon phases were synthesized by laser pyrolysis using $Fe(CO)_5$ vapors and SiH_4 gas as Fe and Si precursors, then passivated and coated with biocompatible agents, such as L-3,4-dihydroxyphenylalanine (L-DOPA) and sodium carboxymethyl cellulose (CMC-Na). The resulting magnetic nanoparticles were characterized by XRD, EDS, and TEM techniques. To evaluate their biocompatibility, doses ranging from 0–200 µg/mL hybrid Fe-Si nanoparticles were exposed to Caco2 cells for 24 and 72 h. Doses below 50 µg/mL of both L-DOPA and CMC-Na-coated Fe-Si nanoparticles induced no significant changes of cellular viability or membrane integrity. The cellular internalization of nanoparticles was dependent on their dispersion in culture medium and caused some changes of F-actin filaments organization after 72 h. However, reactive oxygen species were generated after exposure to 25 and 50 µg/mL of both Fe-Si nanoparticles types, inducing the increase of intracellular glutathione level and activation of transcription factor Nrf2. At nanoparticles doses below 50 µg/mL, Caco2 cells were able to counteract the oxidative stress by activating the cellular protection mechanisms. We concluded that in vitro biological responses to coated hybrid Fe-Si nanoparticles depended on particle synthesis conditions, surface coating, doses and incubation time.

Keywords: hybrid Fe-Si nanoparticles; laser pyrolysis; Caco2 cells; cytotoxicity; oxidative stress

1. Introduction

The biomedical applications of nanomaterials are particularly focused on magnetic nanoparticles (MNPs), due to their attractive properties, such as superparamagnetism and significant saturation magnetization. Thus, they have been successfully tested as contrast agents in magnetic resonance imaging (MRI) [1], drug or bioactive molecule carriers for direct delivery to the disease site [2,3], and hyperthermia [4]. These nanosystems were also used in a wide variety of areas, magnetic separation [5], nanostructured soft/hard magnets [6], heat exchanger or cooling nanofluids [7], magneto-optical controlled wavelength filters [8], magnetorheological fluids as mechanic shock absorbers [6], up to environmental management [3,9]. Given the fact that the physical and chemical properties of MNPs largely depend on their synthesis method and chemical structure, several methods have been developed for synthesizing MNPs with different compositions [10–13].

Unprotected zerovalent iron nanoparticles (NPs) do not occur in nature because such NPs would get quickly oxidized in contact with air or water. The proper strategy to preserve the iron zerovalent nanodomains is their encapsulation in protective shells (carbon, polymers silicon, or iron oxide etc.). In comparison with conventional iron oxide NPs, it has been demonstrated that α-Fe-based NPs with the same particle dimensions exhibit a much greater magnetization and coercivity force at room temperature as the hysteresis loops revealed from magnetometry analyses [14]. Due to these properties, Fe-based NPs might be more active for generation of local hyperthermia than iron oxide NPs. Furthermore, Fe-based NPs used as MRI contrast agents have a much stronger shortening effect on T2 relaxation time than iron oxide NPs [15,16].

In addition, due to their high reactivity in an aqueous environment, the coated zerovalent Fe-based NPs must be studied for the characterization of certain features that are significant for biological applications, such as encapsulation, solubility, size, stability, and biocompatibility. To prevent NPs agglomeration and oxidation, which diminish their magnetism, it is important to chemically stabilize the morphology and magnetism of MNPs, during and after synthesis with non-toxic biocompatible coatings [17,18]. Several studies have focused on the design of new generation of nanoparticle systems with biocompatibility, enhanced dispersibility, internalization, and targeting capabilities improved by surface modifications [15,19]. In this respect, various biocompatible agents, such as polyethylene glycol (PEG)-derived compounds [20,21], alginate [22,23], chitosan [24], dextran [25], heparin [26], L-3,4-dihydroxyphenylalanine (L-DOPA) [27,28], phosphonates or carboxymethyldextran [29], Na carboxymethyl-cellulose (CMC-Na) [30] were used for NPs coatings. Many of those cited polymeric coating agents or other synthetic polymers, as well as the well-known biological molecules—proteins, peptides, lipids, or nucleic acids—can also form various nano-assemblies [31], without the introduction of an inorganic core. Such structures can have similar bio-applications to those of the coated nanoparticles, being useful to compare the biocompatibilities and toxicity of the two types of agents. One of the main targeted application—the drug delivery—was reviewed for the polymeric nanoparticles in [32], based on their properties for a sustained and controlled release, as well as on their small size and biocompatibility with tissues and cells. Even if they "have the potential to improve current disease therapies because of their ability to overcome multiple biological barriers and releasing a therapeutic load in the optimal dosage range", their fate after introduction in living organisms is affected by many factors, such as composition, size, heterogeneity, surface functionality (including targeting ligands), and charge, which thus influence the biodistribution, clearance, and also their toxicity [33]. As examples for such all-organic nanoparticle-based drug delivery systems, we can cite the alginate core–Na sulfosuccinate (AOT) bilayer shell loaded with water-soluble doxorubicin, verapamil hydrochloride, clonidine hydrochloride or diclofenac sodium [34], PLGA (D,L-lactic-co-glycolic acid) nanoparticles for antimalarial artesunate agent delivery in *Plasmodium*-infected albino mice [35], or PAMAM (polyamidoamine) dendrimers as insoluble and nephrotoxic drug amphotericin B carriers [36]. However, the PAMAM dendrimer nanoparticles can also present toxicity related with the surface NH_2 group density, which can be significantly diminished for the case of those terminating with –OH or –COOH [37]. Another type of hydrophilic organic nanoparticle used for diagnosis applications (photoacoustic contrast agent, nanoplatform for positron emission tomography (PET) or magnetic resonance imaging (MRI)) were those based on PEGylated natural melanin reported in [38]. An original approach for the synthesis of polymeric nanoparticles started from diacrylates, such as TEGDA (tetra(ethylene glycol)diacrylate), which undergo both linear polymerization and intrachain reticulation using CRP (controlled/living radical polymerization) [39]). Similar cyclized/knotted nanoparticles (composed from poly[bis(2-acryloyl) oxyethyldisulphide-co-2-(dimethylamino) ethyl methacrylate] supplementary ethylenediamine-conjugated) were successfully used as non-viral gene transfection agents for epidermal keratinocytes (skin cells) [40] based on electrostatic interactions. The same type of interactions involving positive ammonium groups of nanoparticles and negative phosphate groups from DNA (deoxyribonucleic acids), resulted in stable polyplexes that were also reported for high efficiency epidermal gene therapy, yet using biocompatible/low toxic highly branched β-aminoesters having ethylenemorpholine and hydroxypentyl groups linked to nitrogen atoms from the main polymeric chains [41,42]. Those special polymers—obtained from a triacrylate branching combined with polyethoxylated bisphenol diacrylate monomers—were tested both in vitro for biocompatibility on human cervical cancer (HeLa) cells, and in vivo on genetic collaged-defective dystrophic epidermolysis bullosa (RDEB) knockout mice, showing improved transfection efficiency and reduced cytotoxicity [43]. The synthesis of newly modified NPs for biomedical applications requires the evaluation of potential risks and toxicity effects resulting from the interaction between NPs and living cells. Failure of candidate coating can occur in a wide variety of modes, including toxicity [44], foreign body response [45] or instability in the biological milieu of hydrolytic enzymes and generation of inflammatory processes [46].

In vitro models are reliable tools to identify the effects of NPs in the human body, allowing the estimation of their toxicity and biocompatibility. Among other factors, cellular toxicity of NPs depends on the particle size, shape, porosity, surface charge, chemical composition, and colloidal stability [47]. Moreover, the nanoparticle–cell interactions and biological responses differ, depending on the cell type [48]. Many cancer cell models are used to study the biological effects of MNPs. One of them is Caco2 cell line, a human intestinal cell model which has been adopted by many researchers for exploring the toxicity of a range of NPs to the gastrointestinal system. Studies on Caco2 cell line are focused on the in vitro biocompatibility of coated magnetic iron oxide NPs for biomedical applications [49]; the effects of magnetic NPs in hyperthermia [50]; the synergistic interactions between magnetic fluid hyperthermia and the anticancer drugs [51]; the interaction with magnetic iron oxide NPs with different coatings [52]; the effect of NP size and surface charge on their interaction with cells, and the mechanism of NP internalization and toxicity [53]. The Caco2 cell line is preferred, also, because it holds many advantages due to its simplicity and reproducibility of results.

Therefore, it is important to analyze the in vitro interactions of the NPs with a specific cell line. Thus, for MNPs with potential in biomedical applications, one may then proceed towards in vivo validation and biodistribution assays. At the cellular level, the nanoparticle uptake and the mechanism by which they enter the cell has been studied, as it has important implications not only for their fate, but also for their impact on the biological systems.

The aim of present study was to succeed the synthesis of hybrid nanoparticle aggregates containing distinct iron-based and silicon nanophases, and to prove their biocompatibility. Nanopowders were prepared by laser pyrolysis using a new special geometry for the reactive gas mixtures' introduction. Thus, we employed a special nozzle endowed with two close and parallel tubes. $Fe(CO)_5$ vapors carried by a C_2H_4 flow and a separate gas mixture of SiH_4 and Ar were used as Fe and Si donors, respectively. Stabilized suspensions were prepared using synthesized NPs covered with two biocompatible agents: L-DOPA or CMC-Na, in order to evaluate their in vitro biological responses on human colorectal epithelial adenocarcinoma cells (Caco2 cell line). The effect induced in vitro was evaluated on different formulations of L-DOPA and CMC-Na-coated NPs in suspensions, and on individual components by varying the synthesis parameters focused to tailor the composition of Fe-Si nanoaggregates, as well as their magnetic properties and crystalline dimension. According to our results, the biological responses of the hybrid Fe-Si NPs were influenced by both the synthesis parameters and the type of coating/stabilizer. The results revealed that L-DOPA and CMC-Na-coated NPs display a different biological behavior on Caco2 cells, which is of great interest for further biomedical applications.

2. Materials and Methods

2.1. Experimental Set-Up for Laser Pyrolysis

Distinct syntheses of Fe@Fe$_x$O$_y$ and Si@SiO$_x$ core shell nanopowders were already performed using previously described laser pyrolysis protocols [14,54,55]. Briefly, for producing nanosized iron or silicon nanopowders in the typical procedure, the focused continuous wave or pulsed CO$_2$ laser radiation (λ = 10.6 µm) orthogonally crossed the gas flows, emerging through the central inlet tube dedicated for reactive gas mixture: (1) C$_2$H$_4$ and Fe(CO)$_5$ vapors for Fe based nanopowders, or (2) SiH$_4$ in combination with an inert gas or C$_2$H$_4$ for Si-based nanopowders. The confinement of gas precursors toward the flow axis and of the freshly nucleated particles was achieved by a coaxial argon (or other inert gas) flow. Here, we employed a COHERENT Diamond E-400 (Coherent, Santa Clara, CA, USA) CO$_2$ pulsed laser emitting in infrared domain at 10.6 µm with 90 kHz frequency, for the simultaneous synthesis of hybrid nanomaterials with distinct Fe-based and Si nanocrystals, just by approaching the two central gas flows via a nozzle with two parallel nearby inner tubes dedicated for Fe and Si precursors, respectively. In order to control the aggregation process, two different geometries for the reaction product evacuation have been used: (1) a classical one with a cylindrical geometry having a 3 cm^2 cross section placed at 3 mm above the reaction zone, or (2) a tronconical one (narrow escape, similar with the expansion nozzle used in [56]), where the smaller base-endowed with a 0.05 cm^2 hole—was placed at 1.5 mm above the reaction zone, as presented in Figure 1. The second exhaust trajectory generated a quick quenching for the exhaust products (powder and resulted gaseous components). In all experiments (labeled Fe-Si), the Fe(CO)$_5$ (the iron precursor) vapors entrained by ethylene emerged through the first central inlet tubes, while a mixture containing SiH$_4$ and Ar emerged into the reaction chamber through the neighboring second central inlet (see Figure 1). The Fe and Si precursors, and partially, the ethylene, were allowed to dissociate in two distinct but adjacent flames, due to the resonant interactions between the laser beam and both ethylene and silane (having thus the role of laser energy transfer agents or sensitizers) and they transferred the resulted heat via intermolecular collisions to both (Fe-rich and Si-rich, respectively) reactive mixtures.

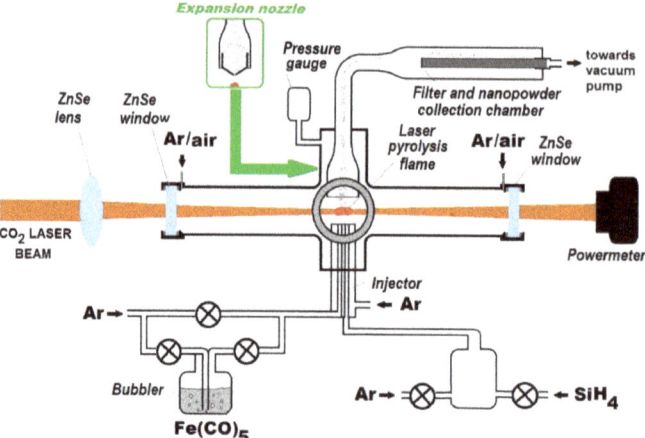

Figure 1. Experimental set-up used for the obtaining of nanometric Fe-Si-based hybrid nanoaggregates by laser pyrolysis followed by a post-irradiation superficial oxidation.

The most relevant samples selected for this study were synthesized using the parameters presented in Table 1. In all cases, an annular external argon flow (2500 sccm) assured the confinement toward the central flow axes. At the end of synthesis, the input gas streams were stopped, the remaining gas extracted with the vacuum pump from both reaction and collection chambers, followed by synthetic air (the oxidizer agent) slowly being introduced in the main chamber through the lateral outlets (located near the IR-transparent windows). This "soft oxidation" treatment ensured the development of an oxidic shell at zerovalent iron surfaces, preventing thus the particles burning upon air exposure [57]. A similar oxidic shell (made from SiO_2) seems also to superficially cover the Si nanoparticles due this treatment.

Table 1. Experimental parameters for the standard/rapid quenching laser-assisted synthesis of Fe-Si-based hybrid nanoparticle aggregates.

Sample/Parameters	Exhaust Geometry	D1 Flow	D2 Flow		Laser Power	Flame Temp. (°C)
		$D_{C_2H_4}/Fe(CO)_5$ (sccm)	D_{SiH_4} (sccm)	D_{Ar} (sccm)	$P_{L/Ar}/P_{L/abs.}$ (W)	
Fe-Si2	normal	60	20	50	115/105	660
Fe-Si3	normal	60	10	40	115/108	620
Fe-Si7	narrow	60	5	55	115/110	540

After the synthesis and superficial oxidation treatment, the morphology and composition of the as prepared NPs were characterized by X-ray diffraction (XRD), energy-dispersive X-ray analysis (EDX), transmission electron microscopy (TEM), and selected area electron diffraction (SAED). Also, their magnetic features were investigated via vibrating sample magnetometry (VSM). Hybrid nanoaggregates might contain two distinct components: a magnetic one due to presence of Fe-based nanodomains, and a non-magnetic one if Si rich nanomaterial co-occur randomly mixed with the first one in the same powder. This fact appears predominantly, when the two parallel inlets are positioned too far apart (more than 2 mm). For this reason, only those samples that separate magnetically more than 95 wt % from a methanol-based suspension were used in the next studies. Also, all three samples selected here (see Table 1) were synthesized using 1.0 mm distance between the two inlet tubes, and they revealed this macroscopic magnetic homogeneity.

2.2. Synthesis and Coating of Hybrid Fe-Si Nanoparticles

As raw materials for the laser pyrolysis synthesis, we employed iron pentacarbonyl (97%) from Sigma-Aldrich (St. Louis, MO, USA) as vapors from volatile liquid and gaseous ethylene (99.999 vol. %), silane (99.99% vol. %), argon (99.9999 vol. %), and synthetic air (having 20% O_2 and 80% N_2 vol. %) from Linde Gas (Timisoara, Romania). For the water-based nanoparticle suspensions' preparation, we employed L-DOPA (3,4 dihydroxy-L-phenylalanine, product code D9628), carboxymethylcellulose sodium salt (low viscosity, product code C5678) and Dulbecco's phosphate buffered saline (PBS, product code D1408), all purchased from Sigma-Aldrich (St. Louis, MO, USA).

The preparation of stabilized suspensions was done according the same procedure as in [27] when L-DOPA was used as stabilizer. As a particularity, Fe-Si nanoaggregates showed a good stability in distilled water (pH ~5.5, due to the atmospheric CO_2 absorption) but their magnetic properties decreased down to 60% in comparison with those dispersed in acetone (a base fluid presumed to be inert, which does not modify the particles magnetic properties). Due to this reason, the homogenized dry mixture of nanopowder and CMC-Na stabilizer was slowly introduced in water under the combined action of the ultrasonic horn disperser (20 mm diameter, Hielscher UIP 1000-hd Ultrasonic Homogenizer, Hielscher Ultrasonics, Teltow, Germany) and a vibrating thin rod during 5 min, and then for the entire suspension, the ultrasonic treatment was continued for 30 min using an external cold water bath, to maintain a temperature around 30 °C. For catechol stabilization, firstly, a 3 g/L L-DOPA hot solution was prepared, then the magnetic powder was added using the vibrating rod and the ultrasonic bath (Labsonic LBS2 from Falc Instruments, Treviglio, Italy), sealed and ultrasonicated on the same bath for 5 h at 70 °C, followed by the same half hour horn ultrasonication, also at 70 °C temperature. Using these procedures, the magnetic saturation of final stabilized suspension dropped only by 15% in comparison with the one made at the same powder concentration, in acetone. In both cases, the nanopowders were suspended and stabilized in distilled water, and then transferred in PBS.

2.3. Characterization of Hybrid Fe-Si Nanoparticles and Resulted Suspensions

The crystalline phase composition of raw nanopowders was evaluated using a PANalyticalX'Pert MPD theta–theta X-ray diffraction (XRD) apparatus (PANalytical, Almelo, Netherlands) using a Cu K-α source (0.15418 nm), while their morphology and structure were examined with a Philips CM 120ST (120 kV) Transmission Electron Microscope (TEM), (Philips, Amsterdam, Netherlands). Energy-dispersive X-ray spectroscopy (EDS) measurements for elemental analysis were performed inside a scanning electron microscope FEI Quanta Inspect S (FEI, Hillsboro, OR, USA) at 10 kV accelerating voltage, using an ELEMENT Silicon Drift Detector from EDAX Co (FEI, Hillsboro, OR, USA). Magnetic hysteresis curves were obtained at room temperature using a vibrating sample magnetometer (VSM) under applied fields up to 1000 kA/m. A Malvern Zetasizer apparatus (Malvern, Worcestershire, UK) was employed for the aqueous media suspended particles mean hydrodynamic size analyses using dynamic light scattering (DLS) method.

2.4. Cell Line Culture and Treatment

The Caco2 cell line, originally derived from a human colorectal adenocarcinoma, was purchased from American Type Culture Collection (ATCC HTB-37, ATCC/LGC Standards GmbH, Wesel, Germany). Human Caco2 cell line is a continuous line of heterogeneous epithelial colorectal adenocarcinoma cells, rapid and easy to culture, and is also used to predict in vivo toxicity [58]. Caco2 cells are approximately 30 to 70 µm, spindle- or polygon-shaped (high cell density), with adherent cells growing as a confluent monolayer.

The cell cultures were grown in 75 cm^2 flasks in complete Minimum Essential Medium (MEM; M0643, Sigma-Aldrich, St. Louis, MO, USA) supplemented with 1% antibiotic–antimycotic mix solution (A5955; Sigma-Aldrich, St. Louis, MO, USA) and 20% fetal bovine serum (10270-106, origin South America, Gibco, by Life Technologies, Carlsbad, CA, USA) and maintained at 37 °C in humidified atmosphere (95%) with 5% CO_2.

To evaluate the biological effect induced in Caco2 cells by hybrid Fe-Si NPs exposure, the cells were seeded in 96 and 24-well plates at a density of 5×10^4 cells/mL and allowed to attach overnight. Then, hybrid Fe-Si NPs and the two stabilizers (L-DOPA and CMC-NA) were serially diluted (0 = control, 12.5, 25, 50, 100, 200 µg/mL for NPs, and 7.5, 15, 30, 60, 120 µg/mL for corresponding concentrations of stabilizers in NPs suspensions) in cell culture medium, and incubated with the cells for 24 and 72 h.

2.5. Cell Viability and IC_{50} Evaluation

Cell viability was measured after cell exposure to nanoparticles by 3-(4,5-dimethylthiazol-2-yl)-2,5-diphenyltetrazolium bromide (MTT) spectrophotometric test [59]. Briefly, the cells were seeded in 96-well plates at a density of 10^4 cells/well/200 µL, and allowed to adhere for 24 h. Hybrid Fe-Si NPs (0–200 µg/mL) and the two stabilizers (0–120 µg/mL) were added into culture media and incubated for 24 and 72 h. After each time interval, the medium with NPs was removed from all wells, and 75 µL of 1 mg/mL MTT solution (M2128, Sigma-Aldrich) was added for 2 h at 37 °C. The formazan produced by MTT reduction in metabolic active cells was solubilized in 150 µL isopropanol, and the absorbance was measured at 595 nm using a FlexStation 3 microplate reader (Molecular Devices, San Jose, CA, USA).

IC_{50} values or inhibitory concentrations were calculated to identify the dose that inhibits 50% of the viability of Caco2 cells. For calculating the IC_{50} values, the treatment concentrations (x) and the viability inhibition rate obtained by the MTT (y) test were used. The data were plotted by linear regression, and the IC_{50} values were estimated using the equation: $Y = a \times X + b$; $IC_{50} = (0.5 - b)/a$.

2.6. Cell Morphology and F-Actin Cytoskeleton Imaging

Morphologic characteristics of Caco2 cells after exposure to NPs were analyzed by optical and fluorescence microscopy. Bright-field representative images with Caco2 cells were acquired by phase contrast microscopy using an inverted microscope Olympus IX73 (Olympus, Tokyo, Japan) and CellSens Dimension imaging software (ver. 1.11, Olympus, Tokyo, Japan). Cell actin cytoskeleton was fluorescently labeled using Alexa Fluor 488 phalloidin dye (A12379, Molecular Probes by Life Technologies, Carlsbad, CA, USA), which binds F-actin filaments with high selectivity, providing a green fluorescence. Briefly, after NPs exposure cells were fixed with 4% paraformaldehyde for 10 min and permeabilized with a solution of 0.1% Triton X-100 in 2% bovine serum albumin for 45 min. Finally, cells were stained for 45 min at room temperature with 150 nM Alexa Fluor 488 phalloidin solution. Images were captured with an inverted fluorescence microscope Olympus IX71 (Olympus, Tokyo, Japan) with Cell^F software (ver. 5.0, Olympus, Tokyo, Japan) using identical settings. Fluorescence intensity of phalloidin-positive cells was quantified by using ImageJ (ver. 1.47q, Bethesda, MD, USA), and the results expressed as background-corrected integrated fluorescence density. Six images for each sample were analyzed and the fluorescence intensity was measured. The graph was represented using the mean fluorescence ± standard deviation.

2.7. Lactate Dehydrogenase (LDH) Assay

The LDH amount released in culture medium was assessed as a measure of cell membrane integrity using the In Vitro Toxicology Assay Kit, Lactic Dehydrogenase-Based (TOX7, Sigma-Aldrich, St. Louis, MO, USA). According to the manufacturer's instructions, volumes of 50 µL of culture supernatants removed from the same 96-well plates used for MTT test, were incubated with 100 µL mix composed from equal parts (1:1:1) of dye, substrate, and cofactor for 30 min in dark. The reaction was stopped by adding 15 µL of 1 N HCl, and the absorbance was read at 490 nm using a microplate reader.

2.8. Measurement of ROS Production

The level of intracellular reactive oxygen species (ROS) generated after exposure to hybrid Fe-Si NPs in Caco2 cells was measured as previously described [60] using 2′,7′-dichlorofluorescein diacetate (H2DCF-DA; Sigma-Aldrich, St. Louis, MO, USA). Only two NPs concentrations were investigated: 25 and 50 µg/mL, selected after cell viability evaluation. The cells were seeded in 96-well plates at a density of 2×10^4 cells/well and after 1 to 4 h of incubation with NPs incubation, ROS production was recorded (as relative fluorescence units, RFU) using a fluorescence microplate reader FlexStation 3 (Molecular Devices, , San Jose, CA, USA) at 485 nm ex./520 nm em. wavelength.

2.9. Protein Extraction

Caco2 cells, harvested from culture flasks, were washed with PBS, trypsinized, and centrifuged at 1500 rpm for 5 min. Cell pellets were washed again, resuspended in 400 µL of PBS, and then sonicated on ice three times, for 30 s each. The total protein extract was centrifuged at 3000 rpm for 10 min at 4 °C. Aliquots of the supernatant were used for further determination. The protein concentration, expressed as mg/mL, was measured by Bradford method, using bovine serum albumin as standard [61].

2.10. Quantification of GSH Content

The intracellular reduced glutathione (GSH) concentration was evaluated using the Glutathione Assay Kit (CS0260, Sigma-Aldrich, St. Louis, MO, USA). Briefly, after treatment with NPs, protein extracts were precipitated with 5-sulfosalicylic acid (1:1) and the supernatants were recovered. A volume of 10 µL from each sample was added in 150 µL assay buffer containing 5,5′-dithiobis(2-nitrobenzoic acid) (DTNB; D8130, Sigma-Aldrich, St. Louis, MO, USA), and incubated for 10 min at room temperature. The 5-thio-2-nitrobenozoic acid (TNB) formed was measured spectrophotometrically at 405 nm. A calibration curve (3.125–200 µM) was similarly prepared using glutathione solution as standard. The results were expressed in nmoles GSH/mg of protein and represented as a ratio of treated cells compared to untreated cells.

2.11. Immunoblotting of Nuclear Factor E2-Related Factor 2 (Nrf-2)

Equal amounts of protein (30 µg) from treated and untreated Caco2 cells were electrophoresed through an SDS-polyacrylamide gel (10% resolving gel) in Tris-glycine buffer at 90 V for 2 h. The proteins were transferred from the SDS-polyacrylamide gel to Immun-Blot PVDF membrane (Bio-Rad, Hercules, CA, USA) using a wet transfer system. Membranes were developed using WesternBreeze Chromogenic Anti-Rabbit Kit (WB7105, Invitrogen, Carlsbad, CA, USA) and rabbit polyclonal primary anti-Nrf-2 antibody (sc-722, Santa Cruz Biotechnology, Heidelberg, Germany) according to the manufacturer's instructions. The protein bands were detected by staining with the BCIP/NBT substrate and visualized with the ChemiDoc Imaging System (Bio-Rad, Hercules, CA, USA). Quantification of bands on Western images was done using the Image Lab software (ver. 5.2, Bio-Rad, Hercules, CA, USA). To normalize Nrf-2 levels, Nrf-2 band intensity was divided by β-actin (A1978, Sigma-Aldrich, St. Louis, MO, USA) band intensity (which serves as reference protein), and represented as percentages of control.

2.12. Statistical Analysis

All tests were performed in triplicate, and data were shown as mean ± standard deviation (SD). The statistical Student's *t*-test was performed for biological tests to analyze significant differences when comparing treated cells with controls. A value of $p < 0.05$ was considered significant.

3. Results and Discussion

3.1. Hybrid Fe-Si Nanoparticles Preparation and Characterization

In the Figure 2, superposed X ray diffractograms of the nanopowders from three selected experiments (two employing large cylindrical gas/particles evacuation geometry—Fe-Si2 and Fe-Si3, and one using the expansion nozzle—Fe-Si7) are presented. The elemental silicon phase can be observed for all powders, but for those synthesized in classical cylindrical geometry, the corresponding peaks are more intense, especially for the Fe-Si2 sample where the highest silane flow was used. Highest Si atomic concentration was found also in the Fe-Si2 sample (see Table 2), confirming the tendency of decreasing the amount of silicon detected in the resulted nanopowders with diminishing SiH_4 flow. The mean silicon crystallite sizes in the nanopowders obtained in this geometry decreased with the diminishing of SiH_4 flow, as can be calculated using Debye–Scherrer formula (17.5 nm for Fe-Si2 vs. 13.3 nm for Fe-Si3). The presence of Fe-based phases, formed by iron pentacarbonyl decomposition under ethylene sensitizer influence, is proved by the identification of Fe_3C (cohenite) peaks, the most intense being those at $2\theta = 45°$. Other phases, such as Fe_3C_7 and αFe, can also be present in small quantities, given that most of their peaks overlap with those of the Fe_3C phase. Even if we used the same ethylene-entrained $Fe(CO)_5$ vapor flow in all three experiments, it seems that the expansion nozzle favorizes their decomposition. Thus, the Fe-Si7 powder exhibits the most intense peak at $2\theta = 45°$, accompanied by smaller peaks at $41°$ and $49°$, all attributed to Fe_3C phase, formed by the ethylene decomposition on the freshly-formed iron clusters resulting from $Fe(CO)_5$ decarbonylation and coalescence, followed by the solubilization of the resulting carbon species. This fact is confirmed by the EDS measurements (see Table 2) which show that the Fe-Si$_7$ samples have the highest iron atomic concentration. A lower intensity peak can be observed for all three samples at $2\theta \sim 36°$, could be attributed to $\gamma Fe_2O_3/Fe_3O_4$ phase, formed by superficial oxidation of iron-based phases during the post-synthesis passivation process.

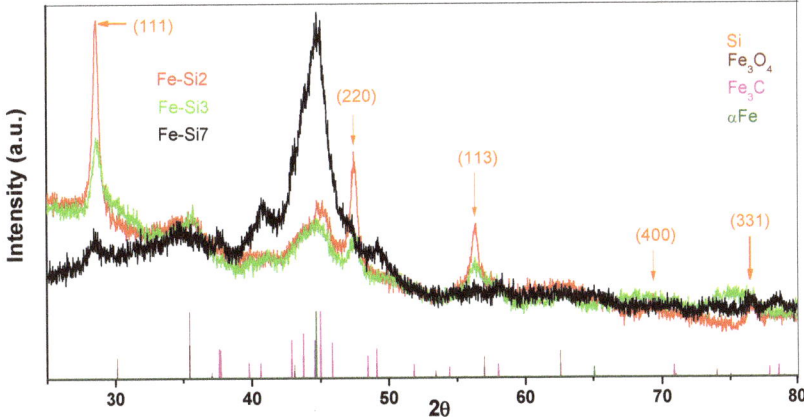

Figure 2. Superposed X-ray diffractograms for the Fe-Si2, Fe-Si3, and Fe-Si7 raw nanopowders, and the reference diffractograms for Fe-based phases.

Table 2. Elemental composition of powders extracted from EDX analyses.

Element/Sample	C (atom %)	O (atom %)	Si (atom %)	Fe (atom %)
Fe-Si2	11.1	23.8	34.3	30.8
Fe-Si3	13.4	33.1	26.7	26.8
Fe-Si7	13.3	26.1	19.9	40.7

Figure 3 contains a series of transmission electron microscopy images from Fe-Si3 and Fe-Si7 samples, showing the round morphology of the observed nanometric particles. The left high-resolution image shows two nanoparticles with diameters around 22–25 nm from the Fe-Si3 powder, where the (031) cohenite crystalline planes—distanced at 2.05 Å—were identified. These nanoparticles are covered with a thin layer of turbostratic (composed from 3 or 4 stacked graphenes distanced at ~3.5 Å) mixed with amorphous carbon. This carbon-based layer can be formed by excess carbon precipitation from the carbon-saturated iron-based NPs upon cooling after the reaction zone. The central high resolution transmission electron microscopy (HR-TEM) image (from Fe-Si7 sample, synthesized with the expansion nozzle) shows a few aggregated nanoparticles deposed onto the amorphous carbon membrane which covers the electron microscope grid. In the upper one, (100) parallel crystalline planes, distanced at 0.31 nm, belonging to silicon phase, can be clearly seen, which extend over 12 nm. In the lower part of same image, another two smaller crystalline zones can be identified, with 0.20 nm interplanar distance, which could be attributed to (031) planes of Fe_3C or to (110) planes of αFe. The third TEM image from the right part of Figure 3 shows the extended fractal aggregates of small (3–5 nm) NPs from the same powder, Fe-Si7. Even at this lower magnification, the core–shell structure of the chained nanoparticles can be clearly noticed.

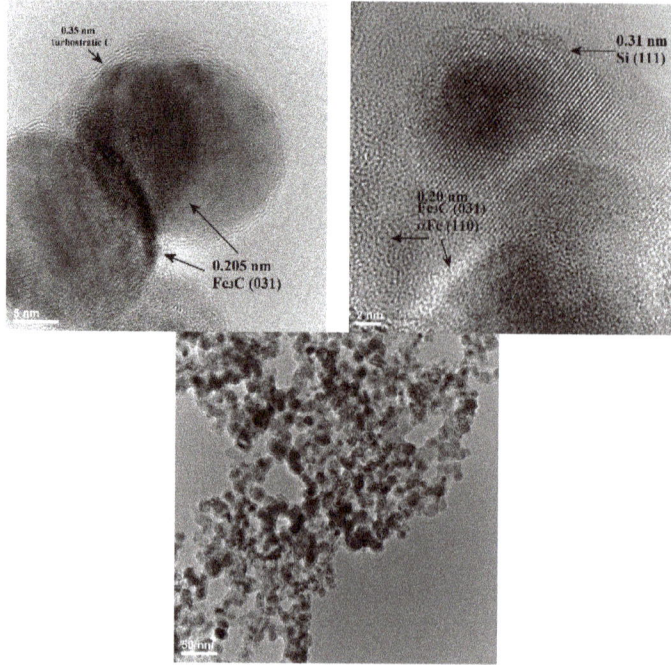

Figure 3. Higher definition (left: Fe-Si3, center: Fe-Si7 samples) and lower definition (right: Fe-Si7 sample) TEM images of nanoparticles from as-synthesized powders.

Table 3 summarizes some of the magnetic parameters of the raw nanopowders, extracted from the room temperature hysterezis magnetization curves. As expected, the highest magnetization (47 emu/g) can be found for the Fe-Si7 sample with the higher Fe and lower Si content. The low values of the coercivity reflect the near superparamagnetic behavior of the NPs, in concordance with their dimensions. The maximum permeability values are of the same size order with those having of Fe-based core and ZnO shells synthesized also by one-step laser pyrolysis, and recently reported by us [36].

Table 3. Magnetic parameters (saturation magnetization, retentivity, coercivity, and maximum permeability) of the raw powders.

Sample	M_s (emu/g)	M_r (emu/g)	H_c (kA/m)	μ_{max} (emu/Oe)
Fe-Si2	21	2.85	5.37	$5.22 \times 10-4$
Fe-Si3	23	3.81	8.84	$7.38 \times 10-4$
Fe-Si7	47	10.53	12.88	$7.87 \times 10-4$

3.2. Coating of Hybrid Fe-Si NPs with L-DOPA or CMC-Na

The dimensional distribution (by number) of polyanionic CMC-Na polyelectrolyte-coated nanoparticle aggregates from the Fe-Si samples is presented in Figure 4. A monomodal asymmetric distribution for Fe-Si2 NPs polyelectrolyte-coated in suspension can be observed, with the mean hydrodynamic size centered at 85.3 nm. However, the scattering intensity counted DLS size distribution from the same suspension (not shown here) reveals a bimodal distribution, which reflects the presence of two distinct populations of aggregates, the smaller having sizes centered around 81 nm, whereas the bigger ones are slightly more than three time larger (centered ~264 nm).

Corroborating those two DLS size distributions, one can conclude that in the CMC-Na-stabilized Fe-Si2 NPs suspension the number of bigger aggregates is very low. The suspension from Fe-Si3 NPs hydrophilized with CMC-Na shows a bimodal distribution (by number), where the smaller nanoparticle aggregates (~70 nm) far outnumber the bigger ones (~230 nm), a situation similar with the previously discussed NPs dispersion. The Fe-Si7 NPs suspended with CMC-Na shows also an asymmetric monomodal size distribution with a reduced "tail" in the 70–90 nm zone, the mean size in this case, being around 67 nm. If we compare the DLS size distributions for all, synthesized suspensions, we can conclude that the CMC-Na agent induces the formation aggregates having smaller sizes than those induced by L-DOPA, and that the use of the expansion nozzle (Fe-Si7 sample) favored also smaller aggregates.

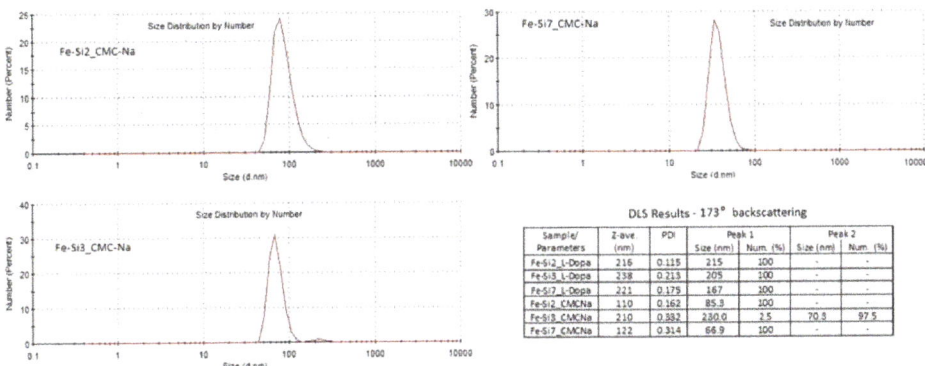

Figure 4. DLS size distribution diagrams of aqueous suspensions containing Fe-Si nanopowders stabilized with CMC-Na and inserted tabulated values of mean hydrodynamic sizes of water-suspended Fe-Si nanoparticle aggregates stabilized with CMC-Na and with L-DOPA.

Since both superficial silicon dioxide and iron oxide formed by passivation of Fe-Si NPs have a hydrophilic behavior, in neutral media they tend to aggregate via hydrogen bonds formation between hydroxyl surface groups. It seems that their coating with CMC-Na polyanionic chains limits the aggregation, and also stabilizes the small aggregates against further coalescence and sedimentation by electrostatic repulsions between negatively charged carboxyl groups.

The successful ultrasonication-assisted L-DOPA coating of laser pyrolysis-synthesized iron oxide nanoparticles in aqueous media was reported by us in [27,62], where a supplementary rhodamine derivate dye labelling was achieved. During this coating procedure, a partial oxidative polymerization of L-DOPA (under the action of dissolved oxygen) to oligomelanins seems to occur, as proven by the darkening of colorless pure L-DOPA solution at the same concentration, which was subjected to an identical sonication treatment. The presence of a conformal coating (~15–20 nm thickness), which also embeds multiple nanoparticles from the Fe-Si3 sample, can be observed in the TEM image from Figure 5a. The chemical anchoring of L-DOPA molecules to the oxidic surfaces of Fe-Si type, in a similar way to that reported for magnetite [63] nanoparticles, occurs via the orthophenolate (catechol) part—see Figure 5b, while the remaining zwitterionic amino acid part assures a high hydrophilicity and electrostatic stabilization at neutral pH. Similar stabilization can also be induced by indole and/or carboxy groups from oligomeric melanins (related with natural eumelanins) resulted by L-DOPA sonication-induced oxidative polymerization as schematically shown in Figure 5b, according to a mechanism also proposed in [64].

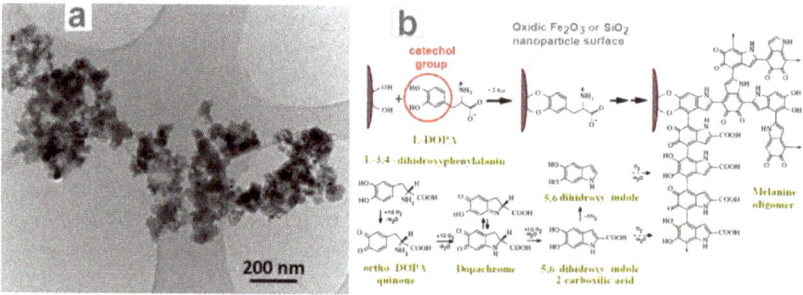

Figure 5. (a) TEM image of L-DOPA coated aggregates of nanoparticle derived from Fe-Si3 sample; (b) Proposed mechanism for L-DOPA attachment and polymerization to oligomelanin on the nanoparticles oxidic surface.

3.3. Biocompatibility Assessment

3.3.1. Cytotoxicity

The new materials developed for biomedical applications require the simultaneous fulfillment of three major conditions: biocompatibility, low toxicity, and biodegradability. Various nanostructures based on iron and silicon have been reported to be highly biocompatible [65–67], and easily metabolized by the body as orthosilicic acid Si(OH)$_4$ or iron ions. The retention of NPs in the body primarily can negatively affect organs, including liver, kidneys, stomach, and intestines.

To assess the biocompatibility of hybrid Fe-Si NPs coated with L-DOPA and CMC-Na, doses ranging from 0–200 µg/mL were exposed to Caco2 cells for 24 and 72 h. Untreated cells and cells treated with the individual components of NPs were used as controls. The results indicated no significant change in Caco2 cell viability exposed to concentrations between 0–100 µg/mL L-DOPA-coated Fe-Si NPs and 0–50 µg/mL CMC-Na-coated Fe-Si hybrid NPs (Figure 6). At the highest dose of 200 µg/mL, NP cell viability decreased after 72 h exposure by 29%, 43%, and 11% in the presence of Fe-Si2_L-DOPA NPs, Fe-Si3_L-DOPA NPs, and, respectively, Fe-Si7_L-DOPA NPs. By comparison, Fe-Si7_CMC-Na NPs (200 µg/mL) were the most toxic, causing a decrease by 73% of cell viability after 72 h of exposure, compared to untreated control. By comparison, the decrease of viability in the Caco2 cells exposed to uncoated NPs was lower, the maximum decrease was induced by 200 µg/mL Fe-Si NPs after 72 h. Surprisingly, the most toxic component for Caco2 cells was L-DOPA which has an IC$_{50}$ value of 81.2 µg/mL. However, the IC$_{50}$ values for the L-DOPA stabilized NPs were higher compared with those stabilized with CMC-Na (Table 4).

By now, L-DOPA and CMC-Na have been used to stabilize various NPs, including iron oxide [68], magnetic Fe-MWCNT [69], Fe@C [70], zinc oxide (ZnO) [71], silica (SiO$_2$), and titania (TiO$_2$) ones [72], as well as anticancer drug carriers [73] etc., but the interactions with cells and tissues were not entirely described and understood.

L-DOPA is an amino acid, precursor of dopamine, biosynthesized naturally by a number of plants and animals. In humans, it is obtained through the metabolic pathway of catecholamines, being biosynthesized directly from L-tyrosine. Some in vitro studies have reported toxic effects of L-DOPA [74,75], whereas others have demonstrated a protective action, similar to the beneficial effects of some dopamine receptor agonists. Furthermore, the results of many in vivo experiments, as well as of clinical trials, did not demonstrate L-DOPA toxicity or remained inconclusive [76]. On the other hand CMC-Na "generally recognized as safe" (GRAS) by the US Food and Drug Administration is widely used in diverse industries including medical applications. The in vitro and in vivo biocompatibility CMC has been demonstrated [22,77] as well as limited biodegradation by glucose residues releasing [78].

In our case, as resulted from Figure 6, NPs coated with CMC-Na presented a higher toxicity compared with those coated with L-DOPA at high doses in Caco2 cells.

Table 4. IC$_{50}$ values (doses that inhibits 50% of the cell viability) calculated after 72 h exposure of Caco2 cells to various doses of hybrid Fe-Si nanoparticles (NPs) and stabilizers ranging from 0–200 µg/mL and 0–120 µg/mL respectively. Data are expressed as mean concentration ± SD (n = 3).

NP Sample	IC$_{50}$ (µg/mL)
Fe-Si2	382.18 ± 10.06
Fe-Si3	383.08 ± 11.86
Fe-Si7	904 ± 15.02
L-DOPA	81.2 ± 4.81
CMC-Na	1339 ± 14.27
Fe-Si2_L-DOPA	355.86 ± 17.23
Fe-Si3_L-DOPA	247.73 ± 14.56
Fe-Si7_L-DOPA	682.37 ± 14.07
Fe-Si2_CMC-Na	219.10 ± 11.83
Fe-Si3_CMC-Na	153.48 ± 8.14
Fe-Si7_CMC-Na	124.10 ± 7.10

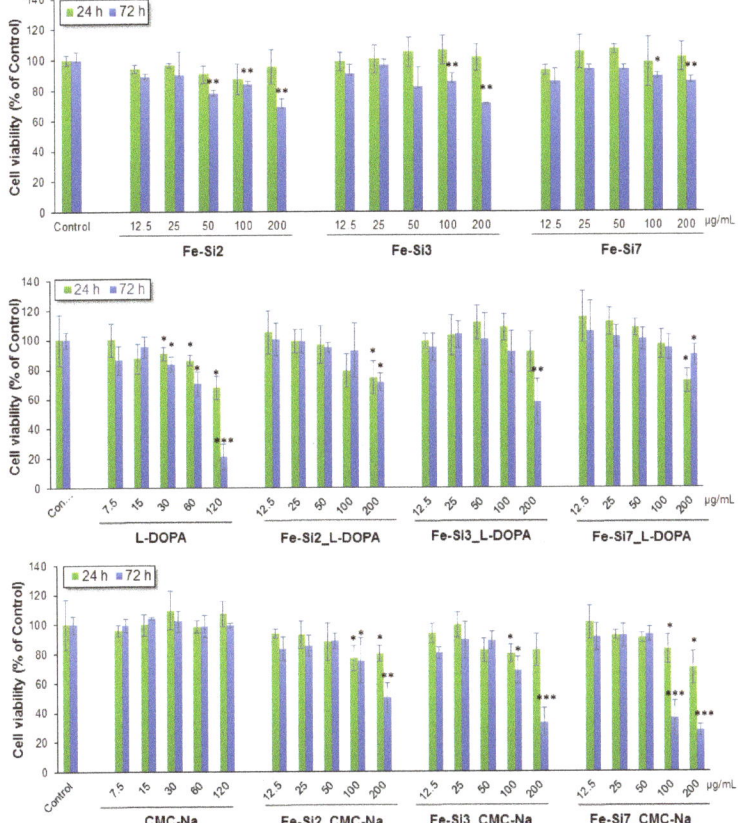

Figure 6. Cell viability of Caco2 cells after 24 and 72 h exposure to different doses (0–200 µg/mL) of hybrid Fe-Si NPs alone and stabilized with L-DOPA and CMC-Na (0–120 µg/mL). Data are expressed as the mean ± SD (n = 3) and represented as percentages of untreated control (100% viability). * $p < 0.05$; ** $p < 0.01$; *** $p < 0.001$ versus untreated control.

The release of lactate dehydrogenase (LDH) into the surrounding culture medium was assessed as a marker for membrane integrity and necrotic events. Upon incubation with all tested suspensions, high activity of LDH was found in the medium of Caco2 cells exposed to stabilized NPs and to L-DOPA (Figure 7). A lower increase of LDH level was also noticed after incubation of Caco2 cells with Fe-Si2, Fe-Si3, and Fe-Si7 NPs compared to untreated control, whereas no release of LDH was observed after cell exposure to Fe-Si7_CMC-Na NPs and CMC-Na alone. These data were in accordance with the results of MTT test and suggest that stabilization of hybrid Fe-Si NPs with L-DOPA and CMC-Na could influence the interaction with Caco2 cells and increases their toxicity at higher doses.

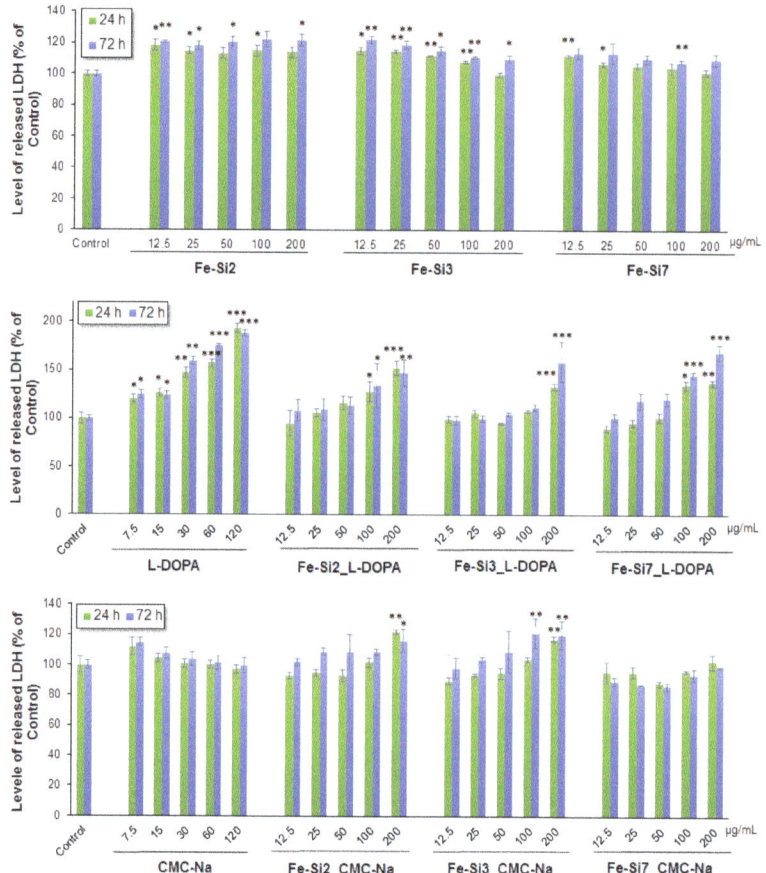

Figure 7. Level of lactate dehydrogenase (LDH) released from Caco2 cells after 24 and 72 h exposure to different doses (0–200 µg/mL) of hybrid Fe-Si NPs alone and stabilized with L-DOPA and CMC-Na (0–120 µg/mL). Data are expressed as the mean ± SD ($n = 3$) and represented as percentages of untreated control (100% viability). * $p < 0.05$; ** $p < 0.01$; *** $p < 0.001$ versus untreated control.

3.3.2. Cell Morphology and Dispersion of NPs in Culture

To study the morphology of treated Caco2 cells, two doses of 25 and 50 µg/mL of Fe-Si NPs were chosen based on cytotoxicity test outcomes. We inspected the filamentous actin cytoskeleton of Fe-Si NP-treated Caco2 cells as a measure of preservation of the overall cellular architecture. Untreated cells showed a regular structure made up of aligned and tightly compacted F-actin or actin bundles (Figure 8a). After incubation of Caco2 cells with each type of NP, no obvious changes in the cortical F-actin system were caused by doses of 25 µg/mL (data not shown). The corresponding morphologic structures remained detectable underneath the plasma membranes of most cells. However, some alterations were noticed in cells exposed for 72 h to 30 µg/mL L-DOPA and 50 µg/mL Fe-Si3, Fe-Si3_CMC-Na, and Fe-Si7_CMC-Na (Figure 8b). Formation of some F-actin aggregates and/or inclusion bodies and a great proportion of actin bundles accumulated on cell periphery were noticed (Figure 8a). By contrast, F-actin cytoskeleton was largely reserved after incubation with Fe-Si7 and Fe-Si7_L-DOPA samples. As stated above, we show that cell viability was not compromised by the presence of the F-actin alterations.

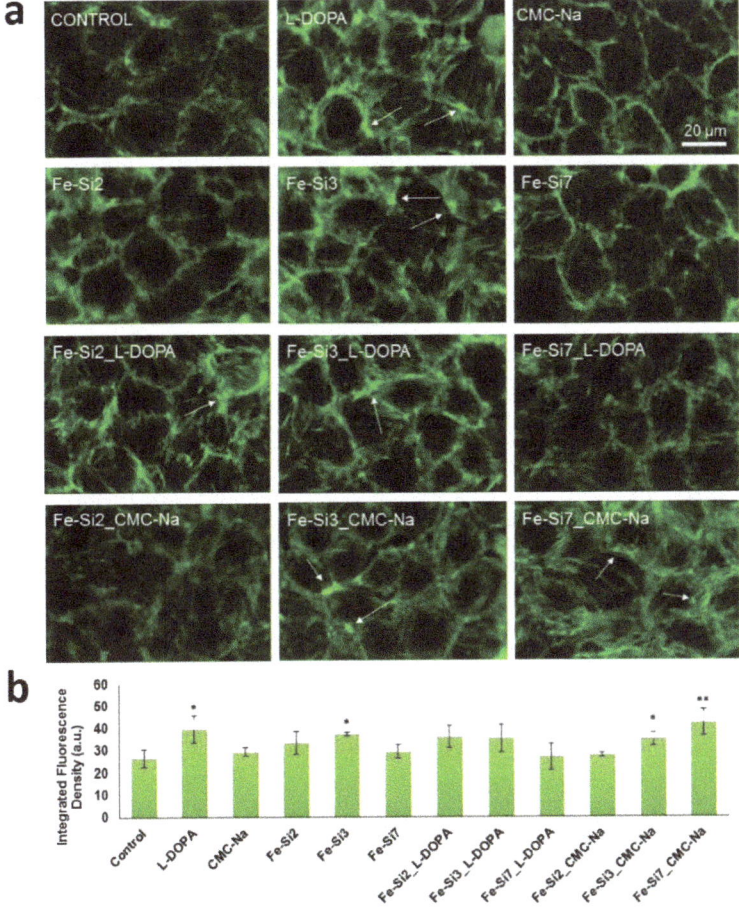

Figure 8. F-actin cytoskeleton in Caco2 cells after exposure for 72 h to 50 µg/mL hybrid Fe-Si NPs. (**a**) Direct immunofluorescence of actin staining by Alexa Fluor 488 phalloidin (green fluorescence). White arrows indicate F-actin aggregation and actin bundles accumulation on cell periphery Magnification: 40×. Control represents untreated cells. Scale bar = 20 µm; (**b**) Quantification of F-actin fluorescence.

The degree of internalization was different between Fe-Si NPs samples. Unstabilized Fe-Si NPs presented a low dispersion in the aqueous suspension, as well as in the culture medium, which hindered the internalization on cellular level. The large aggregates of NPs are impossible to penetrate the cellular membrane, and so the interaction with the cells remained, for the most part, limited to the outer membrane. All stabilized suspensions of NPs were initially well-dispersed solutions, but after their addition in the culture medium, L-DOPA -coated NPs have formed large aggregates, especially the Fe-Si7_L-DOPA sample (Figure 9), probably due to the presence of ionized carboxyl and amino groups that could interact electrochemically between individual NPs and between NPs and amino acids and proteins from the culture media. Figure 9 shows the dispersion of hybrid Fe-Si NPs in the cell culture medium, and their internalization in the Caco2 cell cytoplasm. The Fe-Si NPs stabilized with CMC-Na presented a better dispersion in medium compared with those stabilized with L-DOPA. As it can be seen, no internalization was observed for Fe-Si7_L-DOPA sample.

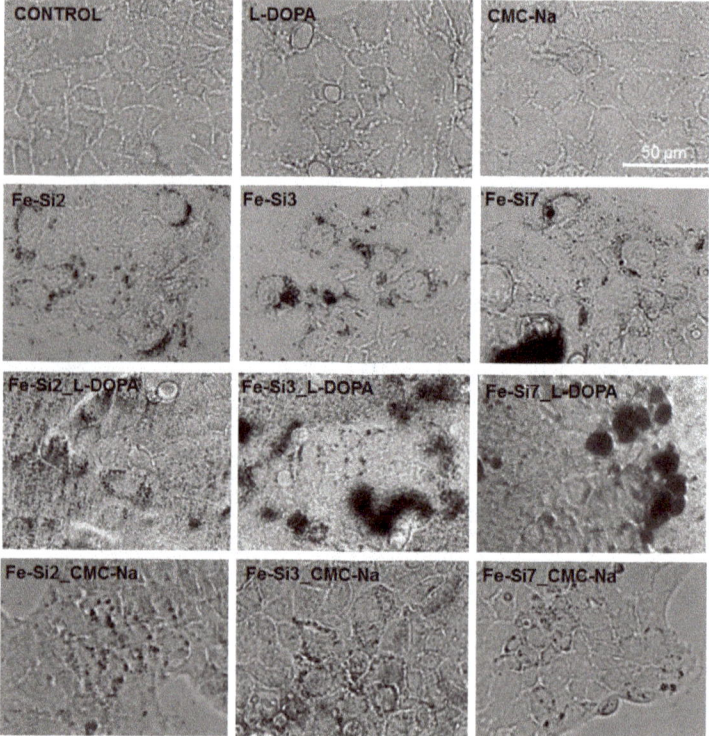

Figure 9. Images representing Caco2 cell morphology after exposure for 72 h to 50 µg/mL hybrid Fe-Si NPs. Bright-field images showing NP dispersion and internalization into the cells. Data are representative of 3 separate experiments with 3 replicates for each experimental condition. Control represents untreated cells. Scale bar = 50 µm.

In a culture medium environment, rich in serum proteins, NPs are covered by the so-called protein corona, which is influenced by the surface properties of the coated NPs in terms of type and amount of absorbed proteins. This protein corona plays an important role in their interaction with the cells and tissues, and thus in biological responses, therapeutic efficiency, and toxicity of NPs [79].

L-DOPA and CMC-Na are chemically different. In the culture medium (pH 7.4), L-DOPA has a neutral charge. According to several protein corona studies, neutral surfaces are prone to adsorb high amount of serum proteins, which can result in higher blood circulation time in vivo [80,81]. Carboxylic acid groups can act as anchor points for addition of secondary molecules by covalent bonding with amine groups, e.g., via carbodiimide chemistry [80].

On the contrary, CMC sodium salt is an anionic derivative of cellulose, negatively charged at neutral pH (pKa of 4.3), in which the hydroxyl groups are partially or fully substituted by carboxymethyl groups (–CH$_2$–COOH). Due to the ionic nature of CMC-Na, it can interact with proteins to form soluble and stable complexes. Also, the polar groups of CMC-Na (–OH, –COOH) can react with metal ions (Fe^{2+}, Fe^{3+}, Ca^{2+}, Mg^{2+}) by electrostatic forces.

The formation of aggregates in cell culture medium favors the absorption of more serum protein onto the NP surface, so the interaction of NPs with cell membrane is quite limited.

In the case of Fe-Si7_L-DOPA sample, the interaction occurred most likely at the cell membrane surface, thus explaining the increased level of LDH, starting with 24 h of incubation with 100 and 200 µg/mL doses. Also, the NP uptake was low. On the contrary, CMC-Na NPs (Fe-Si7_CMC-Na sample) presented a high dispersion in the culture medium and a high internalization in Caco2 cellular cytoplasm occurred (Figure 9). Similar changes were registered for the other CMC-Na coated NP samples. This could indicate that mechanism of toxicity is influenced by the type of coating and degree of dispersion in the culture medium.

3.3.3. Oxidative Stress

The generation of reactive oxygen species (ROS) in Caco2 cells was analyzed up to 4 h of exposure to 25 and 50 µg/mL hybrid Fe-Si NPs. As shown in Table 5, the production of ROS was time-dependent. The unstabilized Fe-Si NPs generated the highest amount of ROS. All samples CMC-Na-coated Fe-Si NPs induced ROS post-exposure at both doses of 25 and 50 µg/mL. In the case of L-DOPA-coated Fe-Si NPs, higher ROS levels were obtained for 25 µg/mL dose. No significant increase of ROS levels was registered in Caco2 cells exposed to Fe-Si7_L-DOPA NPs. Furthermore, a similarity between the results obtained for a dose of 25 µg/mL Fe-Si 2_L-DOPA and Fe-Si2_CMC-Na samples, as well as of Fe-Si3_L_DOPA and Fe-Si3_CMC-Na ones, was observed, which suggests that ROS generation at a low dose of NPs is not influenced by the nature of stabilizer. However, it is clear that a 50 µg/mL dose of L-DOPA-coated Fe-Si NPs induced less ROS compared to CMC-Na-coated Fe-Si NPs. Moreover, we showed that stabilization of Fe-Si NPs with L-DOPA and CMC-Na reduced considerable the ROS production.

According to Zhou et al., studies [82], CMC-Na could play a major role as protective coating by decreasing the toxicity against microorganisms and oxidizing capacity of nanoscale zerovalent iron after suppressing the available oxidants from the surrounding media.

In cancer cells, ROS levels are higher in comparison to normal cells, due to mitochondrial dysfunction, peroxisome activity, increased cellular receptor signaling, increased activity of oxidases, cyclooxygenases, lipoxygenases and thymidine phosphorylase [83]. The high rate of ROS production is counterbalanced by an equally high rate of antioxidant activity in cancer cells to maintain redox balance in order to ensure the cell survival.

Table 5. Intracellular ROS formation in the presence of hybrid Fe-Si NPs in Caco2 cells. Results are expressed as mean relative fluorescence units (RFU) ± SD of three independent experiments. * $p < 0.05$; ** $p < 0.01$ versus control.

Sample	Dose (µg/mL)	ROS Production (RFU)			
		1 h	2 h	3 h	4 h
Control	0	14.26 ± 0.98	18.46 ± 3.45	20.67 ± 1.23	22.15 ± 1.34
Fe-Si2	25	35.45 ± 3.2 **	63.19 ± 5.36 **	78.32 ± 6.49 **	82.37 ± 6.96 **
	50	37.63 ± 2.06 **	67.93 ± 4.92 **	84.08 ± 5.5 **	88.79 ± 5.7 **
Fe-Si3	25	39.59 ± 3.42 **	70.43 ± 6.14 **	88.83 ± 6.38 **	92.41 ± 7.63 **
	50	45.87 ± 10.6 *	81.56 ± 17.35 *	101.3 ± 20.49 *	106.46 ± 22.26 *

Table 5. Cont.

Sample	Dose (µg/mL)	ROS Production (RFU)			
		1 h	2 h	3 h	4 h
Fe-Si7	25	47.58 ± 5.76 **	80.44 ± 9.76 **	93.68 ± 11.33 **	101.24 ± 12.00 **
	50	56.02 ± 8.8 *	91.74 ± 12.63 *	104.05 ± 12.82 **	114.15 ± 14.82 **
L-DOPA	15	11.83 ± 0.48	16.93 ± 0.78	18.73 ± 1.13	20.32 ± 1.04
	30	11.65 ± 0.62	16.63 ± 1.62	18.3 ± 1.99	19.91 ± 2.02
CMC-Na	15	13.04 ± 0.59	19.36 ± 1.06	23.02 ± 1.74	24.43 ± 1.78
	30	11.28 ± 0.62	16.85 ± 0.77	19.73 ± 0.86	21.1 ± 1.00
Fe-Si2_L-DOPA	25	18.39 ± 1.85 *	25.76 ± 2.35 *	29.84 ± 2.99 *	33.03 ± 3.26 *
	50	13.28 ± 1.08	18.23 ± 1.73	21.15 ± 1.89	23.79 ± 1.98
Fe-Si3_L-DOPA	25	19.22 ± 0.42	27.64 ± 0.99 *	32.91 ± 1.67 **	36.36 ± 2.20 **
	50	14.81 ± 2.62	20.19 ± 3.92	22.86 ± 4.26	25.28 ± 4.85
Fe-Si7_L-DOPA	25	19.23 ± 2.47	26.52 ± 3.26	31.17 ± 4.02	35.02 ± 4.70
	50	15.11 ± 1.24	21.23 ± 1.94	24.42 ± 2.23	27.07 ± 2.56
Fe-Si2_CMC-Na	25	16.56 ± 1.50	23.78 ± 2.11*	28.69 ± 2.39*	32.34 ± 2.45 **
	50	15.53 ± 1.69	22.71 ± 2.57	28.36 ± 3.24*	32.68 ± 3.74 *
Fe-Si3_CMC-Na	25	17.51 ± 1.02 *	25.5 ± 1.48 *	31.4 ± 1.82 **	35.9 ± 2.04 **
	50	19.71 ± 0.60 *	29.52 ± 0.95 *	37.7 ± 1.27 **	43.68 ± 1.40 **
Fe-Si7_CMC-Na	25	23.59 ± 3.00 *	39.43 ± 4.53 **	50.29 ± 5.77 **	58 ± 6.61 **
	50	25.23 ± 1.75 *	42.66 ± 3.44 **	56.44 ± 4.65 **	67.36 ± 6.22 **

The concentration of reduced glutathione (GSH), a major component of cellular non-enzymatic antioxidant defense system, increased post-exposure in a time dependent manner. In the first 24 h, no significant variation of the GSH concentration was observed in Caco2 cells exposed to stabilized Fe-Si NPs, but a significant increase was detected in cells exposed to non-stabilized Fe-Si2 and Fe-Si3 NPs, and CMC-Na. After 72 h, its level rose significantly for all types of stabilized NPs, except Fe-Si7_L-DOPA (Figure 10). The highest level of GSH was found in Caco2 cells incubated with 25 µg/mL Fe-Si7_CMC-Na and Fe-Si2_L-DOPA, the percentage increases being 67% and 56% respectively. This suggests the activation of protecting mechanisms by elevating the stock supply of GSH, in order to face the increased ROS production, and thus, preventing the damage of lipids, proteins, and DNA caused by oxidative stress.

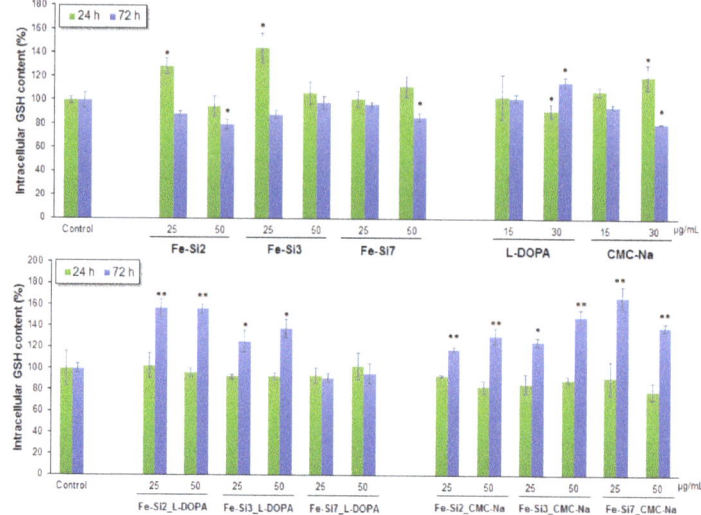

Figure 10. Intracellular GSH content in Caco2 cells after 24 and 72 h exposure to hybrid Fe-Si NPs stabilized with L-DOPA and CMC-Na. Data are expressed as the mean ± SD (n = 3) and represented as percentages of control. * $p < 0.05$; ** $p < 0.01$ versus control.

GSH is a major player in oxidative adaptation of cancer cells which is why it is exploited by researchers as a valid target for cancer targeted therapy [84]. The glutathione level is elevated in cancer cells in order to maintain the redox state and to protect cells from damage induced by free radicals, peroxides, and toxins. Glutathione is a powerful reducing compound, able to react with cellular toxic agents directly or via the reactions catalyzed by the glutathione S-transferase family of enzymes. Studies on NPs toxicity showed that GSH content could vary depending on NP dose. Increased GSH contents were reported by Saddick et al. [85] in brain tissue exposed to 500 µg/L Zn NP, while a significant decrease in GSH content was registered after exposure to 2000 µg/L. Similarly, Hao and Chen (2012) [86] found that GSH increased in the liver, gills, and brain of carp exposed to 0.5 and 5 mg/L of ZnO NPs, and decreased in all tissues of fish exposed to 50 mg/L ZnO NPs. Manke et al. [87] studied oxidative stress as an underlying mechanism for NP toxicity, and postulate that overexpression of antioxidant enzymes is indicative of mild oxidative stress, whereas mitochondrial apoptosis is induced during conditions of severe oxidative stress. According to the abovementioned, we can conclude that a mild oxidative stress was induced by 25 and 50 µg/mL stabilized Fe-Si NPs in Caco2 cells, which results in GSH level increase, and no cell death. During conditions of mild oxidative stress, transcriptional activation of phase II antioxidant enzymes occurs via nuclear factor (erythroid-derived 2)-like 2 (Nrf2) induction, another important mechanism by which cancer cells ensure their antioxidant protection. This transcription factor binds to antioxidant response element (ARE), and activates defensive gene expression, thus increasing the antioxidant proteins levels and protecting against oxidative damage [88]. Normally, Nrf2 interacts with Kelch-like ECH-associated protein 1 (KEAP1), thus leading it to proteasomal degradation. Elevated ROS levels oxidize redox sensitive cysteine residues on KEAP1, which cause the dissociation of KEAP1 from Nrf2, resulting in the increase of active Nrf2 level in the cytoplasm.

The Nrf2 protein expression was assessed in Caco2 cells after exposure for 24 and 72 h to 25 and 50 µg/mL of non-stabilized and stabilized hybrid Fe-Si NPs (Figure 11). In Caco2 cells, the activation of Nrf2 was time-dependent. After 24 h incubation, an increase of Nrf2 level in cells exposed to 25 µg/mL Fe-Si2_L-DOPA, Fe-Si3_L-DOPA, Fe-Si3_CMC-Na, Fe-Si7_CMC-Na samples, and to 50 µg/mL Fe-Si2_CMC-Na, Fe-Si3_L-DOPA, Fe-Si7_CMC-Na samples, compared with untreated control, was noticed. No change was registered for Fe-Si7 and Fe-Si7_L-DOPA samples. These results were in correlation with ROS and GSH levels. After 72 h, the increase of Nrf2 protein expression was significant in cells treated with both doses of all types of NPs. Furthermore, these results were in accordance with the increase of GSH content. By comparison, in cells exposed to the non-stabilized Fe-Si NPs and both stabilizers, the Nrf2 expression was slightly increased in accordance with the low GSH levels.

In this study, we showed that the coating of Fe-Si NPs with L-DOPA or CMC-Na influenced the in vitro biological response in Caco2 cells. The effects of the individual components of the NPs were also investigated in tandem, and were different from those of stabilized Fe-Si NPs, most likely due to their low dispersion in cell culture medium and low internalization into Caco2 cells. According to the cell viability test results, the coating of Fe-Si NPs with L-DOPA increased the biocompatibility of NPs compared to individual components, whereas the capacity of Fe-Si NPs to induce cell death was not changed after coating with CMC-Na. However, instead, this combination reduced significantly the LDH leakage. The coating of hybrid Fe-Si NPs had a great influence on NP dispersion in the cell culture medium and on cellular internalization. The CMC-Na-coated NPs were far better dispersed compared with those stabilized with L-DOPA, which could explain their higher toxicity. Changes of F-actin cytoskeleton organization were highlighted also in the cells treated with CMC-Na-coated NPs, as well as with uncoated NPs and L-DOPA. After treatment with 25 and 50 µg/mL stabilized Fe-Si NPs, ROS were produced in Caco2 cells and a mild oxidative stress was most likely induced. Consequently, the GSH level increased in order to counteract the oxidative stress, which was in accordance with the increased Nrf2 protein expression. Biological data indicated also that Caco2 cells are able to deal with the effects induced by Fe-Si NPs at a dose below 50 µg/mL by activating the scavenging mechanisms against ROS production. Thus, we showed that the Caco2 biological response to Fe-Si NPs displays hormesis, which is an adaptive response of cells to a moderate stress. By comparison, in Caco2 cells treated with unstabilized Fe-Si NPs, a higher amount of ROS was generated, but a lower antioxidant response was induced.

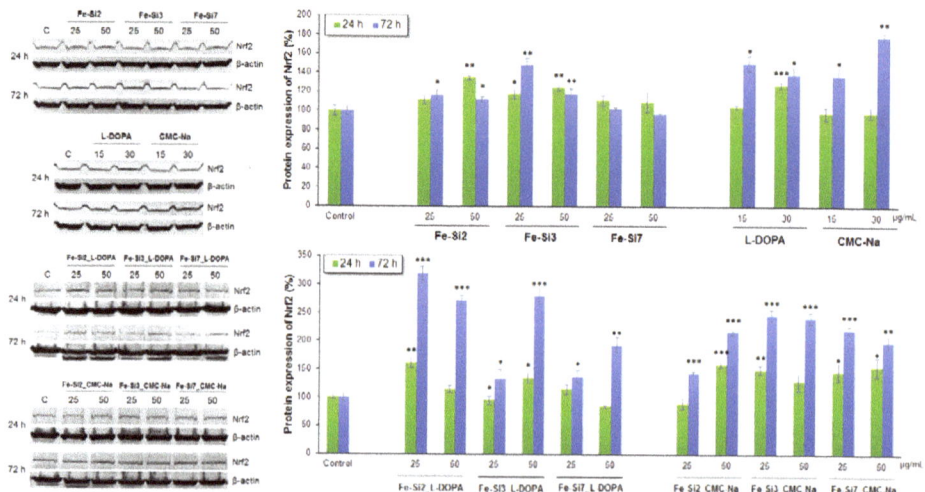

Figure 11. Relative protein expression of Nrf2 in Caco2 cells after 24 and 72 h exposure to 25 and 50 µg/mL of hybrid Fe-Si NPs stabilized with L-DOPA and CMC-Na. The images from the left represent the blot membranes for Nrf2 and β-actin at 24 and 72 h. The graph from the right represents the correspondent quantification of Nrf2 protein bands normalized to β-actin. Each set of samples was related to the untreated control migrated on the same gel. Data are expressed as the mean ± SD (n = 3) and represented as percentages. * $p < 0.05$; ** $p < 0.01$; *** $p < 0.001$ versus untreated control.

Studying of NP toxicity is a significant challenge. Numerous studies have appeared in the literature to differentiate between the toxicity of uncoated and coated NPs, which is extremely difficult, due to the diversity of factors influencing NP toxicity, such as size, shape, surface chemistry, synthesis techniques, coating agents, types of tissues/cells, etc. Similarly with our study, several papers found a higher toxicity of uncoated NPs than coated NPs [89], but some research studies have noticed the toxicity of uncoated NPs to be less than of the coated ones, which was associated with the NP cellular interaction and uptake [90]. Other researchers showed that the coating of iron NPs could decrease the leaching of iron ions and the lysosomal degradation of iron ions, thus reducing the oxidative stress and alterations in iron homeostasis [91,92].

A potential advantage of these new Fe-Si nanoparticle aggregates came from their dual composition: the iron-base phases gives them the sensitivity to magnetic fields which open the path for magnetic-guided/trapped drug delivery or variable-magnetic field-induced hyperthermia and/or heat-controlled drug release, whereas the luminescent nanosized silicon particles allow them to be simultaneously used for bio-labeling. Moreover, the silicon quantum dot toxicity is known to be much lower when compared with classical quantum dots, such as CdSe, CdTe, CdS, ZnS, or ZnSe [93], as proved for PEGylated micelle-encapsulated Si quantum dots synthesized also by laser pyrolysis, allowing them to be used for multiple in vivo applications, such as tumor vasculature targeting, sentinel lymph node, and multicolor near-infrared (NIR) imaging mapping [94]. The possibility of coupling Fe-based magnetic and Si fluorescent nanoparticles in a biocompatible probe was already proved in [95] by co-encapsulation of hydrophobized Fe_2O_3

superparamagnetic NPs and alkyl-capped Si quantum dots in PEGylated phospholipid micelles, yet in this case, those two functions can be uncoupled once the micelle is degraded. In our case, there are some aggregates in which the Fe-based and Si nanoparticles are strongly linked, and more difficult to break apart, which keeps connected, the magnetism and luminescence properties in biological media. However, the problem of luminescence loss in the aqueous-based biological fluids, due to the advanced oxidation of Si nanoparticles, still need to be countered by future studies for the founding of proper capping agents, and also by testing in this direction the CMC-Na and L-DOPA-coated NP aggregates reported in this work.

We think that the knowledge on toxicity of NPs is still limited, and much attention is required on development of new strategies and methods to explore the toxicity of all kind of NPs, in order to keep up with the rapid progress in the synthesis of novel nanomaterials for clinical applications.

4. Conclusions

Magnetic nanopowders containing both Fe-based phases and silicon nanocrystals have been synthesized by one-step laser pyrolysis method, using separate, yet nearby flows of $Fe(CO)_5/C_2H_4$ and SiH_4/Ar, respectively, followed by their gentle oxygen-induced oxidative passivation. Their elemental composition was varied (in the sense of the silicon content decreasing) by keeping constant the Fe precursor flow and diminishing the silane-containing flow. The nanopowders were successfully ultrasonically dispersed in water-based media using two different biocompatible stabilizers: L-DOPA amino acid and Na carboxymethylcellulose polyelectrolyte.

Biological studies showed that L-DOPA-stabilized Fe-Si NPs tend to form aggregates in culture medium, thus minimizing their interaction with the cells, and also toxicity in comparison with those stabilized with CMC-Na that were more dispersed and toxic. However, the Caco2 cells were able to counteract the toxic effects by activating the cellular protection mechanisms. The coated hybrid Fe-Si NPs were found to be biocompatible with colon cancer cells at a dose below 50 µg/mL, and their biological responses were dependent on particle synthesis, surface coating, doses, and incubation time.

Therefore, the next generation of Fe-Si NPs with a biocompatible coating might be, in the future, functionalized with peptides targeting specific cancer cells for imaging studies, as well as local hyperthermia.

Author Contributions: Conceptualization, M.B., F.D. and A.D.; Data curation, M.B. and F.D.; Formal analysis, M.B., F.D., M.A.B. and C.F.; Funding acquisition, M.B. and F.D.; Investigation, M.B., F.D., M.A.B., C.F., A.B. and E.T.; Methodology, M.B., F.D. and M.A.B.; Project administration, M.B. and F.D.; Resources, M.B. and F.D.; Supervision, M.B., F.D., C.F. and A.D.; Validation, M.B., F.D., C.F. and A.D.; Visualization, M.B., C.F. and A.D.; Writing—original draft, M.B., F.D., C.F. and A.D.; Writing—review & editing, M.B., M.A.B., C.F. and A.D.

Funding: This research was funded by Unitatea Executiva pentru Finantarea Invatamantului Superior, a Cercetarii, Dezvoltarii si Inovarii grant number PN-III-P2-2.1-PED-2016-1698 and The APC was funded by Unitatea Executiva pentru Finantarea Invatamantului Superior, a Cercetarii, Dezvoltarii si Inovarii, grant number PN-III-P2-2.1-PED-2016-1698.

Acknowledgments: This work was supported by a grant of the Romanian National Authority for Scientific Research and Innovation, UEFISCDI, project number PN-III-P2-2.1-PED-2016-1698, within PNCDI III program. The authors also acknowledge Oana Marinica for magnetic measurements.

Conflicts of Interest: The authors declare no conflict of interest.

References

1. Hosseini, F.; Panahifar, A.; Adeli, M.; Amiri, H.; Lascialfari, A.; Orsini, F.; Doschak, M.R.; Mahmoudi, M. Synthesis of pseudopolyrotaxanes-coated Superparamagnetic Iron Oxide Nanoparticles as new MRI contrast agent. *Coll. Surf. B Biointerfaces* **2013**, *103*, 652–657. [CrossRef] [PubMed]
2. Xu, H.; Cheng, L.; Wang, C.; Ma, X.; Li, Y.; Liu, Z. Polymer encapsulated upconversion nanoparticle/iron oxide nanocomposites for multimodal imaging and magnetic targeted drugdelivery. *Biomaterials* **2011**, *32*, 9364–9373. [CrossRef] [PubMed]

3. Mohammed, L.; Gomaa, H.G.; Ragab, D.; Zhu, J. Magnetic nanoparticles for environmental and biomedical applications: A review. *Particuology* **2017**, *30*, 1–14. [CrossRef]
4. Franke, K.; Kettering, M.; Lange, K.; Kaiser, W.; Hilger, I. The exposure of cancer cells to hyperthermia, iron oxide nanoparticles, and mitomycin C influences membrane multidrug resistance protein expression levels. *Int. J. Nanomed.* **2013**, *8*, 351–363.
5. Zhuonan, L.; Huihui, Y.; Hao, Z.; Chuanjun, H.; Laifeng, L. Oil-field wastewater purification by magnetic separation technique using a novel magnetic nanoparticle. *Cryogenics* **2012**, *52*, 699–703.
6. Taylor, R.; Coulombe, S.; Otanicar, T.; Phelan, P.; Gunawan, A.; Lv, W.; Rosengarten, G.; Prasher, R.; Tyagi, H. Small particles, big impacts: A review of the diverse applications of nanofluids. *J. Appl. Phys.* **2013**, *113*, 011301. [CrossRef]
7. Peyghambarzadeh, S.M.; Hashemabadi, S.H.; Hoseini, S.M.; Seifi, J. Experimental study of heat transfer enhancement using water/ethylene glycol based nanofluids as a new coolant for car radiators. *Int. Commun. Heat Mass Transf.* **2011**, *38*, 1283–1290. [CrossRef]
8. Liu, T.; Chen, X.; Di, Z.; Zhang, J.; Li, X.; Chen, J. Tunable magneto-optical wavelength filter of long-period fiber grating with magnetic fluids. *Appl. Phys. Lett.* **2007**, *91*, 121116. [CrossRef]
9. Akbarzadeh, A.; Samiei, M.; Davaran, S. Magnetic nanoparticles: Preparation, physical properties, and applications in biomedicine. *Nanoscale Res. Lett.* **2012**, *7*, 144. [CrossRef] [PubMed]
10. El-Dakdouki, M.H.; El-Boubbou, K.; Xia, J.; Kavunja, H.; Huang, X. Methods for Magnetic Nanoparticle Synthesis and Functionalization. In *Chemistry of Bioconjugates*; Narain, R., Ed.; John Wiley & Sons, Inc.: Hoboken, NJ, USA, 2014; pp. 281–314. ISBN 9781118775882.
11. Majidi, S.; Sehrig, F.Z.; Farkhani, S.M.; Goloujeh, M.S.; Akbarzadeh, A. Current methods for synthesis of magnetic nanoparticles. *Artif. Cell Nanomed. Biotechnol.* **2014**, *44*, 722–734. [CrossRef] [PubMed]
12. Kudr, J.; Haddad, Y.; Richtera, L.; Heger, Z.; Cernak, M.; Adam, V.; Zitka, O. Magnetic Nanoparticles: From Design and Synthesis to Real World Applications. *Nanomaterials* **2017**, *7*, 243. [CrossRef] [PubMed]
13. Mosayebi, J.; Kiyasatfar, M.; Laurent, S. Synthesis, Functionalization, and Design of Magnetic Nanoparticles for Theranostic Applications. *Adv. Healthc. Mater.* **2017**, *6*, 1700306. [CrossRef] [PubMed]
14. Kumar, S.; Layek, S.; Pandey, B.; Verma, H.C. Magnetic structure of Fe-Fe oxide nanoparticles made by electrodeposition. *Int. J. Eng. Sci. Technol.* **2010**, *2*, 66–72.
15. Hadjipanayis, C.G.; Bonder, M.J.; Balakrishnan, S.; Wang, X.; Mao, H.; Hadjipanayis, G.C. Metallic Iron Nanoparticles for MRI Contrast Enhancement and Local Hyperthermia. *Small* **2008**, *4*, 1925–1929. [CrossRef] [PubMed]
16. Carvell, J.; Ayieta, E.; Gavrin, A.; Cheng, R.; Shah, V.R.; Sokol, P. Magnetic properties of iron nanoparticle. *J. Appl. Phys.* **2010**, *107*, 103913. [CrossRef]
17. Bychkova, A.V.; Sorokina, O.N.; Rosenfeld, M.A.; Kovarski, A.L. Multifunctional biocompatible coatings on magnetic nanoparticles. *Russ. Chem. Rev.* **2012**, *81*, 1026–1050. [CrossRef]
18. Laurent, S.; Forge, D.; Port, M.; Roch, A.; Robic, C.; Vander Elst, L.; Muller, R.N. Magnetic Iron Oxide Nanoparticles: Synthesis, Stabilization, Vectorization, Physicochemical Characterizations, and Biological Applications. *Chem. Rev.* **2008**, *108*, 2064–2110. [CrossRef] [PubMed]
19. Demirer, G.S.; Okur, A.C.; Kizilel, S. Synthesis and design of biologically inspired biocompatible iron oxide nanoparticles for biomedical applications. *J. Mater. Chem. B* **2015**, *3*, 7831–7849. [CrossRef]
20. Yallapu, M.M.; Foy, S.P.; Jain, T.K.; Labhasetwar, V. PEG-Functionalized Magnetic Nanoparticles for Drug Delivery and Magnetic Resonance Imaging Applications. *Pharm. Res.* **2010**, *27*, 2283–2295. [CrossRef] [PubMed]
21. Illés, E.; Tombácz, E.; Szekeres, M.; Tóth, I.Y.; Szabó, Á.; Iván, B. Novel carboxylated PEG-coating on magnetite nanoparticles designed for biomedical applications. *J. Magn. Magn. Mater.* **2015**, *380*, 132–139. [CrossRef]
22. Ma, H.L.; Qi, X.R.; Maitani, Y.; Nagai, T. Preparation and characterization of superparamagnetic iron oxide nanoparticles stabilized by alginate. *Int. J. Pharm.* **2007**, *333*, 177–186. [CrossRef] [PubMed]
23. Uthaman, S.; Lee, S.J.; Cherukula, K.; Cho, C.S.; Park, I.K. Polysaccharide-Coated Magnetic Nanoparticles for Imaging and Gene Therapy. *Biomed. Res. Int.* **2015**, *2015*, 959175. [CrossRef] [PubMed]
24. Zhu, L.; Ma, J.; Jia, N.; Zhao, Y.; Shen, H. Chitosan-coated magnetic nanoparticles as carriers of 5-fluorouracil: Preparation, characterization and cytotoxicity studies. *Colloid Surf. B* **2009**, *68*, 1–6. [CrossRef] [PubMed]

25. Chen, T.J.; Cheng, T.H.; Chen, C.Y.; Hsu, S.C.; Cheng, T.L.; Liu, G.C.; Wang, Y.M. Targeted Herceptin-dextran iron oxide nanoparticles for noninvasive imaging of HER2/neu receptors using MRI. *J. Biol. Inorg. Chem.* **2009**, *14*, 253–260. [CrossRef] [PubMed]
26. Lee, J.H.; Jung, M.J.; Hwang, Y.H.; Lee, Y.J.; Lee, S.; Lee, D.Y.; Shin, H. Heparin-coated superparamagnetic iron oxide for in vivo MR imaging of human MSCs. *Biomaterials* **2012**, *33*, 4861–4871. [CrossRef] [PubMed]
27. Dumitrache, F.; Morjan, I.; Fleaca, C.; Badoi, A.; Manda, G.; Pop, S.; Marta, D.S.; Huminic, G.; Huminic, A.; Vekas, L.; et al. Highly magnetic Fe_2O_3 nanoparticles synthesized by laser pyrolysis used for biological and heat transfer applications. *Appl. Surf. Sci.* **2015**, *336*, 297–303. [CrossRef]
28. Comănescu, M.V.; Mocanu, M.A.; Anghelache, L.; Marinescu, B.; Dumitrache, F.; Bădoi, A.D.; Manda, G. Toxicity of L-DOPA coated iron oxide nanoparticles in intraperitoneal delivery setting-preliminary preclinical study. *Rom. J. Morphol. Embryol.* **2015**, *56*, 691–696. [PubMed]
29. Costo, R.; Morales, M.P.; Veintemillas-Verdaguer, S. Improving magnetic properties of ultrasmall magnetic nanoparticles by biocompatible coatings. *J. Appl. Phys.* **2015**, *117*, 064311. [CrossRef]
30. Huminic, A.; Huminic, G.; Fleaca, C.; Dumitrache, F.; Morjan, I. Thermal conductivity, viscosity and surface tension of nanofluids based on FeC nanoparticles. *Powder Technol.* **2015**, *284*, 78–84. [CrossRef]
31. Doll, T.A.P.F.; Raman, S.; Dey, R.; Burkhard, P. Nanoscale assemblies and their biomedical applications. *J. R. Soc. Interface* **2013**, *10*, 20120740. [CrossRef] [PubMed]
32. Pinto Reis, C.; Neufeld, R.J.; Ribeiro, A.J.; Veiga, F.; Nanoencapsulation, I. Methods for preparation of drug-loaded polymeric nanoparticles. *Nanomed. Nanotechnol. Biol. Med.* **2006**, *2*, 8–21. [CrossRef] [PubMed]
33. Alexis, F.; Pridgen, E.; Molnar, L.K.; Farokhzad, O.C. Factors affecting the clearance and biodistribution of polymeric nanoparticles. *Mol. Pharm.* **2008**, *5*, 505–515.
34. Chavanpatil, M.D.; Khdair, A.; Patil, Y.; Handa, H.; Mao, G.; Panyam, J. Polymer- surfactant nanoparticles for sustained release of water-soluble drugs. *J. Pharm. Sci.* **2007**, *96*, 3379–3389. [CrossRef] [PubMed]
35. Dauda, K.; Busari, Z.; Morenikeji, O.; Afolayan, F.; Oyeyemi, O.; Meena, J.; Sahu, D.; Panda, A. Poly(D,L-lactic-co-glycolic acid)-based artesunate nanoparticles: Formulation, antimalarial and toxicity assessments. *J. Zhejiang Univ.-Sci. B* **2017**, *18*, 977–985. [CrossRef] [PubMed]
36. Jose, J.; Charyulu, R.N. Prolonged drug delivery system of an antifungal drug by association with polyamidoamine dendrimers. *Int. J. Pharm. Investig.* **2016**, *6*, 123–127. [CrossRef] [PubMed]
37. Naha, P.C.; Mukherjee, S.P.; Byrne, H.J. Toxicology of engineered nanoparticles: Focus on poly(amidoamine) dendrimers. *Int. J. Environ. Res. Public Health* **2018**, *15*, 338. [CrossRef] [PubMed]
38. Fan, Q.; Cheng, K.; Hu, X.; Ma, X.; Zhang, R.; Yang, M.; Lu, X.; Xing, L.; Huang, W.; Gambhir, S.S.; et al. Transferring biomarker into molecular probe: Melanin nanoparticle as a naturally active platform for multimodality imaging. *J. Am. Chem. Soc.* **2014**, *136*, 15185–15194. [CrossRef] [PubMed]
39. Gao, Y.; Zhou, D.; Zhao, T.; Wei, X.; McMahon, S.; O'Keeffe Ahern, J.; Wang, W.; Greiser, U.; Rodriguez, B.J.; Wang, W. Intramolecular cyclization dominating homopolymerization of multivinyl monomers toward single-chain cyclized/knotted polymeric nanoparticles. *Macromolecules* **2015**, *48*, 6882–6889. [CrossRef]
40. Cutlar, L.; Gao, Y.; Aied, A.; Greiser, U.; Murauer, E.M.; Zhou, D.; Wang, W. A knot polymer mediated non-viral gene transfection for skin cells. *Biomater. Sci.* **2016**, *4*, 92–96. [CrossRef] [PubMed]
41. Huang, J.-Y.; Gao, Y.; Cutlar, L.; O'Keeffe-Ahern, J.; Zhao, T.; Lin, F.-H.; Zhou, D.; McMahon, S.; Greiser, U.; Wang, W.; et al. Tailoring highly branched poly(β-amino ester)s: A synthetic platform for epidermal gene therapy. *Chem. Commun.* **2015**, *5*, 8473–8476. [CrossRef] [PubMed]
42. Gao, Y.; Huang, J.-Y.; O'Keeffe Ahern, J.; Cutlar, L.; Zhou, D.G.; Lin, F.-H.; Wang, W. Highly branched poly(β-amino esters) for non-viral gene delivery: High transfection efficiency and low toxicity achieved by increasing molecular weight. *Biomacromolecules* **2016**, *17*, 3640–3647. [CrossRef] [PubMed]
43. Zhou, D.; Gao, Y.; Aied, A.; Cutlar, L.; Igoucheva, O.; Newland, B.; Alexeeve, V.; Greiser, U.; Uitto, J.; Wang, W. Highly branched poly(β-amino ester)s for skin gene therapy. *J. Control. Release* **2016**, *244*, 336–346. [CrossRef] [PubMed]
44. Ertel, S.I.; Ratner, B.D.; Kaul, A.; Schway, M.B.; Horbett, T.A. In vitro study of the intrinsic toxicity of synthetic surfaces to cells. *J. Biomed. Mater. Res.* **1994**, *28*, 667–675. [CrossRef] [PubMed]
45. Morais, J.M.; Papadimitrakopoulos, F.; Burgess, D.J. Biomaterials/tissue interactions: Possible solutions to overcome foreign body response. *AAPS J.* **2010**, *12*, 188–196. [CrossRef] [PubMed]

46. Santerre, J.P.; Woodhouse, K.; Laroche, G.; Labow, R.S. Understanding the biodegradation of polyurethanes: From classical implants to tissue engineering materials. *Biomaterials* **2005**, *26*, 7457–7470. [CrossRef] [PubMed]
47. Gatoo, M.A.; Naseem, S.; Arfat, M.Y.; Dar, A.M.; Qasim, K.; Zubair, S. Physicochemical Properties of Nanomaterials: Implication in Associated Toxic Manifestations. *BioMed Res. Int.* **2014**, *2014*, 498420. [CrossRef] [PubMed]
48. Septiadi, D.; Crippa, F.; Moore, T.L.; Rothen-Rutishauser, B.; Petri-Fink, A. Nanoparticle-Cell Interaction: A Cell Mechanics Perspective. *Adv. Mater.* **2018**, *30*, 1704463. [CrossRef] [PubMed]
49. Foglia, S.; Ledda, M.; Fioretti, D.; Iucci, G.; Papi, M.; Capellini, G.; Lisi, A. In vitro biocompatibility study of sub-5 nm silica-coated magnetic iron oxide fluorescent nanoparticles for potential biomedical application. *Sci. Rep.* **2017**, *7*, 46513. [CrossRef] [PubMed]
50. Rodríguez-Luccioni, H.L.; Latorre-Esteves, M.; Méndez-Vega, J.; Soto, O.; Rodríguez, A.R.; Rinaldi, C.; Torres-Lugo, M. Enhanced reduction in cell viability by hyperthermia induced by magnetic nanoparticles. *Int. J. Nanomed.* **2011**, *6*, 373–380.
51. Lee, J.S.; Rodríguez-Luccioni, H.L.; Méndez, J.; Sood, A.K.; Lpez-Berestein, G.; Rinaldi, C.; Torres-Lugo, M. Hyperthermia induced by magnetic nanoparticles improves the effectiveness of the anticancer drug cis-diamminedichloroplatinum. *J. Nanosci. Nanotechnol.* **2011**, *11*, 4153–4157. [CrossRef] [PubMed]
52. Moersdorf, D.; Hugounenq, P.; Phuoc, L.; Mamlouk-Chaouachi, H.; Felder-Flesch, D.; Begin-Colin, S.; Pourroy, G.; Bernhardt, I. Influence of magnetic iron oxide nanoparticles on red blood cells and Caco-2 cells. *Adv. Biosci. Biotechnol.* **2010**, *1*, 439–443. [CrossRef]
53. Bannunah, A.M.; Vllasaliu, D.; Lord, J.; Stolnik, S. Mechanisms of Nanoparticle Internalization and Transport Across an Intestinal Epithelial Cell Model: Effect of Size and Surface Charge. *Mol. Pharm.* **2014**, *11*, 4363–4373. [CrossRef] [PubMed]
54. Popovici, E.; Dumitrache, F.; Morjan, I.; Alexandrescu, R.; Ciupina, V.; Prodan, G.; Vekas, L.; Bica, D.; Marinica, O.; Vasile, E. Iron/iron oxides core-shell nanoparticles by laser pyrolysis: Structural characterization and enhanced particle dispersion. *Appl. Surf. Sci.* **2007**, *254*, 1048–1052. [CrossRef]
55. Lacour, F.; Guillois, O.; Portier, X.; Perez, H.; HerlinBoime, N.; Reynaud, C. Laser Pyrolysis synthesis and characterization of luminescent silicon nanocrystals. *Physica E* **2007**, *38*, 11–15. [CrossRef]
56. Wegner, K.; Pratsinis, S.E. Scale-up of nanoparticle synthesis in difusion fame reactors. *Chem. Eng. Sci.* **2003**, *58*, 4581–4589. [CrossRef]
57. Veintemillas-Verdaguer, S.; Morales, M.P.; Serna, C.J. Effect of the oxidation conditions on the maghemites produced by laser pyrolysis. *Appl. Organomet. Chem.* **2001**, *15*, 365–372. [CrossRef]
58. Kang, T.; Guan, R.; Chen, X.; Song, Y.; Jiang, H.; Zhao, J. In vitro toxicity of different-sized ZnO nanoparticles in Caco-2 cells. *Nanoscale Res. Lett.* **2013**, *8*, 496. [CrossRef] [PubMed]
59. Mosmann, T. Rapid colorimetric assay for cellular growth and survival: Application to proliferation and cytotoxicity assays. *J. Immunol. Methods* **1983**, *65*, 55–63. [CrossRef]
60. Gavrila-Florescu, L.; Dumitrache, F.; Balas, M.; Fleaca, C.T.; Scarisoreanu, M.; Morjan, I.P.; Dutu, E.; Ilie, A.; Banici, A.M.; Locovei, C.; et al. Synthesis of Fe based core@ZnO shell nanopowder by laser pyrolysis for biomedical applications. *Appl. Phys. A* **2017**, *123*, 802. [CrossRef]
61. Bradford, M.M. A rapid and sensitive method for the quantitation of microgram quantities of protein utilizing the principle of proteindye binding. *Anal. Biochem.* **1976**, *72*, 248–254. [CrossRef]
62. Panariti, A.; Lettiero, B.; Alexandrescu, R.; Collini, M.; Sironi, L.; Chanana, M.; Morjan, I.; Wang, D.; Chirico, G.; Mieserrochi, G.; et al. Dynamic inveistgations of interaction of biocompatible iron oxide nanoparticles with epithelial cells for biomedical applications. *J. Biomed. Nanotechnol.* **2013**, *9*, 1–13. [CrossRef]
63. Hong, P.; Xiao, Z.; Kaixun, H.; Huibi, X. Modification of Fe_3O_4 magnetic nanoparticles by L-DOPA or Dopamine as an enzyme support. *J. Wuhan Univ. Technol.* **2008**, *23*, 480–485.
64. Azari, S.; Zou, L.; Cornelissen, E. Assessing the effect of surface modification of polyamide RO membrane by L-DOPA on the short range physiochemical interactions with biopolymer fouling on the membrane. *Colloid Surf. B* **2014**, *120*, 222–228. [CrossRef] [PubMed]
65. Hasan, M.; Yang, W.; Ju, Y.; Xin, C.; Wang, Y.; Deng, Y.; Mahmood, N.; Hou, Y. Biocompatibility of iron carbide and detection of metals ions signaling proteomic analysis via HPLC/ESI-Orbitrap. *Nano Res.* **2017**, *10*, 1912–1923. [CrossRef]

66. Park, J.H.; Gu, L.; von Maltzahn, G.; Ruoslahti, E.; Bhatia, S.N.; Sailor, M.J. Biodegradable Luminescent Porous Silicon Nanoparticles for In Vivo Applications. *Nat. Mater.* **2009**, *8*, 331–336. [CrossRef] [PubMed]
67. Ruizendaal, L.; Bhattacharjee, S.; Pournazari, K.; Rosso-Vasic, M.; de Haan, L.H.J.; Alink, G.M.; Marcelis, A.T.M.; Zuilhof, H. Synthesis and Cytotoxicity of Silicon Nanoparticles with Covalently Attached Organic Monolayers. *Nanotoxicology* **2009**, *3*, 339–347. [CrossRef]
68. Luna-Martı́nez, J.F.; Reyes-Melo, E.; Gonzalez-Gonzalez, V.; Guerrero-Salazar, C.; Torres-Castro, A.; Sepulveda-Guzman, S. Synthesis and Characterization of a Magnetic Hybrid Material. Consisting of Iron Oxide in a Carboxymethyl Cellulose Matrix. *J. Appl. Polym. Sci.* **2012**. [CrossRef]
69. Sobik, M.; Pondman, K.M.; Erné, B.; Kuipers, B.; ten Haken, B.; Rogalla, H. Magnetic Nanoparticles for Diagnosis and Medical Therapy. In *Carbon Nanotubes for Biomedical Applications. Carbon Nanostructures*; Klingeler, R., Sim, R., Eds.; Springer: Berlin/Heidelberg, Germany, 2011; pp. 85–95. ISBN 978-3-642-14802-6.
70. Fleaca, C.T.; Dumitrache, F.; Morjan, I.; Niculescu, A.M.; Sandu, I.; Iliea, A.; Stamatin, I.; Iordache, A.; Vasile, E.; Prodan, G. Synthesis and characterization of polyaniline_Fe@C magnetic nanocomposite powder. *Appl. Surf. Sci.* **2015**, *374*, 213–221. [CrossRef]
71. Suo, B.; Li, H.; Wang, Y.; Li, Z.; Pan, Z.; Ai, Z. Effects of ZnO nanoparticle-coated packaging film on pork meat quality during cold storage. *J. Sci. Food Agric.* **2017**, *97*, 2023–2029. [CrossRef] [PubMed]
72. Saxena, N.; Naik, T.; Paria, S. Organization of SiO_2 and TiO_2 Nanoparticles into Fractal Patterns on Glass Surface for the Generation of Superhydrophilicity. *J. Phys. Chem. C* **2017**, *121*, 2428–2436. [CrossRef]
73. El-Hag Ali, A.; Abd El-Rehim, A.; Kamal, H.; Hegazy, D.; El-Sayed, A. Synthesis of carboxymethyl cellulose based drug carrier hydrogel using ionizing radiation for possible use as site specific delivery system. *J. Macromol. Sci. Part A Pure Appl. Chem.* **2008**, *45*, 628–634. [CrossRef]
74. Basma, A.N.; Morris, E.J.; Nicklas, W.J.; Geller, H.M. L-DOPA cytotoxicity to PC12 cells in culture is via its autoxidation. *J. Neurochem.* **1995**, *64*, 825–832. [CrossRef] [PubMed]
75. Melamed, E.; Offen, D.; Shirvan, A.; Djaldetti, R.; Barzilai, A.; Ziv, I. Levodopa toxicity and apoptosis. *Ann. Neurol.* **1998**, *44*, S149–S154. [CrossRef] [PubMed]
76. Lipski, J.; Nistico, R.; Berretta, N.; Guatteo, E.; Bernardi, G.; Mercuri, N.B. L-DOPA: A scapegoat for accelerated neurodegeneration in Parkinson's disease? *Prog. Neurobiol.* **2011**, *94*, 389–407. [CrossRef] [PubMed]
77. Jiang, L.Y.; Li, Y.B.; Zhang, L.; Wang, X.J. Preparation and characterization of a novel composite containing carboxymethyl cellulose used for bone repair. *Mater. Sci. Eng. C* **2009**, *29*, 193–198. [CrossRef]
78. Lee, S.Y.; Bang, S.; Kim, S.; Jo, S.Y.; Kim, B.C.; Hwang, Y.; Noh, I. Synthesis and in vitro characterizations of porous carboxymethyl cellulose-poly(ethylene oxide) hydrogel film. *Biomater. Res.* **2015**, *19*, 12. [CrossRef] [PubMed]
79. Zanganeh, S.; Spitler, R.; Erfanzadeh, M.; Alkilany, A.M.; Mahmoudi, M. Protein corona: Opportunities and challenges. *Int. J. Biochem. Cell Biol.* **2016**, *75*, 143–147. [CrossRef] [PubMed]
80. McDonagh, B.H.; Singh, G.; Hak, S.; Bandyopadhyay, S.; Augestad, I.L.; Peddis, D.; Sandvig, I.; Sandvig, A.; Glomm, W.R. L-DOPA-Coated Manganese Oxide Nanoparticles as Dual MRI Contrast Agents and Drug-Delivery Vehicles. *Small* **2016**, *12*, 301–306. [CrossRef] [PubMed]
81. Sakulkhu, U.; Mahmoudi, M.; Maurizi, L.; Salaklang, J.; Hofmann, H. Protein Corona Composition of Superparamagnetic Iron Oxide Nanoparticles with Various Physico-Chemical Properties and Coatings. *Sci. Rep.* **2014**, *4*, 5020. [CrossRef] [PubMed]
82. Zhou, L.; Le Thanh, T.; Gong, J.; Kim, J.-H.; Kim, E.-J.; Chang, Y.-S. Carboxymethyl cellulose coating decreases toxicity and oxidizing capacity of nanoscale zerovalent iron. *Chemosphere* **2014**, *104*, 155–161. [CrossRef] [PubMed]
83. Zhou, D.; Shao, L.; Spitz, D.R. Reactive Oxygen Species in Normal and Tumor Stem Cells. *Adv. Cancer. Res.* **2014**, *122*, 1–67. [PubMed]
84. Ortega, A.L.; Mena, S.; Estrela, J.M. Glutathione in Cancer Cell Death. *Cancers* **2011**, *3*, 1285–1310. [CrossRef] [PubMed]
85. Saddick, S.; Afifi, M.; Abu Zinada, O.A. Effect of Zinc nanoparticles on oxidative stress-related genes and antioxidant enzymes activity in the brain of Oreochromis niloticus and Tilapia zillii. *Saudi J. Biol. Sci.* **2015**, *24*, 1672–1678. [CrossRef]

86. Hao, L.H.; Wang, Z.Y.; Xing, B.S. Effect of sub-acute exposure to TiO$_2$ nanoparticles on oxidative stress and histopathological changes in Juvenile Carp (Cyprinus carpio). *J. Environ. Sci.* **2009**, *21*, 1459–1466. [CrossRef]
87. Manke, A.; Wang, L.; Rojanasakul, Y. Mechanisms of Nanoparticle-Induced Oxidative Stress and Toxicity. *BioMed Res. Int.* **2013**, *2013*, 942916. [CrossRef] [PubMed]
88. Sporn, M.B.; Liby, K.T. NRF2 and cancer: The good, the bad and the importance of context. *Nat. Rev. Cancer* **2012**, *12*, 564–571. [CrossRef] [PubMed]
89. Patil, U.S.; Adireddy, S.; Jaiswal, A.; Mandava, S.; Lee, B.R.; Chrisey, D.B. In Vitro/In Vivo Toxicity Evaluation and Quantification of Iron Oxide Nanoparticles. *Int. J. Mol. Sci.* **2015**, *16*, 24417–24450. [CrossRef] [PubMed]
90. Magdolenova, Z.; Drlickova, M.; Henjum, K.; Runden-Pran, E.; Tulinska, J.; Bilanicova, D.; Pojana, G.; Kazimirova, A.; Barancokova, M.; Kuricova, M.; et al. Coating-dependent induction of cytotoxicity and genotoxicity of iron oxide nanoparticles. *Nanotoxicology* **2015**, *9*, 44–56. [CrossRef] [PubMed]
91. Malvindi, M.A.; de Matteis, V.; Galeone, A.; Brunetti, V.; Anyfantis, G.C.; Athanassiou, A.; Cingolani, R.; Pompa, P.P. Toxicity assessment of silica coated iron oxide nanoparticles and biocompatibility improvement by surface engineering. *PLoS ONE* **2014**, *9*, e85835. [CrossRef] [PubMed]
92. Levy, M.; Lagarde, F.; Maraloiu, V.A.; Blanchin, M.G.; Gendron, F.; Wilhelm, C.; Gazeau, F. Degradability of superparamagnetic nanoparticles in a model of intracellular environment: Follow-up of magnetic, structural and chemical properties. *Nanotechnology* **2010**, *21*, 395103. [CrossRef] [PubMed]
93. Liu, J.; Erogbogbo, F.; Yong, K.-T.; Ye, L.; Liu, J.; Hu, R.; Chen, H.; Hu, Y.; Yang, Y.; Yang, J.; et al. Assessing Clinical Prospects of Silicon Quantum Dots: Studies in Mice and Monkeys. *ACS Nano* **2013**, *7*, 7303–7310. [CrossRef] [PubMed]
94. Erogbogbo, F.; Yong, K.-T.; Roy, I.; Hu, R.; Law, W.-C.; Zhao, W.; Ding, H.; Wu, F.; Kumar, R.; Swihardt, M.; et al. In Vivo Targeted Cancer Imaging Sentinel Limph Node Mapping and Multi-Channel Imaging with Biocompatible Silicon Nanocrystals. *ACS Nano* **2011**, *1*, 413–423. [CrossRef] [PubMed]
95. Erogbogbo, F.; Yong, K.-T.; Hu, R.; Law, W.-C.; Ding, H.; Chang, C.-W.; Prasad, P.N.; Swihardt, M. Biocompatibel Magnetofluorescent Probes: Silicon Quantum Dots Coupled with Superparamagnetic Iron (III) Oxide. *ACS Nano* **2010**, *9*, 5131–5138. [CrossRef] [PubMed]

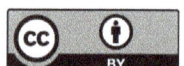

© 2018 by the authors. Licensee MDPI, Basel, Switzerland. This article is an open access article distributed under the terms and conditions of the Creative Commons Attribution (CC BY) license (http://creativecommons.org/licenses/by/4.0/).

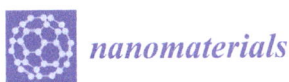

Article

Evaluation of the PEG Density in the PEGylated Chitosan Nanoparticles as a Drug Carrier for Curcumin and Mitoxantrone

Yao Chen, Di Wu, Wu Zhong, Shuwen Kuang, Qian Luo, Liujiang Song, Lihua He, Xing Feng and Xiaojun Tao *

Key Laboratory of Study and Discovery of Small Targeted Molecules of Hunan Province, School of Medicine, Hunan Normal University, Changsha 410013, China; ychen@smail.hunnu.edu.cn (Y.C.); iswudi@smail.hunnu.edu.cn (D.W.); zwu123@smail.hunnu.edu.cn (W.Z.); shwkuang@smail.hunnu.edu.cn (S.K.); luoqian1996@smail.hunnu.edu.cn (Q.L.); song1221@hunnu.edu.cn (L.S.); hlh197@hunnu.edu.cn (L.H.); fengxing@hunnu.edu.cn (X.F.)
* Correspondence: xjtao@hunnu.edu.cn; Tel.: +86-182-2972-2319

Received: 15 May 2018; Accepted: 8 June 2018; Published: 1 July 2018

Abstract: Polyethylene glycolated (PEGylated)curcumin-grafted-chitosan (PCC) conjugates were synthesized with three PEG/chitosan feed molar ratios (1/5, 1/7.5, and 1/10), namely PCC1, PCC2 and PCC3. Chemical structures of these conjugates were characterized by Fourier transform infrared (FTIR) and proton nuclear magnetic resonance (^{1}H NMR). The degrees of substitution (DS) of PEG were 0.75%, 0.45% and 0.33%, respectively, for PCC1, PCC2 and PCC3by ^{1}H NMR analysis. Self-assembled PCC nanoparticles (NPs) were spherical as observed in transmission electron microscope images. Mitoxantrone (MTO)-loaded PCC NPs were prepared to analyze the particle size, zeta potential, drug loading, drug release and in vitro cytotoxicity. The MTO-loaded PCC3 NP (DS = 0.33%) possessed the smallest size (~183.1 nm), highest zeta potential (~+34.0 mV) and the largest loading capacity of curcumin (CUR, ~16.1%) and MTO (~8.30%). The release results showed that MTO-loaded PCC3 NP demonstrated the lowest percentage of MTO release and increased as pH decreased, but the CUR release could only be detected at pH 4.0. In the cytotoxicity study, MTO-loaded PCC3 NP displayed the highest cytotoxicity in HepG2 cell line and the best synergistic effect among the tested NPs. Our results suggest that the DS of PEG has impacts on the structures and functions of PCC NPs: the smaller DS of PEG was associated with the smaller size, the higher zeta potential, the slower drug release, and the higher cytotoxicity of NPs.

Keywords: curcumin; mitoxantrone; synergism; PEG; chitosan nanoparticles

---

1. Introduction

Chemotherapy is one of the main strategies for the treatment of late stage of malignant tumors. Curcumin (CUR), a hydrophobic pigment derived from *Curcuma longa*, has been proposed as a good candidate for adjuvant therapy because of its anti-cancer effects, reversal of cancer cell multidrug resistance, and absence of obvious cytotoxicity in normal tissues [1–3]. However, clinical application of CUR is limited due to its low water solubility and physico-chemical stability [4]. Recently, the combination chemotherapy of CUR and other drugs has attracted increasing attention on improving therapeutic efficacy by signaling different pathways, and suppressing and reversing drug resistance [3,5,6]. Mitoxantrone (MTO), a chemotherapeutic drug, has curative effect on variety of malignant tumors, but its associated cardiac toxicity and myelosuppression create significant health impairments [7,8]. Studies have shown that the combination of MTO and CUR can enhance the MTO efficacy, therefore, may reduce the MTO dose and the side effects [5,9].

Polymeric nanoparticles have been widely used for biomedical applications especially for drug delivery, which can be formed by self-assembly of amphiphilic polymers in water [10]. Use of polymeric nanoparticles for drug delivery provides many advantages for cancer treatment, including increased drug solubility and stability, enhanced permeability and retention (EPR) effect, easy surface modification and environmental stimuli-responsive properties [11,12].

Chitosan (CS) has often been used as the backbone of polymeric nanoparticles because of its basic properties such as good biocompatibility, biodegradability and low toxicity [13–15]. Chitosan nanoparticles (CS NPs) with positive surface charges bind to the negatively charged cell membrane, facilitating cellular uptake [16]. However, CS NPs can be recognized and internalized by macrophages in the reticuloendothelial system (RES) [17,18]. Methoxy polyethylene glycol (PEG) was applied to modify CS as a drug carrier [19,20]. PEG was grafted to CS to block the positive charge on the surface of CS NPs so that the CS NPs may escape phagocytosis of RES cells, prolonging their retention time in blood circulation [21]. The length of PEG with the different Mw can affect the size of PEGylated chitosan nanoparticles and the drug delivery functions [20]. We used 2000 Mw PEG and varied the ratio of PEG grafted to evaluate the characteristics and the biological functions of NPs.

In this study, we designed an amphiphilic conjugate by conjugating CUR with CS as hydrophobic moieties and grafting PEG. In aqueous solution, the amphiphilic conjugate automatically forms water-soluble PEGylated CUR-grafted-CS (PCC) NPs. As MTO is encapsulated, it forms the MTO-loaded PCC NPs (PCCM NPs).

The formation of PCC NPs involves a self-assembly process driven by the direct force of interaction between hydrophobic components and the influence of outer fields such as the template on the surface of NPs. As a result of all factors integrated, the NPs are stabilized under thermodynamic equilibrium [22,23]. We have demonstrated the effects of hydrophobicity in formation of NPs using different degrees of substitution (DS) of cholesterol in pullulan nanoparticles and have reported a method for connecting a hydrophobic molecule to produce an amphiphilic conjugate [24,25]. Excessive substitution of hydrophobic molecules in the core would result in NPs that are too hydrophobic and agglomerate easily, while low substitution is insufficient to drive self-assembly [26]. In the current study, we applied this method to graft CUR to the CS. PEG grafted to the amphiphilic CUR-grafted-CS (CCS) constitutes the hydrophilic part; however, its effects on self-assembly process and formation of the NPs' physical and biological properties have not been studied. We are particularly interested in how the grafted density of PEG correlated with the characteristics and the biological functions of PCCM NPs. Thus, we prepared three of PCCM NPs with different PEG/CS feed ratio and evaluated the correlation between PEG/CS ratio and the NP characteristics, drug potency and the synergism of MTO and CUR in combination. Finally, the effect of pH on drug release from these three PCCM NPs was determined as a proxy for assessing the drug's release under the physiological condition and the acidic microenvironment of cancer.

2. Materials and Methods

2.1. Materials

Chitosan (average molecular weight 20 kDa, degree of deacetylation > 90%) was purchased from Solarbio (Beijing, China). Curcumin, methoxy polyethylene glycol (2000 Da) and mitoxantrone hydrochloride were purchased from Sigma-Aldrich (Shanghai, China). 1-Ethyl-3-(3-dimethylaminopropyl) carbodiimide hydrochloride (EDCI) and 4-dimethylaminopryidine (DMAP) were purchased from Aladdin Reagent Co. Ltd. (Shanghai, China). Dulbecco's modified Eagle Medium (DMEM) was purchased from Gibco (Grand Island, NY, USA). Hepg2 cell line was from Shanghai Institutes for Biological Sciences, Chinese Academy of Sciences (Shanghai, China).

2.2. Synthesis of Polyethylene Glycolated (PEGylated) Curcumin-Grafted-Chitosan (PCC) Conjugates

The synthetic process of CUR-grafted-CS (CCS) and PCC are illustrated in Figure 1.

Synthesis of CCS: First, CUR succinate (CURS) was synthesized based on a previously published method with slight modifications [27]. Next, CCS conjugate was prepared by chemically grafting CURS to CS through amide formation. In brief, 0.065 g succinic anhydride (SA, 0.65 mmol) and 0.08 g DMAP (0.65 mmol) were dissolved in 15 mL dimethyl sulfoxide (DMSO); after heating and stirring at 50 °C for 4 h, 0.2 g CUR (0.54 mmol) was added for heating and stirring for 24 h under N_2 protection to obtain CS. Subsequently, 0.12 g EDCI (0.62 mmol) and 0.075 g NHS (0.65 mmol) were added to the DMSO solution containing the CURS, and stirring was continued at 25 °C for 12 h. At the same time, 0.35 g CS (2.16 mmol) was dissolved in acetate buffer (200 mM, pH 5.0) to get a 0.5% (w/v) solution. Lastly, the CS solution was slowly added to the CURS solution, and these were reacted under N_2 at 25 °C for 48 h. After the reaction, the resulting suspension was added into 200 mL absolute ethanol. The precipitate formed and went through vacuum filtration, then washed with absolute ethanol, tetrahydrofuran and diethyl ether, respectively, and dried to yield CCS conjugate.

Synthesis of PCC: PEG succinate (PEGS) was synthesized as described in [28]. In brief, 0.15 g SA (1.5 mmol) and 0.18 g DMAP (1.5 mmol) were dissolved in 15 mL dry CH_2Cl_2; after heating at reflux for 3 h at 60 °C, 2 g PEG (1.0 mmol) was added for heating and stirring for 24 h. The resulting solution was precipitated by diethyl ether and then filtered. The white powder was dissolved in deionized water after drying, then dialyzed against water for 2 days and the solution was lyophilized. PCC was produced by conjugating the carboxylic acid group of PEGS with the amine group of CS at PEG/CS molar ratios of 1/5, 1/7.5, and 1/10 (PCC1, PCC2, and PCC3) in the presence of EDCI/NHS. Then, 0.2 g PEGS (0.096 mmol), 0.014 g NHS (0.12 mmol) and 0.022 g EDCI (0.012 mmol) were dissolved in 10 mL DMSO and stirred at 25 °C for 4 h. At the same time, CCS (0.08 g, 1/5; 0.12 g, 1/7.5; 0.16 g, 1/10) was dissolved in acetate buffer (200 mM, pH 5.0) to get a 0.5% (w/v) solution. Lastly, the CCS solution was slowly added to the PEGS solution, and these were reacted under N_2 at 25 °C for 48 h. The resulting suspension was washed with CH_2Cl_2/methanol (volume ratio: 4:1) and centrifuged at 8500 rpm for 10 min, the supernatant was removed. The above process was repeated three times and the precipitate was rinsed with deionized water and lyophilized to obtain three of PCC conjugates.

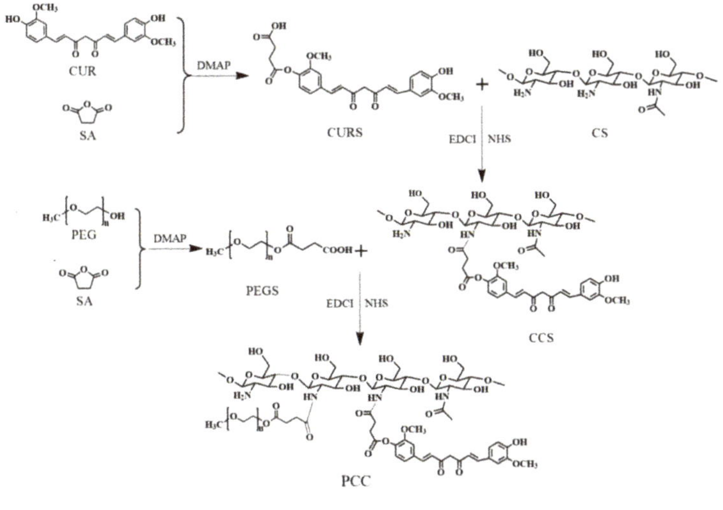

Figure 1. The chemical synthesis of Polyethylene glycolated (PEGylated)curcumin-grafted-chitosan (PCC).

2.3. Fourier Transform Infrared (FTIR), Proton Nuclear Magnetic Resonance (^{1}H NMR) and Ultraviolet (UV-Vis) Spectroscopy

The FTIR spectra for CUR, CS, CCS, PEG and PCC1 were recorded on FTIR spectrometer (Nicolet, TM Nexus 470-ESP, Thermo Fisher Scientific, Waltham, MA, USA) using KBr pellets. The ^{1}H NMR spectra for CUR and PEG were recorded on a 500 MHz NMR spectrometer (BRUKER AVANCE-500, Bruker, Billerica, MA, USA) using DMSO-d6 solvent. The ^{1}H NMR spectra for CS, PCC1, PCC2 and PCC3 were recorded on the same NMR spectrometer using CD_3COOD/D_2O solvent (1%, v/v). CUR was dissolved in methanol to obtain 200 µg/mL solution and PCC conjugates and CS were dissolved in acetic acid (1%, v/v) to obtain 1 mg/mL (w/v) for each solution. Then, the absorbances of these solutions were scanned from 200 nm to 700 nm wavelengths using an UV-Visible spectrophotometer (Shimadzu UV-2550, Kyoto, Japan).

2.4. Preparation PCC Nanoparticles (NPs)

PCC NPs were prepared by dialysis method [25]. Briefly, 5 mg PCC was suspended in 10 mL of 1% acetic acid solution under gentle shaking at 37 °C until it was completely dissolved and then dialyzed against 2000 mL of distilled water for 24 h with 10 exchanges by using a dialysis bag (molecular weight cut-off 8000–14,000 Da) to remove acetic acid. Then, the solution was sonicated using a probe type sonifier at 100 W with pulsing (pulse on 2.0 s, off 2.0 s) for 2 min in an ice water bath. The self-assembled PCC NPs were then filtrated through 0.45 µm-membrane and stored at 4 °C.

2.5. Dynamic Light Scattering (DLS) and Transmission Electron Microscopy (TEM)

The size and zeta-potential of different PCC NPs were determined by DLS (Zetasizer 3000 HS, Malvern Instruments, Malvern, UK). The NPs suspensions were filtered with a 0.45 µm filter, and each batch was analyzed in triplicate. To observe the morphologic features of PCC NPs, one drop of PCC NPs suspension was placed on carbon-coated 300 mesh grids. Then, the grids were air-dried and examined by TEM (Tecnai G2 20 S-Twin, FEI Hong Kong Inc., Hong Kong, China) at an accelerating voltage of 80 KV.

2.6. Preparation and Characterization of Mitoxantrone-loaded PCC NPs (PCCM NPs)

PCC conjugate (20 mg) was suspended in 20 mL of 1% acetic acid solution under gentle shaking at 37 °C until it was completely dissolved. Then, 2 mg MTO was dissolved in 2 mL of DMSO, dropped into the above solutions, dialyzed for 24 h in distilled water using a dialysis bag (molecular weight cut-off 8000–14,000 Da) to remove organic solvent and free MTO, and the PCCM NPs solution was obtained. MTO-loaded PCC1, PCC2 and PCC3 NPs were obtained in the same way and named PCCM1, PCCM2 and PCCM3 respectively.

2.7. Determination of Entrapment Efficiency (EE) and Loading Capacity (LC)

PCCM NPs solution (5 mL) was sonicated for 5 min (pulse on 2.0 s, off 2.0 s) to release the drug from NPs. The absorbances of MTO and CUR in the solution were measured at 608 nm and 425 nm, respectively, by microplate spectrophotometer (UV-384 plus, Molecular Devices, Thermo Fisher Scientific Inc., Waltham, MA, USA) to calculate the drug concentrations. MTO encapsulation efficiency (EE), MTO load capacity (LC_M) and CUR load capacity (LC_C) were calculated as follows:

EE% = (the amount of drug in the nanoparticles)/(the amount of totally added drug) × 100%

LC% = (the amount of drug in the nanoparticles)/(the amount of nanoparticles weight) × 100%

2.8. Determination of Drug Release from PCCM NPs In Vitro

The effect of pH on drug release was measured by a dialysis method as previously described [24]. Briefly, PCCM NPs solution (5 mL) was put into a dialysis bag (8–12 kDa MWCO) and dialyzed in 25 mL of PBS (releasing media) with pH 7.4, 6.8 or 4.0 at 37 °C under 100 rpm shaking. Free MTO was dialyzed under the same conditions. Then, 2 mL of releasing medium was collected for sampling and replaced with an equal volume of the fresh solution at pre-defined time intervals (T_n, n = 0, 0.5, 1, 2, 4, 8, 12, 24 and 48 h). The absorbances of MTO and CUR in the solution were measured by microplate spectrophotometer to determine the concentrations of MTO and CUR released. The percentage rate of drug release (Q%) was calculated as follows:

$$Q\% = \left(C_n \times V + V_n \sum_{t=0}^{n} C_i \right) / (W_{NP} \times LC\%)$$

where W is NPs weight; C_n is the sample concentration at T_n; V is the total volume of release medium; V_n is the sample volume (2 mL); and C_i is the sample concentration at $T_i (i = 0, 0.5, 1, \ldots, n$ h, both V_0 and C_0 are equal to zero).

2.9. Determine PCCM NPs' Cytotoxicity In Vitro

MTT assay was used to determine the drug cytotoxicity by measuring HepG2 cell viability. HepG2 was cultured in DMEM medium supplemented with 10% FBS and 100 U of penicillin–streptomycin in a humidified atmosphere of 95% air and 5% CO_2 incubator at 37 °C. HepG2 cells were seeded at 20,000 cells/well in 96-well plates and incubated overnight. Then, the drug was added and incubated for 24 h. The medium was removed and started MTT assay to determine cell viability. MTT assay was performed according to the manufacturer's protocol. The percentage of cell viability was calculated based on the ratio of the absorbance of drug-treated cells to that of untreated cells. The untreated cell was counted as 100% survival. The dose–effect curves of HepG2 cell viabilities were performed under the treatments of PCCM1, PCCM2 and PCCM3. The MTO concentration in PCCM NPs was determined by the absorbance at 608 nm wavelength and the MTO treatment concentration was fixed at 2, 4, 8, 16 and 32 µg/mL for each PCCM. Because the PCCM NPs contained MTO and CUR, and the loading capacity of CUR and MTO has been determined (Table 1), the CUR concentrations in PCCM NPs were estimated based on the ratio of MTO/CUR loading capacity (Table 2). The PCCM treatment concentration was the sum of MTO and CUR.

Table 1. Characterization of mitoxantrone-loaded PCC NPs (PCCM NPs).

Sample	Feed PEG/CS Molar Ratio	PEG Molar DS	EE%	LC$_M$%	LC$_C$%	Zeta Potential (mV)	Size (nm)	PDI
PCCM1	1/5	0.75%	90.5 ± 2.89	7.42 ± 0.16 *,#	12.3 ± 0.52 *,#	12.8 ± 4.02 *,#	250.2 ± 21.5 *	0.153
PCCM2	1/7.5	0.45%	88.6 ± 1.61	8.14 ± 0.14	14.0 ± 0.87 *	21.2 ± 4.27 *	233.1 ± 19.2 *	0.216
PCCM3	1/10	0.33%	87.3 ± 1.74	8.30 ± 0.24	16.1 ± 0.21	34.0 ± 4.52	183.1 ± 15.6	0.225

Data were expressed as mean ± standard deviation (SD) (n = 3). * indicates the significant difference of PCCM1 and PCCM2 vs. PCCM3 ($p < 0.05$); # indicates the significant difference between PCCM1 and PCCM2 ($p < 0.05$). EE%, encapsulation efficiency of MTO; LC$_C$%, loading capacity of CUR; LC$_M$%, loading capacity of mitoxantrone (MTO); polydispersity index (PDI).

Table 2. The concentrations of mitoxantrone (MTO) and chemotherapy (CUR) in PCCM NPs on the treatments of HepG2 cells.

Drugs	Concentration (µg/mL)				
PCCM NPs-MTO	2.00	4.00	8.00	16.00	32.00
PCCM1-CUR	3.32	6.63	13.26	26.52	53.05
PCCM2-CUR	3.44	6.88	13.70	27.50	55.00
PCCM3-CUR	3.85	7.71	15.40	30.80	61.70

To determine the synergistic effect of MTO and CUR in combination, the dose–effect curves with the individual treatment of free MTO (2, 4, 8, 16, 32 and 64 µg/mL), free CUR (2, 4, 8, 16, 32 and 64 µg/mL) and the combination of both with MTO:CUR ratios at 1:1, 1:1.5 and 1:2 against HepG2 cell viability were performed. In drug preparations, DMSO was used to dissolve free MTO and free CUR to make each stock solution of 32 mg/mL that was further diluted with DMEM medium to achieve the desired concentrations. The percentage of cell viability was calculated based on the ratio of the absorbance of drug-treated cells to that of cells treated equal volume of DMSO. The maximal concentration of DMSO in the experimental medium was less than 0.5% (v/v), which did not affect cell viability.

2.10. Calculation of the Synergistic Effect of MTO and CUR

According to the Chou-Talalay model [29,30], the combination index (*CI*) was computed based on the following equation:

$$CI = \left[\frac{p}{(p+q)EC_{50,\,MTO}} + \frac{q}{(p+q)EC_{50,\,CUR}} \right] EC_{50,\,combination}$$

where p and q represent the unit of drug MTO and CUR, respectively. EC_{50} denotes the drug dose at 50% of cell viability achieved. If $CI<1$, the combination can be described as synergistic, if $CI > 1$, antagonistic, and $CI = 1$, additive. The data for calculating CI are presented in Table S1.

Isobole analysis is another way to quantitatively assess the synergism and antagonism that paired drugs produce. According to Tallarida's dose equivalent principle and Loewe additive model, an isobole is generated, which is a line to define the additive effect of paired drugs [31,32]. In practice, we first acquired the dose-effect curves of free MTO and free CUR and transformed the drug dose in $\log_{10}$ scale, and then applied the following equation to calculate the combined doses of the paired drugs to give a specified effect.

$$\ln \frac{P_x}{1 - P_x} = \alpha + \beta x$$

where x is the $\log_{10}$ dose of a drug (MTO or CUR); P_x is cell viability at $\log_{10}$ dose; $(1 - P_x)$ is the cell death at $\log_{10}$ dose; α is the Y-intercept of linear regression equation and β is the slope. The data for plotting the isobole are illustrated in Table S2. The points on the isobole set the combined CUR and MTO at different ratios to produce a 50% of maximum effect. If the EC_{50} of the paired drug dose is located below the isobole, it indicates a synergistic effect, whereas, above the isobole indicates an antagonistic effect.

2.11. Statistical Analysis

All experiments were performed at least three times in vitro. Results are expressed as mean ± standard deviation (SD), analyzed by Student's *t*-test using software SPSS 19.0. $p < 0.05$ was considered significantly different.

3. Results

3.1. FTIR, ^{1}H NMR and UV-Vis Spectroscopic Analysis

The successful syntheses of these compounds were confirmed by FTIR spectra, as shown in Figure 2. In comparison with CUR (A) and CS (B), the spectrum of CCS (C) remained the N-H bond of amino at 1558 cm^{-1} and the aromatic C=C bonds of CUR (marked with red circle). The spectrum of CCS also revealed the particular peak of amide bond at 1650 cm^{-1} (C=O stretching), and the peak of ester bond at 1720 cm^{-1} (C=O stretching). This result indicated the successful conjugation between CUR and CS. In the spectrum of PCC, peaks at 2887 cm^{-1} (C−H stretching) and 1113 cm^{-1} (C−O stretching) corresponded to the characteristic peaks of PEG. The peak of ester bond was shifted to 1734 cm^{-1}. The FTIR spectra confirmed the chemical structure of PCC.

Figure 3A displayed the ^{1}H NMR spectra of CUR, CS, PEG, PCC1, PCC2 and PCC3. The characteristic peaks 2.8 to 3.1 ppm were assigned to the monosaccharide residue (CH-NH-) protons. In the spectrum of PCC conjugates, the highly enhanced peaks at 3.1~4.0 ppm corresponded to the repeated ethyl group ($-CH_2-CH_2-O-$). The peaks at 2.48 ppm corresponded to the methylene (CH_2) protons in succinate linkers between PEG and CS and between CUR and CS. The peaks at 9.4~9.5 ppm were characteristic peaks of CUR, the other characteristic peaks of CUR were not observed, which might be because PCC conjugates' MW were too high [33]. The results of ^{1}H NMR spectra confirmed the successful synthesis of PCC conjugates. The degree of substitution (DS) of PEG residues per 100 sugar units for CS could be calculated by the ratio between the increased integrity at 3.1–4.0 ppm and the monosaccharide residue (CH–NH–, 2.8–3.1 ppm) and further adjusted with PEG molecular weight to obtain molar substitution degree [28,34]. The DS of obtained PCC1, PCC2 and PCC3 were determined as 0.75%, 0.45% and 0.33%, respectively. The UV-Vis spectra were further used to confirm CUR in PCC conjugates' structure. We used the same concentration in each PCC (1 mg/mL) and scanned the PCC absorbance from 200 nm to 700 nm wavelength. As depicted in Figure 3B, the characteristic peaks at 297 nm and 415 nm belonged to chitosan and CUR, respectively. The absorbances of PCC conjugates displayed the following order: PCC3 > PCC2 > PCC1. Therefore, the UV-Vis spectra demonstrated the presence of CUR and CS in the conjugates. PCC3 was composed of more CUR and CS as compared with PCC1 and PCC2 with the same weight.

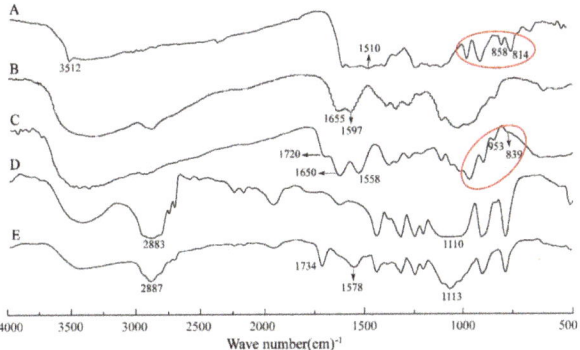

Figure 2. Fourier transform infrared (FTIR) spectra of: Curcumin (CUR) (**A**); Chitosan (CS) (**B**); CUR-grafted-CS (CCS) (**C**); polyethylene glycol (PEG) (**D**); and PEGylated CUR-grafted-CS (PCC) (**E**).

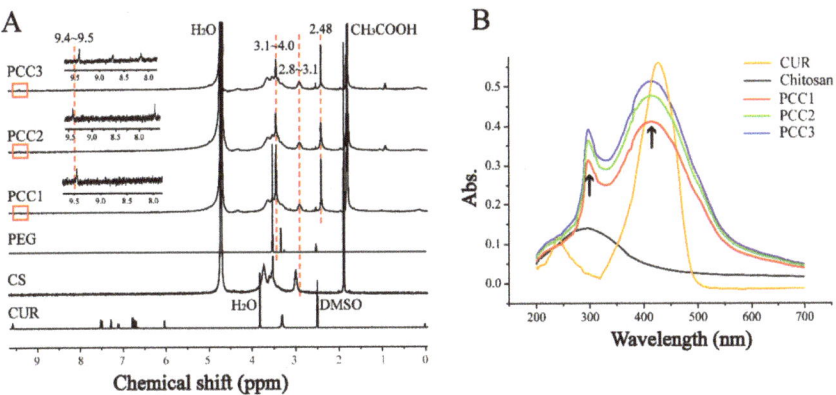

Figure 3. (**A**) Nuclear Magnetic Resonance (^{1}H NMR) spectra for CUR, CS, PEG, PCC1, PCC2 and PCC3; and (**B**) Ultraviolet (UV-Vis) spectra of CUR, CS, PCC1, PCC2 and PCC3.

3.2. Size Distribution, Zeta Potential and Morphology of PCC NPs

The mean distribution size and polydispersity index (PDI) were, respectively, 209.9 nm and 0.076 for PCC1 NP; 177.6 nm and 0.247 for PCC2 NP; and 137.4 nm and 0.267 for PCC3 NP (Figure 4A). The zeta potentials of PCC1, PCC2 and PCC3 NPs were 12.9 ± 4.02 mV, 21.3 ± 4.27 mV and

34.4 ± 9.52 mV, respectively (Figure 4B). As the ratio of PEG/CS decreased, the size of PCC decreased and the zeta potential increased. TEM images show the sphere shape of PCC NPs (Figure 4C–E).

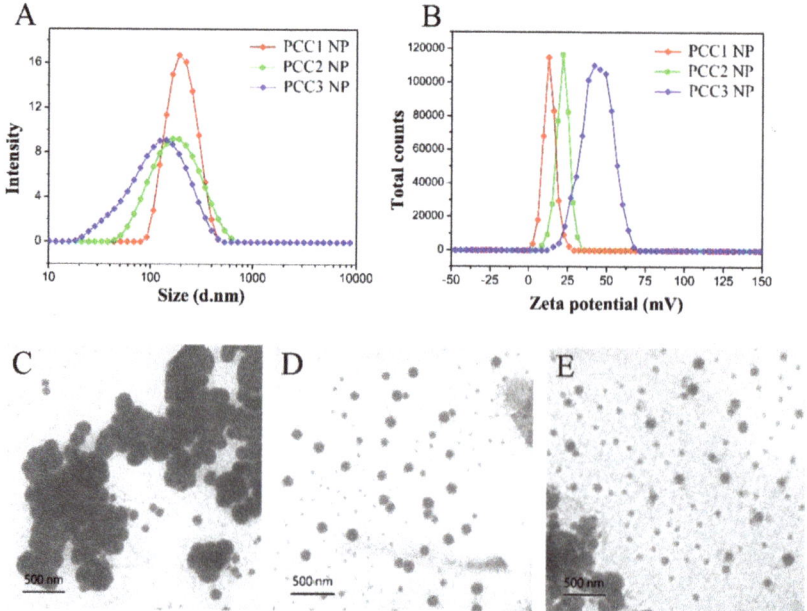

Figure 4. The size distributions (**A**); and zeta potential (**B**) of PCC1, PCC2 and PCC3 NPs. Transmission electron microscopy (TEM) images of: PCC1 NP (**C**); PCC2 NP (**D**); and PCC3 NP (**E**).

3.3. Characterizations of PCCM NPs

Figure 5 schematically illustrates the formation of PCCM NP. As denoted in our design, the hydrophobic molecule CUR was conjugated to the CS polymer and formed the hydrophobic core in the self-assembly process. On the external shell, we varied the ratio of PEG/CS to make three kinds of PCCM NPs and evaluated the properties and biological functions of the NP due to the change of PEG/CS ratio. Characterizations of all of PCCM NPs confirmed our designs, as summarized in Table 1. The PEG/CS ratio in the composition of the external shell significantly affected NPs' properties. Higher degree of PEG grafted on the external shell rendered alarger size distribution, less positive zeta potential and lower drug loading capacity of the NPs (e.g., PCCM1). As the PEG/CS ratio was reduced, all changes of the NPs properties were reversed accordingly (e.g., PCCM2 and PCCM3). The change in PCCM3 was remarkably optimal. It is reasonable to account for the correlations of the PEG/CS and the NPs' characterizations regarding the NPs size, zeta potential and drug loading capacity. The PEG grafted to amino group of the CS could mask the positive charge. More PEG molecules grafted to the CS backbone reduced the area of positively charged CS exposed, which resulted in lowering the zeta potential, or vice versa (Figure 5). In aqueous solution the amphiphilic PCC conjugate formed the micelle with the PEGylated CS hydrophilic chain facing externally. Solvents can mediate aggregation of NPs by H-bonding [22,24]. PCCM with low PEG/CS ratio corresponding to highly positive charges would have more H-bonding connections and result in forming highly compact NPs. As expected, PCCM3 formed in the smallest size, the largest positive zeta potential, but with the highest drug loading capacity. Particularly, the PEG/CS ratio had significant impact on the loading capacity for CUR than that for MTO (Table 1). This was because the assembly of conjugated CUR was directly correlated to the degree of PEG. Since MTO and CUR are hydrophobic molecules, larger amounts of assembled CUR would associate with more MTO being encapsulated. The loading capacities for MTO were indirectly associated with the PEG/CS ratio.

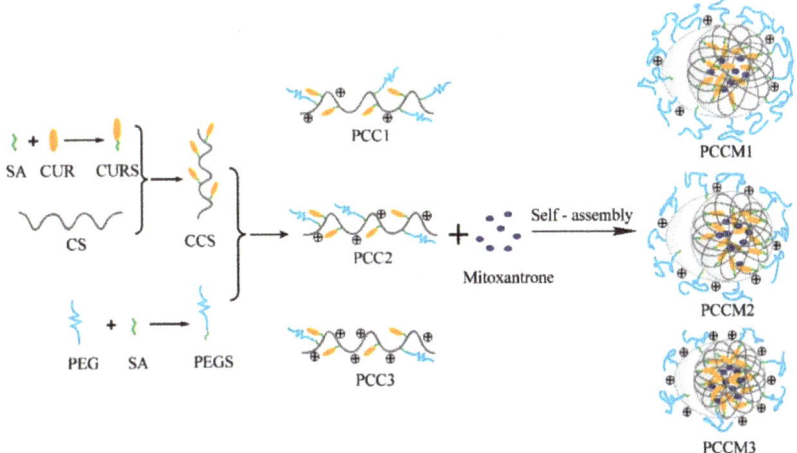

Figure 5. Schematic diagram illustrated the design and self-assembly of PCCM NPs with different density of PEG in each of PCCM.

3.4. Mitoxantrone (MTO) and Curcumin (CUR) Drug Release from PCCM NPs In Vitro

Figure 6 shows the MTO (Figure 6A) and CUR (Figure 6B) release from PCCM NPs at pH 7.4, pH 6.8 and pH 4.0 conditional media. All PCCM NPs exhibited two phases of MTO releasing profile, a rapid release in 10 h followed by a sustained release in 48 h. Free MTO completely released within 8 h under the same conditions. The rapid releasing MTO in the first 10 h probably related to the surface-absorbed MTO [35]. The encapsulated MTO sustained release slowly. Larger sizes of NPs or lower pH conditions were associated with higher percentage of MTO release, displayed in the following order: PCCM1>PCCM2>PCCM3, and the release at pH 4.0 > pH 6.8 > pH 7.4 (Figure 6A). At pH 7.4 conditional medium that mimicked extracellular circulation condition, the MTO release from PCCM3 NP was about 51.54%, which was significantly lower than that from PCCM2 (57.96%) and PCCM1 (61.64%). We anticipated PCCM3 would have the least MTO loss in systemic circulation.

The release of CUR could only be detected at pH 4.0 (Figure 6B). The cumulative release of CUR for 48 h from PCCM1, PCCM2 and PCCM3 was 15.36%, 13.55% and 17.02%, respectively. At pH 6.8 and pH 7.4, the CUR release was close to zero. Therefore, we expect CUR loss was zero in physiological circulation system as long as the NPs were intact. CUR release required breaking the chemical bond between CUR and CS and was exclusively pH dependent, as the CUR released only at pH 4.0 in a time dependent manner. Under the acidic condition such as the microenvironment of cancer cells, acid catalyzed the hydrolysis of amide bonding between CS and CUR and the free CUR gradually diffused out of the NPs. The order of the percentage of CUR release in PCCM NPs was: PCCM3 > PCCM1 > PCCM2. The relatively high level of CUR release in PCCM3 might be related to its larger amount of CUR loaded.

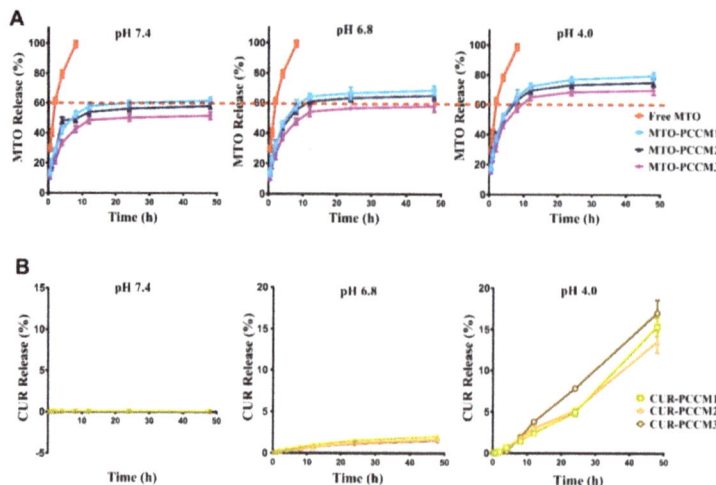

Figure 6. In vitro release profiles of Mitoxantrone (MTO) (**A**) and CUR (CUR) (**B**) from PCCM NPs in pH 7.4, 6.8 and 4.0 conditional media.

3.5. Cytotoxicity Test In Vitro

The treatments of PCCM NPs greatly reduced HepG2 cell viability (Figure 7). PCCM3 displayed the highest level of cytotoxicity while exhibiting the lowest EC$_{50}$ value (14.57 ± 0.78 µg/mL), and the lowest percentage of cell viability (10.82% ± 2.32%) as compared to that of PCCM1 and PCCM2. The biological effects of drugs were dose dependent [36] and correlated with the efficiency of drug endocytosis [37] and, perhaps, the synergism of the drugs in combination [3,38]. We administered uniform MTO concentrations across all PCCM NP treatment groups, but varied the CUR concentrations (Table 2). Among PCCM NPs tested, PCCM3 obtained the highest proportion of CUR (MTO:CUR, 1:1.925), and may partially account for the significantly enhanced cytotoxic effect of PCCM3, as CUR is known to mediate synergistic effects when co-administered with some chemotherapeutic drugs. Moreover, the positively charged of NPs can promote cellular uptake through electrostatic interaction between NPs and cell membrane leading to NPs endocytosis [17,39]. The high positively charged surface of PCCM3 may facilitate NPs endocytosis.

Next, we addressed whether the combination of CUR with MTO could mediate synergistic effect, and, if so, which atios of MTO and CUR would achieve the synergism. We applied the mass-action law model proposed by Chou-Talalay to compute the combination index (*CI*), where *CI* < 1 indicates paired drug effects of synergism; *CI* = 1 indicates additivity; and *CI* > 1 indicates antagonism [30,31]. We generated dose–effect curves using free MTO and free CUR (without NPs encapsulation) to determine the *CI* values of MTO:CUR at 1:1, 1:1.5 and 1:2 (Figure 8A–C). *CI* < 1 was only observed when the MTO:CUR was at 1:2 (CI$_{MTO:CUR\ 1:2}$ = 0.629), whereas, *CIs* > 1 were observed at the other combination ratios (CI$_{MTO:CUR\ 1:1}$ = 1.403, CI$_{MTO:CUR\ 1:1.5}$ = 1.228). A combination ratio of MTO and CUR at 1:2 was critical, at which the synergism was likely achieved. We also used isoboles method to quantitatively assess the synergism and antagonism of the paired drug effects [33]. Based on the doses of MTO and CUR with different combination ratios to achieve 50% of maximum effect, we plotted an isobole that indicated the additive effect of the paired drugs, which allowed us to define the area of super additivity (synergism) or subadditivity (antagonism). Again, only the EC$_{50}$ dose of MTO and CUR at 1:2 combination model was localized below the isobole, suggesting combined MTO and CUR at this ratio would likely produce synergistic effect (Figure 8D). The rationale of the free drug models could be applied to explain the observed results of PCCM NPs. The EC$_{50}$ values of PCCM1, PCCM2 and PCCM3 were 24.39, 21.15 and 14.57 µg/mL and corresponded to the MTO and CUR combination ratios of 1:1.66, 1:1.72 to 1:1.925, respectively. Lower EC_{50} indicates higher the drug potency. The significant increase in the potency of PCCM3 compared to other PCCMs suggested that the MTO/CUR combination ratio in PCCM3 played a critical role in enhancing the drug combination effect toward super additivity.

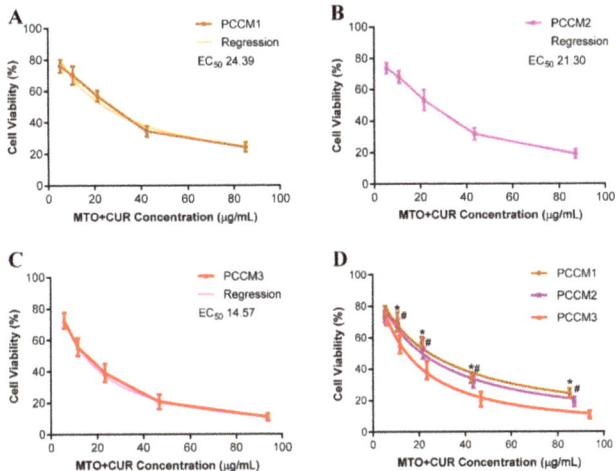

Figure 7. Dose–effect curves and the regressions of: PCCM1 (**A**); PCCM2 (**B**); PCCM3 (**C**); and all PCCM NPs for comparison (**D**). Data represent means ± SD (n = 6). Statistics: * indicates significant differences between PCCM1 and PCCM3 (p < 0.05); # indicates significant differences between PCCM2 and PCCM3 (p < 0.05). There was no significant difference between PCCM1 and PCCM2.

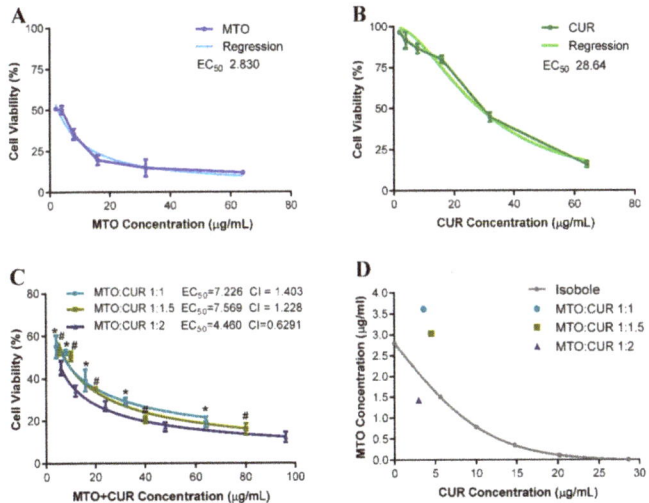

Figure 8. Dose–effect curves and regressions of: free MTO (**A**); and free CUR (**B**); the combination of MTO and CUR at the combination ratio of 1:1, 1:1.5 and 1:2 (**C**); and the isobole (**D**). Data represent means ± SD (n = 6). Statistics: * indicates significant differences between the models of MTO:CUR at 1:1 and 1:2 (p < 0.05); # indicates significant differences between the models of MTO:CUR at 1:1.5 and 1:2 (p < 0.05).

4. Discussion

CUR has been widely considered an adjuvant drug for chemotherapy [3,40,41]. Many studies have reported about the combination of CUR with chemotherapeutic drugs that have demonstrated the enhancement of antitumor effect by CUR and nanonization of CUR that can improve its bioavailability [41–43]. By these methods, CUR was adsorbed on surface of nanoparticles or encapsulated in core of liposomes or micelles. The use of chemically grafting CUR to CS is a novel design that incorporates CUR into NPs structure and allows CUR to be carried. This method offers several advantages: first, the quantity of CUR in the nanocarrier can be regulated because the conjugation of CUR molecules to the CS polymer is a chemical reaction that follows the reaction stoichiometry principle. Once the quantity of CUR is fixed, the proportional MTO molecules associated with CUR by hydrophobic interaction are encapsulated. Secondly, the free drug dose–effect models (Figure 8) suggested that a high proportion of CUR was prerequisite to achieve the synergistic effect in combination with MTO. Relatively, MTO is a highly potent chemotherapeutic drug with adverse cytotoxic side effects and should be kept in low concentration. The design of PCCM NPs is desirable to model CUR and MTO in combination. Using two different approaches to encapsulate two drugs, we can manipulate the drug ratio and ultimately maximize the drug efficacy and the synergism. Thirdly, unloaded CUR required breaking the chemical bonding in acidic conditions. Thus, CUR delivery could be targeted to the tumor cells where the acidic microenvironment was favorable for CUR release.

The strategy of grafting PEG on the NPs surface to escape RES phagocytosis is a sophisticated method [44]. Recently, Yang et al. demonstrated the impact of PEGylation on characterization of CS NPs properties, bioactivities and tissue distributions in vitro and in vivo [20]. Our study used similar methodology for PEGylation and both PEGylated-chitosan NPs displayed comparable results in terms of sizes, zeta potentials and PEG content. Yang's study reported that higher molecular weight and lower grafting rates of PEG resulted in forming smaller and more compact NPs with relatively higher surface charge, which was consistent with our findings. Yang et al. further revealed that PEGylated-CS NPs significantly inhibited macrophage phagocytosis and unspecific interaction with red blood cells. Gref et al. [45] also described that, in PEG concentration above 5%, PEG functioned as a "brush" which effectively shielded the surface charge of the nanoparticles, thereby prolonging the retention time of NPs in circulation and stabilizing NPs structure in vivo. These findings suggest that the PEGylated-CS NPs developed in the current study could be applicable for systemic circulation.

It is well known that synergism or antagonism in a drug pair depends not only on the agonist drug pair, but also on the ratio of the doses. Often, there is a range of dose combinations that are synergistic and other ranges that are either additive or antagonistic [32]. We validated that MTO:CUR at 1:2 is the critical combination ratio to achieve synergistic effect based on the *CI* values and the method of isobolo gram (Figure 8). Most importantly, in this study, we elucidated the rationale of grafted PEG density in the PEGylated CS NPs resulting to alter the drug potency and synergism, and finally presented PCCM3 as the best nanocarrier model for CUR and MTO. PCCM3 with the lowest PEG density (PEG/CS 1:10) and the optimal combination ratio of MTO and CUR that close to 1:2 has demonstrated the best characteristics and the anticancer effects among the three PCCM NPs examined.

5. Conclusions

We successfully fabricated a new design of a drug carrier for MTO and CUR by chemically linked CUR and physically loaded MTO. In evaluating three of PCCM NPs that consisted of different PEG/CS ratio, PCCM NPs with the smallest DS of PEG were determined as the best with regard to their physical properties and the better anticancer effect. Our results established the relationship between physical properties and the biological functions of PCC NPs. We further explained a proper combination ratio of MTO and CUR would achieve synergistic cytotoxicity to cancer cells. Our findings provide new insights in CUR drug carrier development, particularly CUR in combination with the chemotherapeutic drugs for maximizing synergistic effects, thus exhibiting great potential for applications in the combination of CUR and chemotherapeutic drugs for cancer therapy.

Supplementary Materials: The following are available online at http://www.mdpi.com/2079-4991/8/7/486/s1, Table S1: Supplemental data for calculating the combination index, Table S2: Data for plotting the isobole.

Author Contributions: X.T. conceived the project and provided project leadership. Y.C. performed the synthesis of nanoparticle and the characterization experiments and wrote the manuscript. D.W. assisted with the experiments and prepared the manuscript. L.H. and L.S. discussed the project and analyzed data. Q.L., W.Z. and S.K. assisted in preparing experiments and drawing figures. X.F. directed the manuscript and revised it.

Funding: This research was supported by the Hunan Provincial Health Commission General Project (No. B2017073 to X. T.), the Research Foundation of Education Bureau of Hunan Province (No. 14B112 to L.S.), the College students' innovation project fund (No. 2017157 to Y.C, No. 2017030 to S.K.).

Acknowledgments: The authors thank Fong Ming Mo, for study of biological evaluation of the nanoparticles, Mengqi Li for performing experiments and nanoparticle characterization experiments, Chengzhi Wang for cytotoxicity study and Jianyi Lee, for editing manuscript.

Conflicts of Interest: The authors declare no conflict of interest.

References

1. Duan, J.; Mansour, H.M.; Zhang, Y.; Deng, X.; Chen, Y.; Wang, J.; Pan, Y.; Zhao, J. Reversion of multidrug resistance by co-encapsulation of doxorubicin and curcumin in chitosan/poly(butyl cyanoacrylate) nanoparticles. *Int. J. Pharm.* **2012**, *426*, 193–201. [CrossRef] [PubMed]
2. Lu, W.D.; Qin, Y.; Yang, C.; Li, L. Effect of curcumin on human colon cancer multidrug resistance in vitro and in vivo. *Clinics* **2013**, *68*, 694–701. [CrossRef]
3. Xiao, B.; Si, X.; Han, M.K.; Viennois, E.; Zhang, M.; Merlin, D. Co-delivery of camptothecin and curcumin by cationic polymeric nanoparticles for synergistic colon cancer combination chemotherapy. *J. Mater. Chem. B* **2015**, *3*, 7724–7733. [CrossRef] [PubMed]
4. Modasiya, M.K.; Patel, V.M. Studies on solubility of curcumin. *Int. J. Pharm. Life Sci.* **2012**, *3*, 1490–1497.
5. Luty, M.; Kwiecień, E.; Firlej, M.; Łabędź-Masłowska, A.; Paw, M.; Madeja, Z.; Czyż, J. Curcumin augments the cytostatic and anti-invasive effects of mitoxantrone on carcinosarcoma cells in vitro. *Acta Biochim. Pol.* **2016**, *63*, 397. [CrossRef] [PubMed]
6. Yang, M.; Yu, L.; Guo, R.; Dong, A.; Lin, C.; Zhang, J. A modular coassembly approach to all-in-one multifunctional nanoplatform for synergistic codelivery of doxorubicin and curcumin. *Nanomaterials* **2018**, *8*, 167. [CrossRef] [PubMed]
7. Koeller, J.; Eble, M. Mitoxantrone: A novel anthracycline derivative. *Clin. Pharm.* **1988**, *7*, 574–581. [PubMed]
8. Wiseman, L.R.; Spencer, C.M. Mitoxantrone: A review of its pharmacology and clinical efficacy in the management of hormone-resistant advanced prostate cancer. *Drugs Aging* **1997**, *10*, 473–485. [CrossRef] [PubMed]
9. Limtrakul, P.; Chearwae, W.; Shukla, S.; Phisalphong, C.; Ambudkar, S.V. Modulation of function of three ABC drug transporters, p-glycoprotein (ABCB1), mitoxantrone resistance protein (ABCG2) and multidrug resistance protein 1 (ABCC1) by tetrahydrocurcumin, a major metabolite of curcumin. *Mol. Cell. Biochem.* **2007**, *296*, 85–95. [CrossRef] [PubMed]
10. Pridgen, E.M.; Langer, R.; Farokhzad, O.C. Biodegradable, polymeric nanoparticle delivery systems for cancer therapy. *Nanomedicine* **2007**, *2*, 669–680. [CrossRef] [PubMed]
11. Kim, D.; Lee, E.S.; Oh, K.T.; Gao, Z.G.; Bae, Y.H. Doxorubicin-loaded polymeric micelle overcomes multidrug resistance of cancer by double-targeting folate receptor and early endosomal pH. *Small* **2008**, *4*, 2043–2050. [CrossRef] [PubMed]
12. Yan, G.; Li, A.; Zhang, A.; Sun, Y.; Liu, J. Polymer-based nanocarriers for co-delivery and combination of diverse therapies against cancers. *Nanomaterials* **2018**, *8*, 85. [CrossRef] [PubMed]
13. Asamoah-Asare, J. Novel carboxymethyl chitosan-β-cyclodextrin nanoparticles as a drug delivery system; preparation and characterization. *Int. J. Eng. Sci. Res. Technol.* **2014**, *3*, 141–146.
14. Cheung, R.; Ng, T.; Wong, J.; Chan, W. Chitosan: An update on potential biomedical and pharmaceutical applications. *Mar. Drugs* **2015**, *13*, 5156–5186. [CrossRef] [PubMed]

15. Kean, T.; Thanou, M. Biodegradation, biodistribution and toxicity of chitosan. *Adv. Drug Deliv. Rev.* **2010**, *62*, 3–11. [CrossRef] [PubMed]
16. Yue, Z.G.; Wei, W.; Lv, P.P.; Yue, H.; Wang, L.Y.; Su, Z.G.; Ma, G.H. Surface charge affects cellular uptake and intracellular trafficking of chitosan-based nanoparticles. *Biomacromolecules* **2011**, *12*, 2440. [CrossRef] [PubMed]
17. Gorzelanny, C.; Pöppelmann, B.; Pappelbaum, K.; Moerschbacher, B.M.; Schneider, S.W. Human macrophage activation triggered by chitotriosidase-mediated chitin and chitosan degradation. *Biomaterials* **2010**, *31*, 8556–8563. [CrossRef] [PubMed]
18. Jiang, L.Q.; Wang, T.Y.; Webster, T.J.; Duan, H.J.; Qiu, J.Y.; Zhao, Z.M.; Yin, X.X.; Zheng, C.L. Intracellular disposition of chitosan nanoparticles in macrophages: Intracellular uptake, exocytosis, and intercellular transport. *Int. J. Nanomed.* **2017**, *12*, 6383. [CrossRef] [PubMed]
19. Rudzinski, W.E.; Palacios, A.; Ahmed, A.; Lane, M.A.; Aminabhavi, T.M. Targeted delivery of small interfering rna to colon cancer cells using chitosan and pegylated chitosan nanoparticles. *Carbohydr. Polym.* **2016**, *147*, 323–332. [CrossRef] [PubMed]
20. Yang, C.; Gao, S.; Dagnaes-Hansen, F.; Jakobsen, M.; Kjems, J. Impact of peg chain length on the physical properties and bioactivity of pegylated chitosan/sirna nanoparticles in vitro and in vivo. *ACS Appl. Mater. Interfaces* **2017**, *9*, 12203–12216. [CrossRef] [PubMed]
21. Termsarasab, U.; Yoon, I.S.; Park, J.H.; Moon, H.T.; Cho, H.J.; Kim, D.D. Polyethylene glycol-modified arachidyl chitosan-based nanoparticles for prolonged blood circulation of doxorubicin. *Int. J. Pharm.* **2014**, *464*, 127–134. [CrossRef] [PubMed]
22. Boal, A.K.; Ilhan, F.; Derouchey, J.E.; Thurn-Albrecht, T.; Russell, T.P.; Rotello, V.M. Self-assembly of nanoparticles into structured spherical and network aggregates. *Nature* **2000**, *404*, 746. [CrossRef] [PubMed]
23. Grzelczak, M.; Vermant, J.; Furst, E.M.; Liz-Marzán, L.M. Directed self-assembly of nanoparticles. *ACS Nano* **2010**, *4*, 3591–3605. [CrossRef] [PubMed]
24. Tao, X.; Xie, Y.; Zhang, Q.; Qiu, X.; Yuan, L.; Wen, Y.; Li, M.; Yang, X.; Tao, T.; Xie, M. Cholesterol-modified amino-pullulan nanoparticles as a drug carrier: Comparative study of cholesterol-modified carboxyethyl pullulan and pullulan nanoparticles. *Nanomaterials* **2016**, *6*, 165. [CrossRef] [PubMed]
25. Tao, X.; Zhang, Q.; Yang, W.; Zhang, Q. The interaction between human serum albumin and cholesterol-modified pullulan nanoparticle. *Curr. Nanosci.* **2012**, *8*, 830–837. [CrossRef]
26. Tan, Y.L.; Liu, C.G. Self-aggregated nanoparticles from linoleic acid modified carboxymethyl chitosan: Synthesis, characterization and application in vitro. *Colloids Surf. B Biointerfaces* **2009**, *69*, 178–182. [CrossRef] [PubMed]
27. Yang, R.; Zhang, S.; Kong, D.; Gao, X.; Zhao, Y.; Wang, Z. Biodegradable polymer-curcumin conjugate micelles enhance the loading and delivery of low-potency curcumin. *Pharm. Res.* **2012**, *29*, 3512–3525. [CrossRef] [PubMed]
28. Jeong, Y.I.; Kim, D.G.; Jang, M.K.; Nah, J.W. Preparation and spectroscopic characterization of methoxy poly(ethylene glycol)-grafted water-soluble chitosan. *Carbohydr. Res.* **2008**, *343*, 282–289. [CrossRef] [PubMed]
29. Chou, T.C. Drug combination studies and their synergy quantification using the chou-talalay method. *Cancer Res.* **2010**, *70*, 440–446. [CrossRef] [PubMed]
30. Chou, T.C.; Talalay, P. Quantitative analysis of dose-effect relationships: The combined effects of multiple drugs or enzyme inhibitors. *Adv. Enzym Regul.* **1984**, *22*, 27. [CrossRef]
31. Loewe, S. The problem of synergism and antagonism of combined drugs. *Arzneimittel-Forschung* **1953**, *3*, 285. [PubMed]
32. Tallarida, R.J. Quantitative methods for assessing drug synergism. *Genes Cancer* **2011**, *2*, 1003–1008. [CrossRef] [PubMed]
33. Chaoran, X.; Wei, H.; Yaqi, L.; Chao, Q.; Lingjia, S.; Lifang, Y. Self-assembled nanoparticles from hyaluronic acid-paclitaxel prodrugs for direct cytosolic delivery and enhanced antitumor activity. *Int. J. Pharm.* **2015**, *493*, 172–181.
34. Prego, C.; Torres, D.; Fernandezmegia, E.; Novoacarballal, R.; Quiñoá, E.; Alonso, M.J. Chitosan-peg nanocapsules as new carriers for oral peptide delivery. Effect of chitosan pegylation degree. *J. Control. Release* **2006**, *111*, 299. [CrossRef] [PubMed]

35. Yuan, R.; Zheng, F.; Zhong, S.; Tao, X.; Zhang, Y.; Gao, F.; Yao, F.; Chen, J.; Chen, Y.; Shi, G. Self-assembled nanoparticles of glycyrrhetic acid-modified pullulan as a novel carrier of curcumin. *Molecules* **2014**, *19*, 13305–13318. [CrossRef] [PubMed]
36. Zimmer, A.; Katzir, I.; Dekel, E.; Mayo, A.E.; Alon, U. Prediction of multidimensional drug dose responses based on measurements of drug pairs. *Proc. Natl. Acad. Sci. USA* **2016**, *113*, 10442–10447. [CrossRef] [PubMed]
37. Bareford, L.M.; Swaan, P.W. Endocytic mechanisms for targeted drug delivery. *Adv. Drug Deliv. Rev.* **2007**, *59*, 748–758. [CrossRef] [PubMed]
38. Cheah, Y.H.; Nordin, F.J.; Sarip, R.; Tee, T.T.; Azimahtol, H.L.P.; Sirat, H.M.; Rashid, B.A.A.; Abdullah, N.R.; Ismail, Z. Combined xanthorrhizol-curcumin exhibits synergistic growth inhibitory activity via apoptosis induction in human breast cancer cells mda-mb-231. *Cancer Cell Int.* **2009**, *9*, 1. [CrossRef] [PubMed]
39. Gan, Q.; Wang, T.; Cochrane, C.; Mccarron, P. Modulation of surface charge, particle size and morphological properties of chitosan-TPP nanoparticles intended for gene delivery. *Colloids Surf. B Biointerfaces* **2005**, *44*, 65–73. [CrossRef] [PubMed]
40. Ma, W.; Qiang, G.; Ying, L.; Wang, X.; Wang, J.; Tu, P. Co-assembly of doxorubicin and curcumin targeted micelles for synergistic delivery and improving anti-tumor efficacy. *Eur. J. Pharm. Biopharm.* **2016**, *112*, 209–223. [CrossRef] [PubMed]
41. Zhao, X.; Chen, Q.; Liu, W.; Li, Y.; Tang, H.; Liu, X.; Yang, X. Codelivery of doxorubicin and curcumin with lipid nanoparticles results in improved efficacy of chemotherapy in liver cancer. *Int. J. Nanomed.* **2015**, *10*, 257–270.
42. Esfandiarpour-Boroujeni, S.; Bagheri-Khoulenjani, S.; Mirzadeh, H.; Amanpour, S. Fabrication and study of curcumin loaded nanoparticles based on folate-chitosan for breast cancer therapy application. *Carbohydr. Polym.* **2017**, *168*, 14–21. [CrossRef] [PubMed]
43. Peng, S.; Zou, L.; Liu, W.; Li, Z.; Liu, W.; Hu, X.; Chen, X.; Liu, C. Hybrid liposomes composed of amphiphilic chitosan and phospholipid: Preparation, stability and bioavailability as a carrier for curcumin. *Carbohydr. Polym.* **2016**, *156*, 322–332. [CrossRef] [PubMed]
44. Pelaz, B.; Del, P.P.; Maffre, P.; Hartmann, R.; Gallego, M.; Rivera-Fernández, S.; Jm, D.L.F.; Nienhaus, G.U.; Parak, W.J. Surface functionalization of nanoparticles with polyethylene glycol: Effects on protein adsorption and cellular uptake. *ACS Nano* **2015**, *9*, 6996. [CrossRef] [PubMed]
45. Gref, R.; Lück, M.; Quellec, P.; Marchand, M.; Dellacherie, E.; Harnisch, S.; Blunk, T.; Müller, R.H. 'Stealth' corona-core nanoparticles surface modified by polyethylene glycol (peg): Influences of the corona (peg chain length and surface density) and of the core composition on phagocytic uptake and plasma protein adsorption. *Colloids Surf. B Biointerfaces* **2000**, *18*, 301–313. [CrossRef]

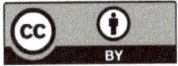

© 2018 by the authors. Licensee MDPI, Basel, Switzerland. This article is an open access article distributed under the terms and conditions of the Creative Commons Attribution (CC BY) license (http://creativecommons.org/licenses/by/4.0/).

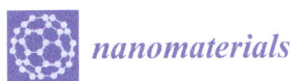

Review

Antimicrobial Effects of Biogenic Nanoparticles

Priyanka Singh [1], Abhroop Garg [1], Santosh Pandit [2], V. R. S. S. Mokkapati [2] and Ivan Mijakovic [1,2,*]

1. The Novo Nordisk Foundation Center for Biosustainability, Technical University of Denmark, 2800 Kgs. Lyngby, Denmark; prisin@biosustain.dtu.dk (P.S.); abhgar@biosustain.dtu.dk (A.G.)
2. Systems and Synthetic Biology Division, Department of Biology and Biological Engineering, Chalmers University of Technology, 41296 Chalmers, Sweden; pandit@chalmers.se (S.P.); ragmok@chalmers.se (V.R.S.S.M.)
* Correspondence: ivan.mijakovic@chalmers.se; Tel.: +46-070-982-8446

Received: 7 November 2018; Accepted: 4 December 2018; Published: 5 December 2018

Abstract: Infectious diseases pose one of the greatest health challenges in the medical world. Though numerous antimicrobial drugs are commercially available, they often lack effectiveness against recently developed multidrug resistant (MDR) microorganisms. This results in high antibiotic dose administration and a need to develop new antibiotics, which in turn requires time, money, and labor investments. Recently, biogenic metallic nanoparticles have proven their effectiveness against MDR microorganisms, individually and in synergy with the current/conventional antibiotics. Importantly, biogenic nanoparticles are easy to produce, facile, biocompatible, and environmentally friendly in nature. In addition, biogenic nanoparticles are surrounded by capping layers, which provide them with biocompatibility and long-term stability. Moreover, these capping layers provide an active surface for interaction with biological components, facilitated by free active surface functional groups. These groups are available for modification, such as conjugation with antimicrobial drugs, genes, and peptides, in order to enhance their efficacy and delivery. This review summarizes the conventional antibiotic treatments and highlights the benefits of using nanoparticles in combating infectious diseases.

Keywords: antibiotics; nanoparticles; biogenic nanoparticles; antimicrobial; antibiotic resistance; multidrug resistant (MDR) microorganisms

1. Introduction

The term 'antibiotic' hails from the word 'antibiosis' (meaning against life). Antibiotics are chemical compounds, which can either kill or inhibit the growth of microorganisms. Antibiotics can be classified as antibacterial, antifungal, and antiviral, depending on their target group. However, generally speaking, the term antibiotic is most commonly used to describe antibacterial compounds [1]. For decades, antibiotics have been used to treat diseases, as well as for providing support in various medical procedures ranging from organ transplant to chemotherapy. Various classes or generations of antibiotics have been developed depending upon developing MDR and their mode of resistance. The widely known antimicrobial mechanism of antibiotics includes, inhibition of enzymes, interference in DNA, RNA and protein synthesis, and disruption of membrane structure [2]. A world without antibiotics is difficult to imagine. However, this could turn into a reality owing to the emergence of antibiotic resistance in microorganisms [3]. As aptly described by González-Candelas et al., 'Antibiotic resistance represents one of the best examples of natural selection in action; and also one of the major hurdles in humankind's fight against infectious diseases' [4]. The development of drug resistance in microorganisms leads to usage of high drug doses, higher toxicity treatments, longer stays in hospitals, and an increase in mortality [5]. There are various factors which contribute towards antibiotic resistance in microorganisms, such as misuse and overuse of antibiotics, their extensive agricultural use, and availability of fewer new antibiotics [6]. Furthermore, the ease of transportation (of affected individuals and food commodities) in today's era helps spreading of pathogenic microorganisms farther and faster around the globe [7].

Apart from the negative social and economic effects on society, antibiotic resistance poses a serious threat of spread of epidemic infections [7]. The World Health Organization (WHO) has declared antimicrobial resistance (AMR) as one of the 'biggest threats to global health' [8]. Around 25,000 deaths per annum have been estimated in the European Union because of AMR [3]. Globally, the estimated number of deaths due to multidrug resistant microorganisms is around 700,000 per year [9]. The possible known mechanisms of antibiotic resistance in bacteria are; (1) reduced uptake of antimicrobial drugs and/or increased efflux of drugs, (2) alterations of antibiotic target, (3) development of drug degrading/modifying enzymes in microorganisms, and (4) formation of biofilm layer which surrounds the bacteria and avoids its exposure to antibiotics [10]. These possibilities ultimately result in either less accumulation of drugs in microbial cells or short intracellular residence of drugs, due to which the therapeutic levels of drugs cannot be easily achieved [11]. Consequently, a higher amount and repeated administration of drugs is required, leading to adverse side effects on human beings and animals.

Pathogenic microorganisms have developed resistance against almost all the types of antibiotics currently being used [12]. Most importantly, there have been no reports on the development of any new antibiotics class in the past few decades. In addition, antibiotics innovation and commercialization is an expensive and long process, which includes discovery of new antibiotics, several clinical trials, and licensing [13]. This situation is compounded by the fact that bacterial resistance can emerge quickly to any new antibiotics, resulting in a reduction in antibiotic use and a decline in sales. Thus, lack of antibiotics development will ultimately result in an increased risk of death from infections following surgeries such as organ transplants or chemotherapy [14]. Therefore, there is an imperative need to develop new drugs to tackle these problems.

To answer these problems, scientists became interested in achieving a rapid diagnostic and targeted therapy by either completely avoiding or modifying the use of conventional antibiotics. This search led to investigating the metals such as silver, copper, zinc, and titanium, which are originally antimicrobial in nature. Metals have been used as antimicrobial agents from centuries. Unlike antibiotics, metals act against microorganisms through several different mechanisms such as membrane disintegration, damage of cellular components (DNA, protein and electron transport chain), and reactive oxygen species (ROS) generation [15]. The emergence of nanotechnology helped in understanding and exploring the unique properties of these metals. Conversion of bulk metal-to-metal nanoparticles demonstrated the enhancement of all the properties of parent metal at nano scale [16]. Transformation of bulk element to nano level, not only reduces its size, but also leads to the formation of different shapes at nano level, such as spherical, triangular, truncated triangle, octahedral, rod, and flower-shaped [17,18]. This variation in geometry facilitates applications in various fields. Especially, it is very advantageous for antimicrobial applications, since the antimicrobial action of nanoparticles is directly proportional to the surface area available for interaction with biological components. Thus, the metallic nanoparticles became one of the most promising choices to overcome the microbial resistance and fight MDR microorganisms [11].

To produce the metallic nanoparticles, several conventional methods have been in use for decades. For instance, physical methods such as melt mixing, laser ablation, physical vapor deposition, sputtering, and chemical methods like thermolysis, photoreduction, microemulsion and sol-gel. These methodologies often result in instability of nanoparticles, attachment of toxic substances on nanoparticle surface, and production of hazardous byproducts. For instance, to produce silver nanoparticles (AgNPs) chemically, a reducing agent (borohydrite), capping agent (starch, polyethyl glycol), and other stabilizing agents are required. By contrast, "green" methodologies have overcome all these limitations [19]. Green methodologies involve biogenic synthesis of metallic nanoparticles by using biological resources such as microorganisms and plants [20–22]. Microorganisms usually exhibit a process called bioreduction, which involves the accumulation of metallic ions in order to reduce their toxicity. Microorganisms bioreduce intracellularly with the help of various reducing species present either inside the cell and on the cell wall, or extracellularly by different metabolites. Plants also possess the reducing capability because of various flavonoids, proteins, and water-soluble biomolecules. The advantages of green synthesis include: (1) production of stable nanoparticles, (2) biocompatible coating on the nanoparticles' surface which provides additional active surface area for interaction in the biological environment, (3) no hazardous byproduct formation, (4) additional reduction or stabilizing agents are not required, which ultimately makes the process economical (Figure 1) [23,24]. The stability and biocompatibility of green nanoparticles corresponds to their capping layer, which usually form during synthesis of biogenic nanoparticles, and originates from the corresponding biological extracts used for synthesis. This layer affects the biological activity of nanoparticles and is useful in long-term stability. Huang et al. demonstrated that nanoparticles formed from microorganisms through nucleation and surface growth could be entrapped by the additional surface (capping layer), often exhibiting excellent stability [25]. Despite the fact that biogenic metallic nanoparticles are biocompatible in nature with high stability and amenable for biomedical applications, a balance between price, process, and scalability is still a considerable challenge. Especially for microorganisms involved in biogenic nanoparticles production, there is a requirement of sophisticated instruments throughout the process for the maintenance, production, and purification of nanoparticles. For instance, freezers are required for microorganisms' preservation, incubators with temperature and shaking control are required for nanoparticle production, and centrifuges are required for purification of nanoparticles. All these heavy instruments required for the complete process of nanoparticle production and purification make the methodology comparatively expensive [26,27]. In the case of plants, the requirement of natural resource management, which includes plant culturing and maintenance, is an important issue that needs to be addressed [28,29]. However, the advantages of biogenic metallic nanoparticles over physiochemically-obtained nanoparticles cannot be over looked for future research and commercialization in the field of antimicrobial applications.

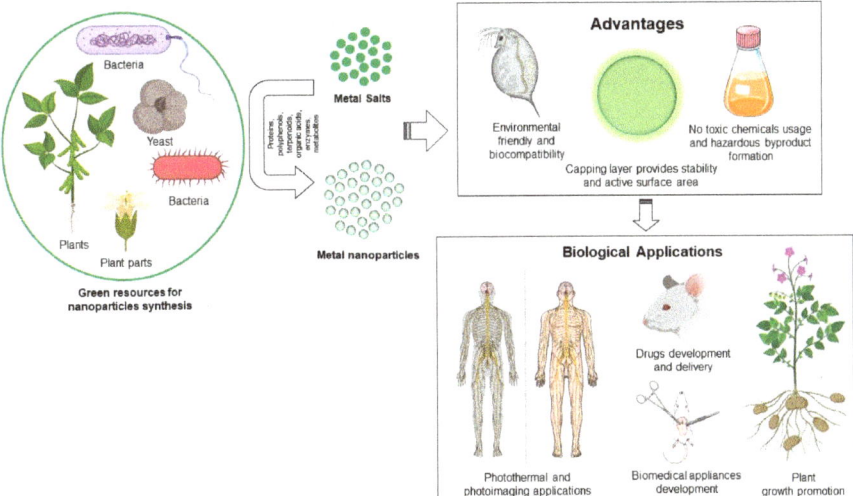

Figure 1. Green synthesis of metallic nanoparticle, their advantages and biological applications.

In this review, we focused on conventional antibiotics, developing drug resistance, nanoparticle development, and overcoming drug resistance problems. We also focused on the biogenicity of metallic nanoparticles and their future perspectives.

2. Microbial Resistance to Antimicrobial Drugs

2.1. Conventional Antibiotics

Penicillin was the first antibiotic to be discovered in 1928, which marked the beginning of the modern era of antibiotics [6]. Antibiotics can be classified on the basis of their mode of action, spectrum of action, or their chemical structure. For example, antibiotics can either be bactericidal (lethal to bacteria) or bacteriostatic (causing growth inhibition of bacteria). The broad-spectrum antibiotics target both the Gram-negative and Gram-positive bacteria, while the narrow spectrum antibiotics target only one of them [30]. Based on their molecular structures, antibiotics can be classified as β-lactams, macrolides, tetracyclines, quinolones, aminoglycosides, sulphonamides, glycopeptides, and oxazolidinones [1].

The β-lactam antibiotics interfere with the cell wall synthesis in bacteria by binding to penicillin binding protein (PBP). The function of PBPs is to cross-link the peptide units in the peptidoglycan layer. Binding of β-lactams to PBPs leads to the inhibition of the latter, and subsequently cell lysis. The β-lactam antibiotics are further divided into penicillins, cephalosporins, monobactams, and carbapenems. In the late 1960s, the emergence of penicillin-resistant bacteria was observed. These bacteria were able to synthesize β-lactamases, enzymes that could degrade β-lactam antibiotics. The discovery of carbapenems circumvented this problem, as this new class of β-lactams was insensitive to the β-lactamases. Amongst all the known β-lactams, carbapenems exhibit the broadest spectrum of activity [1]. Unfortunately, the emergence of carbapenem resistance was also reported in bacteria [31]. Glycopeptides also target the bacterial cell wall synthesis, but in addition to blocking the PBPs, they also inhibit peptidoglycan synthesis [1]. A detailed account of recent developments in glycopeptide antibiotics has been published elsewhere [32]. The macrolides, tetracyclines, aminoglycosides, and oxazolidinones inhibit the bacterial growth by targeting protein synthesis in the cells. Macrolides bind to the 50S ribosomal subunit and inhibit the elongation of mRNA during translation, thus halting protein synthesis [1]. Oxazolidinones also bind to the 50S ribosomal subunit, but unlike the macrolides, inhibit protein synthesis by impeding the formation of 70S translation initiation complex [33]. Together, these two classes form the 50S inhibitors group. Tetracyclines and aminoglycosides, the 30S inhibitors group, bind to the 30S ribosomal subunit denying aminoacyl-tRNAs access to the ribosome and subsequently inhibiting protein synthesis. While macrolides and tetracyclines are typically bacteriostatic, aminoglycosides are broadly bactericidal in their mode of action [1]. Nucleic acid (DNA and RNA) synthesis is fundamental to a cell's survival. Quinolones inhibit bacterial growth by blocking the action of DNA helicases, which are indispensable for unwinding the double helical structure of DNA prior to DNA replication or repair. Additionally, quinolones also interfere with the functions of topoisomerase II and topoisomerase IV in bacteria leading to a negative effect on RNA polymerase, thereby inhibiting RNA synthesis [1]. Sulfonamides structurally mimic para-aminobenzoic acid (PABA), a substrate for the synthesis of folic acid in bacterial cells. Folic acid is indispensable for nucleic acid (DNA) synthesis, thus by competing with PABA and blocking folic acid synthesis; sulfonamides inhibit cell division and cause growth inhibition in bacteria. Unfortunately, resistance to these conventional antibiotics has been reported in bacteria, making it difficult to treat the infections caused by these bacteria [34].

2.2. Developing Resistance to Antimicrobials

Recently-developed multidrug resistant (MDR) microorganisms includes: vancomycin resistant *Staphylococcus aureus* and *Enterococcus* sp. such as *E. faecalis* and *E. faecium* [35], penicillin resistant *Streptococcus pneumonia*, multidrug resistant *Mycobacterium tuberculosis, Salmonella enterica, Pseudomonas aeruginosa, Vibrio cholera, Acinetobacter baumannii*, and carbapenem resistant *Enterobacteriaceae* [9]. Broadly speaking, bacteria develop drug resistance by acquiring the drug resistance genes, which is followed by the expression of these resistance genes, and selection of the cells expressing the resistance genes. The acquisition of resistance genes can occur via horizontal gene transfer (HGT) by transduction, transformation, or conjugation [36]. Another possibility of acquiring the resistance genes is by spontaneous mutation in the existing genes [37]. When a microbe, which already has a drug resistance gene, acquires another type of drug resistance gene, such microbes then become multi drug resistant (MDR). Next, the acquired resistance genes are expressed when the microbes possessing them are exposed to antimicrobial drugs. Finally, a selection pressure for microbes expressing a resistance gene leads to a widespread resistance towards that antimicrobial. This could happen when the microbes are not eliminated completely upon exposure to the drug, resulting in a positive selection pressure for the drug resistant microbes. For example, a positive selection pressure for microbes expressing resistance genes occurs when a patient misses a scheduled dose of the antimicrobial or takes an insufficient number of doses (poor patient compliance). Consequently, the microbes get exposed to the drug but are not completely eliminated. Poor patient compliance plays an even more significant role in developing drug resistance against drugs with short elimination half-lives. Because the time required for removal of these drugs from the host body is short, it is necessary to replenish the drug in short intervals accompanied by a higher number of doses for complete eradication of the microbe [12].

However, administration of an appropriate number of doses at appropriate intervals does not eliminate the positive selection pressure for drug resistance. The clinical outcomes of time-dependent antibiotics are measured as a function of t > MIC (minimum inhibitory concentration), which is defined as the time duration, between the doses, for which the drug concentration in plasma is more than its MIC. Thus, persistent plasma concentration of a time-dependent antibiotic between zero and its MIC for a long time can lead to the development of resistance against the drug. This especially concerns antibiotics with long elimination half-lives such as β-lactams, tetracyclines, and clindamycin [5]. The clinical outcomes of concentration dependent antibiotics are measured as a function of C_{max}/MIC, which is defined as the ratio of maximum drug concentration in plasma to its MIC, per dosing interval. Thus, a drop in C_{max}/MIC value below a target threshold during a dosing interval can lead to the development of resistance against the drug, independent of its elimination half-life. Vancomycin, aminoglycosides, and quinolones are some examples of the concentration-dependent antibiotics [5].

2.3. Mechanisms of Drug Resistance to Antimicrobials

2.3.1. Decreased Uptake and Efflux Pumps

Decreased uptake and increased efflux of a drug does not allow for accumulation of the drug inside the cell to a concentration that is lethal to cells. For this purpose, various bacteria possess resistance genes for specific types of antibiotics. For example, both Gram-positive and Gram-negative bacteria possess the genes for tetracycline efflux pumps TetA, TetB, and TetK. The *tetA* gene is not expressed under native conditions owing to its repression by the repressor protein TetR. Tetracycline binds to TetR, thus inactivating it, which in turn leads to the expression of the *tetA* gene. The TetA efflux pump then flushes out tetracycline, thereby conferring resistance to the bacteria against tetracycline. Other examples of resistance due to increased efflux include resistance against fluoroquinolones in Gram-negative bacteria and resistance against macrolide in Gram-positive bacteria [5]. Examples of decreased uptake of antibiotics include aminoglycoside resistance in Gram-negative bacteria. One of the known vancomycin resistance mechanisms is a thickening of the cell wall [5].

2.3.2. Alteration of Antimicrobial Target

Bacteria can also develop resistance by expressing genes that code for an alternate version of the antibiotic target. These altered substrates usually have lower binding affinity to the antibiotic as compared to the wild type versions, thus decreasing the activity of the antibiotic. For example, resistance against β-lactams in methicillin resistant *Staphylococcus aureus* (MRSA) conferred by *mecA*, which codes for an altered PBP known as PBP2A. The β-lactams have lower binding affinities towards PBP2A than PBP, and therefore, *mecA* confers resistance against all the β-lactams [5,38,39]. Another example is resistance against glycopeptides conferred by the resistance gene *vanA* expressing the enzyme D-alanine-D-lactate ligase. This enzyme modifies the terminal D-ala-D-ala domain of peptidoglycan precursor (target of vancomycin) to D-ala-D-lactate. The affinity of vancomycin towards this modified precursor is about 1000 times lower than the wild type version, thus making the cells expressing *vanA* resistant towards vancomycin [5,40]. Other examples that use this mechanism to develop drug resistance include resistance to sulfonamides in *Escherichia coli*, *Streptococcus pneumoniae*, *Neisseria meningitidis*, resistance to quinolones in Gram-positive and Gram-negative bacteria, and resistance to macrolides, aminoglycosides, and tetracyclines [5,41].

2.3.3. Modification of Antimicrobial Drugs

Bacteria have also been observed to express resistance genes coding for antibiotic modifying enzymes. For example, ACT *N*-acetyltransferase which catalyzes the acetylation of an NH_2 group of aminoglycoside, the APH O-phosphotransferase which catalyzes the phosphorylation of an OH group of aminoglycoside, and ANT O-adenyltransferase which catalyzes the adenylation of an OH group of aminoglycoside. In all these cases, modification of the antibiotic leads to its decreased binding affinity towards its target, the 30S ribosomal subunit, consequently reducing its antimicrobial activity. Modification and inactivation of chloramphenicol by acetyltransferases is the most common mechanism of developing chloramphenicol resistance. Other antibiotics for which such mechanisms of developing drug resistance are observed include β-lactams, tetracyclines, macrolides, quinolones, and streptogramins [5,42].

2.3.4. Production of Competitive Inhibitor

Antibiotic resistance is also acquired by producing a competitive inhibitor of the drug. For example, *S. aureus* and *N. meningitides* produce an increased amount of PABA that competes with sulfonamide for its target, dihydropteroate synthetase, and thus conferring resistance against sulfonamide drugs [5].

2.3.5. Persister Cells

When a small fraction in bacterial population randomly stops or slows down their metabolic activity by expressing the toxin-antitoxin (TA) genes, they become more tolerant to the antimicrobial drug. These cells are known as persisters. Upon exposure to antibiotics, most of the bacterial population is wiped out, leaving behind the persisters. These persisters can cause recurrence of the infection when they resume their metabolic activity [5,36].

2.3.6. Biofilm Formation

Biofilms are formed when bacterial cells immobilize themselves by attaching to a surface such as human tissues and medical implants. It is very difficult to treat the infections associated with biofilms because of the extracellular polymeric substance (EPS) matrix present around the bacterial cells. The EPS matrix is extremely tolerant towards various antibiotics, thus leading to chronic infections in humans [5,43]. The EPS matrix forms a barrier between antibiotics and bacterial cells. The EPS matrix acts a sieve and molecules above a certain size, including antibiotics, cannot pass through it. The antibiotics also get trapped in the EPS matrix because of its negative charge. Furthermore, the EPS matrix contains enzymes that can modify antibiotics and rip them off their antimicrobial activity. It has also been suggested that by reducing the antibiotic concentration below their MIC (and above 0), the EPS matrix could help in development of antibiotic resistance in the bacterial cells [5,44]. Although some antibiotics, such as rifampicin and vancomycin, have been shown to penetrate the EPS matrix, they could not eradicate the slow growing bacterial cells, especially the persister cells [43].

2.3.7. Swarming

Swarming is a type of multicellularity observed in many bacterial species. It happens when groups of highly differentiated cells (swarm cells) come together as a single unit on semisolid surfaces. The planktonic cells become elongated and develop multiple flagella. These swarm cells remain in each other's vicinity and migrate together, like a raft. The swarm cells have been shown to be highly resistant to multiple antibiotics. However, sub culturing the swarm cells in liquid medium causes them to revert back to planktonic cells, as well as restoring their antibiotic susceptibility [5,38].

2.3.8. Intracellular Microbes

Being inside the host cell, the intracellular microbes are shielded from the antimicrobial drugs because of the limited capacity of the drugs to enter the host cell [5].

In recently published reviews, a more detailed account on the mode of action of antibiotics and different mechanisms of resistance against antibiotics is available [34,45].

3. Promising Biogenic Metallic Nanoparticles for Antibacterial Applications

As discussed above, metallic nanoparticles due to their shape-and-size-dependent tunable properties became central focus for many biomedical applications including antimicrobial. Metallic nanoparticles such as silver, copper, titanium, zinc, and iron can be used against MDR microorganisms due to their antimicrobial nature [11,46]. Importantly, biogenic nanoparticles are mainly utilized for antimicrobial applications due to their long-term stability and biocompatibility. The mechanisms behind the antimicrobial effect of these nanoparticles are oxidative stress, metal ion release, and non-oxidative stress occurring simultaneously (Figure 2) [47]. There are several examples where green metallic nanoparticles obtained from microorganisms have been explored for antimicrobial applications against many pathogenic microorganisms. For instance, biogenic AgNPs obtained from *Brevibacterium frigoritolerans* DC2 [48], *Sporosarcina koreensis* DC4 [49], and *Bhargavaea indica* DC1 [18], showed antimicrobial activity against *Vibrio parahaemolyticus*, *Salmonella enterica*, *Bacillus anthracis*, *Bacillus cereus*, *Escherichia coli*, and *Candida albicans*. Copper nanoparticles (CuNPs) obtained from *Sida acuta* showed antimicrobial activity against *Escherichia coli*, *Proteus vulgaris*, and *Staphylococcus aureus* [50]. In addition, these nanoparticles showed enhancement in the antimicrobial efficacy of conventional antibiotics such as lincomycin, oleandomycin, vancomycin, novobiocin, penicillin G, and rifampicin, when applied together. Research on zinc oxide also revealed its antibacterial activity against *S. aureus*, *E. coli*, and *P. aeruginosa* [51]. Thus, the findings suggest that combining the current antibiotics with green metallic nanoparticles can be further helpful for enhancing their antimicrobial activity. Moreover, a comparative study between biological and chemical nanoparticles demonstrated that the biological nanoparticles exert higher antimicrobial effect than the chemically synthesized nanoparticles. For example, Sudhasree et al. proposed that the biological synthesized nickel nanoparticles from *Desmodium gangeticum* are more monodispersed and have higher antioxidant, antibacterial, and biocompatible activities in LLC PK1 (epithelial cell lines) than chemically synthesized nanoparticles. Specifically, in terms of antibacterial activity, they tested both the nanoparticles against *S. aureus*, *K. pneumonia*, *P. aeruginosa*, *V. cholerae*, and *Proteus vulgaris*, and found that chemically synthesized nickel nanoparticles were not at all active against *K. pneumonia*, *P. aeruginosa* and *P. vulgaris*, whereas biological nanoparticles showed antimicrobial activity against these microorganisms. For *S. aureus*, chemical nanoparticles were less active than the biological ones. However, in the case of *V. cholerae*, chemical nanoparticles were more effective [52]. Mohammed et al. also described how biologically synthesized zinc nanoparticles have more antimicrobial potential against *Salmonella typhimurium* ATCC 14028, *B. subtilis* ATCC 6633, and *Micrococcus luteus* ATCC 9341 compared with chemically synthesized zinc nanoparticles [23]. Table 1 provides an overview of several types of biogenic nanoparticles, their source, and any reported antimicrobial activity.

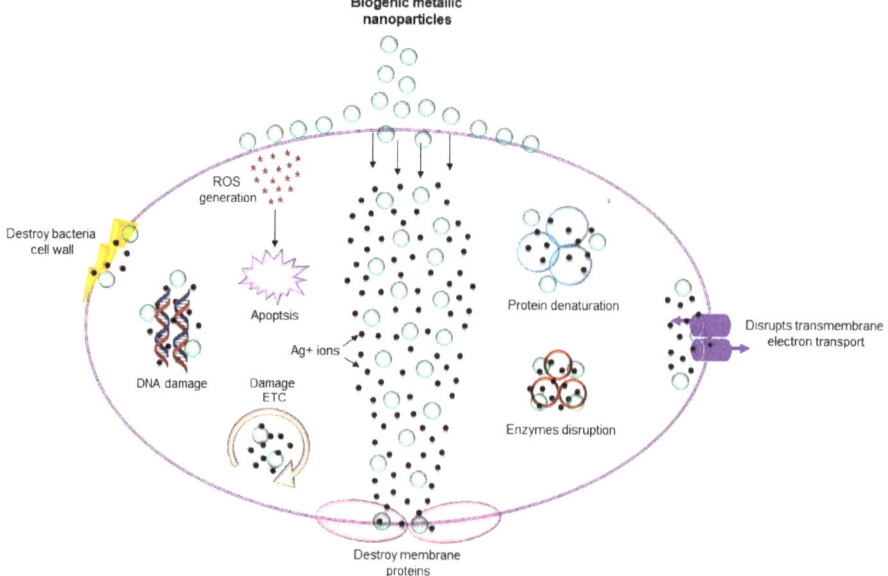

Figure 2. Various mechanism of antimicrobial activity of biogenic metallic nanoparticles. ROS: reactive oxygen species.

However, this list is not exhaustive, and only a few seminal studies are mentioned here. From past few decades, nanoparticles, especially coating of nanosilver, are being used in bone prostheses, dental implants and surgical instruments as an antibacterial preventive measure and as coating on wound dressing to combat the microorganisms in wounds [53,54]. These nanoparticles target the bacterial cells and disturb the crucial function of cell membrane such as membrane respiration and membrane permeability [55,56]. Furthermore, they react with intracellular components such as proteins and nucleic acids, and inhibit cell division and gene transfer [55,56]. There are many reports showing the antimicrobial activity of various nanoparticles, mainly silver, zinc, copper, titanium, magnesium, and gold [57,58]. The mechanism of action of nanoparticles and antibiotics seems to be similar in the case of interference in the synthesis of DNA, RNA, and protein, as well as membrane disruption [2,53,55]. However, most of these metallic nanoparticles exhibit antimicrobial activity through multiple mechanisms, which decrease the possibility of development of resistance against them in microorganisms [56]. To develop resistance towards such nanoparticles, microbial cells would need to acquire multiple simultaneous gene mutations, which is not very probable. Furthermore, synthesizing such nanoparticles by using the green way would result into proteins, polysaccharides, and small bioactive compounds binding to the nanoparticles, which further enhance their antimicrobial activity towards the MDR microorganisms. In this section, we discuss a few metallic nanoparticles that are synthesized by green method(s) and their effect on different pathogenic microorganisms.

3.1. Gold Nanoparticles (AuNPs)

One of the most widely studied biogenic nanoparticles are gold nanoparticles (AuNPs). Predominantly, the shape of the AuNPs is spherical [59], triangular [60], and hexagonal [61], though rod-shaped nanoparticles were also reported in various studies. AuNPs are synthesized either from the whole plant or by the combination of various components that act as reducing agents. Interestingly, the type of extracts that are used as bioreductants defines the size and shape of synthesized nanoparticles. AuNPs synthesized from *Galaxaura elongate* is one important example where a wide range of size (4–77 nm) and shapes (spherical, rod, triangular, hexagonal) of nanoparticles were obtained [62]. Another important discovery is the effect of pH on the size of AuNPs. It was reported that nanoparticles with core size 6 nm and 18 nm were obtained at pH 9 and pH 2 respectively, from mango peel extract [63]. AuNPs are known for their biocompatibility to microbial cells with no bacteriostatic or bactericidal activity. However, antibiotics integrated AuNPs are shown to have strong bactericidal effect against the drug resistant bacteria. The ampicillin bound AuNPs has been shown to damage ampicillin resistant bacteria, including MRSA, *P. aeruginosa*, *Enterobacter aerogenes*, and *E. coli* K-12 sub-strain DH5-alpha [64] by multiple mechanisms. AuNPs-AMP can overwhelm the high concentrations of beta-lactamase expressed by these bacteria and in addition, AuNP-AMP inhibits the transmembrane pump that catalyzes drug efflux from the bacterial cell [64].

3.2. Silver Nanoparticles (AgNPs)

AgNPs have remarkable bactericidal and fungicidal properties, that have been exploited in pharmaceutical industry, paints, ointments, food, fabrics, and packaging industries [65]. Large-scale green synthesis of different shapes and sizes of AgNPs from plants, bacteria, fungi, and yeast has been studied extensively [23]. The basic antibacterial mechanism of AgNPs has been shown to be either due to the release of silver ions or due to the intracellular deposition of nanoparticles [58,66]. The detailed mechanism mainly involves cell membrane damage, disruption of energy metabolism, generation of oxidative stress due to ROS formation, and inhibition of transcription. Silver ions released from AgNPs have been shown to interact with sulfur- and phosphorus-containing groups of proteins in the cell wall and plasma membrane of bacteria [67]. The initial interaction of silver ions with microbial cells starts with the binding of cationic silver with the negatively charged microbial cell, which leads to the formation of multiple pores in the cell membrane and outflow of the intracellular contents. This also causes an electrochemical imbalance in the cells and allows the silver ions to pass through the plasma membrane into the cytoplasm of the bacterial cell and interact with the intracellular components resulting in permanent cell damage [55]. Silver ions also have been shown to inhibit the activity of proteins and enzymes that are essential for ATP production, inhibit respiratory enzymes leading to the production of ROS, damage RNA and DNA, and destabilize and disrupt the outer membrane. Nanoparticles, owing to their small size with large surface area, have a high possibility to cross the peptidoglycan and cell membrane [10,68]. This phenomenon has been described as a rationale for the higher sensitivity of the Gram-negative bacteria towards nanoparticles, as compared to the Gram-positive bacteria having a thicker peptidoglycan layer [19]. The thickness and crosslinking of peptidoglycan in the Gram-positive bacterial cell wall provide more resistance against the penetration of nanoparticles. Many reports with antibacterial activity of AgNPs have correlated their toxicity with size and shape of the particles [69]. The nanoparticles with more surface area have been shown to release silver ions at a higher rate, which is an important factor for high antibacterial activity [70]. Antibacterial activity of AgNPs have been studied against the multidrug resistant bacteria such as *P. aeruginosa*, *E. coli*, *Streptococcus pyogenes*, *S. aureus*, *Klebsiella pneumoniae*, *Salmonella* species, and *Enterococcus* species [71,72]. This bactericidal effect, mostly, is attributed to the inhibition of cell wall synthesis, protein synthesis mediated by the 30S ribosomal subunit, and nucleic acid synthesis. Furthermore, AgNPs have also been shown to enhance the antimicrobial activity of antibiotics such as penicillin G, amoxicillin, vancomycin, clindamycin, and especially erythromycin, against *S. aureus* and *E. coli* [73]. In addition to that, silver carbene complexes encapsulated in nanoparticles have been shown to be effective against multidrug resistant bacteria, including MRSA, multidrug resistant *A. baumannii* (MRAB), *P. aeruginosa*, *Burkholderia cepacia*, and *K. pneumoniae* [74]. The strong bactericidal effect of AgNPs against the multidrug resistant bacteria is mostly due to their multiple mechanisms to disrupt microbial cells. Despite having multiple mechanisms for antibacterial effects, a recent study involving a pretreatment of bacterial cells with sublethal concentration of AgNPs showed lesser membrane damage, lowered levels of intracellular ROS and higher amount of intracellular ATP when bacterial cells were further exposed to ampicillin. This suggests that the pretreatment of bacterial cells with sub-lethal concentrations of AgNPs leads to long-lasting responses that enhance the antibiotic stress resistance in bacteria at multiple levels [75].

3.3. Zinc Oxide Nanoparticles (ZnO-NPs)

Zinc oxide nanoparticles (ZnO-NPs) are synthesized using different biological resources as reducing agents [76]. They are nontoxic, semiconducting material with good photocatalysis and high transparency. ZnO-NPs are synthesized from different parts of plants such as leaves, roots, rhizomes, fruits, flowers, and bark [77]. ZnONPs show a potential antibacterial activity [78] and good photo degradation and have applications in drug delivery [79] and anticancer therapy [80]. ZnO-NPs are also widely tested metallic nanoparticles for their antimicrobial purpose. The wide range of both Gram-positive and Gram-negative bacteria such as *E. coli*, *Listeria monocytogenes*, *Salmonella*, and *S. aureus* have demonstrated sensitivity towards ZnO-NPs [81,82]. ZnO-NPs treatment of bacterial cells leads to ROS generation, lipid peroxidation, membrane leakage of reducing sugars, proteins, DNA, and cell viability [83]. ZnO-NPs has been shown to produce ROS such as super oxide anion and hydrogen peroxide in cells [84,85]. ROS causes membrane leakage of proteins and nucleic acids by enhancing lipid peroxidation on membrane. Additionally, Zn^{+2} ions released from the nanoparticles also damage the cell membrane and interact with intracellular components [86,87]. Recently, ZnO-NPs were shown to inhibit the growth of carbapenem-resistant *A. baumannii* by producing ROS and causing membrane damage, suggesting that ZnO-NPs might be developed as an alternative to carbapenems (beta-lactam) [83].

3.4. Copper Nanoparticles (CuO-NPs)

Cupric oxide nanoparticles (CuO-NPs) gained critical importance due to their applications in anti-microbial activity, pharmaceutical industry, cosmetics, transport, power, and farming [88]. It is relatively easy to produce CuO-NPs by chemical means, but with many disadvantages like low potency, high toxicity, environmentally unfriendliness, and high expense. CuO-NPs are synthesized from various biogenic means like polysaccharides such as pectin, chitosan, alginate, leaf extracts, bacteria and so on. Unlike gold, silver, and other nanoparticles, it has been a challenge to produce stable CuO-NPs due to their proneness to oxidation when exposed to an aqueous medium [89]. Though there are a few reports on CuO-NPs production under inert conditions [90] from copper salts, there are very limited reports that suggest the synthesis of metallic CuO-NPs in noninert conditions. Compared to other nanoparticles, the biogenic synthesis of CuO-NPs is relatively new and ways are being explored to make it with ease and ecofriendly. The mechanism behind the antibacterial activity of CuO-NPs is believed that electrostatic attraction between Cu^{+2} and plasma membrane helps in damaging the membrane and killing cells [91,92]. The Cu^{+2} ions are energetically easier to move across a lipid bilayer and upon being taken up by the cell, lead to ROS production, lipid peroxidation, and protein oxidation [92]. CuO-NPs were shown to have strong antimicrobial activity against both Gram-positive and Gram-negative bacteria [92,93]. The broad-spectrum antimicrobial efficacy of CuO-NPs suggested the possible use in wound healing treatment, such as in bactericidal plasters and bandages, due to its strong bactericidal effect and illegible sensibility of human tissues to copper compounds [94,95].

3.5. Titanium Dioxide Nanoparticles (TiO$_2$-NPs)

Titanium dioxide nanoparticles (TiO$_2$-NPs) possess interesting optical, dielectric, antibacterial, and catalytic properties that makes them interesting for their usage in various catalyst industry [96], sensors [97], biosensors [98], solar cells [99], and as image-contrast agents in medical diagnostics [100]. TiO$_2$-NPs with different morphologies like nanorods and nanotubes are commonly synthesized using different reducing and stabilizing agents [101]. Hydrothermal processing is another approach due to its cost effectiveness and simplicity [102], nevertheless, green routes need to be developed to have a reliable supply in sufficient quantities without any harmful effects on the environment. TiO$_2$-NPs are synthesized from plants [103], fungus [104], and piper betel leaf [105]. TiO$_2$-NPs also exhibit antimicrobial activity by multiple mechanisms suggesting that the possibility of development of resistance by microbial cells against these nanoparticles is very low [10]. TiO$_2$-NPs have been well demonstrated to have bactericidal effect against *E. coli*, *P. aeruginosa*, *S. aureus*, and *E. faecium* [106,107]. One of the mechanisms by which TiO$_2$-NPs kills microorganisms is by generating ROS with the exposure of near to ultra-violet radiation [107]. The generated ROS disrupt the cell membrane interfering with the oxidative phosphorylation, which leads to cell death. A recent report suggested that exposing cells to TiO$_2$ photocatalysis rapidly inactivates the regulatory signaling level, efficiently decreases the coenzyme-independent respiratory chains, lowers ability to take up and transport iron and phosphorous, and lowers the capacity for the biosynthesis and degradation of heme (Fe-S cluster) groups [11,106].

3.6. Magnesium Oxide Nanoparticles

Like other nanoparticles, magnesium oxide nanoparticles (MgO-NPs) also generates the ROS and is the major mechanism behind its antimicrobial activity [70]. Like other nanoparticles, MgO-NPs physically interact with the cell's surface and disrupt the membrane integrity leading to membrane leakage [10]. In addition, they damage the cells by irreversible oxidation of intracellular biomolecules. However, another study demonstrated that MgO-NPs exhibit excellent antibacterial activity in the absence of ROS and lipid peroxidation. The authors suggested that antibacterial activity of MgO-NPs is correlated with the interaction of nanoparticles with the microbial cell membrane, pH change, and release of Mg^{+2} [108]. Furthermore, unlike other nanoparticles, the antimicrobial activity of MgO-NPs has been demonstrated to be due to adsorbing halogen molecules onto the surface of the MgO [10].

4. Concluding Remarks and Future Perspectives

In summary, we would like to conclude that due to poor diagnostics and overdose and incapability of drugs, microorganisms are commonly able to develop resistance against antibiotics. The infections caused by MDR microorganisms are a serious global healthcare issue. To address these problems, biogenic metallic nanoparticles were developed and had proven strong efficacy against various MDR pathogens, either individually or in combination with antibiotics. However, in order to use these nanoparticles for therapeutic applications, some important facts that need to be considered are nanoparticles distribution, their bioavailability, active targeting, and nanoparticles excretion from the body if taken as drug carrier for treating site-specific infections [109].

Owing to the antimicrobial nature of metallic nanoparticles, the applications are not only limited to the biomedical area, but can also be extended to water treatment, textiles, food packaging, cosmetics, agriculture (nanopesticides and nanofertilizers), self-cleaning coatings on mobiles phones, washing machines, and computer keyboards. However, the biogenic nanoparticles have not yet been commercialized for these applications. The true challenge for biogenic nanoparticles is finding the right balance between the production cost, scalability, and their applicability. Hence, in this respect, a great deal of research will be required to focus on economical ways of biogenic nanoparticles development which will make them easily available for all kinds of future applications relevant to either antimicrobial era or other.

Table 1. Overview of several types of biogenic nanoparticles, their source and reported antimicrobial activity.

Origin Plant	NPs Type	Shape of NPs	Size Range of NPs (nm)	Anti-Microbial Effect	References
Phyllanthus amarus	CuO	Spherical	20	Anti-microbial against B. subtilis	[110]
Geranium leaves	Ag	Quasilinear	40	Antimicrobial	[111]
Avena sativa	Au	Rod-shaped	5–20	No data available	[112]
Catharanthus roseus	TiO$_2$	No typical shape	25–110	No data available against bacteria	[113]
Camellia Sinensis	ZnO	Triangular/spherical	30–40	Anti-bacterial	[114]
Bacteria					
Aeromonas hydrophila	ZnO	Spherical	50–70	Aantti-bacterial against P. aeruginosa and A. flavus	[115]
Bacillus mycoides	TiO$_2$	Spherical	40–60	Supress aquatic biofilm growth	[116]
Proteus mirabilis PTCC1710	Au	Spherical	10–20	No reported anti-bacterial activity	[117]
Escherichia coli	CdS	Spherical	2–5	Anti-bacterial against E. coli strain BW25113	[118]
Strains NS2 and NS6	PbS		40–70	Bioremidiation	[119]
Fungus and Yeast					
Volvariella volvacea	Au and Ag	Spherical/hexagonal	20–150	Anti-bacterial	[120]
Aspergillus flavus	TiO$_2$	Oval	60–74	Anti-bacterial against S. aureus	[121]
MKY3	Ag	Hexagonal	2–5	Anti-bacterial against S. aureus and E. coli	[122]

Funding: We acknowledge the financial support from the H.C. Ørsted fellowship, co-funded by Marie Skłodowska Curie, to P.S. and Novo Nordisk Foundation and VINNOVA to I.M.

Conflicts of Interest: The authors declare no conflict of interest.

References

1. Etebu, E.; Arikekpar, I. Antibiotics: Classification and mechanisms of action with emphasis on molecular perspectives. *Int. J. Appl. Microbiol. Biotechnol. Res.* **2016**, *4*, 90–101.
2. Kohanski, M.A.; Dwyer, D.J.; Collins, J.J. How antibiotics kill bacteria: From targets to networks. *Nat. Rev. Microbiol.* **2010**, *8*, 423–435. [CrossRef] [PubMed]
3. Padiyara, P.; Inoue, H.; Sprenger, M. Global Governance Mechanisms to Address Antimicrobial Resistance. *Infect. Dis. Res. Treat.* **2018**, *11*. [CrossRef] [PubMed]
4. González-Candelas, F.; Comas, I.; Martínez, J.L.; Galán, J.C.; Baquero, F. 12–The Evolution of Antibiotic Resistance. In *Genetics and Evolution of Infectious Diseases*, 2nd ed.; Tibayrenc, M., Ed.; Elsevier: London, UK, 2017; pp. 257–284.
5. Pelgrift, R.Y.; Friedman, A.J. Nanotechnology as a therapeutic tool to combat microbial resistance. *Adv. Drug Deliv. Rev.* **2013**, *65*, 1803–1815. [CrossRef] [PubMed]
6. Ventola, C.L. The antibiotic resistance crisis: Part 1: Causes and threats. *P T Peer-Rev. J. Formul. Manag.* **2015**, *40*, 277–283.
7. Baluja, Z.; Nabi, N.; Ray, A. Challenges in Antimicrobial Resistance: An Update. *EC Pharmacol. Toxicol.* **2018**, *6*, 865–877.
8. Davis, M.; Whittaker, A.; Lindgren, M.; Djerf-Pierre, M.; Manderson, L.; Flowers, P. Understanding media publics and the antimicrobial resistance crisis. *Glob. Public Health* **2018**, *13*, 1158–1168. [CrossRef]
9. Betts, J.W.; Hornsey, M.; La Ragione, R.M. Novel Antibacterials: Alternatives to Traditional Antibiotics. *Adv. Microb. Physiol.* **2018**, *73*, 123–169.
10. Blecher, K.; Nasir, A.; Friedman, A. The growing role of nanotechnology in combating infectious disease. *Virulence* **2011**, *2*, 395–401. [CrossRef]
11. Huh, A.J.; Kwon, Y.J. "Nanoantibiotics": A new paradigm for treating infectious diseases using nanomaterials in the antibiotics resistant era. *J. Control. Release: Off. J. Controll. Release Soc.* **2011**, *156*, 128–145. [CrossRef]
12. Teixeira, M.C.; Sanchez-Lopez, E.; Espina, M.; Calpena, A.C.; Silva, A.M.; Veiga, F.J.; Garcia, M.L.; Souto, E.B. Chapter 9—Advances in antibiotic nanotherapy: Overcoming antimicrobial resistance. In *Emerging Nanotechnologies in Immunology*; Shegokar, R., Souto, E.B., Eds.; Elsevier: Boston, MA, USA, 2018; pp. 233–259.
13. Bartlett, J.G.; Gilbert, D.N.; Spellberg, B. Seven ways to preserve the miracle of antibiotics. *Clin. Infect. Dis. Off. Publ. Infect. Dis. Soc. Am.* **2013**, *56*, 1445–1450. [CrossRef] [PubMed]
14. Adeniji, F. Global analysis of strategies to tackle antimicrobial resistance. *Int. J. Pharm. Pract.* **2018**, *26*, 85–89. [CrossRef] [PubMed]
15. Ahn, S.; Singh, P.; Jang, M.; Kim, Y.J.; Castro-Aceituno, V.; Simu, S.Y.; Kim, Y.J.; Yang, D.C. Gold nanoflowers synthesized using Acanthopanacis cortex extract inhibit inflammatory mediators in LPS-induced RAW264.7 macrophages via NF-kappaB and AP-1 pathways. *Colloids Surf. B Biointerfaces* **2018**, *162*, 398–404. [CrossRef] [PubMed]
16. Singh, P.; Singh, H.; Ahn, S.; Castro-Aceituno, V.; Jimenez, Z.; Simu, S.Y.; Kim, Y.J.; Yang, D.C. Pharmacological importance, characterization and applications of gold and silver nanoparticles synthesized by Panax ginseng fresh leaves. *Artif. Cells Nanomed. Biotechnol.* **2017**, *45*, 1415–1424. [CrossRef] [PubMed]
17. Singh, P.; Kim, Y.J.; Wang, C.; Mathiyalagan, R.; Yang, D.C. Microbial synthesis of Flower-shaped gold nanoparticles. *Artif. Cells Nanomed. Biotechnol.* **2016**, *44*, 1469–1474. [CrossRef] [PubMed]
18. Singh, P.; Kim, Y.J.; Singh, H.; Mathiyalagan, R.; Wang, C.; Yang, D.C. Biosynthesis of Anisotropic Silver Nanoparticles by *Bhargavaea indica* and Their Synergistic Effect with Antibiotics against Pathogenic Microorganisms. *J. Nanomater.* **2015**, *2015*, 10. [CrossRef]
19. Singh, P.; Pandit, S.; Garnaes, J.; Tunjic, S.; Mokkapati, V.R.; Sultan, A.; Thygesen, A.; Mackevica, A.; Mateiu, R.V.; Daugaard, A.E.; et al. Green synthesis of gold and silver nanoparticles from Cannabis sativa (industrial hemp) and their capacity for biofilm inhibition. *Int. J. Nanomed.* **2018**, *13*, 3571–3591. [CrossRef]
20. Singh, P.; Kim, Y.J.; Yang, D.C. A strategic approach for rapid synthesis of gold and silver nanoparticles by Panax ginseng leaves. *Artif. Cells Nanomed. Biotechnol.* **2016**, *44*, 1949–1957. [CrossRef]

21. Singh, P.; Kim, Y.J.; Wang, C.; Mathiyalagan, R.; Yang, D.C. The development of a green approach for the biosynthesis of silver and gold nanoparticles by using Panax ginseng root extract, and their biological applications. *Artif. Cells Nanomed. Biotechnol.* **2016**, *44*, 1150–1157. [CrossRef]
22. Singh, P.; Kim, Y.J.; Wang, C.; Mathiyalagan, R.; El-Agamy Farh, M.; Yang, D.C. Biogenic silver and gold nanoparticles synthesized using red ginseng root extract, and their applications. *Artif. Cells Nanomed. Biotechnol.* **2016**, *44*, 811–816. [CrossRef]
23. Singh, P.; Kim, Y.J.; Zhang, D.; Yang, D.C. Biological Synthesis of Nanoparticles from Plants and Microorganisms. *Trends Biotechnol.* **2016**, *34*, 588–599. [CrossRef] [PubMed]
24. Singh, P.; Ahn, S.; Kang, J.P.; Veronika, S.; Huo, Y.; Singh, H.; Chokkaligam, M.; El-Agamy Farh, M.; Aceituno, V.C.; Kim, Y.J.; et al. In vitro anti-inflammatory activity of spherical silver nanoparticles and monodisperse hexagonal gold nanoparticles by fruit extract of *Prunus serrulata*: A green synthetic approach. *Artif. Cells Nanomed. Biotechnol.* **2017**, *46*, 2022–2032. [CrossRef] [PubMed]
25. Abbai, R.; Mathiyalagan, R.; Markus, J.; Kim, Y.J.; Wang, C.; Singh, P.; Ahn, S.; Farh Mel, A.; Yang, D.C. Green synthesis of multifunctional silver and gold nanoparticles from the oriental herbal adaptogen: Siberian ginseng. *Int. J. Nanomed.* **2016**, *11*, 3131–3143.
26. Singh, P.; Kim, Y.J.; Wang, C.; Mathiyalagan, R.; Yang, D.C. Weissella oryzae DC6-facilitated green synthesis of silver nanoparticles and their antimicrobial potential. *Artif. Cells Nanomed. Biotechnol.* **2016**, *44*, 1569–1575. [CrossRef] [PubMed]
27. Jo, J.H.; Singh, P.; Kim, Y.J.; Wang, C.; Mathiyalagan, R.; Jin, C.G.; Yang, D.C. Pseudomonas deceptionensis DC5-mediated synthesis of extracellular silver nanoparticles. *Artif. Cells Nanomed. Biotechnol.* **2016**, *44*, 1576–1581. [CrossRef] [PubMed]
28. Singh, H.; Du, J.; Singh, P.; Yi, T.H. Ecofriendly synthesis of silver and gold nanoparticles by Euphrasia officinalis leaf extract and its biomedical applications. *Artif. Cells Nanomed. Biotechnol.* **2018**, *46*, 1163–1170. [CrossRef] [PubMed]
29. Huo, Y.; Singh, P.; Kim, Y.J.; Soshnikova, V.; Kang, J.; Markus, J.; Ahn, S.; Castro-Aceituno, V.; Mathiyalagan, R.; Chokkalingam, M.; et al. Biological synthesis of gold and silver chloride nanoparticles by Glycyrrhiza uralensis and in vitro applications. *Artif. Cells Nanomed. Biotechnol.* **2018**, *46*, 303–312. [CrossRef] [PubMed]
30. Adzitey, F. Antibiotic Classes and Antibiotic Susceptibility of Bacterial Isolates from Selected Poultry; A Mini Review. *World's Vet. J.* **2015**, *5*, 36–41. [CrossRef]
31. Livermore, D.M.; Warner, M.; Mushtaq, S.; Doumith, M.; Zhang, J.; Woodford, N. What remains against carbapenem-resistant Enterobacteriaceae? Evaluation of chloramphenicol, ciprofloxacin, colistin, fosfomycin, minocycline, nitrofurantoin, temocillin and tigecycline. *Int. J. Antimicrob. Agents* **2011**, *37*, 415–419. [CrossRef]
32. Blaskovich, M.A.T.; Hansford, K.A.; Butler, M.S.; Jia, Z.; Mark, A.E.; Cooper, M.A. Developments in Glycopeptide Antibiotics. *ACS Infect. Dis.* **2018**, *4*, 715–735. [CrossRef]
33. Pandit, N.; Singla, R.K.; Shrivastava, B. Current Updates on Oxazolidinone and Its Significance. *Int. J. Med. Chem.* **2012**. [CrossRef] [PubMed]
34. Dowling, A.; O'Dwyer, J.; Adley, C. *Antibiotics: Mode of Action and Mechanisms of Resistance*; Formatex Research Center: Badajoz, Spain, 2017.
35. Cetinkaya, Y.; Falk, P.; Mayhall, C.G. Vancomycin-resistant enterococci. *Clin. Microbiol. Rev.* **2000**, *13*, 686–707. [CrossRef] [PubMed]
36. Hajipour, M.J.; Fromm, K.M.; Akbar Ashkarran, A.; Jimenez de Aberasturi, D.; Larramendi, I.R.D.; Rojo, T.; Serpooshan, V.; Parak, W.J.; Mahmoudi, M. Antibacterial properties of nanoparticles. *Trends Biotechnol.* **2012**, *30*, 499–511. [CrossRef] [PubMed]
37. Ganjian, H.; Nikokar, I.; Tieshayar, A.; Mostafaei, A.; Amirmozafari, N.; Kiani, S. Effects of Salt Stress on the Antimicrobial Drug Resistance and Protein Pattern of *Staphylococcus aureus*. *Jundishapur J. Microbiol.* **2012**, *5*, 328–331.
38. Jayaraman, R. Antibiotic resistance: An overview of mechanisms and a paradigm shift. *Curr. Sci.* **2009**, *96*, 1475–1484.
39. Deurenberg, R.H.; Stobberingh, E.E. The molecular evolution of hospital- and community-associated methicillin-resistant *Staphylococcus aureus*. *Curr. Mol. Med.* **2009**, *9*, 100–115. [CrossRef]
40. Périchon, B.; Courvalin, P. VanA-Type Vancomycin-Resistant *Staphylococcus aureus*. *Antimicrob. Agents Chemother.* **2009**, *53*, 4580–4587. [CrossRef]

41. Deck, D.H.; Winston, L.G. Sulfonamides, trimethoprim, & quinolones. In *Basic and Clinical Pharmacology*, 12nd ed.; Katzung, B., Masters, S., Trevor, A., Eds.; McGraw-Hill: New York, NY, USA, 2012; pp. 831–838.
42. Poole, K. Mechanisms of bacterial biocide and antibiotic resistance. *J. Appl. Microbiol.* **2002**, *92*, 55S–64S. [CrossRef]
43. Bahar, A.A.; Ren, D. Antimicrobial peptides. *Pharmaceuticals (Basel)* **2013**, *6*, 1543–1575. [CrossRef]
44. Ferreira, C.; Pereira, A.; Melo, L.; Simões, M. Advances in industrial biofilm control with micro-nanotechnology. In *Current Research, Technology and Education Topics in Applied Microbiology and Microbial Biotechnology*; Méndez-Vilas, A., Ed.; Formatex: Badajoz, Spain, 2010; Volume 2.
45. Munita, J.M.; Arias, C.A. Mechanisms of Antibiotic Resistance. *Microbiol. Spectr.* **2016**, *4*. [CrossRef]
46. Fernandez-Moure, J.S.; Evangelopoulos, M.; Colvill, K.; Van Eps, J.L.; Tasciotti, E. Nanoantibiotics: A new paradigm for the treatment of surgical infection. *Nanomed. (Lond.)* **2017**, *12*, 1319–1334. [CrossRef] [PubMed]
47. Zaidi, S.; Misba, L.; Khan, A.U. Nano-therapeutics: A revolution in infection control in post antibiotic era. *Nanomed. Nanotechnol. Biol. Med.* **2017**, *13*, 2281–2301. [CrossRef] [PubMed]
48. Singh, P.; Kim, Y.J.; Singh, H.; Wang, C.; Hwang, K.H.; Farh Mel, A.; Yang, D.C. Biosynthesis, characterization, and antimicrobial applications of silver nanoparticles. *Int. J. Nanomed.* **2015**, *10*, 2567–2577.
49. Singh, P.; Singh, H.; Kim, Y.J.; Mathiyalagan, R.; Wang, C.; Yang, D.C. Extracellular synthesis of silver and gold nanoparticles by *Sporosarcina koreensis* DC4 and their biological applications. *Enzyme Microb. Technol.* **2016**, *86*, 75–83. [CrossRef] [PubMed]
50. Sathiyavimal, S.; Vasantharaj, S.; Bharathi, D.; Saravanan, M.; Manikandan, E.; Kumar, S.S.; Pugazhendhi, A. Biogenesis of copper oxide nanoparticles (CuONPs) using *Sida acuta* and their incorporation over cotton fabrics to prevent the pathogenicity of Gram negative and Gram positive bacteria. *J. Photochem. Photobiol. B Biol.* **2018**, *188*, 126–134. [CrossRef] [PubMed]
51. Pasquet, J.; Chevalier, Y.; Pelletier, J.; Couval, E.; Bouvier, D.; Bolzinger, M.-A. The contribution of zinc ions to the antimicrobial activity of zinc oxide. *Colloids Surf. A Physicochem. Eng. Asp.* **2014**, *457*, 263–274. [CrossRef]
52. Mukherjee, S.; Sushma, V.; Patra, S.; Barui, A.K.; Bhadra, M.P.; Sreedhar, B.; Patra, C.R. Green chemistry approach for the synthesis and stabilization of biocompatible gold nanoparticles and their potential applications in cancer therapy. *Nanotechnology* **2012**, *23*, 455103. [CrossRef]
53. Correa, J.M.; Mori, M.; Sanches, H.L.; da Cruz, A.D.; Poiate, E., Jr.; Poiate, I.A. Silver nanoparticles in dental biomaterials. *Int. J. Biomater.* **2015**, *2015*, 485275. [CrossRef]
54. Burdusel, A.C.; Gherasim, O.; Grumezescu, A.M.; Mogoanta, L.; Ficai, A.; Andronescu, E. Biomedical Applications of Silver Nanoparticles: An Up-to-Date Overview. *Nanomaterials* **2018**, *8*, 681. [CrossRef]
55. Dakal, T.C.; Kumar, A.; Majumdar, R.S.; Yadav, V. Mechanistic Basis of Antimicrobial Actions of Silver Nanoparticles. *Front. Microbiol.* **2016**, *7*, 1831. [CrossRef]
56. Slavin, Y.N.; Asnis, J.; Hafeli, U.O.; Bach, H. Metal nanoparticles: Understanding the mechanisms behind antibacterial activity. *J. Nanobiotechnol.* **2017**, *15*, 65. [CrossRef] [PubMed]
57. Vimbela, G.V.; Ngo, S.M.; Fraze, C.; Yang, L.; Stout, D.A. Antibacterial properties and toxicity from metallic nanomaterials. *Int. J. Nanomed.* **2017**, *12*, 3941–3965. [CrossRef] [PubMed]
58. Hoseinnejad, M.; Jafari, S.M.; Katouzian, I. Inorganic and metal nanoparticles and their antimicrobial activity in food packaging applications. *Critical Rev. Microbiol.* **2018**, *44*, 161–181. [CrossRef] [PubMed]
59. Aromal, S.A.; Vidhu, V.K.; Philip, D. Green synthesis of well-dispersed gold nanoparticles using Macrotyloma uniflorum. *Spectrochim. Acta Part A Mol. Biomol. Spectrosc.* **2012**, *85*, 99–104. [CrossRef] [PubMed]
60. Suman, T.Y.; Rajasree, S.R.; Ramkumar, R.; Rajthilak, C.; Perumal, P. The Green synthesis of gold nanoparticles using an aqueous root extract of *Morinda citrifolia* L. *Spectrochim. Acta Part A Mol. Biomol. Spectrosc.* **2014**, *118*, 11–16. [CrossRef] [PubMed]
61. Sheny, D.S.; Mathew, J.; Philip, D. Synthesis characterization and catalytic action of hexagonal gold nanoparticles using essential oils extracted from *Anacardium occidentale*. *Spectrochim. Acta Part A Mol. Biomol. Spectrosc.* **2012**, *97*, 306–310. [CrossRef] [PubMed]
62. Abdel-Raouf, N.; Al-Enazi, N.M.; Ibraheem, I.B.M. Green biosynthesis of gold nanoparticles using *Galaxaura elongata* and characterization of their antibacterial activity. *Arabian J. Chem.* **2017**, *10*, S3029–S3039. [CrossRef]
63. Yang, N.; WeiHong, L.; Hao, L. Biosynthesis of Au nanoparticles using agricultural waste mango peel extract and its in vitro cytotoxic effect on two normal cells. *Mater. Lett.* **2014**, *134*, 67–70. [CrossRef]

64. Brown, A.N.; Smith, K.; Samuels, T.A.; Lu, J.; Obare, S.O.; Scott, M.E. Nanoparticles functionalized with ampicillin destroy multiple-antibiotic-resistant isolates of Pseudomonas aeruginosa and Enterobacter aerogenes and methicillin-resistant Staphylococcus aureus. *Appl. Environ. Microbiol.* **2012**, *78*, 2768–2774. [CrossRef]
65. Suresh, A.K.; Pelletier, D.A.; Wang, W.; Morrell-Falvey, J.L.; Gu, B.; Doktycz, M.J. Cytotoxicity induced by engineered silver nanocrystallites is dependent on surface coatings and cell types. *Langmuir ACS J. Surf. Colloids* **2012**, *28*, 2727–2735. [CrossRef]
66. Kim, T.; Braun, G.B.; She, Z.G.; Hussain, S.; Ruoslahti, E.; Sailor, M.J. Composite Porous Silicon-Silver Nanoparticles as Theranostic Antibacterial Agents. *ACS Appl. Mater. Interfaces* **2016**, *8*, 30449–30457. [CrossRef]
67. Hindi, K.M.; Ditto, A.J.; Panzner, M.J.; Medvetz, D.A.; Han, D.S.; Hovis, C.E.; Hilliard, J.K.; Taylor, J.B.; Yun, Y.H.; Cannon, C.L.; et al. The antimicrobial efficacy of sustained release silver-carbene complex-loaded L-tyrosine polyphosphate nanoparticles: Characterization, in vitro and in vivo studies. *Biomaterials* **2009**, *30*, 3771–3779. [CrossRef] [PubMed]
68. Lara, H.H.; Ayala-Núñez, N.V.; Ixtepan Turrent, L.D.C.; Rodríguez Padilla, C. Bactericidal effect of silver nanoparticles against multidrug-resistant bacteria. *World J. Microbiol. Biotechnol.* **2010**, *26*, 615–621. [CrossRef]
69. Raza, M.A.; Kanwal, Z.; Rauf, A.; Sabri, A.N.; Riaz, S.; Naseem, S. Size- and Shape-Dependent Antibacterial Studies of Silver Nanoparticles Synthesized by Wet Chemical Routes. *Nanomaterials* **2016**, *6*, 74. [CrossRef] [PubMed]
70. Tang, S.; Zheng, J. Antibacterial Activity of Silver Nanoparticles: Structural Effects. *Adv. Healthc. Mater.* **2018**, *7*, e1701503. [CrossRef] [PubMed]
71. Jinu, U.; Jayalakshmi, N.; Sujima Anbu, A.; Mahendran, D.; Sahi, S.; Venkatachalam, P. Biofabrication of Cubic Phase Silver Nanoparticles Loaded with Phytochemicals from Solanum nigrum Leaf Extracts for Potential Antibacterial, Antibiofilm and Antioxidant Activities Against MDR Human Pathogens. *J. Clust. Sci.* **2017**, *28*, 489–505. [CrossRef]
72. Gopinath, P.M.; Narchonai, G.; Dhanasekaran, D.; Ranjani, A.; Thajuddin, N. Mycosynthesis, characterization and antibacterial properties of AgNPs against multidrug resistant (MDR) bacterial pathogens of female infertility cases. *Asian J. Pharm. Sci.* **2015**, *10*, 138–145. [CrossRef]
73. Shahverdi, A.R.; Fakhimi, A.; Shahverdi, H.R.; Minaian, S. Synthesis and effect of silver nanoparticles on the antibacterial activity of different antibiotics against Staphylococcus aureus and *Escherichia coli*. *Nanomed. Nanotechnol. Biol. Med.* **2007**, *3*, 168–171. [CrossRef] [PubMed]
74. Leid, J.G.; Ditto, A.J.; Knapp, A.; Shah, P.N.; Wright, B.D.; Blust, R.; Christensen, L.; Clemons, C.B.; Wilber, J.P.; Young, G.W.; et al. In vitro antimicrobial studies of silver carbene complexes: Activity of free and nanoparticle carbene formulations against clinical isolates of pathogenic bacteria. *J. Antimicrob. Chemother.* **2012**, *67*, 138–148. [CrossRef]
75. Kaweeteerawat, C.; Na Ubol, P.; Sangmuang, S.; Aueviriyavit, S.; Maniratanachote, R. Mechanisms of antibiotic resistance in bacteria mediated by silver nanoparticles. *J. Toxicol. Environ. Health. A* **2017**, *80*, 1276–1289. [CrossRef]
76. Madhumitha, G.; Elango, G.; Roopan, S.M. Biotechnological aspects of ZnO nanoparticles: Overview on synthesis and its applications. *Appl. Microbiol. Biotechnol.* **2016**, *100*, 571–581. [CrossRef] [PubMed]
77. Ahmed, S.; Annu; Chaudhry, S.A.; Ikram, S. A review on biogenic synthesis of ZnO nanoparticles using plant extracts and microbes: A prospect towards green chemistry. *J. Photochem. Photobiol. B Biol.* **2017**, *166*, 272–284. [CrossRef]
78. Bhuyan, T.; Mishra, K.; Khanuja, M.; Prasad, R.; Varma, A. Biosynthesis of zinc oxide nanoparticles from Azadirachta indica for antibacterial and photocatalytic applications. *Mater. Sci. Semicond. Process.* **2015**, *32*, 55–61. [CrossRef]
79. Ali, K.; Dwivedi, S.; Azam, A.; Saquib, Q.; Al-Said, M.S.; Alkhedhairy, A.A.; Musarrat, J. Aloe vera extract functionalized zinc oxide nanoparticles as nanoantibiotics against multi-drug resistant clinical bacterial isolates. *J. Colloid Interface Sci.* **2016**, *472*, 145–156. [CrossRef] [PubMed]
80. Vimala, K.; Sundarraj, S.; Paulpandi, M.; Vengatesan, S.; Kannan, S. Green synthesized doxorubicin loaded zinc oxide nanoparticles regulates the Bax and Bcl-2 expression in breast and colon carcinoma. *Process. Biochem.* **2014**, *49*, 160–172. [CrossRef]

81. Jones, N.; Ray, B.; Ranjit, K.T.; Manna, A.C. Antibacterial activity of ZnO nanoparticle suspensions on a broad spectrum of microorganisms. *FEMS Microbiol. Lett.* **2008**, *279*, 71–76. [CrossRef]
82. Liu, Y.; He, L.; Mustapha, A.; Li, H.; Hu, Z.Q.; Lin, M. Antibacterial activities of zinc oxide nanoparticles against Escherichia coli O157:H7. *J. Appl. Microbiol.* **2009**, *107*, 1193–1201. [CrossRef]
83. Tiwari, V.; Mishra, N.; Gadani, K.; Solanki, P.S.; Shah, N.A.; Tiwari, M. Mechanism of Anti-bacterial Activity of Zinc Oxide Nanoparticle Against Carbapenem-Resistant Acinetobacter baumannii. *Front. Microbiol.* **2018**, *9*, 1218. [CrossRef] [PubMed]
84. Kumar, A.; Pandey, A.K.; Singh, S.S.; Shanker, R.; Dhawan, A. Engineered ZnO and TiO(2) nanoparticles induce oxidative stress and DNA damage leading to reduced viability of Escherichia coli. *Free Radic. Biol. Med.* **2011**, *51*, 1872–1881. [CrossRef] [PubMed]
85. Horie, M.; Fujita, K.; Kato, H.; Endoh, S.; Nishio, K.; Komaba, L.K.; Nakamura, A.; Miyauchi, A.; Kinugasa, S.; Hagihara, Y.; et al. Association of the physical and chemical properties and the cytotoxicity of metal oxide nanoparticles: Metal ion release, adsorption ability and specific surface area. *Metall. Integr. Biomet. Sci.* **2012**, *4*, 350–360. [CrossRef] [PubMed]
86. McDevitt, C.A.; Ogunniyi, A.D.; Valkov, E.; Lawrence, M.C.; Kobe, B.; McEwan, A.G.; Paton, J.C. A molecular mechanism for bacterial susceptibility to zinc. *PLoS Pathog.* **2011**, *7*, e1002357. [CrossRef] [PubMed]
87. Li, M.; Zhu, L.; Lin, D. Toxicity of ZnO nanoparticles to Escherichia coli: Mechanism and the influence of medium components. *Environ. Sci. Technol.* **2011**, *45*, 1977–1983. [CrossRef] [PubMed]
88. El-Batal, A.I.; El-Sayyad, G.S.; El-Ghamery, A.; Gobara, M. Response Surface Methodology Optimization of Melanin Production by Streptomyces cyaneus and Synthesis of Copper Oxide Nanoparticles Using Gamma Radiation. *J. Clust. Sci.* **2017**, *28*, 1083–1112. [CrossRef]
89. Singh, B.P.; Jena, B.K.; Bhattacharjee, S.; Besra, L. Development of oxidation and corrosion resistance hydrophobic graphene oxide-polymer composite coating on copper. *Surf. Coat. Technol.* **2013**, *232*, 475–481. [CrossRef]
90. El-Batal, A.I.; Al-Hazmi, N.E.; Mosallam, F.M.; El-Sayyad, G.S. Biogenic synthesis of copper nanoparticles by natural polysaccharides and Pleurotus ostreatus fermented fenugreek using gamma rays with antioxidant and antimicrobial potential towards some wound pathogens. *Microb. Pathog.* **2018**, *118*, 159–169. [CrossRef] [PubMed]
91. Hoshino, N.; Kimura, T.; Yamaji, A.; Ando, T. Damage to the cytoplasmic membrane of *Escherichia coli* by catechin-copper (II) complexes. *Free Radic. Biol. Med.* **1999**, *27*, 1245–1250. [CrossRef]
92. Bogdanović, U.; Lazić, V.; Vodnik, V.; Budimir, M.; Marković, Z.; Dimitrijević, S. Copper nanoparticles with high antimicrobial activity. *Mater. Lett.* **2014**, *128*, 75–78. [CrossRef]
93. DeAlba-Montero, I.; Guajardo-Pacheco, J.; Morales-Sanchez, E.; Araujo-Martinez, R.; Loredo-Becerra, G.M.; Martinez-Castanon, G.A.; Ruiz, F.; Compean Jasso, M.E. Antimicrobial Properties of Copper Nanoparticles and Amino Acid Chelated Copper Nanoparticles Produced by Using a Soya Extract. *Bioinorg. Chem. Appl.* **2017**, *2017*, 1064918. [CrossRef]
94. Borkow, G.; Gabbay, J. Putting copper into action: Copper-impregnated products with potent biocidal activities. *FASEB J. Official Publ. Fed. Am. Soc. Exp. Biol.* **2004**, *18*, 1728–1730. [CrossRef]
95. Hostynek, J.J.; Maibach, H.I. Copper hypersensitivity: Dermatologic aspects—An overview. *Rev. Environ. Health* **2003**, *18*, 153–183. [CrossRef]
96. Vamathevan, V.; Amal, R.; Beydoun, D.; Low, G.; McEvoy, S. Photocatalytic oxidation of organics in water using pure and silver-modified titanium dioxide particles. *J. Photochem. Photobiol. A Chem.* **2002**, *148*, 233–245. [CrossRef]
97. Varghese, O.K.; Gong, D.; Paulose, M.; Ong, K.G.; Grimes, C.A. Hydrogen sensing using titania nanotubes. *Sens. Actuators B Chem.* **2003**, *93*, 338–344. [CrossRef]
98. Zhou, H.; Gan, X.; Wang, J.; Zhu, X.; Li, G. Hemoglobin-based hydrogen peroxide biosensor tuned by the photovoltaic effect of nano titanium dioxide. *Anal. Chem* **2005**, *77*, 6102–6104. [CrossRef] [PubMed]
99. Zhang, J.; Li, S.; Ding, H.; Li, Q.; Wang, B.; Wang, X.; Wang, H. Transfer and assembly of large area TiO$_2$ nanotube arrays onto conductive glass for dye sensitized solar cells. *J. Power Sources* **2014**, *247*, 807–812. [CrossRef]
100. Kirillin, M.; Shirmanova, M.; Sirotkina, M.; Bugrova, M.; Khlebtsov, B.; Zagaynova, E. Contrasting properties of gold nanoshells and titanium dioxide nanoparticles for optical coherence tomography imaging of skin: Monte Carlo simulations and in vivo study. *J. Biomed. Opt.* **2009**, *14*, 021017. [CrossRef] [PubMed]

101. Chen, X.; Mao, S.S. Titanium dioxide nanomaterials: Synthesis, properties, modifications, and applications. *Chem. Rev.* **2007**, *107*, 2891–2959. [CrossRef]
102. Mali, S.S.; Betty, C.A.; Bhosale, P.N.; Patil, P.S. Hydrothermal synthesis of rutile TiO$_2$ with hierarchical microspheres and their characterization. *CrystEngComm* **2011**, *13*, 6349–6351. [CrossRef]
103. Sankar, R.; Rizwana, K.; Shivashangari, K.S.; Ravikumar, V. Ultra-rapid photocatalytic activity of *Azadirachta indica* engineered colloidal titanium dioxide nanoparticles. *Appl. Nanosci.* **2015**, *5*, 731–736. [CrossRef]
104. Rajakumar, G.; Rahuman, A.A.; Roopan, S.M.; Khanna, V.G.; Elango, G.; Kamaraj, C.; Zahir, A.A.; Velayutham, K. Fungus-mediated biosynthesis and characterization of TiO$_2$ nanoparticles and their activity against pathogenic bacteria. *Spectrochim. Acta A Mol. Biomol. Spectrosc.* **2012**, *91*, 23–29. [CrossRef]
105. Hunagund, S.M.; Desai, V.R.; Kadadevarmath, J.S.; Barretto, D.A.; Vootla, S.; Sidarai, A.H. Biogenic and chemogenic synthesis of TiO$_2$ NPs via hydrothermal route and their antibacterial activities. *RSC Adv.* **2016**, *6*, 97438–97444. [CrossRef]
106. Foster, H.A.; Ditta, I.B.; Varghese, S.; Steele, A. Photocatalytic disinfection using titanium dioxide: Spectrum and mechanism of antimicrobial activity. *Appl. Microbiol. Biotechnol.* **2011**, *90*, 1847–1868. [CrossRef] [PubMed]
107. Li, Y.; Zhang, W.; Niu, J.; Chen, Y. Mechanism of photogenerated reactive oxygen species and correlation with the antibacterial properties of engineered metal-oxide nanoparticles. *ACS Nano* **2012**, *6*, 5164–5173. [CrossRef]
108. Leung, Y.H.; Ng, A.M.; Xu, X.; Shen, Z.; Gethings, L.A.; Wong, M.T.; Chan, C.M.; Guo, M.Y.; Ng, Y.H.; Djurisic, A.B.; et al. Mechanisms of antibacterial activity of MgO: Non-ROS mediated toxicity of MgO nanoparticles towards *Escherichia coli*. *Small* **2014**, *10*, 1171–1183. [CrossRef] [PubMed]
109. Singh, P.; Pandit, S.; Mokkapati, V.; Garg, A.; Ravikumar, V.; Mijakovic, I. Gold Nanoparticles in Diagnostics and Therapeutics for Human Cancer. *Int. J. Mol. Sci.* **2018**, *19*, 1979. [CrossRef] [PubMed]
110. Singh, K.; Panghal, M.; Kadyan, S.; Chaudhary, U.; Yadav, J.P. Green silver nanoparticles of *Phyllanthus amarus*: As an antibacterial agent against multi drug resistant clinical isolates of *Pseudomonas aeruginosa*. *J. NanoBiotechnol.* **2014**, *12*, 40. [CrossRef]
111. Ordenes-Aenishanslins, N.A.; Saona, L.A.; Duran-Toro, V.M.; Monras, J.P.; Bravo, D.M.; Perez-Donoso, J.M. Use of titanium dioxide nanoparticles biosynthesized by Bacillus mycoides in quantum dot sensitized solar cells. *Microb. Cell Fact.* **2014**, *13*, 90. [CrossRef]
112. Korbekandi, H.; Iravani, S.; Abbasi, S. Production of nanoparticles using organisms. *Crit. Rev. Biotechnol.* **2009**, *29*, 279–306. [CrossRef]
113. Velayutham, K.; Rahuman, A.A.; Rajakumar, G.; Santhoshkumar, T.; Marimuthu, S.; Jayaseelan, C.; Bagavan, A.; Kirthi, A.V.; Kamaraj, C.; Zahir, A.A.; et al. Evaluation of Catharanthus roseus leaf extract-mediated biosynthesis of titanium dioxide nanoparticles against *Hippobosca maculata* and *Bovicola ovis*. *Parasitol. Res.* **2012**, *111*, 2329–2337. [CrossRef]
114. Choi, O.; Deng, K.K.; Kim, N.J.; Ross, L., Jr.; Surampalli, R.Y.; Hu, Z. The inhibitory effects of silver nanoparticles, silver ions, and silver chloride colloids on microbial growth. *Water Res.* **2008**, *42*, 3066–3074. [CrossRef]
115. Chaloupka, K.; Malam, Y.; Seifalian, A.M. Nanosilver as a new generation of nanoproduct in biomedical applications. *Trends Biotechnol.* **2010**, *28*, 580–588. [CrossRef]
116. Liu, H.L.; Dai, S.A.; Fu, K.Y.; Hsu, S.H. Antibacterial properties of silver nanoparticles in three different sizes and their nanocomposites with a new waterborne polyurethane. *Int. J. Nanomed.* **2010**, *5*, 1017–1028.
117. Samadi, N.; Golkaran, D.; Eslamifar, A.; Jamalifar, H.; Fazeli, M.R.; Mohseni, F.A. Intra/extracellular biosynthesis of silver nanoparticles by an autochthonous strain of Proteus mirabilis isolated from photographic waste. *J. Biomed. Nanotechnol.* **2009**, *5*, 247–253. [CrossRef] [PubMed]
118. Mirzajani, F.; Ghassempour, A.; Aliahmadi, A.; Esmaeili, M.A. Antibacterial effect of silver nanoparticles on Staphylococcus aureus. *Res. Microbiol.* **2011**, *162*, 542–549. [CrossRef] [PubMed]
119. Lok, C.N.; Ho, C.M.; Chen, R.; He, Q.Y.; Yu, W.Y.; Sun, H.; Tam, P.K.; Chiu, J.F.; Che, C.M. Proteomic analysis of the mode of antibacterial action of silver nanoparticles. *J. Proteome Res.* **2006**, *5*, 916–924. [CrossRef] [PubMed]

120. Jung, W.K.; Koo, H.C.; Kim, K.W.; Shin, S.; Kim, S.H.; Park, Y.H. Antibacterial activity and mechanism of action of the silver ion in Staphylococcus aureus and *Escherichia coli*. *Appl. Environ. Microbiol.* **2008**, *74*, 2171–2178. [CrossRef] [PubMed]
121. Schreurs, W.J.; Rosenberg, H. Effect of silver ions on transport and retention of phosphate by *Escherichia coli*. *J. Bacteriol.* **1982**, *152*, 7–13. [PubMed]
122. Apte, M.; Sambre, D.; Gaikawad, S.; Joshi, S.; Bankar, A.; Kumar, A.R.; Zinjarde, S. Psychrotrophic yeast *Yarrowia lipolytica* NCYC 789 mediates the synthesis of antimicrobial silver nanoparticles via cell-associated melanin. *AMB Express* **2013**, *3*, 32. [CrossRef]

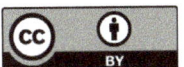

© 2018 by the authors. Licensee MDPI, Basel, Switzerland. This article is an open access article distributed under the terms and conditions of the Creative Commons Attribution (CC BY) license (http://creativecommons.org/licenses/by/4.0/).

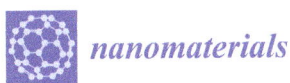

Article

Biosynthesis of Silver Nanoparticles from Oropharyngeal *Candida glabrata* Isolates and Their Antimicrobial Activity against Clinical Strains of Bacteria and Fungi

Mohammad Jalal [1,*,†], Mohammad Azam Ansari [2,*,†], Mohammad A. Alzohairy [3], Syed Ghazanfar Ali [1,†], Haris M. Khan [1], Ahmad Almatroudi [3] and Kashif Raees [4]

1. Department of Microbiology, Jawaharlal Nehru Medical College and Hospital, Aligarh Muslim University, Aligarh 202002, India; syedmicro72@gmail.com (S.G.A.); harismk2003@hotmail.com (H.M.K.)
2. Department of Epidemic Disease Research, Institutes of Research and Medical Consultations (IRMC), Imam Abdulrahman Bin Faisal University, 31441 Dammam, Saudi Arabia
3. Department of Medical Laboratories, College of applied Medical sciences, Qassim University, Qassim 51431, Saudi Arabia; dr.alzohairy@gmail.com (M.A.A.); aamtrody@qu.edu.sa (A.A.)
4. Department of Applied Chemistry, Aligarh Muslim University, Aligarh 202002, India; raeeskashif@gmail.com
* Correspondence: jalalmicro@gmail.com (M.J.); maansari@iau.edu.sa (M.A.A.); Tel.: +91-879-102-668 (M.J.); +966-534-889-655 (M.A.A.)
† These authors contributed equally to this work.

Received: 5 July 2018; Accepted: 20 July 2018; Published: 1 August 2018

Abstract: The objective of the present study was one step extracellular biosynthesis of silver nanoparticles (AgNPs) using supernatant of *Candida glabrata* isolated from oropharyngeal mucosa of human immunodeficiency virus (HIV) patients and evaluation of their antibacterial and antifungal potential against human pathogenic bacteria and fungi. The mycosynthesized AgNPs were characterized by color visualization, ultraviolet-visible (UV) spectroscopy, fourier transform infrared spectroscopy (FTIR), and transmission electron microscopy (TEM). The FTIR spectra revealed the binding and stabilization of nanoparticles with protein. The TEM analysis showed that nanoparticles were well dispersed and predominantly spherical in shape within the size range of 2–15 nm. The antibacterial and antifungal potential of AgNPs were characterized by determining minimum inhibitory concentration (MIC), minimum bactericidal concentration (MBC)/ minimum fungicidal concentration (MFC), and well diffusion methods. The MBC and MFC were found in the range of 62.5–250 µg/mL and 125–500 µg/mL, which revealed that bacterial strains were more susceptible to AgNPs than fungal strains. These differences in bactericidal and fungicidal concentrations of the AgNPs were due to the differences in the cell structure and organization of bacteria and yeast cells. The interaction of AgNPs with *C. albicans* analyzed by TEM showed the penetration of nanoparticles inside the *Candida* cells, which led the formation of "pits" and "pores" that result from the rupturing of the cell wall and membrane. Further, TEM analysis showed that *Candida* cells treated with AgNPs were highly deformed and the cells had shrunken to a greater extent because of their interaction with the fungal cell wall and membrane, which disrupted the structure of the cell membrane and inhibited the normal budding process due to the destruction and loss of membrane integrity and formation of pores that may led to the cell death.

Keywords: *Candida glabrata*; extracellular; mycosynthesis; MIC; MBC; MFC; membrane integrity; TEM; FTIR

1. Introduction

It is worthy to state that the 21st century is the golden era of silver nanotechnology because silver-based materials and silver nanoparticles (AgNPs) are used in textile engineering, waste water treatment and purification, optics, electronics, pharmaceutical industry, as catalysts, optical sensors, and in the medical field as bactericidal, fungicidal, larvicidal, therapeutic, diagnostic, and anticancer agents, in wound dressings, and imaging, etc. [1]. Silver-based materials and AgNPs are also used in the coatings of medical devices, formulation of dental resin composites, coating on water filters, as topical creams to prevent wound infections, as a microbiocidal agent in air sanitizer sprays, respirators, pillows, soaps, laundry detergents, shampoos, socks, wet wipes, washing machines, wall paints, toothpastes, etc. [1–3].

Due to the broad application of AgNPs in various fields, as mentioned above, the demand for large-scale, eco-friendly, non-hazardous, faster, and biocompatible production of AgNPs with specific size, shape, and properties have also been increased. AgNPs can be prepared either by physical, chemical, or biological approaches. The synthesis of AgNPs by physical and chemical methods usually requires expensive equipment, high pressure and temperature, stabilizers, and toxic reducing reagents.

The green routes of synthesis of AgNPs by exploring plant parts and microorganisms, such as bacteria, fungi, algae, etc., has advantages over physical and chemical methods as green approaches are environmentally-friendly, cost-effective, fast, pollution-free, and most importantly, provides non-toxic and biocompatible natural reducing and stabilizing agents. Biosynthesis of AgNPs using various species of filamentous fungi, such as species of *Aspergillus*, *Penicillium*, *Fusarium*, *Trichoderma*, *Verticillium*, *Rhizopus*, *Colletotrichum*, and *Neurospora*, have been well studied and documented [4,5]. Nevertheless, reports on biosynthesis of AgNPs using single-celled yeasts remains limited and a few yeast species, such as yeast strain MKY3 [6], *Saccharomyces boulardii* [7], *S. cerevisiae* [8], *Candida albicans* [9,10], *Candida utilis* [11], and *Candida lusitaniae* [5] have been reported.

Yeast has been chosen for the extracellular biosynthesis of AgNPs because of their better tolerance and metal bioaccumulation property, large scale production, economic viability, convenient downstream processing, and most importantly, fungi produces huge amounts of proteins and enzymes that acts as reducing and stabilizing agents [3,12–14].

The aims of the present work was to achieve: (i) extracellular mycosynthesis of AgNPs using the supernatant of *Candida glabrata* for the first time as reducing and stabilizing agents; (ii) the characterization of mycosynthesized AgNPs using a ultraviolet- visible (UV-Vis) spectrophotometer, fourier transform infrared (FTIR), and transmission electron microscopy (TEM); (iii) the assessment of antibacterial and anticandidal activity of mycosynthesized AgNPs against *Escherichia coli*, *Salmonella typhimurium*, *Klebsiella pneomonaie*, *Shigella flexneri*, *Pseudomonas aeruginosa*, *Staphylococcus aureus*, *C. albicans*, *C. dubliniensis*, *C. parapsilosis*, *C. tropicalis*, *C. krusei*, and *C. glabrata* using agar well diffusion and standard microdilution methods by determining minimum inhibitory concentration (MIC), minimum bactericidal concentration (MBC), and minimum fungicidal concentration (MFC); and (iv) the investigation of a mode of action of AgNPs against *C. albicans* using transmission lectron microscopy (TEM).

2. Materials and Method

2.1. Preparation of Candida Glabrata Supernatant for the Synthesis of Silver Nanoparticles

Candida glabrata were isolated from the oropharyngeal mucosa of patients having oral candidiasis by using a sterile cotton swab. The swabs were then dipped into 5 mL of Sabouraud dextrose broth (SDB) (HiMedia, Mumbai, India) and then 0.1 mL of culture was spread homogenously onto the HiCHROM differential agar (HiMedia, Mumbai India) plates at 37 °C for 48 h. *Candida* spp. were identified by morphology on corn meal agar (CMA), sugar assimilation (SAT), HiCrome agar, and a germ tube test [15]. *C. glabrata* isolates developed characteristic cream to white colonies, whereas *C. albicans* isolates formed light-green colonies. Further, trehalase and maltase tests were performed to confirm the *C. glabrata* isolates [16]. One to two pure colonies of fresh *C. glabrata* cultures were again suspended into 500 mL SDB and incubated for 48–72 h at 28 °C. After incubation, the culture was centrifuged at 12,000 rpm for 10 min and the supernatant was collected and stored at 4 °C for the synthesis of AgNPs. All media was purchased from HiMedia, Mumbai, India.

2.2. Extracellular Mycosynthesis, Sepration and Purification of AgNPs

For the biosynthesis of AgNPs, 20 mL of collected supernatant was added in 1 mM of silver nitrate and then the solution was kept at room temperature overnight. The reduction of silver nitrate into AgNPs showed a change in color of silver nitrate from colorless to brown, which is an indication of the formation of AgNPs. Further, the synthesized AgNPs were separated and isolated by ultracentrifugation as previously described with slight modification [17,18]. To remove excess, unreduced silver ions and other possible impurities from the supernatant, the reaction mixture containing NPs were centrifuged at 14,000 rpm for 20 min with Milli-Q water. The process of centrifugation was repeated at least four times to ensure a better separation of NPs [17]. The particles separated were then resuspended again in ethanol and then centrifugation was further repeated three times [19]. A dark sediment was formed at the bottom of the centrifugal tube. After that, a dried powder of the AgNPs was obtained by freeze-drying [18], and their characterization was performed.

2.3. Characterization of Silver Nanoparticles

The biosynthesized AgNPs were preliminarily characterized by visual observation of the color change of the reaction mixture and then by measuring the absorbance of the colloidal suspension before and after the isolation NPs from the supernatant using UV-Vis spectrophotometer (Perkin-Elmer Lambda 25, Shelton, CT, USA). The preparation of samples for absorbance was accomplished as described in our previous work [20]. Briefly, AgNPs were subjected to mild sonication for 20 min, after which the UV-Vis spectra of AgNPs was monitored in the range of 270–700 nm. Distilled water was used to adjust the baseline [20]. Further, to confirm the presence of protein in the supernatant and their possible role in synthesis and reduction of $AgNO_3$ was carried out by a simple protein-dye binding assay, i.e., Bradford assay (Figure A1). The functional group present in the supernatant that was responsible for the synthesis of AgNPs was analyzed by FTIR (SHIMADZU-8400 spectrometer, Tokyo, Japan) in the range of 400 to 4000/cm. Further, the surface morphology, shape, and size of synthesized AgNPs were characterized by transmission electron microscopy (Joel 2100, Tokyo, Japan).

2.4. Tested Microorganisms

The clinical isolates of fungal and bacterial species, i.e., *C. albicans*, *C. tropicalis*, *C. parapsilosis*, *C. dubliniensis*, *C. krusei*, *C. glabrata*, *S. aureus*, *E. coli*, *P. aeruginosa*, *K. pneomonaie*, *S. typhimurium*, and *S. flexneri* isolated from the oropharyngeal mucosa of the patients used in this study were obtained from the Department of Microbiology, Jawaharlal Nehru Medical College and Hospital, Aligarh Muslim University, India.

2.5. Evaluation of Antimicrobial Activity of Mycosynthesized AgNPs Using a Diffusion Method

The antimicrobial activity of as-synthesized AgNPs against various bacterial isolates, e.g., *S. aureus*, *E. coli*, *S. typhimurium*, *S. flexneri*, *K. pneomonaie*, *P. aeruginosa*, and *Candida* spp., e.g., *C. albicans*, *C. dubliniensis*, *C. parapsilosis*, *C. tropicalis*, *C. krusei*, and *C. glabrata* were examined using a well diffusion method as previously reported [17]. Briefly, a 6 mm diameter well was made on Nutrient and Sabouraud dextrose agar plates previously inoculated with 100 μL of 1×10^6 bacterial and fungal suspension, and then varying concentrations of AgNPs were aseptically filled in the well. The plates were subsequently incubated at 37 °C (Bacteria) and 28 °C (*Candida* spp.) for 24 h, and the antimicrobial activity was analyzed by measuring the diameter of the inhibition zone (mm) around the well.

2.6. Assessment of Antimicrobial Activity of AgNPs by Determining MIC and MBC/MFC

Minimal inhibitory concentration (MIC): The MIC values of mycosynthesized AgNPs against bacterial and *Candida* isolates were assessed using the method described by Ansari et al. [21].

Minimal bactericidal and fungicidal concentration (MBC/MFC): Further, MBC and MFC values of AgNPs against all tested bacteria and *Candida* spp. was examined using a method described in References [17,21].

2.7. Ultrastructural Morphological Changes Caused by AgNPs in C. albicans: TEM Analysis

The morphological and ultrastructure alteration caused by AgNPs in *C. albicans* cells were examined by using transmission electron microscope. The sample preparation and analysis procedures were similar to those described in our previous research work [17].

3. Results and Discussion

3.1. Characterization of Biosynthesized AgNPs

In the present study, *C. glabrata* supernatant was used for the synthesis of AgNPs. After the addition of *C. glabrata* supernatant with 1 mM aqueous solution of silver nitrate, a brownish color was observed, which indicated the extracellular biosynthesis of AgNPs (Figure 1). Previously, it has been reported that the reduction of Ag^+ into AgNPs can be seen very clearly when the color of the solution changes from colorless to brown due to the surface plasmon resonance [6]. Figure 2 shows the UV-Vis spectroscopy of the as-prepared AgNPs in the range of 270–700 nm and a single strong peak was observed at 460.64 nm, which is the characteristic of AgNPs. Bhat et al. [10] reported that the absorption line of biosynthesized AgNPs was 430 nm when the silver nitrate solution was challenged with *C. albicans*.

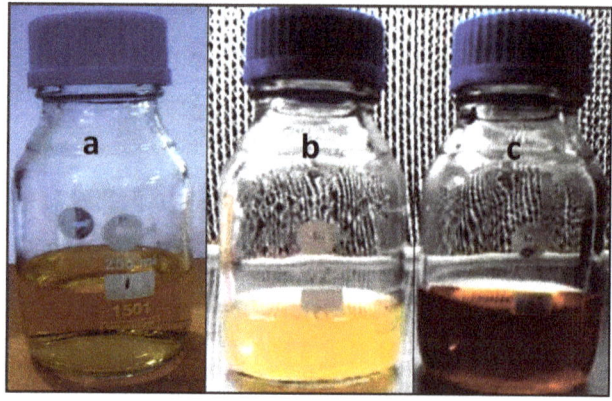

Figure 1. Biosynthesis of AgNPs using an extracellular filtrate of *C. glabrata* after 12 h at room temperature in dark conditions. (**a**) Sterile Sabouraud dextrose broth with $AgNO_3$; (**b**) Cell filtrate without $AgNO_3$; (**c**) Cell filtrate with $AgNO_3$.

FTIR analysis was performed to identify the potential biomolecules and functional groups responsible for the reduction of silver ions to Ag^0 and stabilization of AgNPs [22]. Figure 3 shows a strong absorption line at 3436.03 cm^{-1}, which corresponds to the –OH groups that could arise from carbohydrates present in the supernatant, and the peak at 1636.17 cm^{-1} is due to amides (C–O stretch), i.e., characteristic of the presence of protein and enzymes in the supernatant that confirm the extracellular formation of AgNPs [23]. The peak at 661 cm^{-1} corresponds to C–H (alkane) and C=H bonding (alkene). In a previous study, Bhat et al. [10] found that the protein biomolecules present in the extract of *C. albicans* bind to the synthesized nanoparticles either by free amino or carboxyl groups, and the released extracellular proteins could possibility stabilize the biosynthesized AgNPs.

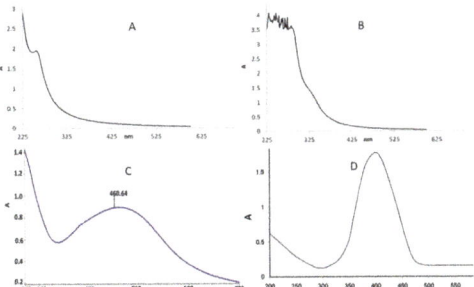

Figure 2. (**A**) UV-visible spectra of 1 mM AgNO$_3$; (**B**) *C. glabrata* supernatant before the addition of AgNO$_3$; (**C**) after addition AgNO$_3$ (biosynthesized AgNPs); and (**D**) commercially available spectra of AgNPs of known size, i.e., 5–16 nm [20].

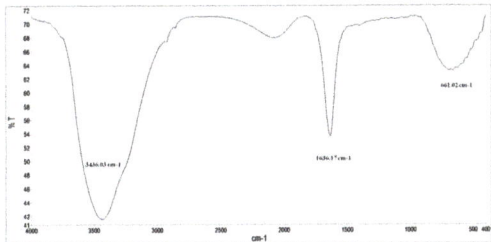

Figure 3. FTIR spectra of AgNPs synthesized by the *C. glabrata* supernatant.

The mechanism of biosynthesis of AgNPs using microorganisms are well understood. It was reported that the biomass or supernatant of microorganisms possibly act as bioreductant and capping agents due to the presence of biomolecules such as proteins, amino acids, enzymes, vitamins, and polysaccharides [10,23]. However, the most widely accepted mechanism for the biosynthesis of AgNPs and other nanoparticles using microbes is mainly due to the presence of enzyme Nicotinamide adenine dinucleotide (NADH) and NADH-dependent nitrate reductase [24–26]. The role of nitrate reductase in the synthesis of AgNPs has been demonstrated by exploring the purified nitrate reductase in vitro for the synthesis of AgNPs and it was found that the reduction of silver ions happens by means of the transfer of electrons from NADH where enzyme NADH-dependent reductase acts as a carrier [24–26].

The TEM micrograph of as-prepared AgNPs exhibited that the synthesized AgNPs were predominantly spherical and oval, well-dispersed, and uniform with a size range of 2–15 nm (Figure 4). Niknejad et al. [8] reported biosynthesis of AgNPs using the yeast *S. cerevisiae* and they found that AgNPs were mainly spherical and polydispersed within the size of 5–20 nm. The size of AgNPs obtained in our study was much smaller than AgNPs synthesized from *Candida utilis*, where the size was 20–80 nm [11]. The image shows both individual and aggregated AgNPs (Figure 4). The particles were well-dispersed and not in direct contact due to capping and stabilization of AgNPs by the proteins around the periphery of the nanoparticles (Figure 4), which further confer the involvement of extracellular proteins and enzymes secreted by *C. glabrata* in the supernatant that acted as reducing and capping agents [22].

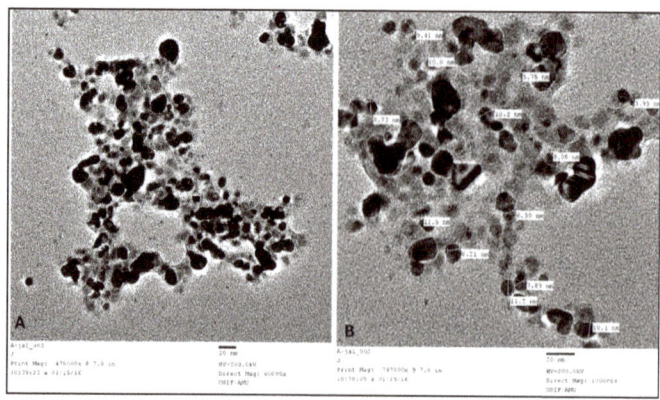

Figure 4. TEM images of AgNPs synthesized by *C. glabrata* supernatant. (**A**): At lower magnification (60,000×); (**B**): at higher magnification (100,000×).

3.2. Antimicrobial Activity of Biosynthesized AgNPs

Antimicrobial activity of biosynthesized AgNPs against human pathogenic microorganisms, i.e., *Candidal* spp. and bacterial spp. was evaluated by agar well diffusion and two-fold microdilution methods. A zone of inhibition test of mycosynthesized AgNPs against tested bacteria and *Candida* spp. at different concentrations are shown in Figures 5 and 6, and it was very clear that AgNPs had an excellent inhibition zone against all strains. The inhibition zone diameter showed that AgNPs were more effective against bacterial strains in comparison to fungi (Figures 5 and 6). No antimicrobial activity has been observed by the *C. glabrata* supernatant. Further, the antimicrobial properties of AgNPs against various bacterial and fungal strains were examined by determining the MIC, MBC, and MFC. The MIC and MBC values for all tested bacterial strains were found in the range of 31.25–125 µg/mL and 62.5–250 µg/mL, respectively (Table 1), whereas the MIC and MFC values for fungal strain was in the range of 62.5–250 µg/mL and 125–500 µg/mL, respectively (Table 2). It was found that AgNPs were bactericidal at low concentration (62.5–250 µg/mL) and fungicidal at high concentration (125–500 µg/mL), which revealed that bacterial strains were more susceptible to AgNPs than fungal strains. In general, it was found that gram-negative and gram-positive bacterial strains showed better antimicrobial activity when compared to fungi *Candida* spp. (Tables 1 and 2). These differences in bactericidal and fungicidal concentrations of the AgNPs were due to the differences in the cell structure and organization of the bacteria and yeast cells. The bacterial cell structure is less complex and they are evolutionarily prokaryotic types, and were therefore unable to fight the toxic effects of AgNPs as effectively as the eukaryotic yeast cells that can resist higher concentrations of AgNPs because of their better cell organization and much more complex structure, and superior detoxification system [27].

Table 1. MIC and MBC values of biosynthesized AgNPs against bacterial strains.

Bacterial Isolates	MIC (µg/mL)	MBC (µg/mL)
Staphylococcus aureus	31	62
Escherichia coli	31	62
Pseudomonas aeruginosa	62	125
Klebsiella pneomonaie	62	125
Salmonella typhimurium	125	250
Shigella flexneri	62	125

Table 2. MIC and MFC values of biosynthesized AgNPs against *Candida strains*.

Fungal Isolates	MIC (µg/mL)	MFC (µg/mL)
Candia albicans	62	125
Candida tropicalis	250	500
Candida parapsilosis	250	500
Candida dubliniensis	125	250
Candida krusei	125	250
Candida glabrata	250	500

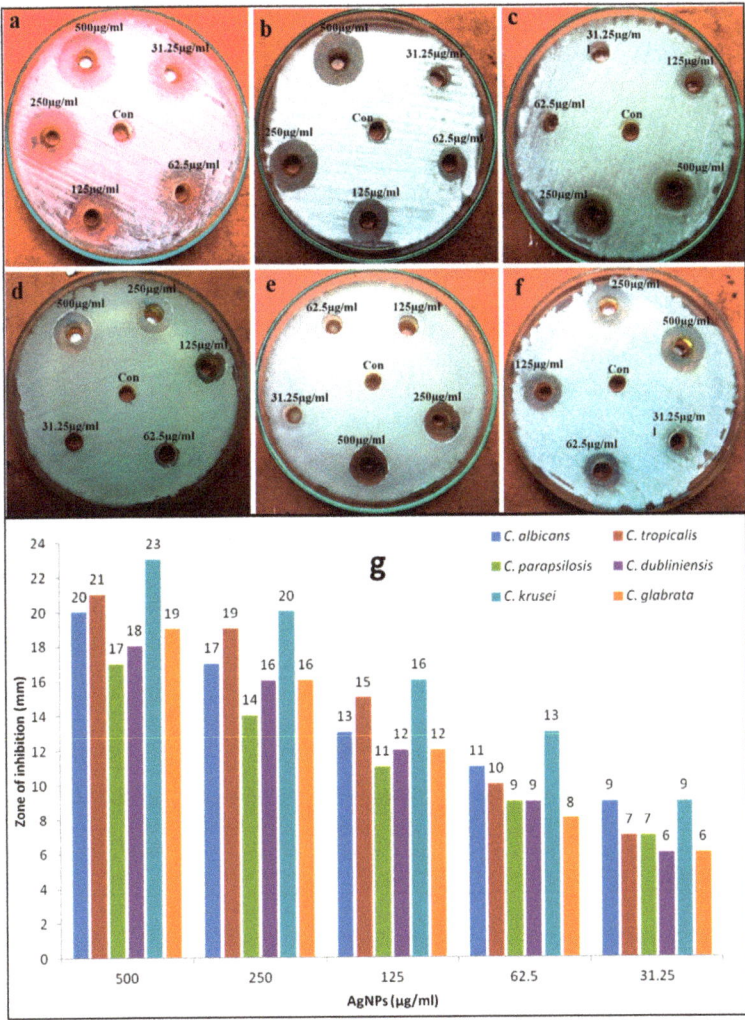

Figure 5. Anticandidal activity of mycosynthesized AgNPs at different concentrations evaluated by agar well diffusion method against different Candida spp.: (**a**) *C. albicans*, (**b**) *C. tropicalis*, (**c**) *C. dubliniensis*, (**d**) *C. glabrata*, (**e**) *C. parapsilosis*, and (**f**) *C. krusei*. Panel (**g**) represents the zone of inhibition (in mm) at different concentrations of AgNPs.

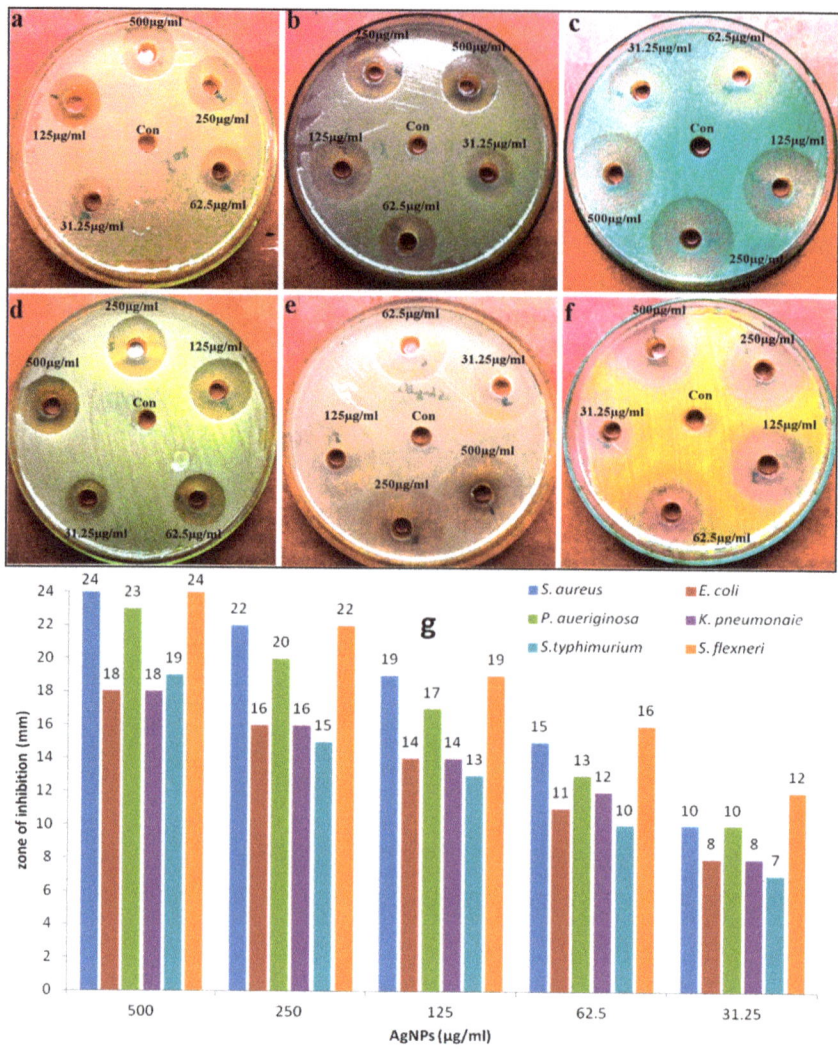

Figure 6. Antibacterial activity of mycosynthesized AgNPs at different concentrations evaluated by agar well diffusion method against different pathogenic bacteria: (**a**) *E. coli*, (**b**) *K. pneomonaie*, (**c**) *P. aeruginosa*, (**d**) *S. typhimurium*, (**e**) *S. flexneri*, and (**f**) *S. aureus*. Panel (**g**) represents the zone of inhibition (in mm) at different concentrations of AgNPs.

3.3. Ultrastructural Changes in C. albicans after Exposure to AgNPs: TEM Analysis

The morphological alteration after exposure to biosynthesized AgNPs in *C. albicans* was investigated using a transmission electron microscope. TEM analysis clearly showed that the untreated *C. albicans* exhibited a normal and well-conserved cell wall that was mainly composed of an outer layer, an intermediate space, and a thin innermost layer of the cell membrane (Figure 7a). However, the *Candida* cells after the AgNP treatment showed an aberrant morphological structure and severe damage that was characterized by the formation of "pits" and "pores" that result in the rupturing of the cell wall and membrane (Figure 7b,c). *Candida* cells treated with AgNPs were highly deformed and the cells had shrunken to a great extent (Figure 7b,c). Further, it was observed that the damaged cells exhibited either complete or localized separation of the membrane from the cell wall (Figure 7b,c). Nasrollahi et al. [28] reported that the antifungal activity of AgNPs was due to the formation of "pits" and "pores" on the surfaces of *C. albicans* and *S. cerevisiae* cells that led to the cell death. It has been observed that AgNPs not only anchor to cells at several sites (Figure 7b,c; black arrows), but they penetrate inside the cells (Figure 7c; red arrows), which could result in cell lysis. In their study, Vazquez-Muñoz et al. found that AgNPs were non-specifically distributed in different regions of the cytoplasm and cell wall, and the mode of action of AgNPs was due to the releasing of silver ions that induced cell death [29]. In the present study, it was observed that the rupturing, disintegration, and detachment of the cell wall and membrane from the cells led to the death of *C. albicans* (Figure 7b,c). Kim et al. found that AgNPs exert an antifungal activity because of their interaction with the fungal cell wall and membrane, which disrupts the structure of the cell membrane and inhibits the normal budding process due to the destruction and loss of membrane integrity, and due to the formation of pores that may led to the cell death [30]. Ishida et al. [31] also reported a similar mode of action of AgNPs against yeast *Cryptococcus neoformans* where they found that the antifungal activity of AgNPs was due to the disruption of the cell wall and cytoplasmic membrane [31]. Hwang et al. [32] found that AgNPs exert an antifungal activity against *C. albicans* due to the production and accumulation of reactive oxygen species (ROS) and free hydroxyl radicals (•OH) inside the cells, which regulates and induces the cell death through mitochondrial dysfunctional apoptosis, release of cytochrome *c*, nuclear fragmentation, DNA damage, and the activation of metacaspases [32].

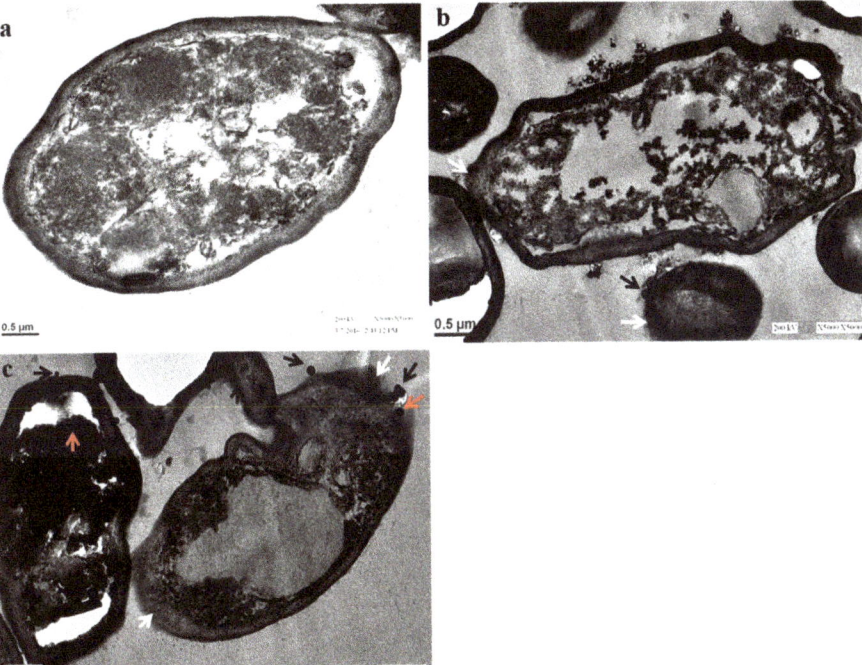

Figure 7. TEM images of *C. albicans*. (**a**) Untreated control cells; (**b**,**c**) Cells treated with 250 μg/mL and 500 μg/mL of AgNPs showing the attachment (black arrows) and penetration of AgNPs inside the cells (red arrows), degradation, destruction, and separation of the outer-most layers of the cell wall and cytoplasmic membrane (white arrows).

4. Conclusions

In this present study, a simple, one-step, safe, rapid, pollutant free, cost-effective, and ecofriendly extracellular silver nanoparticles were prepared using the supernatant of yeast *C. glabrata* as reducing and stabilizing agents for the first time. The synthesized nanoparticles were characterized by UV-visible, TEM, and FTIR spectra. Extracellular synthesis of AgNPs by yeast, i.e., *C. glabrate*, has advantages over mycelium fungi because separation of the particles is much easier and simpler, takes less time without much sophistication, and therefore, extracellular synthesis of AgNPs has importance from the point of view of large-scale production in an environmentally-friendly approach. The extracellular mycosynthesized AgNPs showed excellent antibacterial and antifungal activity against gram-negative and gram-positive pathogenic bacteria and *Candida* spp., respectively. Further, the interaction of AgNPs with *C. albicans* studied by TEM showed the primary attachment and penetration of nanoparticles inside the *Candida* cell that caused the rupturing, disintegration, and detachment of the cell wall and membrane from the cells that led to the death of *C. albicans*. Thus, these mycosynthesized AgNPs may lead to the development of appropriate pharmaceuticals and represent an alternative remedy for the treatment of bacterial and fungal infections, but this needs further in vivo cytotoxic studies before being brought into the market.

Author Contributions: M.A.A. (Mohammad Azam Ansari) and H.M.K. conceived and designed the experiments; M.J. performed the experiments; M.A.A. (Mohammad Azam Ansari) and M.A.A. (Mohammad A. Alzohairy) analyzed the data; H.M.K., S.G.A., A.A. and K.R. contributed reagents/materials/analysis tools; M.A.A. (Mohammad Azam Ansari) wrote the paper. All authors have given approval to the final version of the manuscript.

Funding: This research received no external funding.

Acknowledgments: M.J. is grateful to Maulana Azad National Fellowship, UGC, New Delhi for providing SRF scholarship. The authors are sincerely thankful to USIF, Aligarh Muslim University Aligarh, India and IRMC, Imam Abdulrahman Bin Faisal University, Dammam, Saudi Arabia for providing research facilities. The authors are grateful to Ali Ahmad Khan and Sanjay Sharma, Department of Microbiology J.N. Medical College A.M.U Aligarh for their technical assistance.

Conflicts of Interest: The authors declare no conflict of interest.

Appendix A

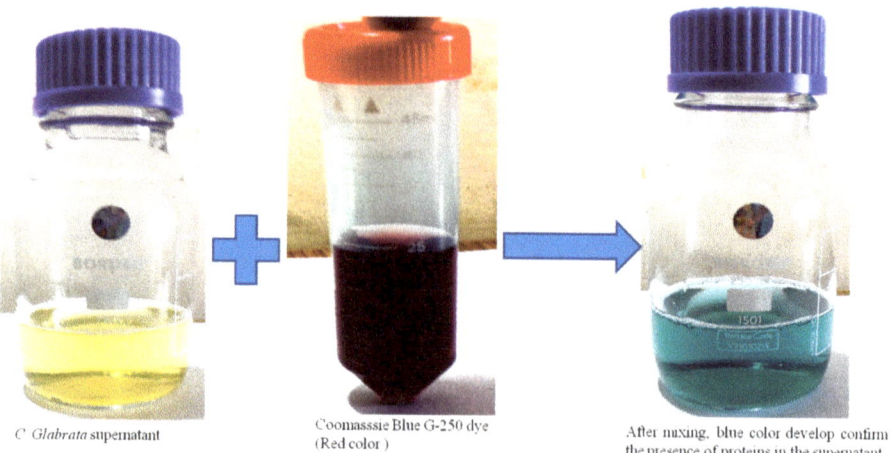

Figure A1. A simple protein-dye binding assay to assess the presence of protein in the supernatant.

References

1. Prabhu, S.; Poulose, E.K. Silver nanoparticles: mechanism of antimicrobial action, synthesis, medical applications, and toxicity effects. *Int. Nano Lett.* **2012**, *2*, 32. [CrossRef]
2. Firdhouse, M.J.; Lalitha, P. Biosynthesis of silver nanoparticles and its applications. *J. Nanotechnol.* **2015**, *2015*. [CrossRef]
3. Velhal, S.G.; Kulkarni, S.D.; Latpate, R.V. Fungal mediated silver nanoparticle synthesis using robust experimental design and its application in cotton fabric. *Int. Nano Lett.* **2016**, *6*, 257–264. [CrossRef]
4. Moghaddam, A.B.; Namvar, F.; Moniri, M.; Tahir, M.P.; Azizi, S.; Mohamad, R. Nanoparticles biosynthesized by fungi and yeast: a review of their preparation, properties, and medical applications. *Molecules* **2015**, *20*, 16540–16565. [CrossRef] [PubMed]
5. Eugenio, M.; Müller, N.; Frasés, S.; Almeida-Paes, R.; Lima, L.M.; Lemgruber, L.; Farina, M.; de Souza, W.; Sant'Anna, C. Yeast-derived biosynthesis of silver/silver chloride nanoparticles and their antiproliferative activity against bacteria. *RSC Adv.* **2016**, *6*, 9893–9904. [CrossRef]
6. Kowshik, M.; Ashtaputre, S.; Kharrazi, S.; Vogel, W.; Urban, J.; Kulkarni, S.K.; Paknikar, K.M. Extracellular synthesis of silver nanoparticles by a silver-tolerant yeast strain MKY3. *Nanotechnology* **2002**, *14*, 95. [CrossRef]
7. Kaler, A.; Jain, S.; Banerjee, U.C. Green and rapid synthesis of anticancerous silver nanoparticles by *Saccharomyces boulardii* and insight into mechanism of nanoparticle synthesis. *Biomed Res. Int.* **2013**, 872940.
8. Niknejad, F.; Nabili, M.; Ghazvini, R.D.; Moazeni, M. Green synthesis of silver nanoparticles: Advantages of the yeast *Saccharomyces* cerevisiae model. *Curr. Med. Mycol.* **2015**, *1*, 17. [PubMed]
9. Atef, A.H.; Mogda, K.M.; Mahmoudc, H.H. Biosynthesis of silver nanoparticles (AgNps) (a model of metals) by *Candida albicans* and its antifungal activity on Some fungal pathogens (*Trichophyton mentagrophytes* and *Candida albicans*). *N. Y. Sci. J.* **2013**, *6*, 27–43.
10. Bhat, M.A.; Nayak, B.K.; Nanda, A. Evaluation of bactericidal activity of biologically synthesised silver nanoparticles from *Candida albicans* in combination with ciprofloxacin. *Mater. Today Proc.* **2015**, *2*, 4395–4401. [CrossRef]
11. Waghmare, S.R.; Mulla, M.N.; Marathe, S.R.; Sonawane, K.D. Ecofriendly production of silver nanoparticles using *Candida utilis* and its mechanistic action against pathogenic microorganisms. *3 Biotech* **2015**, *5*, 33–38. [CrossRef] [PubMed]
12. Azizi, S.; Ahmad, M.B.; Namvar, F.; Mohamad, R. Green biosynthesis and characterization of zinc oxide nanoparticles using brown marine macroalga Sargassum muticum aqueous extract. *Mater. Lett.* **2014**, *116*, 275–277. [CrossRef]
13. Pati, R.; Mehta, R.K.; Mohanty, S.; Padhi, A.; Sengupta, M.; Vaseeharan, B.; Goswami, C.; Sonawane, A. Topical application of zinc oxide nanoparticles reduces bacterial skin infection in mice and exhibits antibacterial activity by inducing oxidative stress response and cell membrane disintegration in macrophages. *Nanomedicine* **2014**, *10*, 1195–1208. [CrossRef] [PubMed]
14. Agarwal, H.; Kumar, S.V.; Rajeshkumar, S. A review on green synthesis of zinc oxide nanoparticles-an eco-friendly approach. *Resour.-Effic. Technol.* **2017**, *3*, 406–413. [CrossRef]
15. Shettar, S.K.; Patil, A.B.; Nadagir, S.D.; Shepur, T.A.; Mythri, B.A.; Gadadavar, S. Evaluation of HiCrome differential agar for speciation of candida. *J. Acad. Med. Sci.* **2012**, *2*, 101.
16. Freydiere, A.M.; Parant, F.; Noel-Baron, F.; Crepy, M.; Treny, A.; Raberin, H.; Davidson, A.; Odds, F.C. Identification of *Candida glabrata* by a 30-second trehalase test. *J. Clin. Microbiol.* **2002**, *40*, 3602–3605. [CrossRef] [PubMed]
17. Jalal, M.; Ansari, M.A.; Shukla, A.K.; Ali, S.G.; Khan, H.M.; Pal, R.; Alam, J.; Cameotra, S.S. Anticandidal green synthesis and antifungal activity of Al2O3 NPs against fluconazole-resistant *Candida* spp isolated from a tertiary care hospital. *RSC Adv.* **2016**, *6*, 107577–107590. [CrossRef]
18. Liu, X.; Kang, J.; Liu, B.; Yang, J. Separation of gold nanowires and nanoparticles through a facile process of centrifugation. *Sep. Purif. Technol.* **2018**, *192*, 1–4. [CrossRef]
19. Yu, W.; Xie, H.; Chen, L.; Li, Y.; Zhang, C. Synthesis and characterization of monodispersed copper colloids in polar solvents. *Nanoscale Res. Lett.* **2009**, *4*, 465. [CrossRef] [PubMed]
20. Ashraf, J.M.; Ansari, M.A.; Choi, I.; Khan, H.M.; Alzohairy, M.A. Antiglycating potential of gum arabic capped-silver nanoparticles. *Appl. Biochem. Biotechnol.* **2014**, *174*, 398–410. [CrossRef] [PubMed]

21. Ansari, M.A.; Khan, H.M.; Khan, A.A.; Sultan, A.; Azam, A.; Shahid, M.; Shujatullah, F. Antibacterial activity of silver nanoparticles dispersion against MSSA and MRSA isolated from wounds in a tertiary care hospital of North India. *Int. J. Appl. Biol. Pharm. Technol.* **2011**, *2*, 34–42.
22. Sanghi, R.; Verma, P. Biomimetic synthesis and characterisation of protein capped silver nanoparticles. *Bioresour. Technol.* **2009**, *100*, 501–504. [CrossRef] [PubMed]
23. Gudikandula, K.; Vadapally, P.; Charya, M.S. Biogenic synthesis of silver nanoparticles from white rot fungi: Their characterization and antibacterial studies. *OpenNano* **2017**, *2*, 64–78. [CrossRef]
24. Ahmad, A.; Mukherjee, P.; Senapati, S.; Mandal, D.; Khan, M.I.; Kumar, R.; Sastry, M. Extracellular biosynthesis of silver nanoparticles using the fungus *Fusarium oxysporum*. *Colloids Surf. B* **2003**, *28*, 313–318. [CrossRef]
25. Kumar, S.A.; Abyaneh, M.K.; Gosavi, S.W.; Kulkarni, S.K.; Pasricha, R.; Ahmad, A.; Khan, M.I. Nitrate reductase-mediated synthesis of silver nanoparticles from AgNO3. *Biotechnol. Lett.* **2007**, *29*, 439–445. [CrossRef] [PubMed]
26. Kalimuthu, K.; Babu, R.S.; Venkataraman, D.; Bilal, M.; Gurunathan, S. Biosynthesis of silver nanocrystals by *Bacillus licheniformis*. *Colloids Surf. B* **2008**, *65*, 150–153. [CrossRef] [PubMed]
27. Panáček, A.; Kolář, M.; Večeřová, R.; Prucek, R.; Soukupová, J.; Kryštof, V.; Hamal, P.; Zbořil, R.; Kvítek, L. Antifungal activity of silver nanoparticles against *Candida* spp. *Biomaterials* **2009**, *30*, 6333–6340. [CrossRef] [PubMed]
28. Nasrollahi, A.; Pourshamsian, K.H.; Mansourkiaee, P. Antifungal activity of silver nanoparticles on some of fungi. *Int. J. Nano Dimens.* **2011**, *1*, 233.
29. Vazquez-Muñoz, R.; Avalos-Borja, M.; Castro-Longoria, E. Ultrastructural analysis of *Candida albicans* when exposed to silver nanoparticles. *PLoS ONE* **2014**, *9*, 108876. [CrossRef] [PubMed]
30. Kim, K.J.; Sung, W.S.; Suh, B.K.; Moon, S.K.; Choi, J.S.; Kim, J.G.; Lee, D.G. Antifungal activity and mode of action of silver nano-particles on *Candida albicans*. *BioMetals* **2009**, *22*, 235–242. [CrossRef] [PubMed]
31. Ishida, K.; Cipriano, T.F.; Rocha, G.M.; Weissmüller, G.; Gomes, F.; Miranda, K.; Rozental, S. Silver nanoparticle production by the fungus *Fusarium oxysporum*: Nanoparticle characterisation and analysis of antifungal activity against pathogenic yeasts. *Mem. Inst. Oswaldo Cruz* **2014**, *109*, 220–228. [CrossRef] [PubMed]
32. Hwang, I.S.; Lee, J.; Hwang, J.H.; Kim, K.J.; Lee, D.G. Silver nanoparticles induce apoptotic cell death in *Candida albicans* through the increase of hydroxyl radicals. *FEBS J.* **2012**, *279*, 1327–1338. [CrossRef] [PubMed]

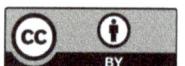

© 2018 by the authors. Licensee MDPI, Basel, Switzerland. This article is an open access article distributed under the terms and conditions of the Creative Commons Attribution (CC BY) license (http://creativecommons.org/licenses/by/4.0/).

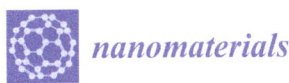

Article

Detection of Histamine Dihydrochloride at Low Concentrations Using Raman Spectroscopy Enhanced by Gold Nanostars Colloids

Eleazar Samuel Kolosovas-Machuca [1], Alexander Cuadrado [1,2], Hiram Joazet Ojeda-Galván [1,3], Luis Carlos Ortiz-Dosal [4], Aida Catalina Hernández-Arteaga [1], Maria del Carmen Rodríguez-Aranda [1], Hugo Ricardo Navarro-Contreras [1], Javier Alda [2,*] and Francisco Javier González [1]

[1] Coordinación para la Innovación y Aplicación de la Ciencia y la Tecnología, Universidad Autónoma de San Luis Potosí, 78210 San Luis Potosí, Mexico; samuel.kolosovas@uaslp.mx (E.S.K.-M.); a.cuadrado@pdi.ucm.es (A.C.); joazet.ojeda@uaslp.mx (H.J.O.-G.); aida.arteaga@uaslp.mx (A.C.H.-A.); carmen.rgz.aranda@gmail.com (M.d.C.R.-A.); hnavarro@uaslp.mx (H.R.N.-C.); javier.gonzalez@uaslp.mx (F.J.G.)

[2] Applied Optics Complutense Group, Faculty of Optics and Optometry, University Complutense of Madrid, Av. Arcos de Jalon, 118, 28037 Madrid, Spain

[3] Instituto de Física Luis Terrazas, Benemerita Universidad Autónoma de Puebla, Av. San Claudio, 18, 72570 Puebla, Mexico

[4] Doctorado Institucional en Ingeniería y Ciencias de Materiales, Universidad Autónoma de San Luis Potosí, 78210 San Luis Potosí, Mexico; ortiz.dosal.lc@gmail.com

* Correspondence: javier.alda@ucm.es; Tel.: +34-91-394-6874

Received: 20 December 2018; Accepted: 22 January 2019; Published: 6 February 2019

Abstract: In this paper, we report a fast and easy method to detect histamine dihydrochloride using gold nanostars in colloidal aqueous solution as a highly active SERS platform with potential applications in biomedicine and food science. This colloid was characterized with SEM and UV–Vis spectroscopy. Also, numerical calculations were performed to estimate the plasmonic resonance and electric field amplification of the gold nanoparticles to compare the difference between nanospheres and nanostars. Finally, aqueous solutions of histamine dihydrochloride were prepared in a wide range of concentrations and the colloid was added to carry out SERS. We found SERS amplified the Raman signal of histamine by an enhancement factor of 1.0×10^7, demonstrating the capability of the method to detect low concentrations of this amine molecule.

Keywords: SERS; histamine; nanostars; nanophotonics; computational electromagnetism

1. Introduction

Surface-enhanced Raman spectroscopy (SERS) is a useful technique for the characterization of small groups of molecules near or bound to plasmonic surfaces. It is powerful, non-destructive, and provides information about the chemical structure and identity of materials [1–5]. These capabilities make possible the wide use of SERS in biosensors for the detection of substances of biological interest and pathogens [5–11], being gold and silver two of the metals that offer better results for this kind of applications [12–15]. The above-mentioned metals in the form of nanoparticles have the advantage that can be used directly, as colloidal solutions, acting as tridimensional plasmonic systems with customized resonances that can be tuned with the size and shape of the dispersed nanoparticles [4,16,17]. Au nanostars have been proven useful for SERS, they also present unique optical and electric properties. Previous groups have reported the synthesis of Au nanostar with a good degree of symmetry control by using a robust solution-phase method [18], or by increasing the seed concentration in the growth solution [19]. Also, the potential of these nanostructures has been evaluated in biomedical applications by functionalizing its surface using a biocompatible polymer [20]. Among many existing anisotropic gold nanostructures star-shaped nanoparticles (gold nanostars) have achieved a huge interest, mainly due their high biocompatibility, chemical stability and unique optical properties, which makes them useful in a wide range of applications in fields such as plasmonics, spectroscopy, biological applications (bioimaging, biosensing, drug delivery), and catalysis [21,22]

Histamine is a relevant biological substance in medicine and food science. It is a biogenic amine that transmits signals from cell to cell in the skin, intestines, and organs of the immune system. Structural differences in the receptor cell membranes are responsible for different responses to histamine among individuals [23,24].

For example, the interaction between histamine and H1 receptors causes a drop in the blood pressure and muscle contractions, and the interaction with H2 receptors is associated with acidic stomach secretions [25,26]. The consumption of food with a high concentration of histamine may result in intoxication with symptoms such as nausea, diarrhea, headache, asthma, angioedema, urticaria, and itch. These reactions are part of the histamine poisoning, or scombroid poisoning [27–30]. The concentration of histamine in food should be less than 10 mg/100 g, while the average concentration in human plasma is around 7.2 nmol/L [27,31] . Hence, the determination of histamine concentration that may be present in certain food products is a safety issue of public concern [32].

Conventional methods for determining the presence and concentration of histamine are high-performance liquid chromatography (HPLC), fluorometry, and detection by enzymes (e.g., enzyme linked immunosorbent assay, ELISA) [31]. HPLC and fluorometry involve slow protocols for derivatizing with o-phtalaldehyde or dansyl chloride. Another drawback of the fluorometric assays is that they require methanol extraction and purification with an anion exchange column as a pretreatment. Furthermore, due to the similarity between the structures of histamine and histidine, the measurement tends to have a low selectivity for histamine [8], even when separated previously by HPLC. In contrast, enzyme-based methods provide rapid detection but require the use of unstable enzymes and very expensive test kits, also they may overestimate the amount of histamine [8].

The detection of histamine in food using SERS techniques has been proved recently and opens the way to improved and more reliable detection techniques [33,34]. Our study describes an alternative approach using gold nanoparticles in colloidal suspension which strongly amplifies the Raman signal of extremely low concentrations of histamine dihydrochloride, which corresponds with the dication of the molecule. Previous results using gold and silver nanoparticles for the detection of biological samples have demonstrated the capabilities of the method when using colloids of nanoprisms [11] or surface bounded nanostars [35]. However, the use of colloids with gold nanostars has not been reported so far. In this contribution, results show that the SERS signal of histamine dihydrochloride can be obtained in a fast and accurate way in an aqueous solution, so the results obtained here contribute to the establishment of a useful and valid method for the detection of this biochemical compound.

2. Methods

2.1. Synthesis of Nanoparticles

The first step to fabricate the gold nanostar colloid is to synthesize gold nanospheres with the Turkevich method [36] and subsequently a second reduction with pH control using a Good's buffer and hidroxilammonium chloride respectively. An aqueous solution of chloroauric acid 2.5 mM is heated to 95 °C, and an aqueous solution of trisodium citrate 2.5 mM ($Na_3C_6H_5O_7$) is added as a reducing agent. This produces a red solution which indicates the formation of gold nanospheres. The second stage of the synthesis consists in growing spikes on the surface of the nanoparticles. The nanospheres solution is added to a 50 mM aqueous solution of 2-[4-(2-hydroxyethyl)piperazin-1-yl] ethanesulfonic acid (HEPES), to control and maintain the pH at a physiological value, and hence the morphology of the nanostructure, and with a 0.1 M aqueous solution of hydroxylammonium chloride ($HONH_3Cl$) as a reducing agent. Finally, the solution is washed with deionized water. The colloid changes from red to blue, signaling the formation of gold nanostars. As Figure 1 shows, generated peaks are distributed on the surface of the nanospheres, generating nanostars measuring around 160 nm in diameter.

2.2. Numerical Simulation

In this work, we have performed numerical simulations of the plasmonic optical response using COMSOL Multiphysics. To simplify the calculations, nanostars with a diameter of 150 nm were considered, the peaks were homogenously distributed on the surface of the sphere as conic protuberances, with a height of 25 nm and a maximum diameter of 31 nm, in accordance with the mean values obtained by the SEM images. For an improved study of the optical response of the nanostar, the initial nanospheres 75 nm in radius have been simulated. We evaluate of the optical response through the extinction efficiency, Q_{ext}, which is calculated as:

$$Q_{ext} = \frac{\int_V \vec{J}\vec{E}dv + \int_S \vec{n}\vec{S}ds}{I_0 \pi D^2/4}, \quad (1)$$

The first part of the numerator is the power loss related with the Joule effect, where $\vec{J}$ and $\vec{E}$ are the induced current density and the electric field along the structure, respectively; and the integration is evaluated within the nanostructure. The second part of the numerator is related to the scattered power, where $\vec{n}$ is the normal vector pointing outwards and $\vec{S}$ is the Poynting vector. In this case, the integration surface is a sphere located in the far field region. Finally, I_0 and D are the incident irradiance and the diameter of the particle, respectively.

2.3. Spectroscopic Measurements

To complete this analysis, the optical responses of both types of nanoparticles were measured through UV–Vis spectroscopy to compare them with the calculated extinction coefficients. We used a Ocean Optics spectrometer (model USB650) (Largo, FL, USA). To perform SERS, histamine dihydrochloride serial 1:10 successive dilutions were prepared from an initial 3 M stock solution until a 3×10^{-7} M one was obtained. From these solutions of histamine, new dilutions were made 1:3 with the nanostars colloid, mixed with deionized water, to give the final mixture of histamine and nanoparticles from 1 M to 1×10^{-7} M. The pH range was maintained in the range of 7.1 to 7.9. The Raman measurements were performed on a Horiba Jobin Ybon XplorRA ONE Raman spectrometer (Irvine, CA, USA) coupled to an Olympus BX41 optical microscope (Ciudad de México, México), using a near-infrared ($\lambda = 785$ nm) Raman laser source with an average power of 20 mW at the sample location. This laser line has the advantage that strongly minimizes the huge fluorescence background typical of biological samples.

3. Results

The synthesis of gold nanostars was successful and 160-nm-diameter structures showing triangular peaks were obtained from gold nanospheres. Figure 1a shows a SEM image of one of the fabricated nanostars. When prepared in colloid form, nanostars coalesce in clusters of several units (see Figure 1b). This is of importance from a spectroscopic point of view because these clusters may distort the maximum peaks of the spectral response.

Through numerical simulations, the spectral response of the nanoparticles used in this work was calculated. The fabrication of gold nanostars uses gold nanospheres as a precursor nanostructure, the plasmonic response of the synthesized nanostructures varied either by increasing the radius of the spheres or by generating small random peaks on its surface. As it happens with the synthesized gold nanoparticles, the spherical geometry is the starting point of the numerical simulations. The nanostar geometry is obtained after adding spikes over the nanosphere surface to resemble the actual shape of gold nanostars.

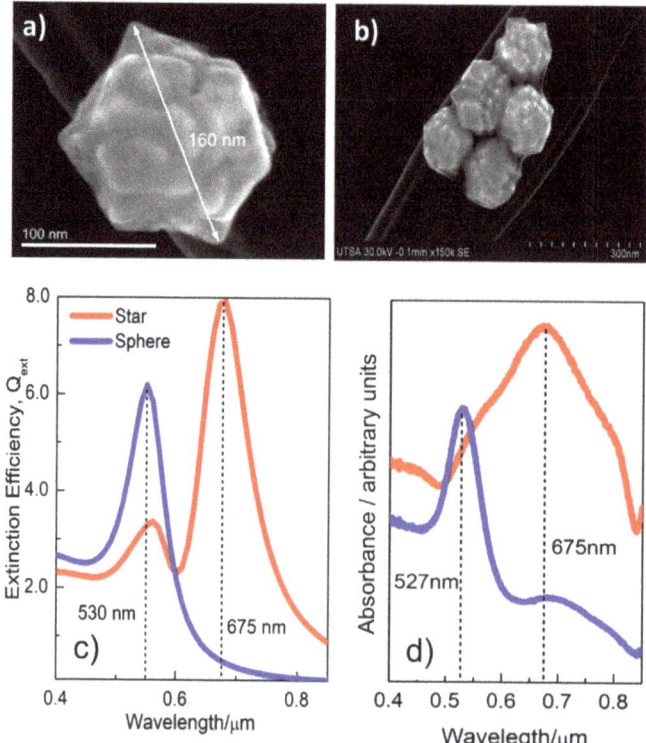

Figure 1. (a) Scanning electron micrograph of a gold nanostar with a diameter of about 160 nm. The diameter distribution shows a median value of 159 nm with a standard deviation of 3 nm. (b) Clustering of gold nanostar that will be present in the colloid. (c) Extinction coefficient evaluated through numerical simulations of both nanospheres (blue) and nanostars (red). (d) Measured spectral absorbance of colloids of nanospheres (blue) and nanostars (red) at a concentration of 2.5 mM.

The numerically calculated optical response of the studied nanostructures is shown in Figure 1c and expressed in terms of the extinction coefficient of the structure. According to Mie theory, gold nanospheres (blue line) show a plasmonic resonance located at 530 nm. This response is red-shifted towards 550 nm for the nanostar, but now the importance of this resonance is smaller than the main peak at 675 nm related with the presence of the protuberances. This main response depends on the height and maximum diameter values of the peaks of the nanostars. To complete this analysis, the optical responses of both types of nanoparticles were measured through UV–Vis spectroscopy to compare them with the calculated extinction coefficients. The absorption spectra are given in Figure 1d. The nanosphere colloid (blue line) presents the expected plasmonic resonance at 530 nm, according to the simulation shown in Figure 1c. As predicted by computational electromagnetism, the optical response of the nanostar (red line) has a resonance centered at 675 nm, and shows broader bandwidth. This effect can be explained considering the morphology variation of the generated nanostars, as well as their size distribution in the sample, and the presence of clusters (see Figure 1b). It is shown that the nanostars have a resonance closer to the wavelength of the incident laser (785 nm), hence, the amplification will be larger for nanostars.

The signal obtained from Raman spectroscopy is proportional to the fourth power of the modulus of the electric field. Therefore, moderate field enhancements, although spatially confined, provide large amplification factors of the Raman response. Figure 2 shows the spectral field enhancement factor for nanostars. We may see that the maximum of it appears at a wavelength $\lambda_{max} = 675$ nm. Our experimental setup excites the Raman spectra using an excitation laser operating at $\lambda_{exc} = 780$ nm, where the field enhancement is about ×80, that is good enough to generate a Raman signal amplification of around 4×10^7. Through computational electromagnetism we have evaluated the near field distribution around nanostars when the incidence is having an amplitude of 1 V/m. Therefore, the obtained electric field also represents the field enhancement map of the structure. The results for λ_{max}, and λ_{exc} are shown in Figures 2b and 2c respectively. As expected, the electric field is located near the tip of the peaks, achieving a strong enhancement. For comparison, we have evaluated the electric field map generated by a nanosphere (see Figure 2d). In this case, the electric near field has a dipolar distribution, resulting in a field enhancement factor of ×7.4. These results express the goodness of nanostars with respect to nanospheres, because higher field enhancement will strongly increases the capability to detect a Raman shift.

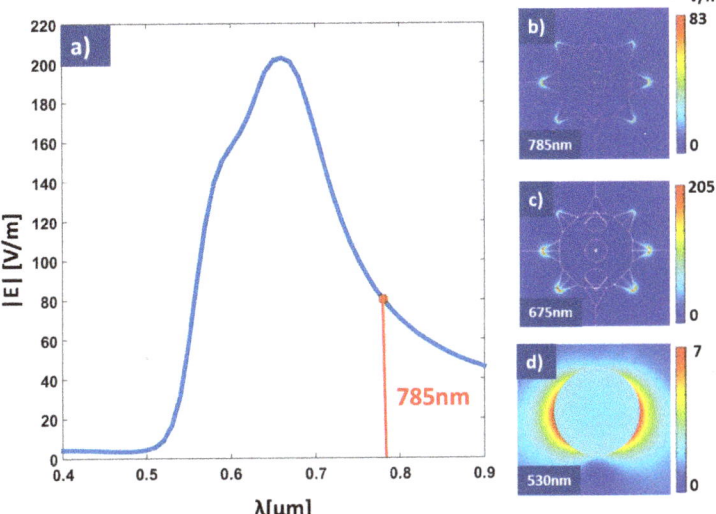

Figure 2. (a) Spectral field enhancement for the nanostar geometry. Our fabricated structures shows its maximum of the field enhancement($\lambda_{max} = 675$ nm) slightly shifted from the wavelength of the excitation source of our Raman spectrometer ($\lambda_{exc} = 785$ nm). (b–d) Near field maps for the nanostar and nanosphere geometries at different wavelengths. (b,d) are evaluated at the maximum response wavelength for each geometry, and (c) is for the excitation wavelength. As far as the input plane wave is having an electric field amplitude of 1 V/m, the near field map also represents the field enhancement.

Using the model described in the supplementary material in [37] we calculated a SERS enhancement factor (EF) of 1.0×10^7 for the band at 1260 cm^{-1}. This result is somewhat larger than those obtained for a silver film over nanosphere (AgFON) from Wen-Chi Lin et al. (4.3×10^6) [38] and far larger than that obtained from molecularly imprinted polymers by Fang Gao et al. (1.0×10^4) [27]. This also applies even for the values reported in refs. [39,40], being our EF value closer to 1.91×10^7, recently reported [41]. As the spectral positions of the bands in Raman and SERS measurements are nearly unchanged, it is reasonable to conclude that the EF produced by the nanostructure is predominantly responsible for the high SERS signal intensity.

Raman spectrum of powder histamine dihydrochloride is shown in Figure 3a as a reference. The Raman shift spectra of most of the vibrational modules of the histamine in solid state and the histamine dihydrochloride coincide. The Raman peaks are compared with Raman vibrational modules of histamine of previous works (Table 1) [38,42,43], and the vibrational modules are found at the same Raman shifts, detecting peaks related to histamine.

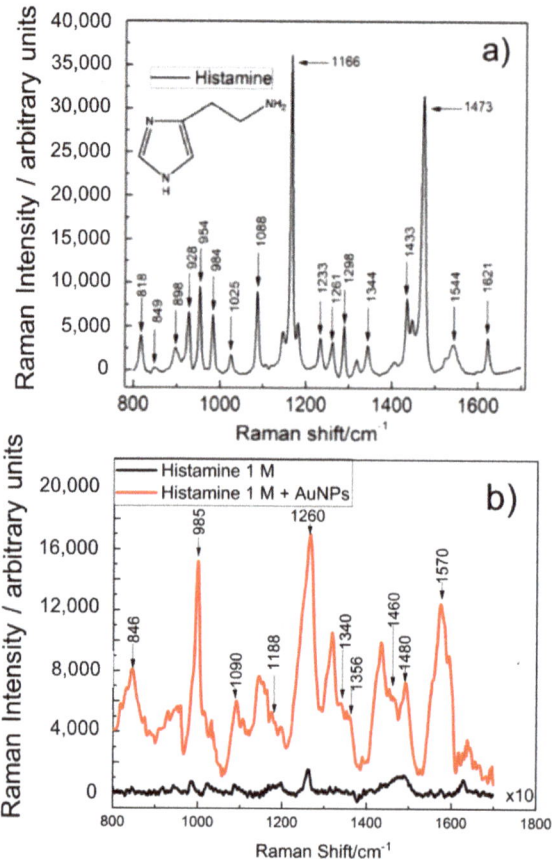

Figure 3. (a) Raman spectrum of powder histamine after baseline correction using Vancouver algorithm, where the modes observed correspond with the work reported by Collado et al. [42]. (b) Raman spectra of histamine 1 M with (red) and without AuNPs (black).

Once the nanostars were added to the different solutions of histamine dihydrochloride an increase in the intensity was observed allowing the identification of the characteristic Raman peaks of the histamine molecule that correspond to the vibrational modes of the imidazole ring. Figure 3b and Table 1 allows the identification of these vibrations at low concentrations. For example, the 846 cm^{-1} corresponds to a bending in the plane of the imidazole ring or in the side chain of the molecule (ring A, wagging C), the peak at 985 cm^{-1} corresponds to a flexion of the plane of the imidazole ring (v(N1-H), v(C2-H)), some other peaks around 1260 cm^{-1} correspond to flexions in the plane of the NH, and bending in the plane of CH respectively: Sy(N3-H), Sy(C4-H), v(C2-H), and v(N1-H) [38,42,43]. These results show how, even at very low concentrations (10^{-7} M), it is still possible to identify histamine thanks to the SERS technique using gold nanostar colloids (see top spectrum at Figure 4).

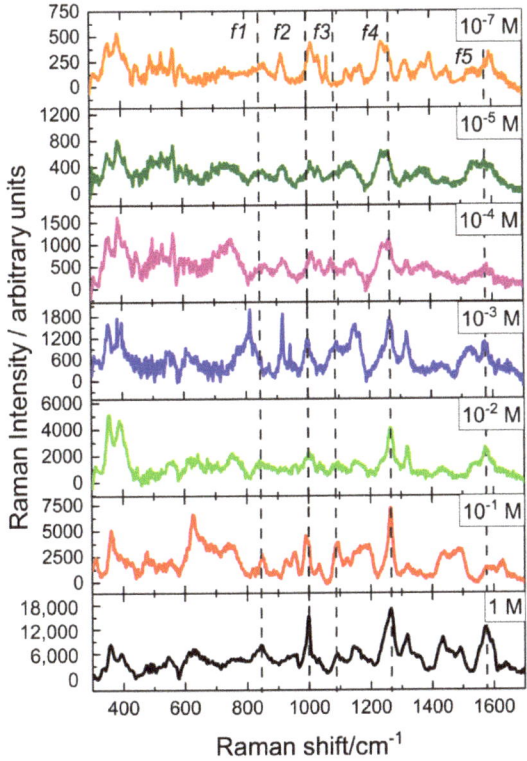

Figure 4. Raman spectra of the vibrational resonances of the histamine dication molecule at several concentrations. All the solutions include gold nanoparticles. Dashed vertical lines corresponde with characteristic peaks of the histamine molecule. Figure 5 will focus our attention on the *f*4 resonance around $\kappa = 1265$ cm^{-1}.

After performing SERS on different solutions of histamine dihydrochloride, it is observed that the addition of the gold nanostructures increases the intensity of the Raman spectrum (see Figure 3b). This is due to the surface plasmon resonance at the nanostars that produces larger enhancement of the electric fields that subsequently amplify the emitted light from irregular points (gaps, sharp edges, etc.) [1]. Figure 4 shows the Raman spectra for several concentrations of histamine, from 1 M to 10^{-7} M. A lower concentration means weaker signal. However, the characteristic peaks of the histamine spectrum are revealed allowing its identification. To prove this result, we have made an analysis of the resonance around $\kappa = 1265$ cm^{-1} (see Figure 5). This Raman shift is representative of the histamine spectra. Around this wavenumber, the phonon modes in the collected Raman spectra were decomposed into Lorentzian lineshapes. Raman spectra were analyzed by first removing the background contribution using a linear function, then, the Lorentzian curves profiles have been used for the fitting procedure of the experimental Raman spectra. This fitting applies a Levenberg–Marquardt least-squares-based iterative algorithm to optimize the parameters of the Lorentzian functions (center, height, and FWHM). These obtained spectra and Lorentzian components are shown in Figure 5a, and the importance of the Lorentzian component centered at $\kappa = 1265$ cm^{-1} is presented in Figure 5 as a function of the molarity of the sample. We may see how the Lorentzian at $\kappa = 1265$ cm^{-1} remains relevant at every concentration, revealing the presence of histamine in the sample.

Table 1. Comparison in wavenumber, κ (cm^{-1}) of our measurements (first column) with previously published works: Lin et al. [38] (second column), and Torreggiani et al. [43]. Mode notation: ν = stretching; sy = symmetric; τ = twisting

κ (cm^{-1})	κ (cm^{-1}) [38]	κ (cm^{-1}) [43]	Assignment
846			ring A, wagging C
895			ν (N3-H)
950			ring A
985		980	ν (N1-H), ν (c2-H)
1028	1024.73	1005	sy (C5-H), τ (C2-H), ν (C1-H)
1090	1084.05	1088	sy (N3-H), sy (C5-H)
1188			wagging C, ν (C2-H)
1260		1270	ring breathing
1340			τ (C1-H), ν (N1-H)
1356	1358.07		translation C, ν (C1-H), ν (N1-H)
1438		1435	
1460	1455.46		ν (C4-H), sy (N3-H)
1480			sy (C5-H), sy (N3-H)
1570	1567.61	1579	ν (N3-H)
1629		1618	

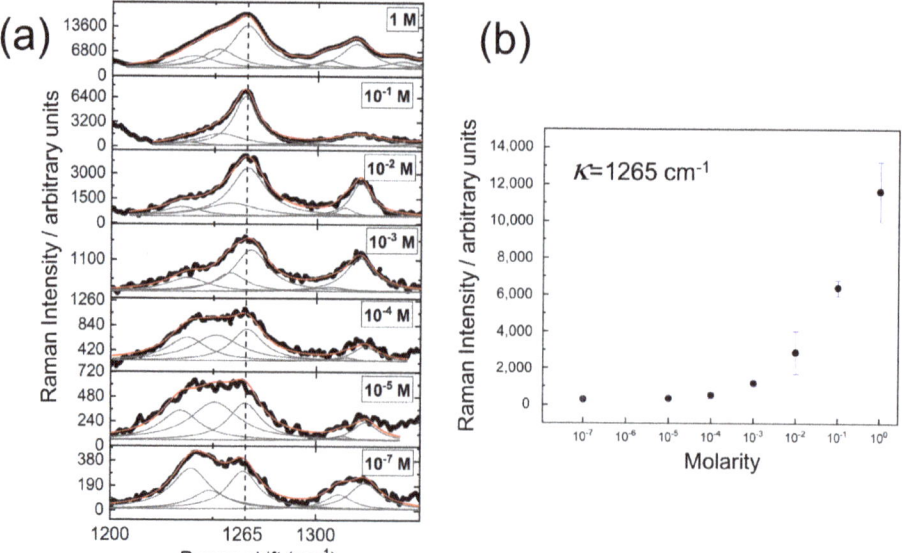

Figure 5. (a) Detail of the Raman spectra around $\kappa = 1265$ cm^{-1} (represented as a dashed vertical line). The gray lines under the curve correspond with the Lorentzian lineshapes obtanied after fitting. The red line represents the results obtained from this decomposition. This fitting has been done for several molarity values from 1 M to 10^{-7} M. The case of $M = 10^{-6}$ has not been prepared nor measured. (b) Relative intensity of the $\kappa = 1265$ cm^{-1} Lorentzian peak as a function of molarity. The error bars represent the variability between samples.

4. Conclusions

As result of the comparison between the extinction coefficient evaluated from simulation and the measured optical response of nanoparticles, we positively demonstrated the capability of numerical simulations to deal with nanostructures intended to interact with molecules. Because of their reliability, these tools can help speed-up the selection of geometries of nanoparticles in biochemical applications.

The detection and identification of histamine being a serious concern in safety regulations of the food industry, and some other areas of biomedicine, requires the availability of reliable analytical tools. In this contribution, we have demonstrated that Raman spectroscopy amplified by surface plasmon resonance allows qualitative analysis of histamine at extremely low concentrations (as low as 10^{-7} M) in aqueous dilutions. The resonance takes place at the field-enhancement location of gold nanoparticules having a nanostars geometry and prepared as a colloid. This colloid was added to solutions of histamine dihydrochloride at various concentrations. A simulation was performed with a finite element method to calculate the spectral extinction coefficient, and the field-enhancement due to the nanoparticles. Spectroscopic measurements have proved that spectral absorption fits well with the numerically obtained results supporting the reliability of the simulations. According with the computational evaluation of the field enhancement, an increase was observed in the spectral intensity, as well as an amplification of the characteristic Raman peaks of the histamine molecule. The SERS enhancement factor is 1×10^7, which indicates the potential application of the proposed method, allowing lower limits of detection of the molecule.

In summary, this work proposes a reliable method for the detection of histamine in concentrations as low as 10^{-7} M, which is a concentration suitable for food quality control applications (concentrations of $\approx 10^{-4}$ M). Further work and refinement of the technique are needed to detect histamine at even lower physiological concentration ($\approx 10^{-9}$ M) using the above-mentioned method.

Author Contributions: E.S.K.-M. and L.C.O.-D. conceived the presented idea and developed the theory, E.S.K.-M. also compared the numerical simulations with experimental results. A.C. and J.A. performed the numerical simulations and interpreted the numerical and experimental results. H.J.O.-G. and A.C.H.-A. carried out the nanoparticle synthesis and H.J.O.-G. also characterized them with scanning electon microscopy. M.d.C.R.-A. designed and performed the experiments and characterized the histamine with Raman spectroscopy. H.R.N.-C. and F.J.G. designed and directed the project. All the authors participate and helped in the final writing of the paper.

Funding: F.J. González would like to acknowledge support from project 32 of "Centro Mexicano de Innovación en Energía Solar", and from Consejo Nacional de Ciencia y Tecnología (CONACyT) México through the Terahertz Science and Technology National Lab (LANCYTT). Additional funding has been obtained from FAI-UASLP, as well as access to Laboratorio Nacional de Análisis Físicos, Químicos y Biológicos-UASLP, and Laboratorio Nacional de Ciencia y Tecnología Terahertz (LANCYTT). A.C. Hernández-Arteaga and H.J. Ojeda-Galván acknowledge the financial support of CONACyT through Ph.D. and postdoctoral scholarships during the course of this research.

Conflicts of Interest: The authors declare no conflict of interest. The funding agencies had no role in the design of the study; in the collection, analyses, or interpretation of data; in the writing of the manuscript, or in the decision to publish the results.

References

1. Sharma, B.; Frontiera, R.R.; Henry, A.I.; Ringe, E.; Duyne, R.P.V. SERS: Materials, applications, and the future. *Mater. Today* **2012**, *15*, 16–25. [CrossRef]
2. Kneipp, K.; Wang, Y.; Kneipp, H.; Perelman, L.T.; Itzkan, I.; Dasari, R.R.; Feld, M.S. Single Molecule Detection Using Surface-Enhanced Raman Scattering (SERS). *Phys. Rev. Lett.* **1997**, *78*, 1667–1670. [CrossRef]
3. Willets, K.A.; Van Duyne, R.P. Localized Surface Plasmon Resonance Spectroscopy and Sensing. *Annu. Rev. Phys. Chem.* **2007**, *58*, 267–297. [CrossRef] [PubMed]
4. Kneipp, K.; Kneipp, H.; Itzkan, I.; Dasari, R.R.; Feld, M.S. Ultrasensitive Chemical Analysis by Raman Spectroscopy. *Chem. Rev.* **1999**, *99*, 2957–2976. [CrossRef] [PubMed]
5. Stiles, P.L.; Dieringer, J.A.; Shah, N.C.; Van Duyne, R.P. Surface-Enhanced Raman Spectroscopy. *Ann. Rev. Anal. Chem.* **2008**, *1*, 601–626. [CrossRef] [PubMed]

6. Jeanmaire, D.L.; Duyne, R.P.V. Surface raman spectroelectrochemistry: Part I. Heterocyclic, aromatic, and aliphatic amines adsorbed on the anodized silver electrode. *J. Electroanal. Chem. Interfacial Electrochem.* **1977**, *84*, 1–20. [CrossRef]
7. Lazcka, O.; Campo, F.J.D.; Munoz, F.X. Pathogen detection: A perspective of traditional methods and biosensors. *Biosens. Bioelectron.* **2007**, *22*, 1205–1217. [CrossRef] [PubMed]
8. Velusamy, V.; Arshak, K.; Korostynska, O.; Oliwa, K.; Adley, C. An overview of foodborne pathogen detection: In the perspective of biosensors. *Biotechnol. Adv.* **2010**, *28*, 232–254. [CrossRef] [PubMed]
9. Jung, J.; Cheon, D.; Liu, F.; Lee, K.; Seo, T. A Graphene Oxide Based Immuno-biosensor for Pathogen Detection. *Angew. Chem.* **2010**, *122*, 5844–5847. [CrossRef]
10. Sekhon, S.S.; Kim, S.G.; Lee, S.H.; Jang, A.; Min, J.; Ahn, J.Y.; Kim, Y.-H. Advances in pathogen-associated molecules detection using Aptamer based biosensors. *Mol. Cell. Toxicol.* **2013**, *9*, 311–317. [CrossRef]
11. Izquierdo-Lorenzo, I.; Alda, I.; Sanchez-Cortes, S.; Garcia-Ramos, J.V. Adsorption and Detection of Sport Doping Drugs on Metallic Plasmonic Nanoparticles of Different Morphology. *Langmuir* **2012**, *28*, 8891–8901. [CrossRef]
12. Otsuka, H.; Nagasaki, Y.; Kataoka, K. PEGylated nanoparticles for biological and pharmaceutical applications. *Adv. Drug Deliv. Rev.* **2012**, *64*, 246–255. [CrossRef]
13. Grabar, K.C.; Freeman, R.G.; Hommer, M.B.; Natan, M.J. Preparation and Characterization of Au Colloid Monolayers. *Anal. Chem.* **1995**, *67*, 735–743. [CrossRef]
14. Bozzini, B.; D'Urzo, L.; Lacitignola, D.; Mele, C.; Sgura, I.; Tondo, E. Investigation into dynamics of Au electrodeposition based on analysis of SERS spectral time series. *Trans. IMF* **2009**, *87*, 193–200. [CrossRef]
15. Bozzini, B.; Gaudenzi, G.P.D.; Mele, C. A SERS investigation of the electrodeposition of Ag-Au alloys from free-cyanide solutions—Part II. *J. Electroanal. Chem.* **2004**, *570*, 29–34. [CrossRef]
16. El-Zahry, M.R.; Mahmoud, A.; Refaat, I.H.; Mohamed, H.A.; Bohlmann, H.; Lendl, B. Antibacterial effect of various shapes of silver nanoparticles monitored by SERS. *Talanta* **2015**, *138*, 183–189. [CrossRef] [PubMed]
17. García-Cámara, B.; Algorri, J.F.; Cuadrado, A.; Urruchi, V.; Sánchez-Pena, J.M.; Serna, R.; Vergaz, R. All-Optical Nanometric Switch Based on the Directional Scattering of Semiconductor Nanoparticles. *J. Phys. Chem. C* **2015**, *119*, 19558–19564. [CrossRef]
18. Niu, W.; Chua, Y.A.A.; Zhang, W.; Huang, H.; Lu, X. Highly Symmetric Gold Nanostars: Crystallographic Control and Surface-Enhanced Raman Scattering Property. *J. Am. Chem. Soc.* **2015**, *137*, 10460–10463. [CrossRef]
19. Dacarro, G.; Pallavicini, P.; Bertani, S.M.; Chirico, G.; D'Alfonso, L.; Falqui, A.; Marchesi, N.; Pascale, A.; Sironi, L.; Taglietti, A.; et al. Synthesis of reduced-size gold nanostars and internalization in SH-SY5Y cells. *J. Colloid Interface Sci.* **2017**, *505*, 1055–1064. [CrossRef]
20. Navarro, J.R.G.; Manchon, D.; Lerouge, F.; Blanchard, N.P.; Marotte, S.; Leverrier, Y.; Marvel, J.; Chaput, F.; Micouin, G.; Gabudean, A.M.; et al. Synthesis of PEGylated gold nanostars and bipyramids for intracellular uptake. *Nanotechnology* **2012**, *23*, 465602. [CrossRef] [PubMed]
21. Liu, T.M.; Yu, J.; Chang, C.A.; Chiou, A.; Chiang, H.K.; Chuang, Y.C.; Wu, C.H.; Hsu, C.H.; Chen, P.A.; Huang, C.C. One-step shell polymerization of inorganic nanoparticles and their applications in SERS/nonlinear optical imaging, drug delivery, and catalysis. *Sci. Rep.* **2014**, *4*, 5593. [CrossRef]
22. Huang, W.S.; Sun, I.W.; Huang, C.C. Promotion of SERS and catalytic activities with bimetallic and ternary concave nanolayers. *J. Mater. Chem. A* **2018**, *6*, 13041–13049. [CrossRef]
23. Black, J.W.; Duncan, W.A.M.; Durant, C.J.; Ganellin, C.R.; Parsons, E.M. Definition and Antagonism of Histamine H2-receptors. *Nature* **1972**, *236*, 385–390. [CrossRef]
24. Bodmer, S.; Imark, C.; Kneubühl, M. Biogenic amines in foods: Histamine and food processing. *Inflamm. Res.* **1999**, *48*, 296–300. [CrossRef]
25. Maintz, L.; Novak, N. Histamine and histamine intolerance. *Am. J. Clin. Nutr.* **2007**, *85*, 1185–1196. [CrossRef]
26. Rahmani, H.; Ingram, C. Histamine controls food intake in sheep via H1 receptors. *Small Rumin. Res.* **2007**, *70*, 110–115. [CrossRef]
27. Gao, F.; Grant, E.; Lu, X. Determination of histamine in canned tuna by molecularly imprinted polymers-surface enhanced Raman spectroscopy. *Anal. Chim. Acta* **2015**, *901*, 68–75. [CrossRef]
28. Stratton, J.E.; Hutkins, R.W.; Taylor, S.L. Biogenic Amines in Cheese and other Fermented Foods: A Review. *J. Food Prot.* **1991**, *54*, 460–470. [CrossRef]

29. Kovacova-Hanuskova, E.; Buday, T.; Gavliakova, S.; Plevkova, J. Histamine, histamine intoxication and intolerance. *Allergol. Immunopathol.* **2015**, *43*, 498–506. [CrossRef]
30. de Cerio, O.G.D.; Barrutia-Borque, A.; Gardeazabal-García, J. Scombroid Poisoning: A Practical Approach. *Actas Dermo-Sifiliográficas (Engl. Ed.)* **2016**, *107*, 567–571. [CrossRef]
31. Harsing, L.G.; Nagashima, H.; Duncalf, D.; Vizi, E.S.; Goldiner, P.L. Determination of Histamine Concentrations in Plasma by Liquid Chromatography/electrochemistry. *Clin. Chem.* **1986**, *32*, 1823–1827.
32. Cinquina, A.; Longo, F.; Cali, A.; Santis, L.D.; Baccelliere, R.; Cozzani, R. Validation and comparison of analytical methods for the determination of histamine in tuna fish samples. *J. Chromatogr. A* **2004**, *1032*, 79–85. [CrossRef]
33. Janci, T.; Mikac, L.; Ivanda, M.; Marusic Radovcic, N.; Medic, H.; Vidacek, S. Optimization of parameters for histamine detection in fish muscle extracts by surface-enhanced Raman spectroscopy using silver colloid SERS substrates. *J. Raman Spectrosc.* **2016**, *48*, 64–72, [CrossRef]
34. Janci, T.; Valinger, D.; Kljusuric, J.G.; Mikac, L.; Vidacek, S.; Ivanda, M. Determination of histamine in fish by Surface Enhanced Raman Spectroscopy using silver colloid SERS substrates. *Food Chem.* **2017**, *224*, 48–54. [CrossRef]
35. Lai, C.H.; Wang, G.A.; Ling, T.K.; Wang, T.J.; Chiu, P.-K.; Chau, Y.F.C.; Huang, C.C.; Chiang, H.P. Near infrared surface-enhanced Raman scattering based on star-shaped gold/silver nanoparticles and hyperbolic metamaterial. *Sci. Rep.* **2017**, *7*, 5446. [CrossRef]
36. Kimling, J.; Maier, M.; Okenve, B.; Kotaidis, V.; Ballot, H.; Plech, A. Turkevich Method for Gold Nanoparticle Synthesis Revisited. *J. Phys. Chem. B* **2006**, *110*, 15700–15707. [CrossRef]
37. Childs, A.; Vinogradova, E.; Ruiz-Zepeda, F.; Velazquez-Salazar, J.J.; Jose-Yacaman, M. Biocompatible gold/silver nanostars for surface-enhanced Raman scattering. *J. Raman Spectrosc.* **2016**, *47*, 651–655. [CrossRef]
38. Lin, W.C.; Tsai, T.R.; Huang, H.L.; Shiau, C.Y.; Chiang, H.P. SERS Study of Histamine by Using Silver Film over Nanosphere Structure. *Plasmonics* **2012**, *7*, 709–716. [CrossRef]
39. Rodríguez-Lorenzo, L.; Álvarez Puebla, R.A.; de Abajo, F.J.G.; Liz-Marzán, L.M. Surface Enhanced Raman Scattering Using Star-Shaped Gold Colloidal Nanoparticles. *J. Phys. Chem. C* **2010**, *114*, 7336–7340. [CrossRef]
40. Nalbant Esenturk, E.; Hight Walker, A.R. Surface-enhanced Raman scattering spectroscopy via gold nanostars. *J. Raman Spectrosc.* **2009**, *40*, 86–91. [CrossRef]
41. Zhang, W.; Liu, J.; Niu, W.; Yan, H.; Lu, X.; Liu, B. Tip-Selective Growth of Silver on Gold Nanostars for Surface-Enhanced Raman Scattering. *ACS Appl. Mater. Interfaces* **2018**, *10*, 14850–14856. [CrossRef]
42. Collado, J.A.; Ramírez, F.J. Vibrational spectra and assignments of histamine dication in the solid state and in solution. *J. Raman Spectrosc.* **2000**, *31*, 925–931. [CrossRef]
43. Torreggiani, A.; Tamba, M.; Bonora, S.; Fini, G. Raman and IR study on copper binding of histamine. *Biopolymers* **2003**, *72*, 290–298. [CrossRef]

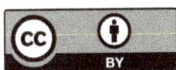

© 2019 by the authors. Licensee MDPI, Basel, Switzerland. This article is an open access article distributed under the terms and conditions of the Creative Commons Attribution (CC BY) license (http://creativecommons.org/licenses/by/4.0/).

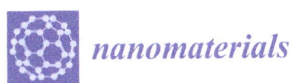

Article

Facile Ag-Film Based Surface Enhanced Raman Spectroscopy Using DNA Molecular Switch for Ultra-Sensitive Mercury Ions Detection

Xiujie Liu [1], Mengmeng Liu [1], Yudong Lu [2,*], Changji Wu [2], Yunchao Xu [1], Duo Lin [1], Dechan Lu [2], Ting Zhou [2] and Shangyuan Feng [1,*]

1. Key Laboratory of Optoelectronic Science and Technology for Medicine of Ministry of Education, Fujian Provincial Key Laboratory of Photonics Technology, Fujian Normal University, Fuzhou 350007, China; m18396517281@163.com (X.L.); MM_liu@163.com (M.L.); m13512027287_1@163.com (Y.X.); linduo1986@163.com (D.L.)
2. Fujian Key Laboratory of Polymer Materials, College of Chemistry and Materials Science, Fuzhou 350007, China; 18060489009@163.com (C.W.); 18149544204@163.com (D.L.); zt1102801305@163.com (T.Z.)
* Correspondence: luyd@fjnu.edu.cn (Y.L.); syfeng@fjnu.edu.cn (S.F.); Tel.: +86-591-8348-9919 (S.F.)

Received: 1 July 2018; Accepted: 1 August 2018; Published: 6 August 2018

Abstract: Heavy metal pollution has long been the focus of attention because of its serious threat to human health and the environment. Surface enhanced Raman spectroscopy (SERS) has shown great potential for metal detection owing to many advantages, including, requiring fewer samples, its minimal damage to specimen, and its high sensitivity. In this work, we proposed a simple and distinctive method, based on SERS, using facile silver film (Ag-film) combined with a DNA molecular switch, which allowed for the highly specific detection of heavy metal mercury ions (Hg^{2+}). When in the presence of Hg^{2+} ions, the signals from Raman probes attach to single-stranded DNA, which will be dramatically enhanced due to the specific structural change of DNA strands—resulting from the interaction between Hg^{2+} ions and DNA bases. This SERS sensor could achieve an ultralow limit of detection (1.35×10^{-15} M) for Hg^{2+} detection. In addition, we applied this SERS sensor to detect Hg^{2+} in real blood samples. The results suggested that this SERS platform could be a promising alternative tool for Hg^{2+} detection in clinical, environmental, and food inspection.

Keywords: surface-enhanced Raman spectroscopy (SERS); Ag-film; Hg^{2+} ions detection; SERS sensor

1. Introduction

Great attention has been paid to heavy metal pollution in our living environment, especially from mercury ions, which can accumulate in the human body [1,2], thus endangering human health. In general, heavy metal can accumulate through food and water, and is easily enriched via the skin and digestive tract, which can lead to damages to the nervous system, cardiovascular system, and the liver [3,4]. The clinical manifestations of chronic mercury poisoning were mainly neurological symptoms, such as headaches, dizziness, and ataxia [5,6]. Therefore, it is of great significance to develop a highly specific and ultrasensitive sensor for detecting the content of Hg^{2+} ions in blood, water, and food samples. At present, there are many traditional methods used to analyze Hg^{2+} ions in samples, such as cold-vapor atomic absorption spectrometry (CV-AAS) [7], the dithizone colorimetric method [8], atomic emission spectrometry [9], and inductively coupled plasma mass spectrometry (ICP-MS) [10]. However, these methods have some deficiencies, such as expensive instruments, complex sample preprocessing, high cost, and vulnerability to the interference of other metal ions. Therefore, it is necessary to develop a more simple, convenient, and sensitive method for the detection of Hg^{2+} ions.

Surface enhanced Raman spectroscopy (SERS) technology is a very powerful trace detection tool that not only has most of the advantages of Raman spectroscopy, which can provide abundant structural information of chemical molecules, real-time and in-situ detection, but also has high sensitivity, simple sample treatment, and high accuracy [11,12]. Fleischmann and Van Duyne et al. found that the Raman signals of the pyrimidine molecules adsorbed on the rough surface of the silver electrode was greatly enhanced [13,14]. With the use of SERS, the Raman signal can be dramatically enhanced by up to 10^{14} times, as compared to normal Raman spectroscopy [15], because of its electronic resonance between optical fields and surface plasmons [16]. Many noble metals, for example, Au, Ag, or Cu can engender strong electromagnetic enhancements [17]. Subsequently, on this basis, a variety of enhanced substrates were developed, such as nanoparticles of different shapes that included nanospheres [18], nanorods [19], nanowires [20], and so on. SERS could overcome the shortcoming of Raman spectra's low sensitivity and achieve rich structural information that is hard to obtain by conventional Raman spectroscopy. What is more, it can effectively analyze and represent the adsorption orientation, the variation of adsorption state, and the interface information of the compound at the interface [21,22]. With the rapid development of laser technology, nanotechnology, and computer technology, SERS has been widely applied in the material analysis, biomedicine [23], food safety, and in environmental monitoring [11,24]. It should be noted that although mercury, showing a high toxicity to the human body, has been definitively prohibited, it was still widely distributed in water, soil, ambient air, and even food and cosmetics [25,26]. Through breathing, the skin, and the digestive system, it is accumulated and enriched in the organs, especially in the lung, liver, and brain [27,28]. In recent years, the trace detection of heavy metal ions has attracted more and more attention. Several groups have proposed various methods for detecting Hg^{2+}, which is based on different SERS substrates. Liu's group has developed a one-step, room temperature, and colorimetric method by using oligonucleotide-tethered AuNPs probes and a linker oligonucleotide with a number of T-T mismatches, resulting in the formation of particle aggregates accompanied colorimetric responses with the addition of Hg^{2+} into the solution [29]. Yang et al. have provided an approach for the visual and fluorescent sensing of Hg^{2+} in aqueous solution, which is based on the Hg^{2+}-induced conformational change of a thymine (T)-rich single-stranded DNA (ssDNA), and the difference in electrostatic affinity between ssDNA and double stranded (dsDNA) with gold nanoparticles [30]. His group used the resultant Ag–Au NPs@Si as a substrate for detecting Hg^{2+} ions with a low detection limit of 100 fM, and had a good linear relationship [31]. Herein, we developed a new method with more power to detect Hg^{2+} ions with a low detection limit of 1.35×10^{-15} M in human blood samples.

Since mercury ions (Hg^{2+}) can specifically form a strong and stable thymine-Hg^{2+}-thymine complex (T-Hg^{2+}-T) with thymine bases (T) [29,30], the oligonucleotide probes can be designed based on this principle to detect mercury ions. For the first time, the functionalized silver film was used as a SERS substrate for Hg^{2+} ions detection. Herein, a facile SERS substrate was prepared for Hg^{2+} detection by silver mirror reaction (SMR), which was one of the most effective technologies for preparing micro-nanometallic materials, and has the features of cost-effectiveness, high uniformity, simplicity of operator, and so on [32,33]. By taking the advantages of the specific binding of oligonucleotides and silver-based Raman-active substrate, in this work, we proposed a simple and highly specific method to detect the content of Hg^{2+} ions in complex biomatrices, and aim to overcome the drawbacks of traditional detection methods of Hg^{2+} ions, such as poor specificity and sensitivity.

2. Materials and Methods

2.1. Materials and Reagents

Silver nitrate ($AgNO_3$), ammonium hydroxide ($NH_3 \cdot H_2O$), glucose ($C_6H_{12}O_6$), absolute ethyl alcohol (C_2H_6O), Rhodamine 6G (R6G), glass slides (0.5 cm × 0.5 cm), sodium chloride (NaCl), Phosphate-buffered solution (PBS, PH = 7), and DNA probe (Cy5-TTCTTTCTTGGGGTTGTTTGTT-SH) were purchased from the Sangon Biotech (Shanghai, China). $CaCl_2$, $CuCl_2$, $MnCl_2$, $AlCl_3$, $ZnCl_2$,

NiCl$_2$, CdCl$_2$, FeCl$_3$, MgSO$_4$, and HgCl$_2$, were analytical reagents and had not been further purified. The standard solutions of Hg^{2+} ions were diluted by deionized water. The blood samples were obtained from the Fujian Province Tumor Hospital, Fuzhou, China. All of the chemical regents were analytical grade, and all solutions were prepared with ultrapure water.

2.2. Instrumentation

The SERS spectra was obtained using a confocal Raman micro-spectrometer (Renishaw, London, UK) under the excitation of a 785 nm laser in the range of 400–1800 cm^{-1}, which was performed by using the software package WIRE 2.0 (Renishaw, London, UK). The laser power that we chose was about 5 mW, employing typically 10 s exposure time, and a 2 cm^{-1} resolution of the Raman spectra. We used a microscope with a Leica ×20 objective to obtain the spectral signal in posterior scattering geometry. The wavelength was calibrated by using the 520 cm^{-1} vibration band of the silicon wafer. Scanning electron microscopy (SEM) images were taken with a JSM-6380LV scanning electron microscope (JEOL, Tokyo, Japan).

2.3. Preparation of Samples

2.3.1. The Preparation of Silver Ammonium Solution

The concrete steps were as follows. The ammonia solution was added in the 3 mL 2 wt% silver nitrate solution, drop by drop, to prepare the silver ammonia solution. A brown precipitate was first produced, and ammonia was continuously added dropwise until the precipitate completely dissolved [34]. Then, a drop of 6 wt% glucose solution was added and shaken.

2.3.2. The Preparation of Standard Solutions of DNA Probe (Cy5-α-SH) and Rhodamine 6G (R6G)

Firstly, the PBS buffer solution was used as a solvent to dissolve the DNA probe (Cy5-α-SH) and prepared the solution with a concentration of 100 µM. Then, the initial concentration was diluted to the concentration of 1 µM and was used in this experiment.

In addition, weighing R6G powder was dissolved in deionized water and was transferred to a volumetric flask, setting to a constant volume and shaking. The concentration of the solution was 10^{-4} M and was stored for later use.

2.3.3. The Formulation of Standard Solutions of Hg^{2+}

Briefly, Hg^{2+} solution was prepared with ultrapure water at an initial concentration of 10^{-3} M. The solution was then shaken completely to form a highly dispersed solution. Following this, the solution was diluted to a concentration from 10^{-6} to 10^{-15} M.

2.3.4. Preparation of Human Plasma Samples

After 12 h of overnight fasting, a single 3 mL peripheral blood sample was obtained from the study subjects between 7:00 a.m.–8:00 a.m. with the use of coagulant. Blood cells were removed by centrifugation at 2000 rpm for 15 min to obtain the blood plasma.

2.4. Preparation of SERS Substrate

2.4.1. Cutting and Cleaning of the Slides

First of all, sheet glass was cut into small pieces of 0.5 cm in length and width (0.5 × 0.5 cm). The prepared small pieces of glass were degreased, soaked with chromic acid for more than 2 h, and then washed with ultrapure water, followed by an ultrasound for 30 min in anhydrous ethanol and washed with ultrapure water 5–6 times.

2.4.2. Synthesis of the Silver Film

The treated small glass flakes were put into the prepared silver ammonium solution. The reaction time was 15 min and the temperature was 70 °C, which was the most significant aspect of accurately controlling the reduction reaction time and temperature. As a result, a layer of silver was deposited on the slide. It was taken out of the glass, washed 4–5 times with ultrapure water, and dried in a slow nitrogen flow to prepare for the next modification with the DNA probes.

2.5. Reproducibility Detection of SERS Substrate

Firstly, R6G was used as the target molecules, and the prepared standard solution, was randomly dripped on the substrate of Ag-film. After drying, it was placed under a microscope to collect the Raman spectrum by a ×20 objective.

In addition, the reproducibility of the substrate of Ag-film was verified by using the DNA probe as the target molecules, and the SERS substrates of the assembled probe chain, were immersed in the standard solution of Hg^{2+} with a concentration of 10^{-8} M. After drying in a gentle nitrogen flow, a ×20 objective was used to collect the corresponding SERS spectra.

2.6. Construction of Probes for Detection of Mercury Ions (Hg^{2+})

The prepared substrate constructed the SERS sensor that specifically responded to Hg^{2+} by conjugating with single-stranded DNA (Cy5-α-SH). The assembly process was as follows. The prepared SERS substrates were immersed in the assembly buffer (PH = 7.0) for 12 h, which contained 1 µM DNA probes (Cy5-α-SH) with a double labeling of dye molecules Cy5 and thiol molecules, and 10 mM phosphoric acid solution. Then, the substrates were placed in phosphate buffered saline solution, including 0.1 M NaCl, overnight to ensure that sufficient stem-loop DNA self-assembled with the silver film via Ag-S bonds. Next, the substrates were again washed five times with phosphate buffered solution (PBS) and dried with a gentle nitrogen flow.

2.7. Detection of Mercury Ions (Hg^{2+})

The assembled substrates were immersed in the standard solution with different concentrations of Hg^{2+} for 120 min, and taken out and washed 3 times. After drying, a SERS measure was performed to obtain the corresponding Raman spectra by using a 785 nm laser with a power of 5 mW, and the control baseplates were also observed and detected by a Leica ×20 objective.

2.8. Detection of Hg^{2+} Ions in Blood Samples

The blood samples were collected from the Fujian Province Tumor Hospital. Firstly, the blood was taken from healthy volunteers, and the blood plasma was obtained by centrifugation. The main components of plasma include 90–92% of water, and the other 10% are mainly solute plasma proteins. The obtained plasma interacted with the assembled substrate for 2 h, taken out and washed 3 times, and then dried under nitrogen to perform SERS detection. Next, we added the standard solution of Hg^{2+}, with the concentration of 50 nM and 100 nM, to the plasma samples by the standard addition method. Finally, the assembled substrates were immersed in the prepared plasma samples, and then a SERS measurement was performed. Each sample was measured 3 times to obtain an average.

3. Results and Discussion

The proposed SERS sensor was based on the specific binding feature of the T-Hg^{2+}-T coordination, and the Cy5-labeled DNA strands (Cy5-α-SH) can be self-assembled on the silver film substrate via Ag-S bonds [6,29]. In this study, DNA strands were used as a switch for the Raman signal, which indirectly indicated whether there were mercury ions (Hg^{2+}) in the analyte, as shown in Figure 1. The SERS substrate of the Hg^{2+} sensor was the Ag film with a uniform surface via silver mirror reaction. Next, the probe chains were modified on the substrate. Briefly, the substrates were immersed in the solution of the probe chains, then removed and dried. Here, the principle of the probe molecule chains, as a signal switch to detect Hg^{2+} ions, was that, in the absence of Hg^{2+} ions, the DNA probes showed an "open" conformation (signal-off), and Cy5-tagged enzyme strands were far away from the substrate, thus producing a weak Raman signal. However, in the presence of the Hg^{2+} ions, the former "open" structural conformation would change into a "hairpin" structure, which was formed by Hg^{2+} ions bonding with thymine bases (T) [30,35]. This conformational change resulted in a shorter distance between Cy5 labeled molecules and the surface of the Ag-film, leading to a strong Raman signal (signal-on). We also investigated the effect of the concentration of single-stranded DAN and the space occupied by the probes of the stem-loop structure on the experiment. He's group [36,37] employed gold nanoparticles (AuNPs), decorated with a silicon nanowire array (SiNWAr), for surface-enhanced Raman scattering (SERS) substrates to detect Hg^{2+}. By comparing the relationship between fluorescence intensity and the corresponding concentration of Cy5-ssDNA, we can observe that, with the increase of Cy5 modified single-stranded DNA from 0 to 1 µM, fluorescence intensity gradually enhances and tends to be a saturated value. Similarly, the size range of the synthesized Ag-film substrate in our experiment was at the micro-nanometer level and obviously exhibited a three-dimensional spatial configuration, which was formed by silver clusters in the shape of a polyhedron at the top. In addition, the size of the substrate they used was the same as ours (0.5 × 0.5 cm), and therefore, the concentration of ss-DNA was 1 µM in our experiment when assembling DNA molecules on an Ag-film substrate. We predicted that there was enough space for the ss-DNA to form a "hairpin" structure on a SERS substrate. In the experiment, the sensitivity of the analysis system would be affected by the length of the DNA strands and the number of T-T mismatched bases. Yang's group proposed a method for visual and fluorescence sensing of Hg^{2+} in aqueous solution, and also made a corresponding study of the length of single-stranded DNA and the number of T-T mismatched bases with the interaction of Hg^{2+} ions [30]. By comparing the fluorescence response of a different number of the T-T mismatch sites to the different concentrations of Hg^{2+}, the DNA chains of the 7 mer T-T mismatch sites had the most significant responses to the fluorescence of Hg^{2+}. In addition, comparing the fluorescence response of single-stranded DNA with different chain lengths to different concentrations of Hg^{2+}, it was found that the corresponding fluorescence of Hg^{2+} was decreased with the increase of chain length. Importantly, the greatest advantage of the DNA strand of the 7 mer T-T mismatch sites was that they were more sensitive to the low concentration of Hg^{2+} ions—so, the DNA strand currently used is optimal.

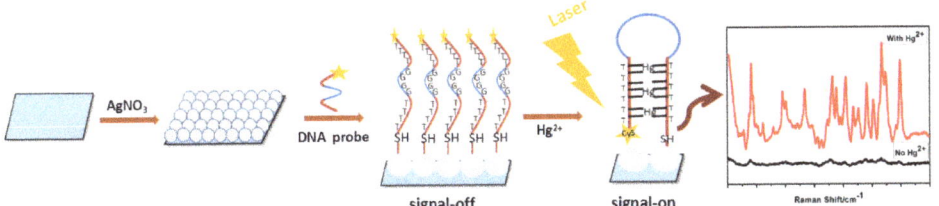

Figure 1. Schematic illustration of the mechanism of the surface-enhanced Raman scattering (SERS) sensor for the detection of mercury ions (Hg^{2+}), based on the T-Hg^{2+}-T coordination.

In our experiment, the Ag film was synthesized by silver mirror reaction and was used as a SERS substrate. The Ag film formed was analogous to a 3-D spatial structure, which was evidently demonstrated in the scanning electronic microscopy (SEM) image (Figure 2a). Close examination revealed that there were many nano-cavities and nano-gaps formed by the stacking of closely adjacent nanoparticles. Many papers have shown an extremely strong local field enhancement in the gap between two closely spaced silver nanoparticles [38,39]. Therefore, the 3-D Ag-film substrates may generate a lot of effective hot spots and a strong SERS response for DNA detection. In addition to this, our method is characterized by the features of cost-effectiveness and facile synthesis, as well as being easy to repeat. The spatial morphology is evidently demonstrated in the scanning electronic microscopy (SEM) image (Figure 2a).

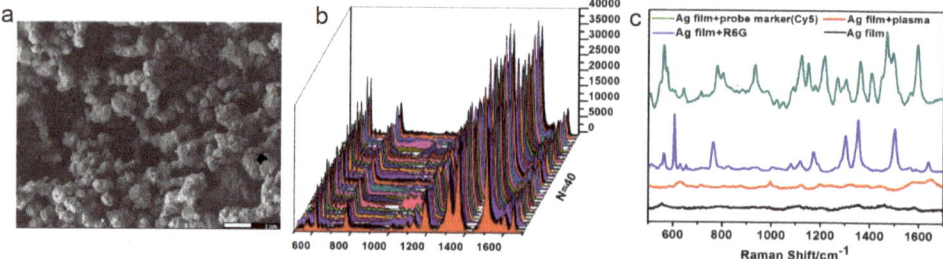

Figure 2. (a) The SEM image demonstrating the morphology of the Ag-film substrate. (b) SERS spectra of R6G with a concentration of 10^{-4} M were collected from 40 random points on the resultant substrates. (c) The spectral signal of plasma detected on a silver-film substrate (red), SERS spectra of R6G (10^{-4} M) distributed on silver film substrate (blue), spectrum of the Cy5 reporter (green), and background signal of the synthesized Ag film substrate (black).

The SERS technology has the advantages of high accuracy, easy operation, and simple sample pretreatment [11,12]. Therefore, SERS detection plays an active role in the rapid detection of trace level and heavy metal ions. However, the reproducibility of SERS detection is a common problem that has plagued researchers. In order to evaluate and verify the Ag film-based substrate used in our experiments, we used R6G as target molecules on the synthesized substrates, and SERS measurements were performed from 40 random spots. The resulting SERS spectra are shown in Figure 2b, which clearly presents a relatively uniform Raman spectrum, and the Relative standard deviation (RSD) value of the Raman spectrum of R6G was 15.1%—by selecting a Raman peak of R6G at 1362 cm^{-1}. Typically, the SERS spectra of R6G, with a concentration of 10^{-4} M, was measured on a prepared silver film substrate (the blue line), as shown in Figure 2c, the red line is the spectral signal of plasma detected on an Ag-film substrate showing that the plasma has a lesser background interference signal on the silver film, and the green line was the spectrum of SERS reporter Cy5. The background signal of this substrate is the black line, showing that the synthesized Ag film had little background interference, enabling a reliable SERS detection using this substrate.

By utilizing this Cy5 labeled, single-stranded DNA, with SERS sensor as a signal switch, we measured different concentrations of Hg^{2+} ions in the standard solution; a series of SERS spectra of Hg^{2+} ions with concentrations from 1.0×10^{-14} to 1.0×10^{-6} M could be obtained. Importantly, we were able to clearly observe the characteristic peaks of Cy5 reporters (Figure 3a). According to the principle of T-Hg^{2+}-T coordination [29,35], when there was no mercury ions, the signal switch was in the "closed state", so the SERS signal of the Cy5 reporters was very weak—as shown by the black line in Figure 3a. However, when the Hg^{2+} ions were presented, in the measured solution, the signal switch was "turned on" and the SERS signal of the Cy5 was immensely enhanced. Furthermore, with the concentration of the Hg^{2+} ions increasing gradually, the SERS intensity of Cy5 was increased simultaneously, which can thus be used as an indicator for the concentration of the Hg^{2+} ions. In order to accurately demonstrate the effect of concentrations of Hg^{2+} ions on the SERS intensity, we monitored the intensity of the SERS peak at 1595 cm^{-1} (assigned to C=N stretching modes). As shown in Figure 3b, the SERS intensity of Cy5 at 1595 cm^{-1} was increased from 2153.6 to 14,478.8 (a.u.), and the concentration of Hg^{2+} gradually increased from 10 fM to 1 µM. The standard curve was achieved as $y = 1575.7x + 24{,}019$, it should be noted that the calculated correlation coefficient was $R^2 = 0.9991$, indicating that it exhibited a good linear relationship between the logarithm of concentration of Hg^{2+} and SERS intensity of the probe, and the limit of detection (LOD) for Hg^{2+} was 1.35×10^{-15} M. We adopted a method of signal-to-noise ratio (S/N) of approximately 3:1, which was generally considered to be acceptable for estimating the limit of detection (LOD). Taking the standard solution of Hg^{2+} with a concentration of 10^{-14} M as an example, the SERS intensity of the 1595 cm^{-1} peak, and the background baseline, were selected to calculate, and the LOD was 1.35×10^{-15} M. Compared with other reports based on the mechanism of T-Hg^{2+}-T coordination [30,40], a much lower LOD for mercury ions using SERS measurement can be obtained using this novel sensor with single-stranded DNA as a signal switch. The LOD obtained was seven orders of magnitude lower, as compared to the defined limit (10 nM) in drinkable water by the United States Environmental Protection Agency (USEPA). At a higher magnification of the SEM image, as shown in Figure 2a, we can clearly observe that the size range of the synthesized silver film substrate was at the micro-nanometer level and obviously exhibited a three-dimensional spatial configuration that was formed by silver nanoparticles and silver clusters in the shape of a polyhedron at the top [41,42]. It is well known that a powerful and effective SERS substrate was attributed to the huge amount of micro-/nanoscale structures of polyhedral and nanoscale junctions [38,39], which thereby formed a great deal of SERS "hot spots" that enhanced the intensity of the electromagnetic field, resulting in the tremendous enhancement of the SERS signal. It was precisely for this reason that the limit of detection (LOD) for Hg^{2+} ions in our experiments can be as low as 1.35×10^{-15} M. In addition, we also made a standard curve of the SERS intensity of Cy5 at 1362 cm^{-1} (attributed to the methine chain deformation of Cy5) with logarithmic Hg^{2+} concentrations from 10^{-14} to 10^{-6} M, and the correlation coefficient was $R^2 = 0.9990$. By comparing the correlation coefficients of the two peak positions, we can draw a conclusion that the values of R^2 were almost the same, and it also proved that the correlation between the SERS intensity and concentrations of Hg^{2+} ions is good.

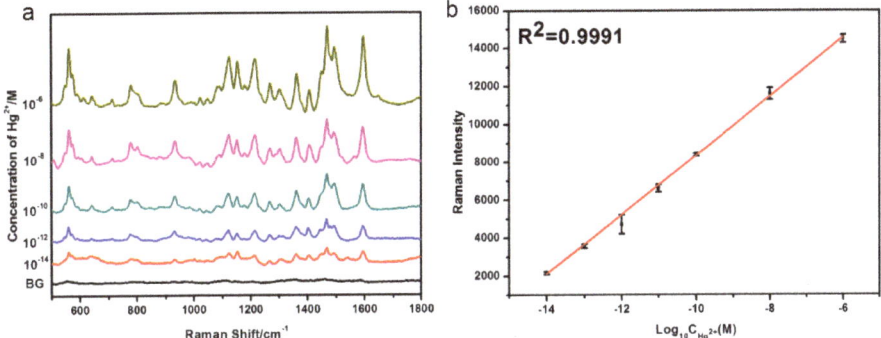

Figure 3. (**a**) SERS spectra of Cy5 with different concentrations of Hg^{2+} in distilled water ranging from 1.0×10^{-14} to 1.0×10^{-6} M (BG = blank control), (**b**) standard curve of Raman intensity of Cy5 at 1595 cm^{-1} with logarithmic Hg^{2+} concentrations from 10^{-14} to 10^{-6} M.

To evaluate the reproducibility of the Hg^{2+} sensor, after modifying the DNA probes on the Ag-film substrates, we used the standard solution of Hg^{2+} with a concentration of 10^{-8} M to immerse the substrate, and then measured the SERS spectrum at ten randomly selected spots. The RSD value was 7.5%, from a comparison of the intensity of the Raman peaks at 1362 cm^{-1} in Figure 4a, which bring reliable SERS detection. In addition, in order to verify the stability of the sensor, we placed the substrate in the air for three days where it interacted with a standard solution of Hg^{2+} at a concentration of 10^{-8} M. Figure 4b shows the SERS signals of the labeled molecule from substrates, exposed to the common air environment for zero days and three days, and we can clearly see that the Raman signals did not significantly attenuate. Consequently, we can conclude that the SERS sensor exposed to air over a short time could not lead to an obvious attenuation of SERS signals. This can be explained as follows. Under mild oxidizing conditions, the formation of a silver oxide layer after 20 h of exposure time was not detected by X-ray photoelectron spectroscopy (XPS). Then, by using UV to detect again, the relevant data showed no significant shift in the surface plasmon bands of immobilized Ag NPs after three days of exposure to environmental air [43,44]. Sukhishvili's group followed the idea that molecular oxygen does not oxidize silver under ambient conditions, and the ozone is considered to be the main oxidant for starting the oxidation process of silver. In addition, studies on the change of plasma absorption bands show that chemical enhancement was the main reason for the attenuation of SERS signals by exposure to ambient air. However, in our experiment, since there was no direct contact between the labeling molecule and the SERS substrate after the formation of the "hairpin" structure [31,45], the enhancement effect of the SERS signals mainly depend on the electromagnetic enhancement, and not the chemical enhancement. Therefore, in the mild environment of the laboratory, silver oxidation has little effect on the detection results within a short time.

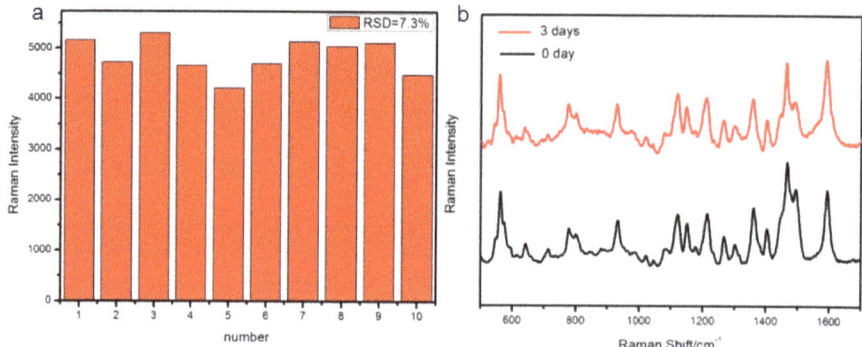

Figure 4. (a) Relative standard deviation (RSD) of specific Raman modes at 1362 cm^{-1} of the 10 random points; and, (b) SERS signals of the labeled molecule (Cy5) on the functionalized Ag-film substrates under the exposure to the common air environment for 0 days and 3 days.

To verify the high selectivity and specificity of this SERS sensor, we also measured other metal ions using this sensor. By comparing the SERS intensity of the 1362 cm^{-1} peaks for the Cy5-labeled molecules, as shown in Figure 5, the strong Raman signal can only be observed in the presence of Hg^{2+} ions, rather than any other metal ions. The mixture of ions showed a smaller Raman intensity than the Hg^{2+} only. This is explainable. In the experiment, when Hg^{2+} ions were detected separately, the concentration was 10 nM and the volume was 200 µL, and the amount of Hg^{2+} ions substance (n) was 2×10^{-10} mol. However, the concentration of Hg^{2+} used in the preparation of the mixed solution was 10 nM and the volume was 60 µL, the n of Hg^{2+} was 6×10^{-11} mol. The n of Hg^{2+} ions in the mixed solution was only one third of the original. The less amount of Hg^{2+} ions, the less Raman-labeled molecules can be detected, thus the intensity of the Raman spectrum will be reduced. It should be noticed that the spectral intensity of Hg^{2+} was still distinctly stronger than in other metal ions, even though the concentration of other interference metal ions was 100 times higher than the Hg^{2+} ions. This demonstrated that this sensor was highly selective for Hg^{2+} ions because Hg^{2+}, and probe chains, had considerable binding affinity to form the stable T-Hg^{2+}-T complexes.

To evaluate the practicability of this method, we used it to detect the Hg^{2+} ions in real human blood samples. The method we used was the standard addition method. We measured the content of Hg^{2+} ions in the blood of a healthy person, and the prepared blood samples added the standard solutions of Hg^{2+} ions with different concentrations. The SERS measurement for each specimen was repeated three times. The related statistics are shown in Table 1. The resulting recovery rate for Hg^{2+} ions was 91–104%, showing a remarkable recovery rate. The results showed that this method has good prospects and applicability for the detection of Hg^{2+} in body fluid.

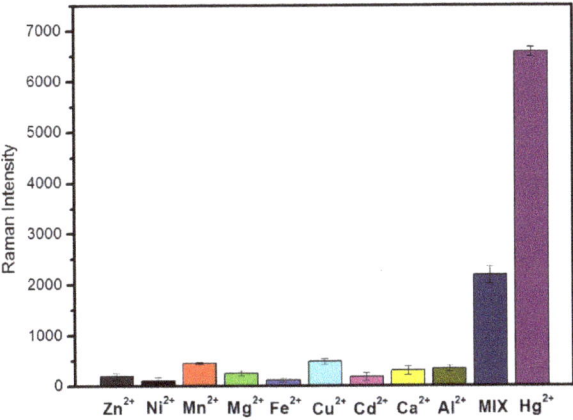

Figure 5. Specificity of the SERS sensor for Hg^{2+} detection. The concentration of Hg^{2+} was 10 nM and other interference metal ions were 1 μM. Additionally, all metal ions were mixed together, including the Hg^{2+} ions (mix).

Table 1. Determination results of Hg^{2+} in human blood samples.

Sample	Spiked Concentration (nM)	Detected Concentration (Mean ± SD, nM, n = 3)	Recovery (%)
Original blood	0	$(2.0 \times 10^{-4}) \pm 1.67$	
blood sample 1	50	48.89 ± 1.37	91–104
blood sample 2	100	97.66 ± 6.6	95–101

4. Conclusions

In summary, an ultra-sensitive, highly specific SERS sensor was developed for detecting Hg^{2+} ions in solution, and in complex human body fluids, using single-stranded DNA as the signal switch. In the presence of Hg^{2+} ions, there was a transformation from an "open" single-strand of DNA, to a "hairpin" configuration via the T-Hg^{2+}-T coordination. Additionally, using the silver mirror reaction, we prepared a highly efficient SERS substrate, which was characterized with a homogeneous 3D micro-nano structure, thus achieving enormous "hotspots". Results show that this sensor has both high sensitivity (a limit of detection of 1.35×10^{-15} M) and specificity for Hg^{2+} detection. Even for real blood samples, this sensor still presented a high performance for Hg^{2+} detection, demonstrating the great potential of this senor for heavy metal ions detection in real human biofluids.

Author Contributions: Data curation, X.L.; Formal analysis, X.L., C.W. and D.L.; Funding acquisition, Y.L. and S.F.; Investigation, M.L., Y.X., D.L. and T.Z.; Resources, S.F.; Writing-review & editing, S.F.

Funding: National Natural Science Foundation of China (No. 61575043), the scientific research innovation team construction program of Fujian Normal University (No. IRTL1702), strait united fund (No. U1605253), the program for Changjiang Scholars and Innovative Research Team in University (No. IRT1115), Natural Science Foundation of Fujian Province of China (Nos. 2016J01292, 2015J01436), and the program for new century excellent talent in Fujian Province University (No. J1-1160).

Acknowledgments: This work was supported by Fujian Province Tumor Hospital, P. R. China, Department of Radiation Oncology, the Teaching Hospital of Fujian Medical University, Fujian Cancer Hospital & Fujian Medical University Cancer Hospita, Fuzhou, Fujian, 350122, China. The authors thank Yao Lin for improving the English.

Conflicts of Interest: The authors declare that there are no conflict of interest.

References

1. Järup, L. Hazards of heavy metal contamination. *Br. Med. Bull.* **2003**, *68*, 167–182. [CrossRef] [PubMed]
2. Zahir, F.; Rizwi, S.J.; Haq, S.K.; Khan, R.H. Low dose mercury toxicity and human health. *Environ. Toxicol. Pharmacol.* **2005**, *20*, 351–360. [CrossRef] [PubMed]
3. Tchounwou, P.B.; Ayensu, W.K.; Ninashvili, N.; Sutton, D. Environmental exposure to mercury and its toxicopathologic implications for public health. *Environ. Toxicol.* **2003**, *18*, 149–175. [CrossRef] [PubMed]
4. Liu, J.; Chen, Y.; Wang, W.F.; Feng, J.; Peng, S.; Ma, S.; Chen, H.; Chen, X. Effective synthesis of highly fluorescent nitrogen doped carbon nanoparticles for selective sensing of Hg^{2+} in food and cosmetics samples. *RSC Adv.* **2016**, *6*, 89916–89924. [CrossRef]
5. Kim, H.N.; Ren, W.X.; Kim, J.S.; Yoon, J. Fluorescent and colorimetric sensors for detection of lead, cadmium, and mercury ions. *Chem. Soc. Rev.* **2012**, *43*, 3210–3244. [CrossRef] [PubMed]
6. Xu, Z.; Lan, T.; Huang, X.; Dong, C.; Ren, J. A sensitive assay of mercury using fluorescence correlation spectroscopy of gold nanoparticles. *Luminescence* **2015**, *30*, 605–610. [CrossRef] [PubMed]
7. Serafimovski, I.; Karadjova, I.; Stafilov, T.; Cvetković, J. Determination of inorganic and methylmercury in fish by cold vapor atomic absorption spectrometry and inductively coupled plasma atomic emission spectrometry. *Microchem. J.* **2008**, *89*, 42–47. [CrossRef]
8. Takahashi, Y.; Danwittayakul, S.; Suzuki, T.M. Dithizone nanofiber-coated membrane for filtration-enrichment and colorimetric detection of trace Hg(II) ion. *Analyst* **2009**, *134*, 1380. [CrossRef] [PubMed]
9. Matusiewicz, H.; Fish, J.; Malinski, T. Electrochemical preconcentration of metals using mercury film electrodes followed by electrothermal vaporization into an inductively coupled plasma and determination by atomic emission spectrometry. *Anal. Chem.* **1987**, *59*, 2264–2269. [CrossRef] [PubMed]
10. Townsend, A.T.; Miller, K.A.; Mclean, S.; Aldous, S. The determination of copper, zinc, cadmium and lead in urine by high resolution ICP-MS. *J. Anal. At. Spectrom.* **1998**, *13*, 1213–1219. [CrossRef]
11. Li, J.F.; Zhang, Y.J.; Ding, S.Y.; Panneerselvam, R.; Tian, Z.Q. Core-Shell Nanoparticle-Enhanced Raman Spectroscopy. *Chem. Rev.* **2017**, *117*. [CrossRef] [PubMed]
12. Ma, P.; Liang, F.; Yang, Q.; Wang, D.; Sun, Y.; Wang, X.; Gao, D.; Song, D. Highly sensitive SERS probe for mercury(II) using cyclodextrin-protected silver nanoparticles functionalized with methimazole. *Microchim. Acta* **2014**, *181*, 975–981. [CrossRef]
13. Fleischmann, M.; Hendra, P.J.; Mcquillan, A.J. Raman spectra of pyridine adsorbed at a silver electrode. *Chem. Phys. Lett.* **1974**, *26*, 163–166. [CrossRef]
14. Jeanmaire, D.L.; Duyne, R.P.V. Surface raman spectroelectrochemistry: Part I. Heterocyclic, aromatic, and aliphatic amines adsorbed on the anodized silver electrode. *J. Electroanal. Chem. Interfacial Electrochem.* **1977**, *84*, 1–20. [CrossRef]
15. Feng, S.; Zheng, Z.; Xu, Y.; Lin, J.; Chen, G.; Weng, C.; Lin, D.; Qiu, S.; Cheng, M.; Huang, Z. A noninvasive cancer detection strategy based on gold nanoparticle surface-enhanced raman spectroscopy of urinary modified nucleosides isolated by affinity chromatography. *Biosens. Bioelectron.* **2017**, *91*, 616–622. [CrossRef] [PubMed]
16. Kneipp, J.; Kneipp, H.; Kneipp, K. SERS—A single-molecule and nanoscale tool for bioanalytics. *Chem. Soc. Rev.* **2008**, *37*, 1052–1060. [CrossRef] [PubMed]
17. Stiles, P.L.; Dieringer, J.A.; Shah, N.C.; Van Duyne, R.P. Surface-enhanced Raman spectroscopy. *Annu. Rev. Anal. Chem.* **2008**, *1*, 601–626. [CrossRef] [PubMed]
18. Frens, G. Controlled Nucleation for the Regulation of the Particle Size in Monodisperse Gold Suspensions. *Nat. Phys. Sci.* **1973**, *241*, 20–22. [CrossRef]
19. Murphy, C.J.; Sau, T.K.; Gole, A.M.; Orendorff, C.J.; Gao, J.; Gou, L.; Hunyadi, S.E.; Li, T. Anisotropic Metal Nanoparticles: Synthesis, Assembly, and Optical Applications. *J. Phys. Chem. B* **2005**, *109*, 13857–13870. [CrossRef] [PubMed]
20. Wiley, B.; Sun, Y.; Xia, Y. Synthesis of silver nanostructures with controlled shapes and properties. *Acc. Chem. Res.* **2007**, *40*, 1067–1076. [CrossRef] [PubMed]
21. Otto, A.; Mrozek, I.; Grabhorn, H.; Akemann, W. Surface-enhanced Raman scattering. *J. Phys. Condens. Matter* **1992**, *4*, 1143. [CrossRef]
22. Campion, A.; Kambhampati, P. Surface-enhanced Raman scattering. *Chem. Soc. Rev.* **1998**, *27*, 241–250. [CrossRef]

23. Feng, S.; Chen, R.; Lin, J.; Pan, J.; Chen, G.; Li, Y.; Cheng, M.; Huang, Z.; Chen, J.; Zeng, H. Nasopharyngeal cancer detection based on blood plasma surface-enhanced Raman spectroscopy and multivariate analysis. *Biosens. Bioelectron.* **2010**, *25*, 2414–2419. [CrossRef] [PubMed]
24. Lin, D.; Feng, S.; Pan, J.; Chen, Y.; Lin, J. Colorectal cancer detection by gold nanoparticle based surface-enhanced Raman spectroscopy of blood serum and statistical analysis. *Opt. Express* **2011**, *19*, 13565–13577. [CrossRef] [PubMed]
25. Lin, C.Y.; Yu, C.J.; Lin, Y.H.; Tseng, W.L. Colorimetric sensing of silver(I) and mercury(II) ions based on an assembly of Tween 20-stabilized gold nanoparticles. *Anal. Chem.* **2010**, *82*, 6830–6837. [CrossRef] [PubMed]
26. Boening, D.W. Ecological effects, transport, and fate of mercury: A general review. *Chemosphere* **2000**, *40*, 1335–1351. [CrossRef]
27. Clarkson, T.W.; Magos, L.; Myers, G.J. The toxicology of mercury-current exposures and clinical manifestations. *N. Engl. J. Med.* **2003**, *349*, 1731–1737. [CrossRef] [PubMed]
28. Li, S.; Xu, L.; Ma, W.; Kuang, H.; Wang, L.; Xu, C. Triple Raman Label-Encoded Gold Nanoparticle Trimers for Simultaneous Heavy Metal Ion Detection. *Small* **2015**, *11*, 3435–3439. [CrossRef] [PubMed]
29. Xue, X.; Wang, F.; Liu, X. One-Step, Room Temperature, Colorimetric Detection of Mercury (Hg^{2+}) Using DNA/Nanoparticle Conjugates. *J. Am. Chem. Soc.* **2008**, *130*, 3244–3245. [CrossRef] [PubMed]
30. Wang, H.; Wang, Y.; Jin, J.; Yang, R. Gold nanoparticle-based colorimetric and "turn-on" fluorescent probe for mercury(II) ions in aqueous solution. *Anal. Chem.* **2008**, *80*, 9021. [CrossRef] [PubMed]
31. Zhu, Y.; Jiang, X.; Wang, H.; Wang, S.; Wang, H.; Sun, B.; Su, Y.; He, Y. A Poly Adenine-Mediated Assembly Strategy for Designing Surface-Enhanced Resonance Raman Scattering Substrates in Controllable Manners. *Anal. Chem.* **2015**, *87*, 6631–6638. [CrossRef] [PubMed]
32. Cheng, M.L.; Yang, J. Seed-mediated growth method for electroless deposition of AgNPs on glass substrates for use in SERS measurements. *J. Raman Spectrosc.* **2010**, *41*, 167–174. [CrossRef]
33. Sun, W.; Chen, G.; Zheng, L. Electroless deposition of silver particles on graphite nanosheets. *Scr. Mater.* **2008**, *59*, 1031–1034. [CrossRef]
34. Saito, Y.; Wang, J.J.; And, D.A.S.; Batchelder, D.N. A Simple Chemical Method for the Preparation of Silver Surfaces for Efficient SERS. *Langmuir* **2002**, *18*, 2959–2961. [CrossRef]
35. Mor-Piperberg, G.; Tel-Vered, R.; Elbaz, J.; Willner, I. Nanoengineered electrically contacted enzymes on DNA scaffolds: Functional assemblies for the selective analysis of Hg^{2+} ions. *J. Am. Chem. Soc.* **2010**, *132*, 6878–6879. [CrossRef] [PubMed]
36. Sun, B.; Jiang, X.; Wang, H.; Song, B.; Zhu, Y.; Wang, H.; Su, Y.; He, Y. A Surface-Enhancement Raman Scattering Sensing Strategy for Discriminating Trace Mercuric Ion (II) from Real Water Samples in Sensitive, Specific, Recyclable and Reproducible Manners. *Anal. Chem.* **2015**, *87*, 1250–1256. [CrossRef] [PubMed]
37. Wei, X.; Su, S.; Guo, Y.; Jiang, X.; Zhong, Y.; Su, Y.; Fan, C.; Lee, S.T.; He, Y. A molecular beacon-based signal-off surface-enhanced Raman scattering strategy for highly sensitive, reproducible, and multiplexed DNA detection. *Small* **2013**, *9*, 2493–2499. [CrossRef] [PubMed]
38. Hwang, J.S.; Chen, K.Y.; Hong, S.J.; Chen, S.W.; Syu, W.S.; Kuo, C.W.; Syu, W.Y.; Lin, T.Y.; Chiang, H.P.; Chattopadhyay, S. The preparation of silver nanoparticle decorated silica nanowires on fused quartz as reusable versatile nanostructured surface-enhanced Raman scattering substrates. *Nanotechnology* **2010**, *21*, 025502. [CrossRef] [PubMed]
39. Shin, S.; Lee, J.; Lee, S.; Kim, H.; Seo, J.; Kim, D.; Hong, J.; Lee, S.; Lee, T. A Droplet-Based High-Throughput SERS Platform on a Droplet-Guiding-Track-Engraved Superhydrophobic Substrate. *Small* **2017**, *13*, 1602865. [CrossRef]
40. Wu, X.; Tang, L.; Ma, W.; Xu, L.; Liu, L.; Kuang, H.; Xu, C. SERS-active Au NR oligomer sensor for ultrasensitive detection of mercury ions. *RSC Adv.* **2015**, *5*, 81802–81807. [CrossRef]
41. Li, T.; Zhu, K.; He, S.; Xia, X.; Liu, S.; Wang, Z.; Jiang, X. Sensitive detection of glucose based on gold nanoparticles assisted silver mirror reaction. *Analyst* **2011**, *136*, 2893. [CrossRef] [PubMed]
42. Shen, L.; Ji, J.; Shen, J. Silver mirror reaction as an approach to construct superhydrophobic surfaces with high reflectivity. *Langmuir* **2008**, *24*, 9962–9965. [CrossRef] [PubMed]
43. Han, Y.; Lupitskyy, R.; Chou, T.M.; Stafford, C.M.; Du, H.; Sukhishvili, S. Effect of Oxidation on Surface-Enhanced Raman Scattering Activity of Silver Nanoparticles: A Quantitative Correlation. *Anal. Chem.* **2011**, *83*, 5873–5880. [CrossRef] [PubMed]

44. Waterhouse, G.I.N.; Bowmaker, G.A.; Metson, J.B. Oxidation of a polycrystalline silver foil by reaction with ozone. *Appl. Surf. Sci.* **2001**, *183*, 191–204. [CrossRef]
45. Yu, S.; Wang, H.; Jiang, X.; Sun, B.; Song, B.; Su, Y.; Yao, H. Ultrasensitive, Specific, Recyclable, and Reproducible Detection of Lead Ions in Real Systems through a Polyadenine-Assisted, Surface-Enhanced Raman Scattering Silicon Chip. *Anal. Chem.* **2016**, *88*, 3723–3729.

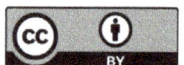

© 2018 by the authors. Licensee MDPI, Basel, Switzerland. This article is an open access article distributed under the terms and conditions of the Creative Commons Attribution (CC BY) license (http://creativecommons.org/licenses/by/4.0/).

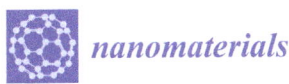

Article

Biocompatible Nanocomposite Implant with Silver Nanoparticles for Otology—In Vivo Evaluation

Magdalena Ziąbka [1,*], Elżbieta Menaszek [2], Jacek Tarasiuk [3] and Sebastian Wroński [3]

[1] Department of Ceramics and Refractories, Faculty of Materials Science and Ceramics, AGH University of Science and Technology, 30-059 Krakow, Poland
[2] Department of Cytobiology, Collegium Medicum, Faculty of Pharmacy, UJ Jagiellonian University, 30-001 Krakow, Poland; elzbieta.menaszek@uj.edu.pl
[3] Department of Condensed Matter Physics, Faculty of Physics and Applied Computer Science, AGH University of Science and Technology, 30-059 Krakow, Poland; tarasiuk@agh.edu.pl (J.T.); wronski@fis.agh.edu.pl (S.W.)
* Correspondence: ziabka@agh.edu.pl

Received: 9 August 2018; Accepted: 25 September 2018; Published: 27 September 2018

Abstract: The aim of this work was to investigate of biocompatibility of polymeric implants modified with silver nanoparticles (AgNPs). Middle ear prostheses (otoimplants) made of the (poly)acrylonitrile butadiene styrene (ABS) and ABS modified with silver nanoparticles were prepared through extrusion and injection moulding process. The obtained prostheses were characterized by SEM-EDX, micro-CT and mechanical tests, confirming their proper shape, good AgNPs homogenization and mechanical parameters stability. The biocompatibility of the implants was evaluated in vivo on rats, after 4, 12, 24 and 48 weeks of implantation. The tissue-healing process and cytotoxicity of the implants were evaluated on the basis of microscopic observations of the materials morphology after histochemical staining with cytochrome c oxidase (OCC) and acid phosphatase (AP), as well as via micro-tomography (ex vivo). The in vivo studies confirmed biocompatibility of the implants in the surrounding tissue environment. Both the pure ABS and nanosilver-modified ABS implants exhibited a distinct decrease in the area of granulation tissue which was replaced with the regenerating muscle tissue. Moreover, a slightly smaller area of granulation tissue was observed in the surroundings of the silver-doped prosthesis than in the case of pure ABS prosthesis. The kinetics of silver ions releasing from implants was investigated by ICP-MS spectrometry. The measurement confirmed that concentration of the silver ions increased within the implant's immersion period. Our results showed that middle ear implant with the nanoscale modification is biocompatible and might be used in ossicular reconstruction.

Keywords: nanocomposites; medical devices; middle ear prosthesis; silver nanoparticles; biocompatibility; thermoplastic polymer

1. Introduction

The need to replace or reconstruct ossicles has led to the development of surgical techniques enabling innovative prostheses implantation. New structural and material possibilities have improved the design and preparation of prostheses so as to make them vary in size, shape and the applied material. Nowadays, it is common knowledge that a well-designed material may result in a more advantageous postoperative response. Moreover, proper modifications of the chemical composition change the parameters and functions of mechanical prostheses.

The ossicular chain reconstruction may be carried out with either partial ossicular replacement prosthesis (PORP) or total ossicular replacement prosthesis (TORP). Unfortunately, many ossicular chain reconstructions—using either PORPs or TORPs—still fail. There are various factors determining the success of the operations, such as the proper length of the prosthesis, stability of implantation, recurring illnesses, risk of inflammation, and reaming out the ear to provide passage of air [1,2]. Another important factor is the presence of either anatomic incus or stapes that facilitate the stability of the prosthesis fixation. Despite the possible difficulties and complications, both partial [3–5] and total prostheses [6] are effective in ossicular chain reconstructions.

The research conducted for the last 40 years has thoroughly described the requirements set for materials used in laryngological surgeries. The most important issue is the optimal quality of sound transmission that is influenced by various biological, acoustic and mechanical factors. As far as the biomechanical functions of the device are concerned, the mechanical properties of the implant material are key factors. Still, it is possible to tailor the material to specific needs depending on the implantation site, the size of the implant and the manner of manufacturing. The materials for middle ear prostheses do not face precise strength requirements. Yet it is common knowledge that the implant material should have such mechanical properties so as to best resemble the tissue it is supposed to substitute. It is a challenge to design a perfect material, considering the complex structure and the chain of auditory ossicles, as well as the wide spectrum of Young's modulus for particular elements (e.g., ligaments, muscles, joint and bones) which ranges from 0.049 MPa (for ligaments) to 14 GPa (for bones) [7]. The transmission of high-frequency sound depends on such parameters as the surface of the prosthesis, its stiffness (rigidity), Young modulus, Kirchhoff modulus, friction and the implant's density and weight (mass) [8–10]. Although the lightness of the structure is connected with the type and size of the implant, the essential factor is the material of the prosthesis. In order to provide the best quality of high-frequency transmission, the implants ought to be as light as possible—the higher specific gravity of the implant, the lower its high-frequency sensitivity [11]. Apart from the sound transmission of the middle ear implant, the biological functions of the material are a key requirement in medical applications.

The mechanical properties of the material dedicated for ear implants are also clearly defined. The biomaterial is supposed to sustain its shape, constant measurements, proper elasticity and rigidness for the longest possible period of time. The material should be also resistant to changing loads and prove its high resilience in fatigue tests. Additionally, middle ear prostheses must be capable of making micro movements between the eardrum and middle-ear chamber.

Polymeric/(poly)acrylonitrile butadiene styrene (ABS) materials play a significant role in bone surgery and laryngology [12]. There were a few reasons for selecting high ABS as a material for prototype implants. First of all, it is very convenient to obtain complex shapes by means of injection moulding. ABS polymers can be modified with silver nanoparticles, obtaining the following advantages: bactericidal efficacy against *Staphylococcus aureus* and *Escherichia coli*, slight but visible cytotoxicity against fibroblasts (ensuring better implant-bone fixation without scarring), no cytotoxic activity against osteoblasts, advantageous mechanical properties, fatigue stability, high homogenization of nanosilver in the polymer matrix and a high level of silver ions released into the environment [13]. All the previously mentioned factors proved Ag-modified ABS to be a very promising material for a prototype of the middle ear implant.

The potential for the use of nanoparticles in surgery is huge. Antibacterial properties of silver nanoparticles are used in urology, implantology and dentistry, as well as to treat burns or other chronic wounds [14,15]. For instance, catheters can be coated with silver nanoparticles to endow them with antibacterial properties and prevent surface biofilm formation [16]. In the surgery of ossicular replacement prosthesis, none of the implants possess bactericidal properties. Nowadays, the range of commercially available materials used for bone reconstruction is impressive. On the market, the most popular group of materials used for such prostheses are metals (titanium), ceramic (hydroxyapatite), polymers (PTFE-teflon) and some composites (HAPEX) [17]. According to the literature reports, the titanium prostheses display better biostability and biocompatibility in comparison to allogenic grafts. The titanium implants sustain proper stiffness and they are efficient in sound transmission and lightweight, which is a vital factor in the postoperative assessment [18]. The ossicular chain reconstructions are often performed with hydroxyapatite prostheses, as an alternative to auto- and homografts. They are popular mainly due to the biological aspect. It is one of the main components of bones and teeth and it forms a stable implant/tissue bonding without the fibrous layer around the prosthesis. Hydroxyapatite also stimulates the cell proliferation and is highly biocompatible [19]. The negative feature, however, is the formation of a big mass in the relatively small middle ear cavity [20]. Teflon is used to obtain partial ossicular replacement prosthesis, ventilation tubes and drains, incus and stapes prostheses (piston type) usually with a platinum wire. Due to its hydrophobicity and low surface energy teflon is especially popular for the stapes prostheses [21]. One of the most popular materials for the ossicle chain reconstruction is HAPEX. It is composed of 40% synthetic hydroxyapatite (HAp) and 60% high-density polyethylene (HDPE). In the stress tests, HAPEX has proven to be a stable implant/bone bonding. Fibrous tissue formation was observed on the implant surface and the implant/bone border, in some cases a thin epithelium layer outside was also observed [22].

In our case, the whole prosthesis is made of a thermoplastic polymer (ABS), which makes it lightweight. It is also possible to adjust the implant's length. The round shape of the head plate minimizes the risk of tympanic membrane damage. The openwork construction of prosthesis (antenna) allows its easy placement in the middle ear and creates an opportunity to manually form a desired shape, according to the particular ossicular chain damages. Moreover, the mechanical properties, such as Young's modulus, are similar to the bone. Additionally, the cheap manufacturing method makes the product competitive in the scope of general costs of treatment. The novelty is also the antibacterial function of the plastic prosthesis. This medical device is similar to the titanium prosthesis in shape but, up to now, it has never been manufactured by injection moulding and extrusion. Therefore, antimicrobial polymers are highly demanded as a strategy to avoid otitis media infections.

The perfect prosthesis material should be biocompatible with the surrounding tissues, it cannot result in acute immunological, toxic, or allergic reactions [23]. Moreover, it should not display mutagenic or carcinogenic effects. From the biological point of view, especially in the case of chronic middle ear infection, the material's stability in the environment is an essential quality too. The material should neither degrade nor facilitate the further inflammation process [24,25]. It should be endowed with proper wettability value to facilitate the epithelial cells proliferation, which guarantees the successful adaptation of the implant.

According to the correct sequence of biological research, the implant material should first undergo the in vitro cytotoxicity testing procedures. Then it should be tested on animals to describe an interaction with the soft tissue and, preferably, also in the environment corresponding to the one of the middle ear [26].

In this work, the medical devices made of nanocomposite with antibacterial silver nanoparticles have been described as valid tools for otolaryngology. The biocompatibility of these devices has been tested in vivo. Our results showed that this micro-device with the nanoscale modification is biocompatible and very promising as a novel middle ear prosthesis.

2. Materials and Methods

2.1. Material Manufacturing

The otoimplants were manufactured by means of extrusion and injection moulding method, using the Multiplas machine (Multiplas Enginery Co., LTD, Taiwan) fitted with a special steel moulding form. The two types of the implants were injected: (poly)acrylonitrile butadiene styrene (ABS) and ABS with the addition of 0.1 wt. % silver nanoparticles (AgNPs). The silver was developed at the Intercollegiate Faculty of Biotechnology, University of Gdansk and Medical University of Gdansk manufacture according to Banasiuk et al. 2016 [27]. The size and shape of nanoparticles were estimated via SEM and TEM [27]—they were characterized as spherical and measuring below 50 nm in diameter (Figure 1). The AgNPs were agglomerated as an aqueous environment evaporated during the procedure of sample preparation for SEM and nanoparticles started to aggregate.

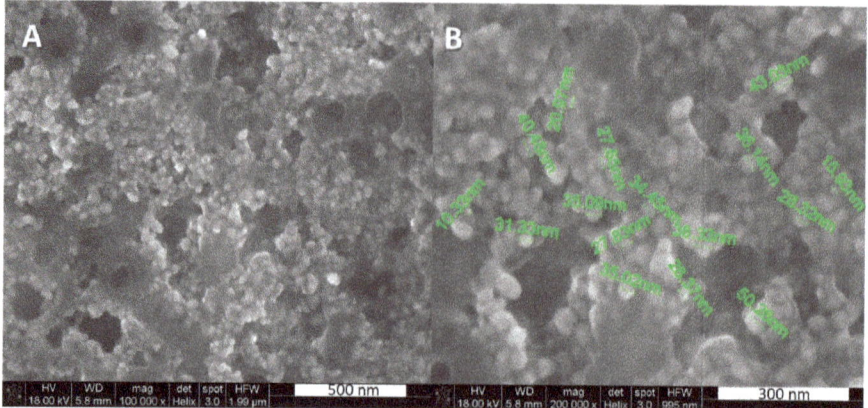

Figure 1. SEM images showing the silver nanoparticles, (**A**) silver nanoparticles (AgNPs), scale 500 nm, (**B**) AgNPs with visible diameter, scale 300 nm.

The procedure of obtaining the prostheses according to Ziąbka et al. 2017 [28] consisted of a few steps. First, the granulate was prepared and dried in the laboratory dryer at 80 °C for 6 h. Next, the nanosilver particles were incorporated and homogenized with polymer granules in the plasticizing chamber using a 0.8 m-long screw. Subsequently, the material was injected into the steel moulding form, cooled and extracted. The injection parameters were selected and adapted for the process according to the characteristic data sheet of the polymer manufacturer (injection temperature in three zones—240 °C, injection pressure—80 kg cm^{-2}, flow—70%).

The shape of our otoimplant (Figure 2) does not vary significantly from the other prostheses, as it has to replace ossicular chain bones and easily fit in the middle ear. However, we have enhanced some of its parts to simplify the surgical procedure. The shape we developed is surgically handy, ensuring the precise implantation in the middle ear.

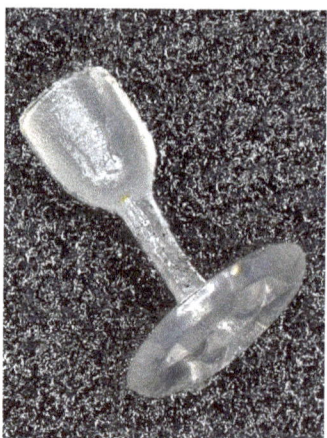

Figure 2. The middle ear implant—otoimplant.

The prosthesis consists of the three elements: A "cup" which is placed on the head of the stapes, a "piston"—joining the cup and an "antenna"—the implant base which bends on the tympanic membrane. The openwork construction of the antenna determines the implant weight and expedites the implantation.

2.2. Material Evaluation

Scanning Electron Microscopy

The SEM-Quanta FEG-250 scanning electron microscope (FEI, Eindhoven, The Netherlands) was used to perform a detailed examination of the otoimplants microstructure. The measurements and observations were conducted in high vacuum conditions, with a back scattered electron detector (BSE), with the accelerated voltage of 10–18 kV. The microstructure observations were conducted on two kinds of the implants—one was made of pure ABS and the other of ABS modified with silver nanoparticles. All the samples were coated with a carbon layer.

Additionally, the microstructure of these implants was investigated using the Nova Nano SEM 200 scanning electron microscope (FEI, Eindhoven, The Netherlands) coupled with a Genesis XMX-ray microanalysis system (EDAX, Tilburg, The Netherlands). The measurements and observations were conducted in low vacuum conditions with a secondary electron detector (SE), the accelerated voltage was 10–18 kV. The samples were coated with a carbon layer.

2.3. Implantation Procedure

The procedure of implantation was performed at the Animal Facility of the Faculty of Pharmacy CM UJ Krakow (the consent no 251/2015 issued by the 1st Local Ethical Committee on Animal Testing in Krakow). The experiment was performed according to the PN ISO 10993-6 guidelines [29]. The male adult Wistar rat (*Rattus norvegicus*) was chosen as a research model. The animals were kept in standard conditions at the stable temperature of about 20 °C and the 12:12 h light cycle.

The middle ear prostheses made of pure ABS and silver-doped ABS were sterilized at a low temperature gas plasma (the Sterrad 120 apparatus) using hydrogen peroxide vapour in the double-cycle (2 × 45 min) and implanted into the rats' gluteus muscles. The animals were divided into four groups for 30, 90, 180 and 360-day cycles, 5 rats in each batch. Prior to the surgery, the animals were sedated with the intraperitoneal injection (Ketamine + Xylazine: 100 mg/kg + 10 mg/kg animal body weight) and the implantation area was shaved and disinfected with iodine. Next, a small incision was made in the skin and the underlying muscle to create a small pouch (3–4 mm deep) where the implant was inserted. Then the double stitching was applied (degradable PDS II Johnson & Johnson Intl) to complete the surgery. The implantation procedure is presented in Figure 3.

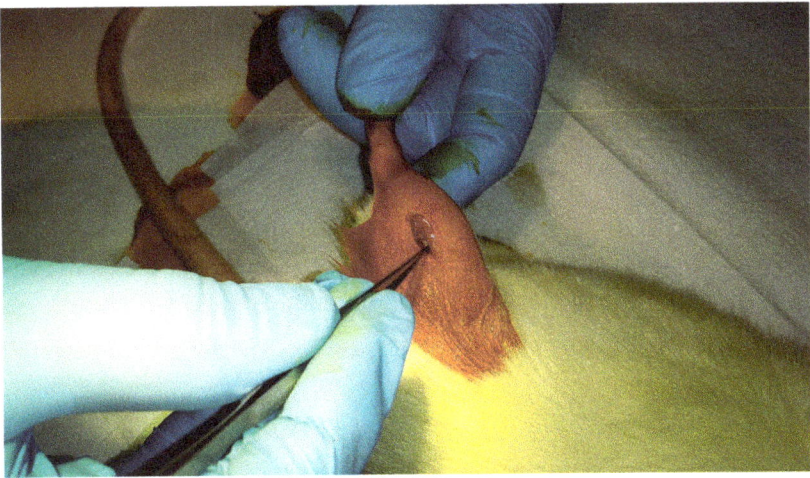

Figure 3. Implantation procedure of middle ear prosthesis into the rats' gluteus muscle.

2.4. In Vivo Examination

After a set period of time (30, 90, 180 or 360 days) the rats were decapitated, then the tissue samples were extracted and prepared (frozen in liquid nitrogen, cut into 9 μm-thick slices with a cryostat microtome—Shandon, Thermo Sci., GB) for histoenzymic and microstructural assessment. Additionally, the lymph glands adjacent to the implant site were extracted for further examinations. The histoenzymic reactions such as cytochrome c oxidase (OCC) and acid phosphatase (AP) were performed to identify the response to a foreign body and to assess the healing process. Slides performed for the AP activity were also stained with Mayer's hematoxylin for better visualization of tissue structure. The observations were conducted using an optical microscope (Olympus BH2, Tokyo, Japan, objective 4–20×) and images were taken with a digital camera. In each series, the tissue samples containing the pure ABS implant and the ABS/AgNPs implant were extracted and immersed into formalin for the further micro-CT study. The samples of blood were harvested for CRP (C Reactive Protein) examination as well.

2.5. C Reactive Protein Measurement

Blood was collected directly from the heart of 5 rats decapitated after 30 days of implantation. The C reactive protein (CRP) concentration in blood serum was measured by an immunoturbidimetric method using the Cobas 8000 machine (Roche Hitachi, Mannheim, Germany).

2.6. Micro-CT Observation

The rats' muscle tissues containing the implants of the two kinds (pure ABS and ABS/AgNPs) were harvested and fixed in 4% buffered formalin to perform the Micro-CT observations. The tests were performed 30, 90, 180 and 360 days after the implantation. All the samples were scanned in wet conditions at room temperature using a Nanotom 180N device (GE Sensing & Inspection Technologies Phoenix X-ray Gmbh, Grasbrunn, Germany). The micro-CT system provided a unique spatial and contrast resolution due to the installed ultra-high performance nanofocus X-ray tube (180 kV/57 W) and the tungsten target with a diamond window. The working parameters of the X-ray tube were $I = 200$ μA and $V = 70$ kV. The magnification was set to 6.7, which corresponds to 7.5 μm resolution. Each projection was averaged from five expositions taking 500 ms for each. The total number of projections was 1800. The reconstruction of the scanned implants was performed with the aid of proprietary GE software datos X ver. 2.1.0 using the Feldkamp algorithm for cone beam X-ray CT. The post-reconstruction data treatments, such as denoising, thresholding and visualization, were run in VG Studio Max.

2.7. ICP-MS

The pure polymer otoimplants and silver-doped otoimplants were incubated at 37 °C in 50 mL of UHQ water for one year. The ions release observations were also carried out on bigger samples (10 mm in diameter) due to the low concentration. The silver ions concentration was also examined in the blood harvested from the rats' hearts one month after the implantation. The in vitro release of silver ions was studied by means of inductively coupled plasma mass spectrometry (ICP-MS), using the ICP-MS Perkin-Elmer Plasma 6100 spectrometer. Prior to performing ICP-MS analysis, so as to prohibit the silver ions (Ag^+) reduction into metallic silver, the filtered samples were acidified with nitric acid, up to the final concentration of 0.1 mol/L. The silver concentration values of the investigated samples were determined using ICP-MS at m/z 107, applying the external standard calibration procedure.

2.8. Mechanical Tests

The mechanical parameters were established during the uniaxial stretching, using the universal testing machine Inspekt Table Blue 5 kN (Hegewald & Peschke GmbH, Nossen, Germany) and the intelligent testing software LabMaster. The tested samples were shaped as paddles made of ABS polymer and the silver-modified composite. Their measurements are compliant with PN-EN ISO 527-1 norm [30]. In order to perform the tensile strength test, the paddles were placed in the grips of the testing machine and the tensile force F was applied. The measuring speed of the upper grip of the machine was 50 mm/min and the measuring length of the paddles was 40 mm. The measuring accuracy of elongation was 0.01 mm, and of the force—0.5 N with the nominal range of the cylinder—5000 N. The obtained force-deformation graph made it possible to establish such parameters as Young's modulus E, tensile strength σ and elongation at the maximum εFmax force.

2.9. Statistical Analysis

The results were analyzed using the one-way analysis of variance (ANOVA) with Duncan post hoc tests, performed with Statistica 13.1 (Dell Inc., Round Rock, TX, USA) software. The results were considered statistically significant when $p < 0.05$.

3. Results and Discussion

3.1. Microstructure Observation of Middle Ear Prosthesis

The observations of the implants' microstructure using the SEM method and micro-CT reconstruction confirmed the proper prosthesis shape obtained in the injection moulding process (Figure 4B–D). All the prostheses elements (the cup, the piston and the antenna) were of a homogeneous and consistent structure in comparison to the 3D model prepared in the Solidworks (Figure 4A).

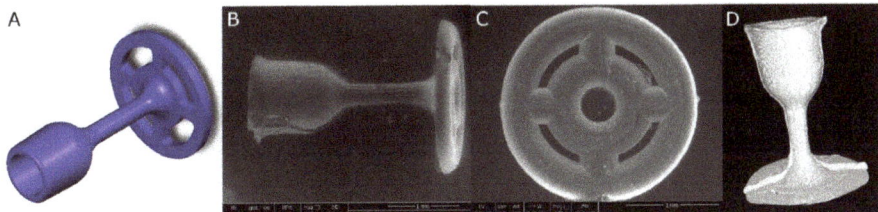

Figure 4. Middle ear prosthesis, (**A**) 3D model, (**B,C**) SEM images showing the implant from different sides, (**D**) prosthesis 3D reconstruction after micro-CT scanning.

An innovative solution is the openwork construction of the antenna that allows easier implantation and determines the weight of the implant. Initially, the complex mould shape and the small size of the medical device caused many difficulties. However, the well-thought-out injection moulding conditions and the efficient silver nanoparticles dispersion in the polymer matrix resulted in developing laryngological implants. Moreover, the implants were obtained in accordance with the design assumptions and the connection of the individual elements was proper. It is common knowledge that good dispersion and strong interfacial interactions between the nanoparticles and the polymer matrix are critical to engineering a strong composite. Therefore, it is a challenge to obtain the sufficient dispersion of hydrophobic fillers in a polymer matrix. Although various surfactants are widely used as they enhance dispersion, their cytotoxicity limits the biomedical applications [31]. Therefore, in our research, we decided against using any surfactants or toxic chemicals.

3.2. Ex Vivo Investigations of Tissue-Implants Samples

All the rats not only survived the procedure but the in vivo tests did not reveal any postoperative complications or external symptoms of inflammation, e.g., reddening and irritation in both types of implants. After the 30-day postoperative period, the fur was growing back on the implantation site, whereas after 3 months the spot was fully covered in hair (Figure 5). There were no signs of scars or stitching left. Having removed the skin, the tissue with the area of surgery was visible. After

30 days a so-called "lens"—the place where the tissue collapsed—was easy to identify. From 90 days of implantation, the tissue looked absolutely ordinary. No macroscopic differences were to be observed between the two types of implants.

The internal organs of the rats were examined too. No changes in morphology were noted in kidneys, spleen, liver or intestines. The tissue samples were extracted for further microscopic and histochemical observations.

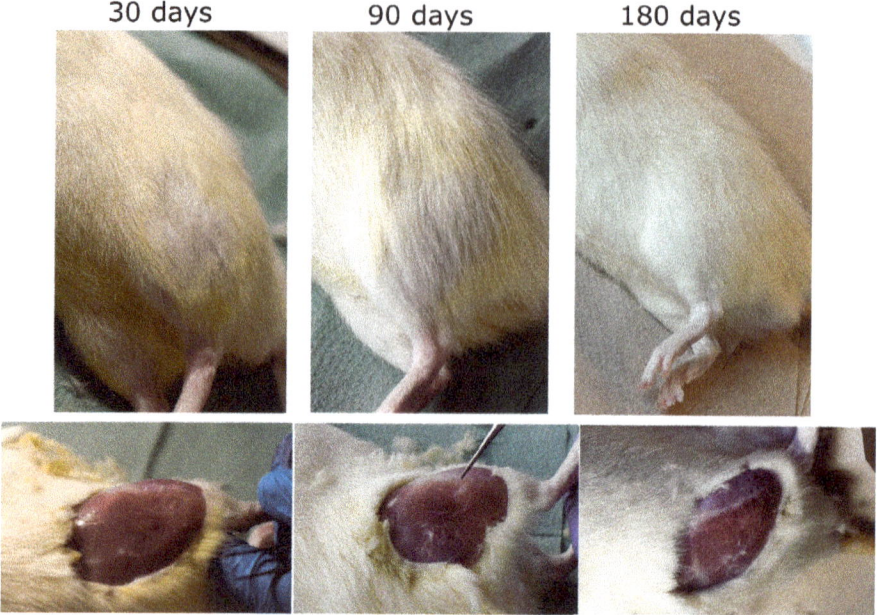

Figure 5. Implantation site after 30 days (**left**), 90 days (**center**) and 180 days for otoimplant/AgNPs.

3.3. Histochemical Analysis

The in vivo histochemical tests (OCC and AP) conducted on the animals answered the questions concerning the cytotoxicity of the implanted material. OCC is an enzyme with high sensitivity to xenobiotics and its normal activity shows that the presence of an implant or ions released from its surface does not inhibit the metabolism of surrounding tissues. AP activity tests were carried out to demonstrate the intensity of inflammation caused by the presence of the implant in the tissue. The surgical insertion of the material resulted in an immunological response—first, it was the reaction to the surgery itself, then to the implanted material. In our study, moderate inflammation was observed around both types of implants (Figure 6). The presence of immune cells (granulocytes, macrophages and lymphocytes) involved in healing processes and the rejection of a foreign body was observed. As a result, the granulation phenomenon took place. The granulation tissue was being gradually replaced by the regenerating muscles and—subsequently—with the mature fully-developed muscles. The scar tissue formed only in the place of surgical incisions.

In some cases, there was an acute inflammatory infiltration. It is worth noting that both kinds of implants (ABS and ABS/AgNPs) led to similar immunological reactions, i.e., a lownumber of mast cells and eosinophiles. The observed inflammation resulted from the tissue damage and was the natural response to a foreign body. The local inflammation was observed around the prosthesis in the tissue samples obtained a month after the surgery and sectioned for histochemical analysis (Figure 6).

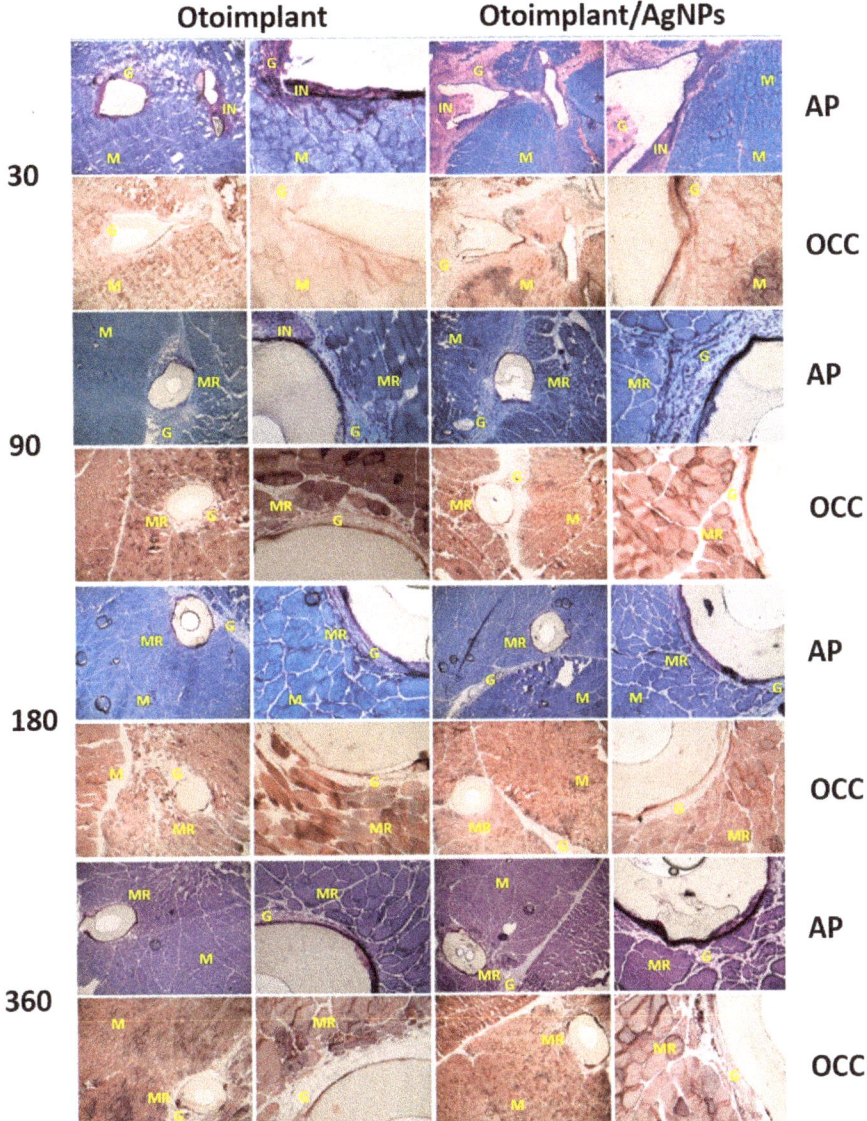

Figure 6. Cross-sections of tissues with otoimplant (on the **left**) and otoimplant/AgNPs (on the **right**) after 30, 90, 180 and 360 days of implantation in the rats' muscles, acid phosphatase (AP) and cytochrome c oxidase (OCC) staining, objective 4, 20×. NOTE: The following symbols are used to describe the tissue cross-sections: M—muscle tissue, G—granulation tissue, IN—inflammatory infiltration, MR—regenerating muscle.

The C Reactive Protein tests (CRP) did not show any local inflammatory findings, as the AgNPs prostheses were too small to cause a negative response in blood. No inflammation or toxic effect was observed, which means that the concentration level of bioactive particles was safe. The mean value of CRP acute protein concentration was below the lower reference value in all the five investigated cases. CRP values in the investigated group were determined to be below 1 (reference value < 5.0). These values proved the lack of inflammation signals in the tested blood after 30 days of the implantation, which confirmed that the low concentration of silver ions could not affect the metabolic parameters of the blood. Therefore, no more CRP tests were conducted for longer experimental series. The elevated CRP, beyond being a biomarker of inflammation, may reflect the molecular disease mechanisms. For example, the CRP production by hepatocytes—the main source of the acute-phase reactant—appears to be regulated primarily by the proinflammatory cytokines interleukin (IL)-6 and IL-1. Furthermore, CRP itself has the ability to activate the complement system and enhance phagocytosis via opsonization [32].

During the studies, it became evident that the tissue response to the implant is largely dependent on the prosthesis shape. The acute inflammatory infiltration was observed more frequently in the antenna part than in the cup part of the implant. It seemed that the elaborate antenna design constricted the flow of juvenile tissues into its interior, thus the proper tissue growth was hindered in the inner part of the implant (Figure 7).

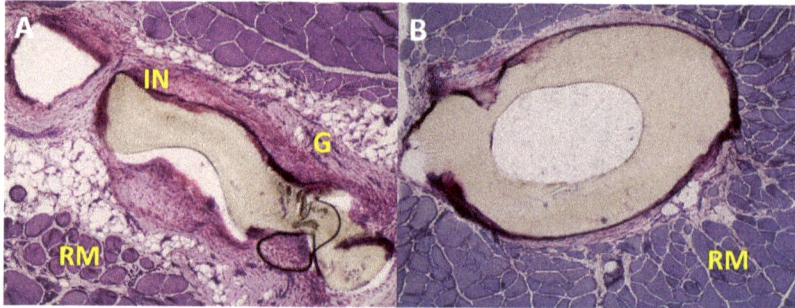

Figure 7. Exemplary images of the tissue around otoimplant after 360 days after the implantation. AP staining, magnification 10×. The images show the differences in the reconstruction of tissues around the implant parts: the antenna (**A**) and the cup (**B**).

During the first month, the inflammation occurred mainly due to the surgical procedures and the implant presence. The implant instability—as it could still move inside the pouch in the rat muscle—might have been another reason for the inflammation. During the recovery the muscles were active and their constrictions would push the prosthesis outwards. The irritation of the muscle tissue was also caused by the obvious firmness and rigidity of the foreign body as well as the diversified shape of the implant. Still, despite the complex and gossamer design of the antenna, after 90 postoperative days, the granulation cells emerged in the spaces between the antenna elements.

The microscopic observations led to the conclusion that the inflammatory reaction was weaker for the samples extracted after the 3-month implantation than for samples after 30 days of implantation. There was a significant decrease in the granulation tissue area for otoimplant/AgNPs prosthesis. (Figure 8). The regenerating muscle tissue was present at the implantation site and the first visible differences were noted between the two implant types after three months. The continuing inflammation was connected with the surgery and the presence of the foreign body, regardless of the material properties. The tissues far from the implantation site were a properly ordered mosaic, typical for skeletal muscles.

The implants were surrounded by the granulation tissuebut in some places were in close contact with the regenerating muscle tissue. However, in the case of the AgNPs-modified otoimplant the granulation tissue area was visibly smaller and it was getting replaced by the regenerating muscle tissue, thus suggesting that the presence of silver nanoparticles facilitated the healing process.

The inflammation diminished significantly around the implant after 180 days of the implantation. In the case of both the otoimplant and the silver-doped otoimplant, the granulation tissue areas diminished. However, the area of granulation tissue seemed to be slightly smaller for the Ag-modified prosthesis.

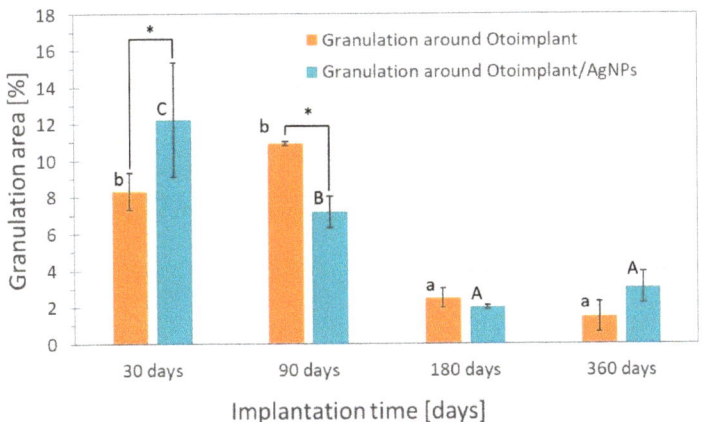

Figure 8. Granulation area for otoimplant and otoimplant/AgNPs measured after 30, 90, 180 and 360 days of the implantation. Statistically significant differences ($p < 0.05$) between otoimplant and otoimplant/AgNPs after specific implantation time are indicated by *; between different implantation times for otoimplant and otoimplant/AgNPs—by a–b and A–C, respectively.

After 360 days of the implantation, the granulation remained on a constant level in comparison to the measurement after 180 days. To prove that silver nanoparticles may accelerate healing processes the area of granulation was measured in the Image J program and presented in a diagram as the results of the average values (Figure 8).

The in vitro tests revealed more numerous population of living cells and thus—lower cytotoxicity of the Ag-modified implants. The results indicated that the small number of nanosilver particles released into the surrounding tissue not only had a bactericidal effect but also stimulated the osteoblast proliferation, promoting better osteointegration [33–35].

A remarkable number of regenerating muscle fibres emerged in close proximity to the implant during the postoperative month. Such a phenomenon proved the healing process to be in progress, as the granulation tissues were being gradually replaced by the regenerating muscle fibres. Moreover, the presence of a small amount of the granulation tissue and the regenerating fibres adhering to the prosthesis confirmed not only the better muscle reconstruction but also more promising eventual osteointegration. The observed high OCC enzyme activity in the tissue directly around the implant proved the lack of biomaterial cytotoxicity. The regenerating muscle tissue was characterized by the proper morphology and the mature muscles displayed the desired mosaic arrangement.

During the experiment a small capsule of the connective tissue was revealed close to the implant, resulting from the fast proliferation of fibroblasts. It was an adverse phenomenon, possibly leading to the implant encapsulation and constriction. It is worth noting that the connective tissue overgrowth influences the proper bone/implant fixation; thus, it should be limited or eliminated in the middle ear implantations where the surrounding environment are bone structures [36,37]. Although the tested prostheses are supposed to reconstruct the bones, it was purposeful to conduct the experiments on the muscles, as soft tissues reveal more severe immunological reaction to a foreign body [38].

3.4. Micro-CT Observations

The micro-CT results confirmed that the muscle tissue regeneration was faster for the implants modified with silver nanoparticles (Figure 9). It was particularly evident in the course of time, after longer implantation periods. Thirty days after the operation there was definitely more granulation tissue around the Ag-doped implant than around the pure polymer implant. In both types of prostheses, the muscles were damaged during the surgery so they did not resemble the proper mosaic. However, after 90 days the correct reconstruction of the muscles was noticeable for both types of implants. The micro-CT after 30 days revealed the bigger granulation area of the otoimplant/AgNPs samples, which confirmed the results of histochemical observations obtained at the same time (Figure 8). Three months after the operation it was observed that the area of granulation tissue was decreasing rapidly for the silver-modified implant. In the case of the non-modified implant, the area of granulation tissue was also higher in comparison to the results taken after 30 days. After 180 days, the micro-CT reconstruction revealed that tissue rebuilding was less evident for the otoimplant/AgNPs. However, having analyzed histochemical results along with the Image J evaluation and the micro-CT reconstruction, it may be assumed that after 360 days of the implantation the tissue area around AgNPs enriched implant was comparable to the one after 180 days. The micro-CT showed granulation tissue together with other tissues, therefore, it was necessary to compare the micro-CT results to the histochemical reactions. The CT results were less specific than the histochemical tests. The micro-computed tomography offered more comprehensive and accurate information than traditional methods [39,40]. The 3D visualization based on micro-CT allowed us to observe the implant behaviour in the tissue via the ex vivo imaging. Therefore, the ex vivo observations clearly showed how the muscles surrounding the implants were regenerating with time and both the composition of the implant material and the prosthesis shape facilitated the muscle tissue regeneration. Silver nanoparticles accelerated the healing process. Both the micro-CT imaging and microscopic observations confirmed that the regeneration around the cup was much faster than around the antenna whose complex structure hindered the process. The natural reaction of the muscles to the foreign object also made the implant unstable. The prosthesis of an unusual shape and certain density and stiffness irritated the surrounding tissue.

The histochemical tests and micro-CT proved the AgNPs-modified implant to be better integrated with the regenerated muscle tissue than the pure ABS prosthesis. The images of otoimplant/AgNPs in subsequent time intervals showed that tissue around the implant was growing with the passage of time.

3.5. Silver Ions Release by Modified Implants

The results obtained by the observation of implant tissue samples (Figures 6–9) were then compared to the release of silver from AgNPs-implants over one year of incubation in water. Figure 10 shows that the Ag^+ release depended on the immersion time, increasing as a function of time. However, the highest increase was observed during the first month of incubation. The gradual silver ions decrease was observed from the 3rd month on, whereas between the 6th and 12th month the release was only marginal.

The similar behaviour was expected in the in vivo studies. The gradual release of silver seemed to be an advantageous phenomenon, since the Ag-modified implant was surrounded by the juvenile muscle tissue without the separating granulation layer. The research also proved that the amount of silver released into the tissue was safe and probably advantageous for the faster muscle regeneration. The literature has reported silver nanoparticles to be nontoxic to humans and very effective against bacteria, viruses, and other eukaryotic micro-organisms at very low concentrations and without side effects. Jeong S.H. et.al. [41] proved that for the silver nanoparticles in the content of 0.1% materials exhibit excellent antibacterial effect (bacterial reduction of 99.9%), but for the micron-sized silver in the content above > 0.5 the antibacterial activity was determined as good. A variety of dressings that contain and release silver ions at the wound surface provide controlled release of ions through a slow but sustained release mechanism, which prevents toxicity yet ensures delivery of a therapeutic dose of silver ions to the wound [42].

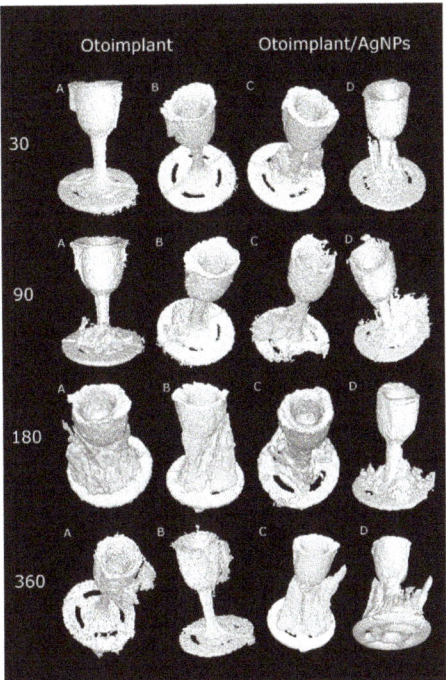

Figure 9. Volume reconstructions showing otoimplant (**A,B**—different orientation of prosthesis) and otoimplant/AgNPs (**C,D**—different orientation of prosthesis) after 30, 90, 180 and 360 days of the implantation in rats muscles, surrounding granulation tissue visible.

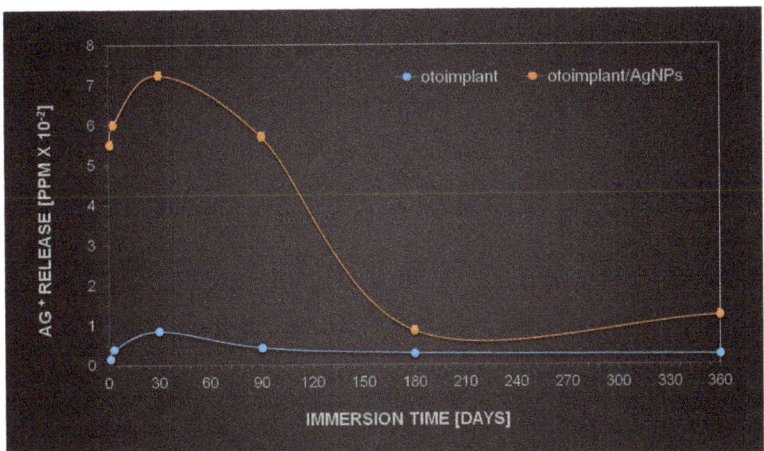

Figure 10. Kinetics of silver ions release during one-year incubation in UHQ water.

There was no strong polymer—filler interactions between AgNPs and the polymer matrix in the nanocomposite networks. This phenomenon loosened the molecular packing of polymeric chains near the nanoparticles and caused an increase in free volume in the nanocomposite networks [43]. The aqueous medium easily diffused into the empty areas and led to the Ag oxidation. Therefore, the water diffusion in the composite sample was expected to result in the higher Ag$^+$ release [44]. The long-term release seemed to be an important factor in regard to practical applications. The subsequent release of silver ions occurred in the interior part of the specimen where water had to cross the diffusion barrier, which inhibited the oxidation process. Conversely, in some cases, polymers could be porous enough to allow water to pass through the polymer and, subsequently, the silver nanoparticles could diffuse out of the polymer [45]. Such a mechanism could be responsible for the prolonged antibacterial efficiency. On the other hand, Helttunen et al. [46] as well as McShan et al. [47] proved that the extensive release of silver from the Ag$^+$ or AgNPs-doped materials was environmentally hazardous and toxic to humans. On the contrary, our long-time observations revealed no toxicity. The research proved that using nanoparticles as active components in composite materials instead of conventional chemical products, e.g., ethanol or bleach, provided the long-lasting bactericidal efficiency with no toxic effect [48]. Therefore, the assumed level of silver concentration in our implant revealed antibacterial efficacy, yet it was not toxic to animals and humans.

3.6. Physicochemical Properties of Prostheses

The scanning electron microscopy observation showed that the surface of both otoimplant and otoimplant/AgNPs was smooth (Figure 11). Silver nanoparticles observed as a light area on SEM images were homogenously distributed in the polymer matrix. The double-cycle injection moulding and extrusion were applied to limit the aggregation of silver nanoparticles. Therefore, the size of nanoparticles remained the same after their integration into polymer. However, even such a precise technology could lead to the prevalence of small aggregates (red square on SEM images proved by EDX spectrum). The observations performed after one year of incubating the samples in deionized water (36 °C) revealed no changes on the surface and in the cross-section. SEM images of the cross-section of polymeric and composite implants showed some porous microstructure (marked with arrows), which could facilitate the silver ions release.

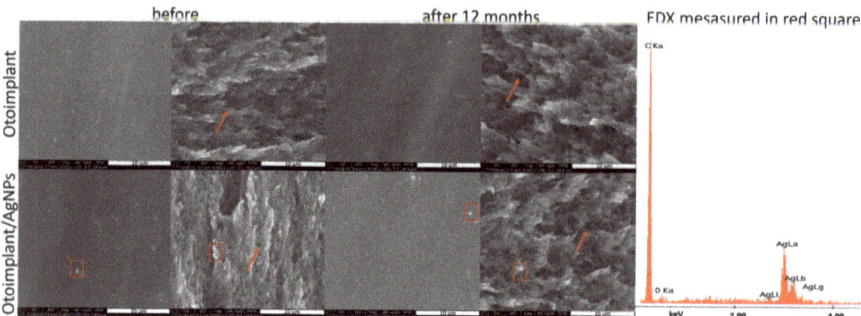

Figure 11. SEM images showing the otoimplant and otoimplant/AgNPs before and after 12 months incubation, surface and cross-section were collected alternately from left to right. On the right—the EDX spectrum collected in the point of the thick red square indicated the presence of AgNPs.

As it was proved in our previous work [28], the long-term bactericidal effect was sustained by the gradual release of silver due to the efficient dispersion of its nanoparticles in the polymer matrix. On the other hand, the surfaces of both the pure implant and implant modified with AgNPs were smooth, which inhibited the bacteria colonization. It is well-known from the literature that the increased roughness facilitates adhesion of osteoblasts to the material surface [49,50]. Higher roughness parameters promote adhesion of bacteria, microbial proliferation and formation of biofilms, which may lead to inflammatory processes, cell necrosis and even rejection of the implanted material [51]. Our assumption was to minimize the bacteria colonization thanks to a remarkably smooth surface. Even if bacteria attached to the porous surface, the gradual silver ions release would guarantee antibacterial efficacy. The conducted mechanical tests proved that the force-elongation curves were similar for both groups of materials—the pure polymers and the composites. Such results suggested that the proposed technology of obtaining polymeric paddles by means of extrusion and injection moulding did not impoverish the mechanical properties of the tested materials. Young's modulus and tensile strength (Figure 12) remained at the same level both for the samples before and after the incubation in deionized water. The addition of 0.1 wt. % of AgNPs did not change tensile strength but slightly decreased Young's modulus of the composite samples. Therefore, AgNPs had no negative effects on the mechanical properties of ABS. In addition, low concentrations of nanoparticles eliminated agglomeration adversely affecting the material's properties. Moreover, the mechanical properties of composites depended on the amount and size of incorporated nanoparticles. Namely, smaller nanoparticles were more effective against bacteria [52]. However, when the AgNPs were smaller than 3 nm, they were more cytotoxic than larger particles—25 nm [15]. On the other hand, the particles measuring 50 nm or more increased the flexural strength of the composite containing 0.2 wt. % of AgNPs. The 40 nm particles did not affect the mechanical parameters of these composites [53]. The findings proved that the mechanical properties of the otoimplant did not change after the incorporation of AgNPs even after the 12-month incubation. Such results suggested that our prosthesis would be stable in clinical performance.

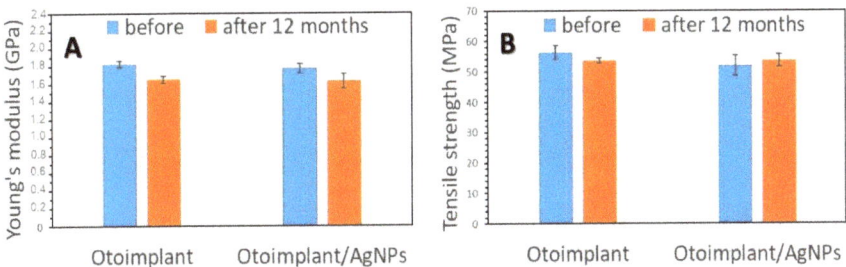

Figure 12. Young's modulus (**A**) and tensile strength (**B**) of otoimplant and otoimplant/AgNPs before and after 12-month incubation in deionized water.

4. Conclusions

Nanotechnology offers great opportunities to improve properties of medical devices. Our in vivo research has proven that the prosthesis made of ABS enriched with silver nanoparticles is biocompatible with the surrounding tissue. Moreover, the AgNPs incorporated into the polymer medical devices ensure a long-lasting antibacterial effect combined with the lack of inflammation or toxic reaction. The addition of silver nanoparticles accelerates the healing process, which is crucial to the length of convalescence after the ossicle chain reconstruction. The microstructural observations as well as mechanical tests have proven the biostability of both prostheses. The low concentration addition of AgNPs to the polymer matrix does not alter the material's mechanical and microstructure properties. The obtained results are the promising basis for further research on the implant prototype that may become an alternative to the devices already available on the medical market.

Author Contributions: M.Z. planned the experiment, prepared the samples, carried out the assessment of physicochemical and biological properties, prepared all figures, discussed the results and wrote the article. E.M. planned and performed in vivo tests. J.T. and S.W. performed micro-CT measurements.

Funding: This research was founded by the National Centre for Research and Development grant no: LIDER/154/L-6/14/NCBR/2015.

Conflicts of Interest: The authors declare no conflict of interest.

References

1. Sheehy, J.L. TORPs and PORPs: Causes of failure—A report on 446 operations. *Otolaryngol. Head Neck Surg.* **1984**, *92*, 583–587. [CrossRef] [PubMed]
2. Dornhoffer, J.L.; Gardner, E. Prognostic Factors in Ossiculoplasty: A Statistical Staging System. *Otol. Neurotol.* **2001**, *22*, 299–304. [CrossRef] [PubMed]
3. Krueger, W.W.; Feghali, J.G.; Shelton, C.; Green, J.D.; Beatty, C.W.; Wilson, D.F.; Thedinger, B.S.; Barrs, D.M.; McElveen, J.T. Preliminary ossiculoplasty results using the Kurz titanium prostheses. *Otol. Neurotol.* **2002**, *23*, 836–839. [CrossRef] [PubMed]
4. Gardner, E.K.; Jackson, C.G.; Kaylie, D.M. Results with titanium ossicular reconstruction prostheses. *Laryngoscope* **2004**, *114*, 65–70. [CrossRef] [PubMed]
5. Murphy, T.P. Hearing results in pediatric patients with chronic otitis Media after ossicular reconstruction with partial ossicular replacement prostheses and total ossicular replacement prostheses. *Laryngoscope* **2000**, *110*, 536–544. [CrossRef] [PubMed]
6. Begall, K.; Zimmermann, H. Rekonstruktion der gehorknochelchenkette mit titan-Implantaten. ergebnisse einer multicenter-Studie. *Laryngorhinootologie* **2000**, *79*, 139–145. [CrossRef] [PubMed]
7. Zhao, F.; Koike, T.; Wang, J.; Sienz, H.; Meredith, R. Finite element analysis of the middle ear transfer functions and related pathologies. *Med. Eng. Phys.* **2009**, *31*, 907–916. [CrossRef] [PubMed]
8. Zahnert, T.; Bornitz, M.; Huttenbrink, K.B. Calculation and experiments on the influence of prosthesis couplin to the middle ear transfer function. In Proceedings of the 3rd Symposium on Middle Ear Mechanics in Research and Otology: Matsuyama, Ehime, Japan, 9–12 July 2003; World Scientific: Singapore, 2003; pp. 83–90.
9. Meister, H.; Mickenhagen, A.; Walger, M.; Dück, M.; Wedel, H.; Stennert, E. Standardisierte Messungen der Schallübertragung verschiedener Mittelohrprothesen. *HNO* **2000**, *48*, 204–208. [PubMed]
10. Meister, H.; Walger, M.; Mickenhagen, A.; Stennert, E. Messung der Schwingungseigenschaften von Mittelohrimplantaten mit einem mechanischen Mittelohrmodell. *HNO* **1998**, *46*, 241–245. [CrossRef] [PubMed]
11. Meister, H.; Walger, M.; Mickenhagen, A.; Wedel, H.; Stennert, E. Standardized measurements of the sound transmission of middle ear implants using a mechanical middle ear model. *Eur. Arch. Otorhinolaryngol.* **1999**, *256*, 122–127. [CrossRef] [PubMed]
12. Suaste-Gómez, E.; Rodríguez-Roldán, G.; Reyes-Cruz, H.; Terán-Jiménez, O. Developing an ear prosthesis fabricated in polyvinylidene fluoride by a 3D printer with sensory intrinsic properties of pressure and temperature. *Sensors* **2016**, *16*, 332. [CrossRef] [PubMed]
13. Kittler, S.; Greulich, C.; Diendorf, J.; Köller, M.; Epple, M. Toxicity of silver nanoparticles increases during storage because of slow dissolution under release of silver ions. *Chem. Mater.* **2010**, *22*, 4548–4554. [CrossRef]
14. Shrikant, M. Nanotechnology for Surgeons. *Indian J. Surg.* **2013**, *75*, 485–492.
15. Acosta-Torres, L.S.; Mendieta, I.; Nuñez-Anita, R.E.; Cajero-Juárez, M.; Castaño, V.M. Cytocompatible antifungal acrylic resin containing silver nanoparticles for dentures. *Int. J. Nanomed.* **2012**, *7*, 4777–4786.
16. Roe, D.; Karandikar, B.; Bonn-Savage, N.; Gibbins, B.; Roullet, J.B. Antimicrobial surface functionalization of plastic catheters by silver nanoparticles. *J. Antimicrob. Chemother.* **2008**, *61*, 869–876. [CrossRef] [PubMed]
17. Ziąbka, M. A review of materials used in middle ear prosthetics. *Ceram. Mater.* **2018**, *70*, 65–85.
18. Hales, N.W.; Shakir, F.A.; Saunders, J.E. Titanium middle ear prostheses in staged ossiculoplasty: Does mass really matter? *Am. J. Otolaryngol. Head Neck Med. Surg.* **2007**, *28*, 164–167. [CrossRef] [PubMed]
19. Kobayashi, T.; Gyo, K.; Shinohara, T.; Yanagihara, N. Ossicular reconstruction using hydroxyapatite prostheses with interposed cartilage. *Am. J. Otolaryngol.* **2002**, *23*, 222–227. [CrossRef] [PubMed]
20. Ocak, E.; Beton, S.; Meço, C.; Dursun, G. Titanium versus Hydroxyapatite prostheses: Comparison of hearing and anatomical outcomes after ossicular chain reconstruction. *Turk. Arch. Otorhinolaryngol.* **2015**, *53*, 15–18. [CrossRef] [PubMed]
21. Mangham, C.A., Jr. Titanium CliP piston versus platinum-ribbon Teflon piston: Piston and fenestra size affect air–bone gap. *Otol. Neurotol.* **2008**, *29*, 8–12. [CrossRef] [PubMed]
22. Meijer, A.G.; Segenhout, H.M.; Albers, F.W.; van de Want, H.J. Histopathology of biocompatible hydroxylapatite-polyethylene composite in ossiculoplasty. *ORL* **2002**, *64*, 173–179. [CrossRef] [PubMed]

23. Pathan, F.; Satpathy, S.; Bhalekar, S.; Sudarshan, K. Tragal cartilage versus polytetrafluoroethylene (TEFLON) partial ossicular replacement prosthesis (PORP): A comparative study of outcomes of ossiculoplasty. *Int. J. Innov. Res. Med. Sci.* **2016**, *1*, 2455–8737.
24. Ovsianikov, A.; Chichkov, B.; Adunka, O.; Pillsbury, H.; Doraiswamy, A.; Narayan, R.J. Rapid prototyping of ossicular replacement prostheses. *Appl. Surf. Sci.* **2007**, *253*, 6603–6607. [CrossRef]
25. Maassen, M.M.; Lowenheim, H.; Pfister, M.; Herberhold, S.; Jorge, J.R.; Baumann, I.; Nusser, A.; Zimmermann, R.; Brosch, S.; Zenner, H.P. Surgical-handling properties of the titanium prosthesis in ossiculoplasty. *ENT Ear Nose Throat J.* **2005**, 142–149.
26. Beutner, D.; Hüttenbrink, K.B. Passive and active middle ear implants. *GMS Curr. Top. Otorhinolaryngol. Head Neck Surg.* **2009**, *8*, 1–19.
27. Banasiuk, R.; Frackowiak, J.E.; Krychowiak, M.; Matuszewska, M.; Kawiak, A.; Ziąbka, M.; Lendzion-Bielun, Z.; Narajczyk, M.; Królicka, A. Synthesis of antimicrobial silver nanoparticles through a photomediated reaction in an aqueous environment. *Int. J. Nanomed.* **2016**, *11*, 315–324.
28. Ziąbka, M.; Dziadek, M.; Menaszek, E.; Banasiuk, R.; Królicka, A. Middle ear prosthesis with bactericidal efficacy—In vitro investigation. *Molecules* **2017**, *22*, 1681. [CrossRef] [PubMed]
29. *PN-EN ISO 10993–10996: 2016, Biological Evaluation of Medical Devices. Tests for Local Effects after Implantation*; International Organization for Standardization: Geneva, Switzerland, 2016.
30. *Polish Norm PN-EN ISO 527–1. Plastics. Determination of Mechanical Properties at Static Stretching. General Rules*; International Organization for Standardization: Geneva, Switzerland, 2012.
31. Kumar, S.; Raj, S.; Kolanthai, E.; Sood, A.K.; Sampath, S.; Chatterjee, K. Chemical functionalization of graphene to augment stem cell osteogenesis and inhibit biofilm formation on polymer composites for orthopedic applications. *ACS Appl. Mater. Interfaces* **2015**, *7*, 3237–3252. [CrossRef] [PubMed]
32. Pearlea, A.D.; Scanzello, C.R.; George, S.; Mandl, L.A.; DiCarlo, E.F.; Peterson, M.; Sculco, T.P.; Crow, M.K. Elevated high-sensitivity C-reactive protein levels are associated with local inflammatory findings in patients with osteoarthritis. *Osteoarthr. Cartil.* **2007**, *15*, 516–523. [CrossRef] [PubMed]
33. Ziąbka, M.; Mertas, A.; Król, W.; Chłopek, J. Preliminary biological evaluation of polyoxymethylene/nanosilver composites. *Eng. Biomater.* **2009**, *12*, 196–199.
34. Hardes, J.; Streitburger, A.; Ahrens, H. The influence of elementary silver versus titanium on osteoblasts behaviour in vitro using human osteosarcoma cell lines. *Sarcoma* **2007**. [CrossRef] [PubMed]
35. Kramer, S.J.; Spadaro, J.A.; Webster, D.A. Antibacterial and osteoinductive properties of demineralized bone matrix treated with silver. *Clin. Orthop. Relat. Res.* **1981**, *161*, 154–162. [CrossRef]
36. Stieve, M.; Hedrich, H.J.; Battmer, R.D.; Behrens, P.; Muller, P.; Lenarz, T. Experimental middle ear surgery in rabbits: A new approach for reconstructing the ossicular chain. *Lab. Anim.* **2009**, *43*, 198–204. [CrossRef] [PubMed]
37. Turck, C.; Brandes, G.; Krueger, I.; Behrens, P.; Mojallal, H.; Lenarz, T.; Stieve, M. Histological evaluation of novel ossicular chain replacement prostheses: An animal study in rabbits. *Acta Oto-Laryngol.* **2007**, *127*, 801–808. [CrossRef] [PubMed]
38. Ooms, E.M.; Egglezos, E.A.; Wolke, J.G.; Jansen, J.A. Soft-tissue response to injectable calcium phosphate cements. *Biomaterials* **2003**, *24*, 749–757. [CrossRef]
39. Elian, N.; Bloom, M.; Dard, M.; Cho, S.C.; Trushkowsky, R.D.; Tarnow, D. Radiological and micro-computed tomography analysis of the bone at dental implants inserted 2, 3 and 4 mm apart in a minipig model with platform switching incorporated. *Clin. Oral Implants Res.* **2012**, *25*, e22–e29. [CrossRef] [PubMed]
40. Schaad, L.; Hlushchuk, R.; Barré, S.; Gianni-Barrera, R.; Haberthür, D.; Banfi, A.; Djonov, V. Correlative imaging of the murine hind limb vasculature and muscle tissue by microct and light microscopy. *Sci. Rep.* **2017**, *7*, 41842. [CrossRef] [PubMed]
41. Jeong, S.H.; Yeo, S.Y.; Yi, S.C. The effect of filler particle size on the antibacterial properties of compounded polymer/silver fibers. *J. Mater. Sci.* **2005**, *40*, 5407–5411. [CrossRef]
42. Zilberman, M.; Elsner, J.J. Antibiotic-eluting medical devices for various applications. *J. Control. Release* **2008**, *130*, 202–215. [CrossRef] [PubMed]
43. Makvandi, P.; Nikfarjam, N.; Sanjani, N.S.; Qazvini, N.T. Effect of silver nanoparticle on the properties of poly(methyl methacrylate) nanocomposite network made by in situ photoiniferter-mediated photopolymerization. *Bull. Mater. Sci.* **2015**, *38*, 1625–1631. [CrossRef]

44. Kumar, R.; Munstedt, H. Silver ion release from antimicrobial polyamide/silver composites. *Biomaterials* **2005**, *26*, 2081–2088. [CrossRef] [PubMed]
45. Kong, H.; Jang, J. Antibacterial properties of novel poly(methyl methacrylate) nanofiber containing silver nanoparticles. *Langmuir* **2008**, *24*, 2051–2056. [CrossRef] [PubMed]
46. Helttunen, K.; Moridi, N.; Shahgaldian, P.; Nissinen, M. Resorcinarene bis-crown silver complexes and their application as antibacterial langmuir−blodgett films. *Org. Biomol. Chem.* **2012**, *10*, 2019–2025. [CrossRef] [PubMed]
47. McShan, D.; Ray, P.C.; Yu, H. Molecular toxicity mechanism of nanosilver. *J. Food Drug Anal.* **2014**, *22*, 116–127. [CrossRef] [PubMed]
48. Marassi, V.; Di Cristo, L.; Smith, S.G.J.; Ortelli, S.; Blosi, M.; Costa, A.L.; Reschiglian, P.; Volkov, Y.; Prina-Mello, A. Silver nanoparticles as a medical device in healthcare settings: A five-step approach for candidate screening of coating agents. *R. Soc. Open Sci.* **2018**, *5*, 171113. [CrossRef] [PubMed]
49. Yamashita, D.; Machigashira, M.; Miyamoto, M.; Takeuchi, H.; Noguchi, K.; Izumi, Y.; Ban, S. Effect of surface roughness on initial responses of osteoblast-like cells on two types of zirconia. *Dent. Mater. J.* **2009**, *28*, 461–470. [CrossRef] [PubMed]
50. Solá-Ruiz, M.F.; Pérez-Martínez, C.; Martín-del-Llano, J.J.; Carda-Batalla, C.; Labaig-Rueda, C. In vitro preliminary study of osteoblast response to surface roughness of titanium discs and topical application of melatonin. *Med. Oral Patol. Oral Cir. Bucal* **2015**, *20*, e88–e93. [CrossRef] [PubMed]
51. Zhu, X.; Radovic-Moreno, A.F.; Wu, J.; Langer, R.; Shi, J. Nanomedicine in the management of microbial infection—Overview and perspectives. *Nano Today* **2014**, *9*, 478–498. [CrossRef] [PubMed]
52. Köroğlu, A.; Şahin, O.; Kürkçüoğlu, I.; Dede, D.Ö.; Özdemir, T.; Hazer, B. Silver nanoparticle incorporation effect on mechanical and thermal properties of denture base acrylic resins. *J. Appl. Oral Sci.* **2016**, *24*, 590–596. [CrossRef] [PubMed]
53. Oyar, P.; Sana, F.A.; Durkan, R. Comparison of mechanical properties of heat-polymerized acrylic resin with silver nanoparticles added at different concentrations and sizes. *J. Appl. Polym. Sci.* **2018**, *135*, 45807. [CrossRef]

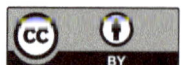

© 2018 by the authors. Licensee MDPI, Basel, Switzerland. This article is an open access article distributed under the terms and conditions of the Creative Commons Attribution (CC BY) license (http://creativecommons.org/licenses/by/4.0/).

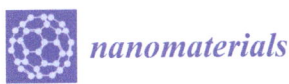

Article

Colloidal Lignin Particles as Adhesives for Soft Materials

Maija-Liisa Mattinen [1,*], Guillaume Riviere [1], Alexander Henn [1], Robertus Wahyu N. Nugroho [1], Timo Leskinen [1], Outi Nivala [2], Juan José Valle-Delgado [1], Mauri A. Kostiainen [3] and Monika Österberg [1]

[1] Bioproduct Chemistry, Department of Bioproducts and Biosystems, School of Chemical Engineering, Aalto University, P.O. Box 16300, FI-00076 Aalto, Espoo, Finland; guillaume.riviere@aalto.fi (G.R.); karl.henn@aalto.fi (A.H.); robertus.nugroho@aalto.fi (R.W.N.N.); timo.leskinen@aalto.fi (T.L.); juanjose.valledelgado@aalto.fi (J.J.V.-D.); monika.osterberg@aalto.fi (M.Ö.)
[2] VTT Technical Research Centre of Finland Ltd., P.O. Box 1000, FI-02044 VTT Espoo, Finland; outi.nivala@helsinki.fi
[3] Biohybrid Materials, Department of Bioproducts and Biosystems, School of Chemical Engineering, Aalto University, P.O. Box 16100, FI-00076 Aalto, Espoo, Finland; mauri.kostiainen@aalto.fi
* Correspondence: maija.mattinen@outlook.com or maija-liisa.mattinen@aalto.fi; Tel.: +358-50-302-3511

Received: 4 November 2018; Accepted: 29 November 2018; Published: 3 December 2018

Abstract: Lignin has interesting functionalities to be exploited in adhesives for medicine, foods and textiles. Nanoparticles (NPs) < 100 nm coated with poly ($_L$-lysine), PL and poly($_L$-glutamic acid) PGA were prepared from the laccase treated lignin to coat nanocellulose fibrils (CNF) with heat. NPs ca. 300 nm were prepared, β-casein coated and cross-linked with transglutaminase (Tgase) to agglutinate chamois. Size exclusion chromatography (SEC) and Fourier-transform infrared (FTIR) spectroscopy were used to characterize polymerized lignin, while zeta potential and dynamic light scattering (DLS) to ensure coating of colloidal lignin particles (CLPs). Protein adsorption on lignin was studied by quartz crystal microbalance (QCM). Atomic force microscopy (AFM) was exploited to examine interactions between different polymers and to image NPs with transmission electron microscopy (TEM). Tensile testing showed, when using CLPs for the adhesion, the stress improved ca. 10 and strain ca. 6 times compared to unmodified Kraft. For the β-casein NPs, the values were 20 and 8, respectively, and for the β-casein coated CLPs between these two cases. When NPs were dispersed in adhesive formulation, the increased Young's moduli confirmed significant improvement in the stiffness of the joints over the adhesive alone. Exploitation of lignin in nanoparticulate morphology is a potential method to prepare bionanomaterials for advanced applications.

Keywords: lignin; nanoparticle; protein; nanocellulose; fibril; enzyme; heat; self-assembly; cross-link

1. Introduction

Technologies focusing on the preparation of adhesives utilizing natural polymers such as proteins and cellulosics for medical, textile and food applications are emerging research fields [1–3] However, biorefinery industry produces also lignin by-product, which is still underutilized, even though this aromatic, antioxidative and antimicrobial biopolymer could be an interesting raw material for many value-added applications [4].

Nanocellulose can be produced by several methods [5–8]. It is a lightweight, transparent and biodegradable polymer. Hence, nanocellulose fibrils (CNF) as well as bacterial nanocellulose (BC) are excellent raw materials for tissue regeneration and replacement [9–12]. Major challenges for the exploitation of CNF include the ability to disperse colloidal material with different formulations. Surface functionalization of the fibrils could be an attractive method to improve stability, functionality and compatibility of the nanomaterial with selected matrices. For example, poly (L-lysine, PL) coated wax particles assembled on CNF surface yield hydrophobic fibrils [13]. Furthermore, capability to obtain tight bonding between tissue edges to prevent bleeding with excellent gas barrier properties and to achieve strong mechanical strength for the sealant, are crucial properties for the medical adhesives to support wound healing and tissue deformation during the recovery [14–16].

Due to excellent solubility and biocompatibility, regenerated silk proteins have been used in medical applications such as textiles, implants and materials for controlled drug release. Deposition of silk fibrin on polymeric surfaces is a remarkable challenge [2]. Enzymatic cross-linking with transglutaminase (Tgase, EC 2.3.1.13) catalyzing cross-links between glutamines and lysines has been used to stabilize proteins against chemicals and proteases [17]. Furthermore, Tgase has been used to graft silk proteins onto damaged wool fibers to improve strength of the surfaces and to degrease felting shrinkage during washing [18].

Foods such as edible coatings are nearby medical applications. Food packages based on petroleum-based raw materials are not biodegradable. They have poor oxygen barrier properties possibly leaching harmful compounds into foods. Water-soluble edible coatings based on dairy proteins could be excellent alternatives for these packages. Protein coatings have good gas barrier properties and no bad flavor or taste [19–21]. For example, nanospheres prepared from caseins form opaque films and could be used to coat foods as well as biological tissues [22]. However, poor water resistance and mechanical strength of the casein coatings needs to be improved to meet full applicability of the nanomaterial in above applications [19].

Silkworm adhesive is an excellent biomimetic model for the preparation coatings for nanoparticulate bonding agents [23] since many technologies for tissue engineering and surgery rely on nanoparticle (NP) based adhesion [24]. Strong and rapid adhesion between hydrogels is feasible at room temperature by spraying hard NPs on the surfaces and bringing them into contact. Tight adhesion between the soft materials is based on the NPs' ability to adsorb tightly onto surfaces, where they act as connectors between polymer chains dissipating energy under stress [24]. Thus, tailored colloidal lignin particles (CLPs) prepared from technical lignin could be interesting nanomaterials to be used as additives in adhesives and coatings. Different CLPs could be produced in the laboratory and semi-industrial scale [25–36]. Enzymatic cross-linking could be an attractive method to increase porosity of NPs in addition to stability improvement against organic solvents [37–39]. Including small molecules in the hydrophobic core of CLPs antioxidant and antimicrobial property of the particles could be enhanced [40,41]. Specificity of the particles could be tailored via surface modification [34,42–44].

In this contribution, tiny CLPs including bilayer polypeptide modifications were prepared from Kraft using self-assembling to tailor CNF surfaces with heat treatment. Furthermore, larger protein coated CLPs were prepared and enzymatically cross-linked for adhering skin tissue (chamois). Finally, water-soluble adhesive formulation was used to demonstrate effect of various NPs for the adhesion of soft chamois specimens. It was concluded that nanoparticle architecture could be an interesting general platform for the preparation technical lignin-based nanobiomaterials for advanced applications.

2. Materials and Methods

2.1. Chemicals

Reagent grade chemicals and solvents for the CLP preparation and modifications were purchased from Sigma-Aldrich (Steinheim, Germany). Water soluble Pritt adhesive (Henkel AG & Co, Düsseldorf, Germany) was purchased from a department store in Finland. Throughout the study, Milli-Q water was used in the aqueous solutions.

2.2. Proteins

Mixture of serum proteins (pI 5.2–7.8), casein from bovine milk (mixture of α-, β-, λ- and κ-subunits), gelatin (MW 47 kDa, pI 7.0–9.0), bovine serum albumin (BSA, 66 kDa, pI 4.8–5.6) and purified β-casein (MW 24 kDa, pI 4.6–5.1) were purchased from Sigma-Aldrich (Germany). For analyses, gelatin was dialyzed (cut-off 21 kDa) and freeze-dried. Due to low solubility, β-casein was first dissolved in H_2O and vortexed at room temperature following dilution with H_2O (1 mg mL^{-1}) and pH adjustment (pH 3.0). After 2 h, the solution was vortexed, ultrasonicated and filtrated. Collagen IV (Col IV) from human placenta (Sigma Aldrich, USA) was treated according to Goffin et al. [45] PL peptide (0.1 m-% in H_2O *w/v*, MW 150–300 kDa, pI 9.0) and sodium salts of poly(L-glutamic acid, PGA) peptides (MW 50–100 kDa and 15–50 kDa) diluted with water (1 mg mL^{-1}) were ordered from Sigma-Aldrich (Germany). Chamois for the adhesion experiments was purchased from Biltema (Espoo, Finland).

2.3. Enzymes

Low redox *Melanocarpus albomyces* laccase (MaL, pH-range 5.0–7.5) was overproduced in *Trichoderma reesei*. High redox *Trametes hirsuta* laccase (ThL, pH-range 4.5–5.0) was produced in its native host following chromatographic purification [46,47]. The reactivities of the enzyme preparations were determined against 2.2-azinobis-(3-ethylbenzothiazoline)-6-sulfonate (ABTS) at pH 4.5 in 25 mM Na-succinate buffer [46] using Perkin Elmer Lambda 45 spectrophotometer (USA) at 436 nm (ε = 29.300 M^{-1} cm^{-1}). For ThL (3.5 mg mL^{-1}), the activity was 5270 nkat mL^{-1} and, for MaL (8.1 mg mL^{-1}), it was 2050 nkat mL^{-1}. Tgase (pH-range 4–9) [17] was purchased from Activa MP Ajinomoto (Japan). After further purification, the enzyme activity (8764 nkat mL^{-1}) was determined as previously described [48].

2.4. Nanocellulose

The preparation of CNF exploited in this study was described by Valle-Delgado et al. [49] CNF was produced using mechanical fibrillation of never-dried, bleached Kraft hardwood birch pulps obtained from Finnish pulp mills using a high-pressure fluidizer (Microfluidics M-110Y) from Microfluidics Int. Co. (Westwood, MA, USA). No pre-treatments were used prior to fibrillation. The number of passes through the microfluidizer was 12 and the final dry matter content was 1.35 wt-%. The operating pressure was 2000 bar. The average width of the fibrils was 8–9 nm, length several micrometers and a zeta potential ca. −3 mV. CNF thin films for the CLP coatings were prepared on the silica plates as recently described [49].

2.5. Preparation of CLPs

Lignin nanoparticles were prepared from Lignoboost^{TM} purchased from Domtar plant (Plymouth, NC, USA) with minor changes in the procedure [25]. First, lignin (2 g) was dissolved in the mixture of THF and H_2O (3:1, *v/v*). Then, H_2O was added in the filtrated solution, filtrated again and finally dialyzed (Spectra/Por® 1, RC dry dialysis tube, 6–8 kDa) for removal of THF. Concentration of the CLP dispersion was ca. 1.5 mg mL^{-1}, average particle size ca. 300 nm and zeta potential ca. −33 mV.

For the preparation of tiny CLPs, lignin was enzymatically oxidized using low and high redox potential laccases. Powdered lignin (1 g) was dissolved in 0.1 M NaOH (700 mL) under constant magnetic stirring at pH 12.5. Then HCl (1 M) was slowly added to adjust the pH 6.0 and 8.0 for the ThL and MaL treatments, respectively. Then, the solution was transferred into a 1 L measuring flask. Due to low reactivity of ThL in alkaline reaction conditions, pH 8.0 was omitted for this enzyme. Then, lignin solutions (330 mL) were oxidized with laccases (500 nkat g^{-1}) and magnetically stirred (20 h). The enzymatic reactions were terminated using acid precipitation (1 M HCl). The supernatant (pH 2) was removed using ultracentrifugation (Optima^{TM} L Series, rotor type 70 Ti, Beckman Coulter, Bromma, Sweden) at 6000 rpm (G-force 1000) for 20 min at 25 °C. The precipitate was collected with H_2O (pH 5.5) and dried (80 °C) prior preparation of tiny CLPs.

After lignin oxidation, the method modified from Lievonen et al. [25] was used to prepare CLPs below 100 nm. Enzymatically treated lignin (0.5–1 mg mL^{-1}) and the references (2.1 mg mL^{-1}) were solubilized in THF:H_2O (3:7, *v/v*) and the mixture was stirred (3 h) following filtration with 0.7 μm

Whatman GF/F (Sigma-Aldrich, Germany). Then, H$_2$O was fast poured into the solution under constant stirring following vigorous mixing (15 min). THF was removed the solution using dialysis (cut-off: 6–8 kDa) under constant flux for 3 days. The aqueous CLP dispersion was filtrated and characterized as previously described [25].

2.6. Adsorption of Proteins on Lignin

Adsorption of model proteins on lignin surface was studied by quartz crystal microbalance with dissipation (QCM-D, Q-Sense E4, Sweden) at different pHs [42]. For the analysis, golden plates were oxidized with UV-light (10 min), spin-coated with polystyrene (PS) and lignin (WS 650, Laurell Technologies Corp., North Wales, PA, USA) [50]. PS was dissolved in toluene (0.5 mg mL^{-1}) applied twice (50 µL) and dried at 80 °C (30 min). Lignin was coated from the dioxane-H$_2$O mixture (85:15 v/v, 0.5 mg mL^{-1}) and applied four times on a plate and dried as above. Spin-coating sequence was 300 rpm (3 s), 1000 rpm (5 s) and finally 2000 rpm (30 s). Protein samples were dissolved in water (10 µg mL^{-1}) at 40 °C and filtrated. For the pH optimization of the β-casein adsorption, it was dissolved in the buffers (50 mM, 0.1 mg mL^{-1}): pH 3.0 and 5.0 (citrate), 6.5 (phosphate), 7.4 (PBS) and 8.5 (Tris-HCl). Then, lignin films were stabilized with the buffers (1 h) and exposed to β-casein adsorption (100 µL min^{-1}, 25 °C) until stable baseline was detected following rinsing with the buffer (30 min). Masses of the adsorbed β-casein were calculated from the frequencies according to Johannsmann et al. [51]. After β-casein adsorption on lignin film at the optimized pH, the protein coating was cross-linked with Tgase using enzyme dosages 5, 25 and 50 nkat in the measuring cell (40 µL).

2.7. Coating CLPs with Proteins

Surfaces of CLPs (1 mg mL^{-1}) were coated with β-casein at pH 3.0 using β-casein to CLP mass ratio of 0.00001 to 1. Extent of surface charge modifications and changes in the average particle size of CLPs were analyzed after stabilization of the samples at room temperature overnight. Bilayer protein coated CLPs were prepared by modifying only slightly negatively charged particles first with PL and then with acidic of sodium salts of PGA. In the end of the experiment excess of PGA was added in the solution to ensure maximal coverage of single PL coated CLPs and presence of large amounts of carboxylic acid groups for the esterification reaction, crucial for CNF coating.

2.8. Stabilization of Protein Coated CLPs

Surfaces of β-casein coated CLPs were enzymatically stabilized using Tgase. To avoid cross-linking and aggregation of the particles, the enzyme dosage was optimized. In the reactions, Tgase activities varied 5–40 nkat g^{-1}. After overnight incubation at room temperature, the enzyme activity was terminated using ultracentrifugation (5000 rpm, 30 min). Supernatant was removed and the precipitate, cross-linked β-casein coated CLPs, were redispersed in H$_2$O at pH 3 and pH 7.5 for the stability studies.

2.9. Physicochemical Characterization of CLPs

Average particle sizes and zeta potential values of CLP dispersions were analyzed using a Zetasizer (Malvern, Nano-ZS90 instrument, Malvern, UK). The zeta potential values were calculated from the electrophoretic mobility data using Smoluchowski model. Three scans were collected for zeta potential and five scans for the average particle size measurement using dynamic light scattering (DLS) to evaluate the reproducibility of the measurements.

2.10. SEC

Polymerization of lignin by laccases was studied by aqueous high-performance gel permeation size exclusion chromatography (HP-GPC/SEC). For the analyses, enzymatically polymerized and cross-linked lignins including molecular weight standards (194 Da to 0.1 kDa) were dissolved in NaOH

(0.1 M) in two concentrations (0.1 and 0.5 mg mL^{-1}). Weight-average molar mass (MW) of the samples were analyzed by Agilent 1260 Infinity (Agilent Technologies, Espoo, Finland) equipped with a UV detector operating at 280 nm as previously [39,52].

2.11. FTIR

Fourier-transform infrared (FTIR) spectra of the lignin samples were recorded using Thermo Nicolet iS50 FTIR spectrometer with iS50 ATR-crystal (Thermo Fisher Scientific, Vantaa, Finland). Analysis of the spectral area (3800–600 cm^{-1}) was carried out as duplicate measurements with 32 scans from each sample and averaged prior normalization, which was based on peak area using Excel (Microsoft, Espoo, Finland).

2.12. AFM

Atomic force microscopy (AFM) was used to characterize spherical morphology and roughness of CLP surfaces before and after protein coating and enzymatic cross-linking to evaluate aggregation between NPs after the treatments. For the imaging, 10 µL of CLP dispersion was pipetted on a freshly cleaved mica sheet and dried overnight at ambient temperature. All samples were imaged in tapping mode in ambient air using a Multimode 8 AFM equipped with a Nanoscope V controller from Bruker Corporation, Santa Barbara, CA, USA). NCHV-A probes with a fundamental resonance frequency of 320–370 kHz, a nominal spring constant of 40 N m^{-1}, and a tip radius below 10 nm were used for imaging. At least three sample areas were imaged from the same mica sheet without further processing of the images except flattening using Nanoscope Analysis 8.15 software from Bruker (USA).

Furthermore, AFM was used to measure adhesion energies between Col IV and lignin, Col IV and gelatin as well as Col IV and casein. For the force measurements the tip less silicon cantilever (CSC38/No Al coating, MicroMasch, Tallinn, Estonia) with a normal spring constant of 40 N m^{-1} was used to study the interactions. Prior to force measurements, the nominal spring constant was determined analyzing the thermal vibration spectra using Sader method [53]. The biomaterial-coated probe was prepared with same method as previously [54]. Adsorption of Col IV onto the colloidal probe was performed in several steps. First, the collagen solution (1 mg mL^{-1}) was placed in ice-filled beaker and thawed by sonication (2 × 10 min). Then, the glass probe was surface modified with 5 vol-% 3-aminopropyl triethoxysilane (APTES) dissolved in ethanol to improve physical adsorption of protein on the glass probe (45 min). Unreacted APTES was rinsed with ethanol and dried. The APTES-modified probe was glued with an optical adhesive (Norland Products, Inc., Cranbury, New Jersey, USA) on the free-end of the cantilever with 3D micromanipulator following UV curing (15 min) at the wavelength of 365 nm. After gluing, the colloidal probes modified with APTES were mounted on metallic disc facilitated with double-side tape and few drops of collagen solution were spin-coated (40 s) at 1000 rpm. The collagen-coated probes were dried overnight and rinsed with Milli-Q water before use. The neat glass probe was used a reference.

AFM force measurements were performed using a Multimode 8 AFM NanoScope V controller coupled with a Pico Force (PF) scanner from Bruker (USA) in a liquid mode. The colloidal probe was mounted on the liquid cell and subsequently inserted into the AFM head. Few drops of PBS buffer (pH 7.4) were injected onto sample film and equilibrated (10 min) before the force measurements. The rate of the approach and retraction of the colloidal probe towards the surface was 2 µm s^{-1}. At least three random locations were probed to ensure the homogeneity of the film surface. The deflection sensitivity was determined from a freshly cleaved mica surface. The recorded data were converted to the profiles of normalized force and the separation distances, where D = 0 was adjusted to be at the maximum applied load [55]. The measured force profiles were compared to the DLVO theory [56,57]. and the adhesion energy was calculated through the integration over the adhesion area. For the proteins (Col IV), the Hamaker constant for calculation of van der Waals forces was 7.5 × 10^{-21} J [58].

2.13. TEM

FEI Tecnai 12 (Hope, CA, USA) operating at 120 kV was used to obtain transmission electron microscopy (TEM) images from the CLP dispersions. For the imaging, 3 µL of the sample was applied on a carbon film supported grid and incubated (2 min). The excess of the solvent was removed by blotting the side of the grid onto paper. Imaging was performed in the brightfield mode with slight under focus.

2.14. Sample Preparation

Chamois specimens washed with acetone and dried with filter paper were cut to narrow strips (3.5 cm × 1.0 cm) following stabilization in the standard conditions (25 °C, 50% humidity). The area used for adhesion was 1 cm^{-2}. In addition to aqueous NP dispersions (CLP, β-casein and CLP coated with β-casein) in 1 mg mL^{-1} concentration, Tgase (100 nkat cm^{-2}) was used for curing β-casein coated CLPs joints. Furthermore, NPs (1 mg mL^{-1}) were dispersed in diluted water-soluble adhesive (10 mg mL^{-1}) to study the effect of the NPs on the adhesion in the agglutinative formulation. Lignin dissolved in THF (1 mg mL^{-1}) and diluted adhesive formulation (H$_2$O:THF, 99:1, v:v) in 10 mg mL^{-1} concentration were used as references. After sticking the specimens with NP dispersions (50 µL and 100 µL), the samples where kept under a metal plate (ca. 200 g) in the standard conditions for 3 days prior to tensile testing (MTS400, MTS Systems Corporation, Eden Prairie, MN, USA).

Tiny and bilayer protein coated CLPs (mass ratio 1 g g^{-1} lignin) were linked on the CNF surfaces using esterification reaction between the carboxylic acid groups with hydroxyls of CNF [49,59]. For the analysis, two drops of modified CLP dispersions were coated (4000 rpm, 1 min) on the CNF surface using a spin-coater from Laurell Technologies Corp., (North Wales, PA, USA). Heated up to 105 °C (10 min) following 5 min treatment at 155 °C. To remove unbound particles, CNF surfaces were rinsed with H$_2$O and dried under nitrogen flow.

3. Results and Discussion

3.1. Tailoring CLP Surfaces with Proteins

Proteins adsorb on lignin surface. The extent of the interactions depends on the physicochemical properties of the biomolecule resulting from the three-dimensional (3D) structure and amino acid composition of the protein [42,50]. To show potential to exploit actual by-product from industry, purified β-casein, previously used in wood [60] and food [21] adhesives was used a model protein for the surface functionalization of CLPs.

3.1.1. β-Casein

Adsorption of β-casein on lignin surface was studied at pH 7.4 using QCM-D (Figure S1A). Gelatin, serum proteins and PL, commonly used to coat tissues to improve cell adhesion [61], were studied for comparison. Positively charged gelatin (47 kDa, pI 7.0–9.0) at pH 7.4 adsorbed better on lignin surface than smaller negatively charged β-casein (24 kDa, pI 4.6–5.1). Adsorption of serum proteins and polypeptide (PL) were weaker. The increase in dissipation was considerably higher at similar frequency values for the β-casein coating compared to other proteins, indicating that the coating is softer and contains more water (Figure S1B).

For the coating of individual CLPs with β-casein, protein adsorption on lignin surface was examined at pH range 3.0–8.5 (Figure 1). It was the highest at pH 3.0 due to positive charge of β-casein in the acidic reaction conditions. A similar adsorbed mass was observed at pH 8.5, but in this case negatively charged β-casein formed particles (ca. 300 nm) that adsorbed on the lignin surface together with the polymeric protein. This is further confirmed when comparing the increase in dissipation (Figure S1C). The dissipation is much higher for layers adsorbed at alkaline pH compared to pH 3.5, indicating that these layers are more loosely bound and contain more water due to the nanoparticulate morphology. The formation of β-casein NPs depends on the pH, time, mixing, protein and salt concentration [20].

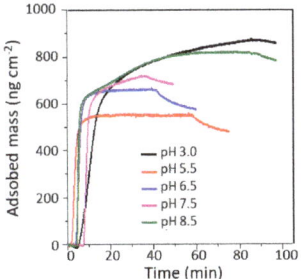

Figure 1. Adsorption of β-casein on lignin thin film at different pH observed using QCM-D.

Hence, pH 3.0 was selected for the coating CLPs with β-casein for further experiments. Figure 2a shows the zeta potential of the CLPs varying from negative (ca. −25 mV) to positive (ca. 25 mV) value when β-casein concentration increased. During the coating, CLPs aggregated when the surface charge of the particles was close to zero (CLP—protein ratio ca. 0.01), as shown in Figure 2b. On the other hand, once clearly positively charged, the protein-coated CLP dispersions were stable for weeks. Large-scale all atom MD simulations [62] have shown that aromatic residues contribute significantly to the protein adsorption on hydrophobic surfaces via strong π–π stacking interactions between $p2$-carbons. The basic residues such as arginine and lysine play equally strong role for the adsorption. The effect of proline residues has been demonstrated recently [42].

In Figure 2 are shown representative TEM images from single CLPs (Figure 2c) including β-casein coated CLPs (Figure 2d) confirming that after protein adsorption, and enzymatic cross-linking (Figure 2e) CLPs remain individual spherical NPs and the aggregation of the particles is minor. During sample preparation on the carbon grid, some of the particles moved close to each other due to water evaporation during drying. The corresponding AFM images are shown in Figure 2f–h and Figure S2A–D. When CLPs were coated with β-casein, very small protein particles could be detected from the background of TEM (Figure 2d) and AFM (Figure S2B,D) images, not visible in the references (Figure 2f,i–k and Figure S2A,C). Apparently, some of these particles adsorbed on CLP surface along with polymeric β-casein since several protruding points (ca. 40 nm) could be imaged from the CLP surfaces by AFM (Figure S2B,D).

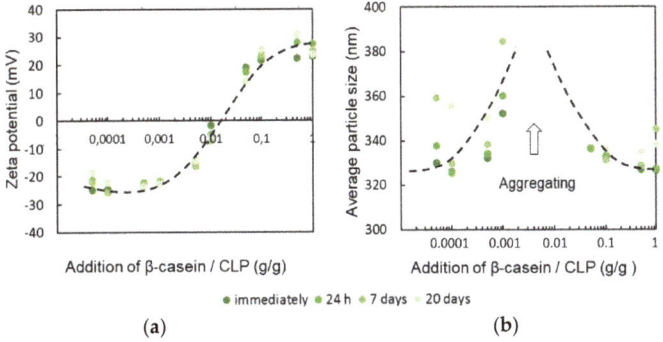

Figure 2. *Cont.*

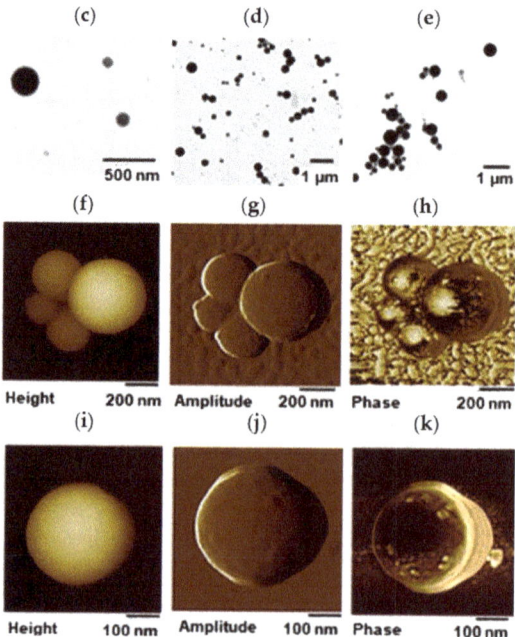

Figure 2. Coating CLPs with β-casein (pH 3.0) evidenced using zeta potential (**a**) and DLC (**b**) measurements as a function of time. TEM images measured from unmodified CLPs (**c**), β-casein coated CLPs (**d**) and β-casein coated CLPs cross-linked with Tgase (**e**). In (**f,g,h**) are shown representative AFM images from enzymatically stabilized CLPs and in (**i,j,k**) are presented the corresponding references.

3.1.2. Poly(L-glutamic acid)

Feasibility to coat CLP surfaces using selected proteins to maximize specific interactions with the substrate such as CNF surface was evaluated. Thus, negatively charged CLPs were first coated with positively charged PL following modification with PGA containing large number of carboxylic acid groups for the esterification reaction with hydroxyls on nanocellulose surface via fast heat treatment. It was hypothesized that tiny CLPs below 100 nm in size coat single CNF fibrils better than larger particles since the typical width for the nanocellulose fibrils is ca. 5–20 nm and the length several micrometers. The average molecular masses of enzymatically polymerized and cross-linked lignin used for tiny CLP preparation are shown in Figure 3 and the characterization using FTIR spectroscopy in Tables S1–S3. In general, the changes in the FTIR spectra between the references and laccase treated samples were minor due to heterogeneous cross-linking reactions and residual moisture in the samples slightly interfering the interpretation of the spectra.

The appearance of the CLP dispersions at pH 6.0 are shown in Figure S3. The average particle sizes for CLPs prepared from enzymatically oxidized lignin were below 100 nm (Table 1). For the references, the particle size was half of that obtained according to the method of Lievonen at al. [25]. In both cases, the zeta potentials were on the same order of magnitude as previously described [25]. The increased molecular weight, higher hydrophobicity of the polymerized and cross-linked lignin as well as lower concentration enabled tight packing of enzymatically oxidized lignin fast mixing promoting tiny NP CLP formation. In the laccase-catalyzed reactions, the cross-links are formed in lignin via different radical reactions. Enzymatic initiation of the radicalization starts from the phenolic hydroxyl groups of lignin following condensation of the free radicals to covalent chemical bonds [37,38,46,47,63]. The representative AFM images of the different CLPs (Figure S4) verify the spherical and smooth surface structure of the NPs stable for several weeks (Table S4), as evident from the TEM images (Figure S5). Solid lignin NPs 10–30 nm in size can be produced using mechanical shearing [32] and are also potential modifiers for CNF surfaces.

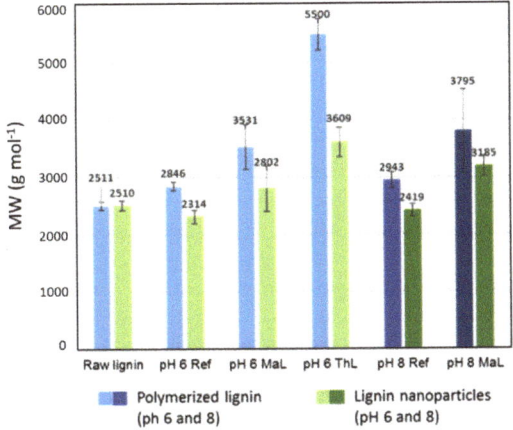

Figure 3. Average molecular masses and standard deviations of the enzymatically oxidized and polymerized lignins. Molecular masses were analyzed also for the CLPs prepared from the enzymatically treated lignins. The smaller values of dissolved CLPs are most likely due to slower solubility of CLPs in alkaline reaction conditions than powdered lignin.

Table 1. Characterization of CLPs prepared from laccase-treated lignin.

Sample	Average Size (nm)	Zeta Potential (mV)	PDI
pH 6.0			
Reference	131 ± 1	−30 ± 1	0.27
MaL-treatment	75 ± 1	−25 ± 1	0.40
ThL-treatment	82 ± 2	−33 ± 1	0.40
pH 8.0			
Reference	125 ± 1	−22 ± 1	0.25
MaL-treatment	65 ± 1	−30 ± 1	0.25
ThL-treatment	-	-	-

(-) Not determined. The enzyme is not reactive at alkaline reaction conditions.

Bilayer protein coated tiny CLPs (ca. 131 nm) are shown in Figure S6. Significant increase in the average particle size from ca. 200 nm to ca. 400 nm confirmed coating of the NPs with small PGA (15–50 kDa). When using larger PGA (150–300 kDa), the effect on the average particle size and extent of the surface coating was minor. Apparently, shorter polymer chain is more desirable for the modification of CLP surfaces over large ones. However, in the both cases, zeta potential values decreased from ca. 40 mV to 30 mV, verifying dual coating of CLPs. In Figure S7A,B are shown adsorption of PL peptide on the intact CLP surface following adsorption of low and high molecular weight PGA confirming the above conclusions.

In the body, NP-specific protein coronas are formed on hard inorganic NPs in minutes comprising hundreds of proteins. Adsorption of serum proteins on lignin (Figure S1A,B) show that CLP surfaces could be tailored accordingly to increase cellular interaction. Compared to hard NPs, soft CLPs are presumably safer since undesirable penetration of the elastic NPs through the biological membranes is minor. Low cytotoxicity [31,64] and resistance for the enzymatic hydrolysis increase potential to exploit CLPs in value-added applications in medicine and cosmetics [2,20].

3.2. Stability of β-Casein Coated CLP

3.2.1. Effect of Enzymatic Cross-Linking

Tailoring CLP surfaces with β-casein allows further modification of the particles with cross-linking enzymes [65]. In vitro studies have shown that Tgase can cross-link proteins in a gel in minutes [17,48]. Hence, to improve stability of β-casein coated CLPs at physiological pHs, for example in stomach (pH 1.0–3.0), duodenum (pH 4.8–8.2) and blood (pH 7.4), Tgase was used to cross-link the β-casein coating. Figure S8A shows the increase in the average particle size of CLPs as a function of enzyme dosage. Particles cross-linked with high enzyme dosage above 20 nkat g^{-1} aggregated immediately because covalent bonds were also formed between the individual particles. The zeta potential values (Figure S8B) decreased after 24-h incubation and, after seven-day treatment, extensive cross-linking of the NPs was detected by eye. Reasonable enzyme dosage for the cross-linking only β-casein coating was found to be 15 nkat g^{-1}. Prior to pH stability studies of the enzymatically cross-linked particles, Tgase activity was removed from the dispersions using ultra-centrifugation (Figure S9). After the treatment, some of the unbound β-casein adsorbed on CLP surfaces increasing the average particle size by ca. 40 nm. Then, the particles were stable for several weeks.

Elasticity of the enzymatically cross-linked β-casein coating was studied by QCM-D (Figure S10A,B). After adsorption of β-casein on lignin film until a stable baseline was observed (Figure S1), Tgase (2 min) was injected into the chamber following cross-linking (10 min) of the protein film. When using the low enzyme dosage (5 nkat), loosely bound β-casein was washed away. However, at the same time, the cross-linking reaction proceeded to a certain extent since a sharp decrease in dissipation was detected due to the formation of elastic networked protein coating. Instead, when using higher enzyme dosages in the measuring cell (25 and 50 nkat), first a small amount of unbound β-casein was removed (tiny increase in the frequency signal). After that, a sharp drop in the frequency was detected due to enzyme adsorption on the β-casein surface. The cross-linking reaction proceeded as in the case of low enzyme dosage. During the enzymatic reaction (10 min), the frequency increased slightly, verifying an accompanied loss of small molecule reaction product (-NH_3^+) [66] as well as decreased water binding capacity of the cross-linked protein coating. Tgase injection following stabilization of the cross-linking reaction was repeated three times until stable baseline was observed.

Figure 2c–h shows representative TEM and AFM images of β-casein coated CLPs cross-linked with Tgase. Compared to CLPs coated with β-casein (Figure S2B,D) the surfaces of cross-linked particles were smoother. From the corresponding TEM images (Figure 2d,c), it is evident that also small protein particles in the background were cross-linked to larger particles. Regarding the applicability of the enzymatically stabilized protein coated CLP dispersions, polymerization of free β-casein to nanosized particles [65] improves homogeneity and stability of the dispersion.

3.2.2. Effect of pH

Understanding dispersion properties is essential for the exploitation CLPs in adhesive formulations. CLPs are stable in wide pH range [25]. However, due to better electrostatic stability in alkaline conditions, the reactivity of CLPs is much higher than in acidic conditions [39,63]. For medical, cosmetic and food applications, it is pivotal that tailored CLPs are stable in physiological conditions.

Figure 4a,b shows the average particle sizes and zeta potential values for β-casein coated CLPs at pH 3.0 and 7.4 as a function of time. In acidic dispersion, NPs started to aggregate after four-day incubation, which was evident also from the more positive zeta potential values. After 25 days, protein-coated particles precipitated. At pH 3.0, β-casein was positively charged, but CLP surface was nearly neutral, promoting aggregation of the coated CLPs. At slightly alkaline dispersion (pH 7.4), the stability of β-casein coated CLPs was excellent. The average particle sizes and zeta potential values remained nearly unchanged for 25 days.

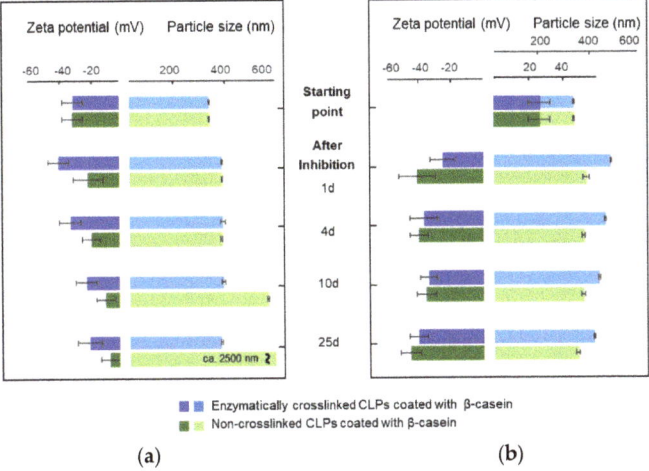

Figure 4. Stability of β-casein coated and enzymatically cross-linked CLPs at (**a**) pH 3.0 and (**b**) pH 7.4 evidenced using average particle size and zeta potential measurements. In both cases, the protein coating following enzymatic cross-linking was performed at 3.0. Enzyme activity was removed using ultracentrifugation following redispersion of the particles at above pH.

To improve stability of the β-casein coated CLPs at pH 3.0, the optimized Tgase dosage (15 nkat g^{-1}) was used to cross-link the surfaces of the particles. The stability of cross-linked protein coated CLPs was excellent compared to the non-cross-linked particles (Figure 4a). The average particle sizes remained nearly unchanged for 25 days. Instead, the zeta potential values became slightly more positive due to some instability of CLPs, as explained above. Instead, at pH 7.4 (Figure 4b), the zeta potential values were stable for weeks, but the average particle sizes increased during the first day after enzyme inhibition and solvent exchange. Then, the cross-linked protein coated CLPs were stable for weeks.

3.3. Adhesive Interactions

AFM force measurement was used to compare strength of the interactions between lignin and model proteins (Figure 5). Col IV is the main component of the skin and, therefore, understanding the interactions of Col IV with other proteins and lignin could be exploited in wound healing and other biomedical applications.

Long-range attractive interactions were detected when Col IV surface was brought into contact with casein and gelatin (Figure 5a), while no meaningful adhesions were detected when the neat glass surface was used (Figure 5b). The force interactions between Col IV and lignin were three times larger than the ones between Col IV and model proteins (Figure 5c) with adhesion energy being 0.0102 ± 0.0006 nJ m^{-1}. Interestingly, the adhesion energy between Col IV and casein as well as Col IV and gelatin was nearly identical at pH 7.4, evident also from the overlapping retraction force profiles (Figure 5a). At high salt concentration, the repulsions detected from the approach force profiles was much longer-ranged than predicted by DLVO theory for pure electrostatic double-layer repulsion (Figure 5d). This reveals that steric repulsions dominate [67]. Based on the approach force profiles separation distance between Col IV and gelatin pair is nearly twofold compared to that of Col IV and casein, while Col IV and lignin was placed in between. Even though casein show lower adhesion energy with Col IV, it is an attractive protein to coat CLPs compared to poorly soluble gelatin having high tendency to aggregate, as recently demonstrated [42]. Thus, purified β-casein containing many reactive sites for enzymatic cross-linking and stabilization is an excellent coat protein for CLPs enabling also fast curing enzymatic means [65].

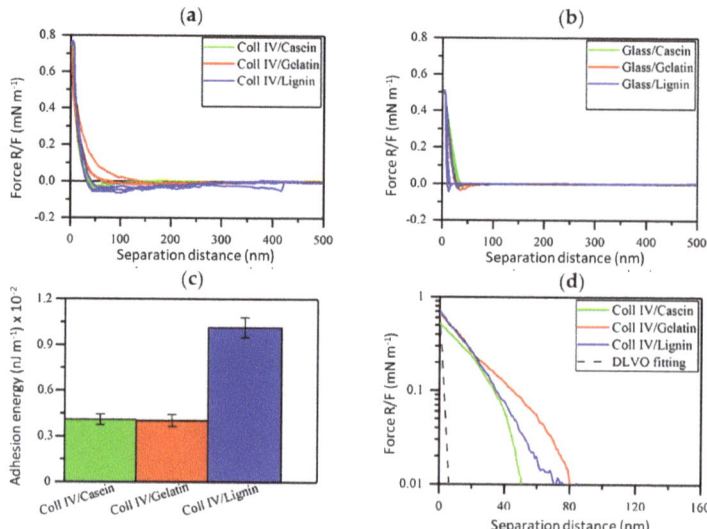

Figure 5. AFM force profiles. Interaction between (**a**) Col IV probe and other proteins and lignin. (**b**) Interaction of the model surfaces with a neat glass probe. (**c**) Corresponding histograms of mean adhesion energy of above interactions including standard deviation. (**d**) DLVO fitting of the data presented in (**b**). The gray dashed line represents the DLVO fitting for PBS (150 mM) at pH 7.4. All force profiles were normalized with the radius of the probe.

3.4. Applications

Chamois specimens and CNF were used model soft matrixes to demonstrate effect of tailored CLPs to adhere soft materials. Furthermore, enzymatic and chemical heat treatment were exploited for fast covalent curing of the agglutinations.

3.4.1. Agglutination of Chamois Specimens with CLPs

Figure 6a show the chamois leather specimen including CLP dispersion used for adhesion. Tensile testing was used to measure the strength of adhesive joints until break down. The representative stress–strain curves for various NP formulations are shown in Figure 6b,c.

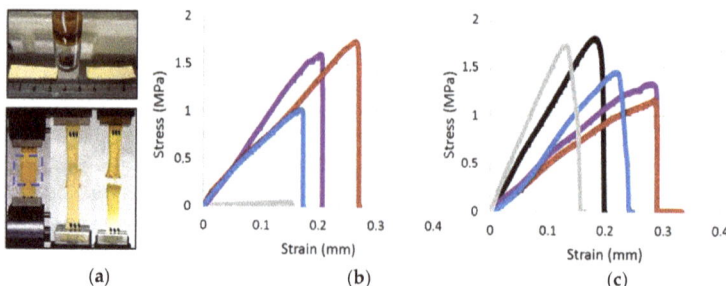

Figure 6. Tensile testing. (**a**) Two chamois specimens to be adhered with CLP dispersion (above). Adhered strips subjected to a controlled tension until failure (below). (**b**) Representative stress–strain curves for the CLPs used for adhesion including the corresponding references. (**c**) Representative stress–strain curves for the same samples as in (**b**) dispersed in water-soluble adhesive. ●CLPs (blue), ●β-casein NPs (red), ●CLPs coated with β-casein (purple), ●commercial adhesive (black), ●polymeric lignin dissolved in THF (grey).

Figure 7a shows the effect of different NPs for adhering protein matrix that was significantly better than that of lignin and commercial water-soluble adhesive. When the number of NPs doubled, the agglutination of the specimens was more than twofold stronger, which was evident from the measured stress values. The differences between the type of the soft material, i.e., lignin or protein, used for the NP preparation was apparent when high NP concentration was used. Adhesive property of β-casein NPs on protein matrix was the highest and for CLPs only half of that. Effect of β-casein coated CLPs on the adhesion was between these two cases showing potential as a method to prepare functional low-cost β-casein NPs from lignin via self-assembly. The tensile strain (Figure 7b) measured from the corresponding samples followed the same order as the stress values. However, the differences between the samples were smaller. When β-casein coated CLPs were used for adhering, the strain values were rather similar between two different quantities. In the case of large number of NPs, the repeatability was poor, presumably due to instability of the β-casein coating at pH 3.0, as explained above. Regarding to the references, lignin powder dissolved in THF and diluted adhesive, the agglutination of the specimens was minor compared to that of NPs. Due to rough, hairy surface of chamois, the NPs spread, adsorbed and penetrated on the soft material better than the thick adhesive formulation, efficiently dissipating energy and retarding fracture of the joints under stress.

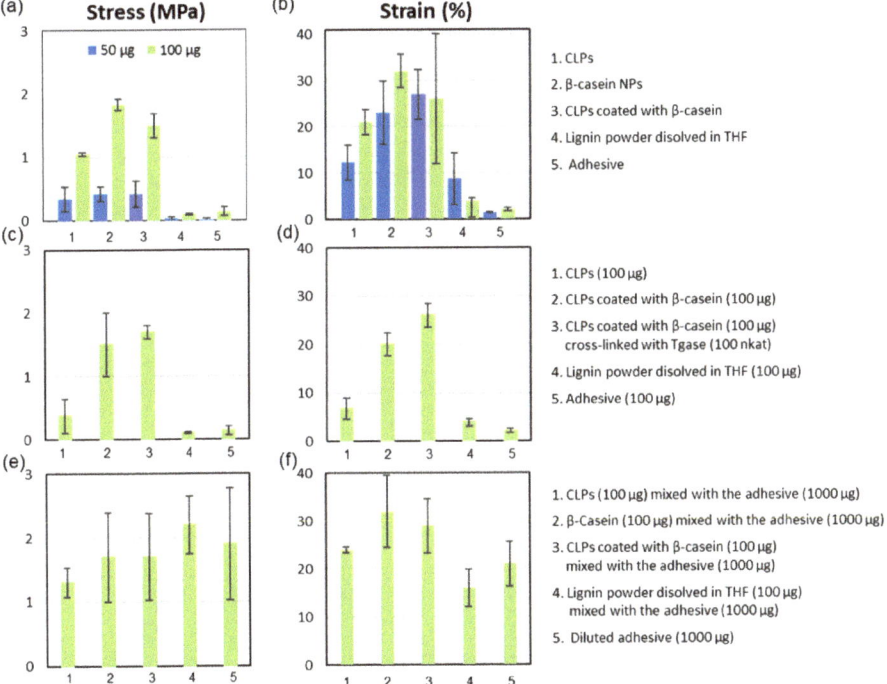

Figure 7. Comparison between tensile stress–strain histograms. (a,b) Different CLPs including the references at two quantities. (c,d) Effect of Tgase catalyzed cross-linking on the adhesion. (e,f) Various NPs including the references dispersed in diluted water-soluble adhesive.

Figure 7c,d shows the increased stress and strain values when β-casein coated CLPs were covalently linked to chamois specimens using low Tgase dosage (100 nkat). Increasing the enzyme activity, the strength of the adhesion could be increased [47,62]. These results suggest that protein coated CLPs could also be linked to biological matrixes using enzymes enabling fast curing in moist environments essential for the medical applications. In such seals, CLPs remain single nanoparticles retaining their physicochemical properties since the covalent linkages are formed via protein coating. It is also plausible that cross-links were formed between amine groups in lysine side-chains and the acyl group derived from the carboxylic acid groups present in CLPs due to side reactions of Tgase [17]. If CLPs are coated with tissue specific proteins, the potential rejection reactions could be diminished during the wound healing, yielding small scars important for cosmetic applications. Accordingly, it is presupposed that CLP formulations could be exploited for the preparation of edible coatings for foods.

Furthermore, to study potential to use CLPs as additive in adhesive formulations, NPs and the references were dispersed in the water-soluble adhesive (Figure 7e,f). Unexpectedly, the stress value was the largest (ca. 5%) for the dispersion containing lignin powder compared to that of diluted adhesive. Mixing protein NPs in the adhesive formulation decreased stress value ca. 3%, and for the unmodified CLPs ca. 7%. In the case of tensile strain measurement, the results were opposite. For CLPs, β-casein NPs and β-casein coated CLPs, the tensile strain improved ca. 5%, 12% and 10%, respectively. For lignin powder, the elasticity of the adhesive joint degreased ca. 5% compared to the diluted adhesive.

Figure 8 shows histograms of Young's modulus for various NPs. The values doubled for the specimens adhered with high number of NPs regardless of the type of the polymer used for the adhesion. Instead, when the NPs were dispersed in the adhesive formulation, the differences between the raw materials became visible. In the case of CLPs, Young's modulus increased (ca. 70 kPa), but, for the protein-based NPs it degreased (ca. 43 kPa), showing more elastic agglutination due to softer structure of the particles and improved compatibility with the substrate. In the adhesive formulation, the Young's modulus was the highest for the polymeric lignin showing much stronger adhesive joint, likely due to varying chemical reactions and interactions between the adhesive components and the substrate. Furthermore, interactions between lignin and protein matrix differ from the ones between CLPs and the substrate. In aqueous dispersion, hydrophobic groups are buried inside the CLPs' hydrophilic groups locating on the surfaces of NPs. Furthermore, the instability of lignin complicated the analyses. The results obtained in the adhesive formulation should be critically considered. Young's modulus determined for the diluted adhesive was between that of CLPs and lignin powder.

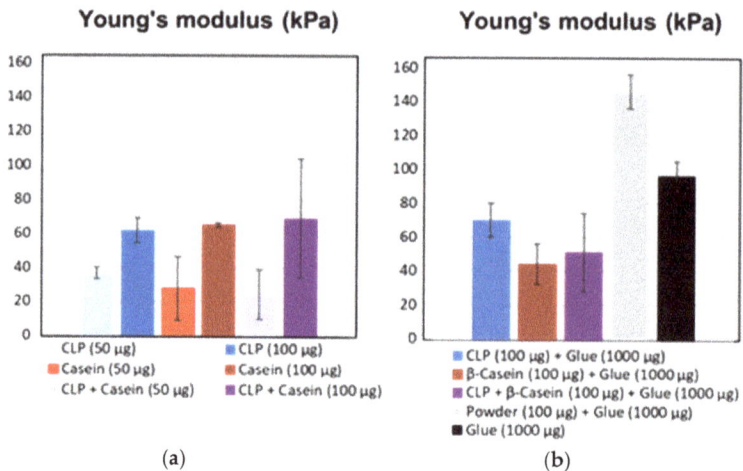

Figure 8. Young's modulus for (a) CLPs, β-casein and CLPs coated with β-casein using two quantities. (b) Corresponding histograms for the NPs dispersed in diluted adhesive including the references.

These results show that, when using NP prepared from soft natural matter (technical lignin, proteins and their combinations), it is possible to obtain strong elastic agglutinations between soft surfaces, as evidenced recently [24,68,69]. The type of biopolymer affects significantly the strength, flexibility and elongation of the joint. Studies with soybean-based adhesives containing polymeric lignin pointed out that protein–lignin ratio is the most critical parameter affecting the adhesive interactions [70,71]. In textiles, enzymatic cross-linking has been used to strengthen lignin-containing adhesives [72]. Apparently, exploitation of technical lignin in nanoparticulate morphology in stable dispersion for adhering is an interesting approach for many lignin applications reviewed [73].

3.4.2. Grafting CLPs on CNF Surfaces

Feasibility to coat CNF with varying sized CLPs was also investigated. Figure 9a shows nanocellulose fibrils spin coated with several layers of tiny CLPs (ca. 75 nm). Covalently linked CLPs clearly follow the fibrous morphology of nanocellulose, changing the surface properties of the hydrophilic polymer to that of more hydrophobic lignin surface. Linking of the NPs was obtained via esterification reaction between carboxylic acid groups of lignin and hydroxyl groups of CNF surface via heat treatment [49]. After washing with H_2O for the removal of unbound CLPs, the fibers accumulated to some extent, however, CLPs remaining linked on the CNF surfaces due to covalent linkages. Hence, it is proposed that CNF modified with CLPs could be excellent bionanomaterials for tissue repairing, having improved stability in body fluids, culture media and resistance against enzymatic hydrolysis.

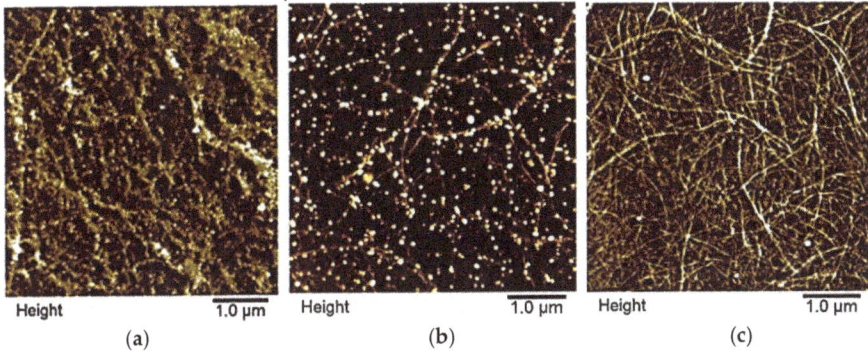

Figure 9. CNF surfaces coated with CLPs: (**a**) Tiny CLPs; (**b**) PL and PGA coated CLPs; and (**c**) reference.

It was also shown that CNF surfaces (Figure 9b) could be coated accordingly with protein coated CLPs using heat treatment. To increase the reactivity between CNF and protein coated CLPs, nanoparticles were modified first with positively charged PL and then with negatively charged PGA containing large number of carboxylic acid groups. CLPs coated only with PL could not be linked on the slightly negative CNF surface to the same extent. In that case, surface modification of CNF, e.g., via carboxylation to increase negative charges on the surface, is a prerequisite. After the heat treatment, the average particle sizes of the modified CLPs clearly decreased (Figure S6A and Figure 9b) due to the formation of covalent linkages between carboxylic acids in PGA and hydroxyls in CLP. After washing with water, most of the bilayer coated CLPs remained on the CNF surface. Feasibility for the bilayer protein coating of CLPs was demonstrated also using QCM-D under identical reaction conditions (Figure S7A,B). PL peptide was first adsorbed to CNF film following adsorption of CLPs yielding intact lignin nanoparticulate surface. Then, PL and PGA (15–50 and 50–100 kDa) were adsorbed on the surface that was finally washed with water. As shown in Figures S6 and S7, it was evident that small PGA adsorbed on CLP surface better than large PGA.

Current polymeric tissue adhesives are often unstable in physiological pH requiring complex in vivo analytical systems for the control of the polymerization and cross-linking reactions. Furthermore, they are often toxic [6,69]. Coating fibers with specific CLPs could be an effective way to improve mechanical strength. Adhesives based on nanobridging via hard inorganic NPs [16] as well as colloidal mesoporous silica (CMS) particles [68] have been proposed as alternatives for traditional medical adhesives. Since the adhesion energy is proportional to the surface area of NPs, enzymatically cross-linked CLPs [39] with tailored functionalities could be potential additives for medical adhesives following enzymatic or thermal treatment for fast curing shown above. Additionally, porous structure of CLPs enables quicker decomposition in biological media than inorganic NPs preventing undesirable accumulation in the body. Due to strong autofluorescence of lignin, it is an attractive raw material enabling sensitive real time detection crucial for the development of image-guided procedures for clinical applications.

4. Conclusions

Development of green technologies [74,75] for the preparation of bio(nano)materials [76] from the forest process side-streams such as adhesives and coatings [77,78] is increasing constantly. Different CLPs prepared and modified to adhere chamois and to modify CNF surface could be potential additives for various formulations to be exploited for wound sealing, edible coatings and fiber modification for textiles to improve adhesion, hydrophobicity, antimicrobial and antioxidative properties of the coatings. Since the cross-linking methods are fast and feasible in the moist environment, clinical fluorescence imaging of aromatic CLPs is possible. Furthermore, it was concluded that, when using tissue specific proteins, e.g., hydrolyzed from collagen, sericins extracted from silk and caseins fractionated from the dairy side-streams, compatibility of the NPs with the substrates could be enhanced. Compared to NPs prepared solely from proteins, the costs of the raw materials are remarkably lower. Apparently, these results pave the way for the exploitation of technical lignin in multiple forms.

Supplementary Materials: The electronic supplementary data associated with this article is available online at http://www.mdpi.com/2079-4991/8/12/1001/s1. Figure S1: Adsorption of proteins on lignin thin films analyzed by QCM-D, Figure S2: AFM images of β-casein coated CLPs, Figure S3: CLP dispersions prepared from laccases treated lignins, Figure S4: AFM height images from CLPs prepared from laccase treated lignin at pH 6, Figure S5: TEM images from CLPs prepared from enzymatically treated lignin one month after preparation, Figure S6: Average particle size and zeta potential of CLPs as a function of PL−CLP mass ratio, Figure S7: Adsorption of PL, PGA and CLPs on slightly negatively charged CNF analyzed by QCM-D, Figure S8: β-Casein coating and enzymatic stabilization of the particles with Tgase, Figure S9: Variation of stabilized CLPs in size after removal of enzyme activity using ultracentrifugation, Figure S10: Elasticity of enzymatically cross-linked β-casein coating, Tables S1–S3: Characterization of laccase treated lignins by FTIR, Table S4: Effect of time on the average particle size, zeta potential and polydispersity (PDI) of CLPs prepared from different lignins at starting concentration 0.5 g L^{-1}.

Author Contributions: M.-L.M. supervised the work including writing of the final version of the manuscript. Furthermore, she was responsible for the adsorption, coating and stabilization studies, TEM imaging as well as planning of the application studies. G.R. prepared and characterized CLP dispersions using different physicochemical methods such as AFM, SEC and FTIR spectroscopy. R.W.N.N. and T.L. carried out the AFM retraction force measurements. A.H. carried out the adhesion experiments with various NPs and chamois specimens using tensile testing. O.N. purified and characterized enzymes used in the study at VTT. J.J.V.-D. conducted the AFM imaging. M.A.K. and M.Ö. provided facilities, scientific discussion and guidance for the study. All authors contributed to the production of the manuscript.

Funding: This research was funded by the Academy of Finland (TaBioMat, *Tailored* biomass derived self-assembling *building blocks for bionanomaterial applications*, grant number 276696). Furthermore, this work has received funding from the Bio Based Industries Joint Undertaking under the European Union's Horizon 2020 research and innovation programme under grant agreement No 720303 (Zelcor project).

Acknowledgments: MSc students Anni Pyysing, Helena Båtsman, Teemu Kemppainen, Ari Ruotsalainen, Mustafa Çan, Andrey Vinogradov (Aalto University, JOIN-E3000 Life science technologies project course, coated lignin nanoparticles for biomaterial applications, Finland) and MSc student Zhenxing Yan (Aalto University, Finland) are acknowledged for the laboratory assistance.

Conflicts of Interest: There are no conflicts to declare.

References

1. Fu, J.; Su, J.; Wang, P.; Yu, Y.; Wang, Q.; Cavaco-Paulo, A. Enzymatic processing of protein-based fibers. *Appl. Microbiol. Biotechnol.* **2015**, *99*, 10387–10397. [CrossRef] [PubMed]
2. Ngo, H.-T.; Bechtold, T. Surface modification of textile material through deposition of regenerated silk fibroin. *J. Appl. Polym. Sci.* **2017**, *134*, 45098–45109. [CrossRef]
3. Hemmilä, V.; Adamopoulos, S.; Karlsson, O.; Kumar, A. Development of sustainable bio-adhesives for engineered wood panels—A Review. *RSC Adv.* **2017**, *7*, 38604–38630. [CrossRef]
4. Esposito, D.; Antonietti, M. Redefining biorefinery: The search for unconventional building blocks for materials. *Chem. Soc. Rev.* **2015**, *44*, 5821–5835. [CrossRef] [PubMed]
5. Klemm, D.; Kramer, F.; Moritz, S.; Lindström, T.; Ankerfors, M.; Gray, D.; Dorris, A. Nanocelluloses: A new family of nature-based materials. *Angew. Chem. Int. Ed.* **2011**, *50*, 5438–5466. [CrossRef] [PubMed]
6. Eichhorn, S.J.; Dufresne, A.; Aranguren, M.; Marcovich, N.E.; Capadona, J.R.; Rowan, S.J.; Weder, C.; Thielemans, W.; Roman, M.; Renneckar, S.; et al. Review: Current international research into cellulose nanofibers and nanocomposites. *J. Mater. Sci.* **2010**, *45*, 1–33. [CrossRef]
7. Xu, X.; Liu, F.; Jiang, L.; Zhu, J.Y.; Haagenson, D.; Wiesenborn, D.P. Cellulose nanocrystals vs. Cellulose nanofibrils: A comparative study on their microstructures and effects as polymer reinforcing agents. *ACS Appl. Mater. Interfaces* **2013**, *5*, 2999–3009. [CrossRef]
8. Abe, K.; Iwamoto, S.; Yano, H. Obtaining cellulose nanofibers with a uniform width of 15 nm from wood. *Biomacromolecules* **2007**, *8*, 3276–3278. [CrossRef]
9. Bhattacharya, M.; Malinen, M.M.; Lauren, P.; Lou, Y.-R.; Kuisma, S.W.; Kanninen, L.; Lille, M.; Corlu, A.; Guen-Guillouzo, C.; Ikkala, O.; et al. Nanofibrillar cellulose hydrogel promotes three-dimensional liver cell culture. *J. Control. Release* **2012**, *164*, 291–298. [CrossRef]
10. Lou, Y.-R.; Kanninen, L.; Kuisma, T.; Niklander, J.; Noon, L.A.; Burks, D.; Urtti, A.; Yliperttula, M. The use of nanofibrillar cellulose hydrogel as a flexible three-dimensional model to culture human pluripotent stem cells. *Stem Cells Dev.* **2014**, *23*, 380–392. [CrossRef]
11. Petersen, N.; Gatenholm, P. Bacterial cellulose-based materials and medical devices: Current state and perspectives. *Appl. Microbiol. Biotechnol.* **2011**, *91*, 1277–1286. [CrossRef] [PubMed]
12. Lin, N.; Dufresne, A. Nanocellulose in biomedicine: Current status and future prospect. *Eur. Polym. J.* **2014**, *59*, 302–325. [CrossRef]
13. Forsman, N.; Lozhechnikova, A.; Khakalo, A.; Johansson, L.-S.; Vartiainen, J.; Österberg, M. Hydrophobic simple and sustainable coating of CNF films and cellulosic textiles based on layer-by-layer deposition of poly-L-lysine and natural wax particles. *Carbohydr. Polym.* **2017**, *173*, 392–402. [CrossRef]
14. Oliveira, C.; Santos, C.; Bezerra, F.; Bezerra, M.; Rodrigues, L. Utilization of Cyanoacrylates Adhesives in Skin suture. *Rev. Bras. Cir. Plást.* **2010**, *25*, 573–576. [CrossRef]
15. Peng, H.; Shek, P. Novel wound sealants: Biomaterials and applications. *Expert Rev. Med. Devices* **2010**, *7*, 639–659. [CrossRef] [PubMed]
16. Meddahi-Pelle, A.; Legrand, A.; Marcellan, A.; Louedec, L.; Letourneur, D.; Leibler, L. Organ Repair, Hemostasis, and In Vivo Bonding of Medical Devices by Aqueous Solutions of Nanoparticles. *Angew. Chem. Int. Ed.* **2014**, *53*, 6369–6373. [CrossRef]
17. Yokoyama, K.; Nio, N.; Kikuch, Y. Properties and applications of microbial transglutaminase. *Appl. Microbiol. Biot.* **2004**, *64*, 447–454. [CrossRef]
18. Cortez, J.; Anghieri, A.; Bonner, P.; Griffin, M.; Freddi, G. Transglutaminase mediated grafting of silk proteins onto wool fabrics leading to improved physical and mechanical properties. *Enzyme Microb. Technol.* **2007**, *40*, 1698–1704. [CrossRef]
19. Arvanitoyannis, I.S.; Dionisopoulou, N.K. *Irradiation of Food Commodities. Techniques, Applications, Detection, Legislation, Safety and Consumer Opinion*, 1st ed.; Arvanitoyannis, I.S., Ed.; Academic Press: London, UK, 2010; pp. 609–634, ISBN 13 978-0128101919.
20. Bonnaillie, L.; Aburto, L.; Tunick, M.; Mulherin, J.; Du, M.; Kwoczak, R.; Akkurt, S.; Tomasula, P. Advances in food packaging films from milk proteins. In Proceedings of the 252nd National Meeting & Exposition of ACS, AGFD: Division of Agricultural and Food Chemistry, Philadelphia, PA, USA, 21–25 August 2016; p. 327816.

21. Bonnaillie, M.L.; Tomasula, P.M. Application of Humidity-Controlled Dynamic Mechanical Analysis (DMA-RH) to Moisture-Sensitive Edible Casein Films for Use in Food Packaging. *Polymers* **2015**, *7*, 91–114. [CrossRef]
22. Zhang, F.; Ma, J.; Xu, Q.; Zhou, J.; Simion, D.; Carmen, G.; Wang, J.; Li, Y. Hollow Casein-Based Polymeric Nanospheres for Opaque Coatings. *ACS Appl. Mater. Interfaces* **2016**, *8*, 11739–11748. [CrossRef]
23. Stewart, R.J.; Wang, C.S.; Shao, H. Complex coacervates as a foundation for synthetic underwater adhesives. *Adv. Colloid Interface Sci.* **2011**, *167*, 85–93. [CrossRef]
24. Rose, S.; Prevoteau, A.; Elziére, P.; Hourdet, D.; Marcellan, A.; Leibler, L. Nanoparticle solutions as adhesives for gels and biological tissues. *Nature* **2014**, *505*, 382–385. [CrossRef]
25. Lievonen, M.; Valle-Delgado, J.J.; Mattinen, M.-L.; Hult, E.-L.; Lintinen, K.; Kostiainen, M.A.; Paananen, A.; Szilvay, G.R.; Setälä, H.; Österberg, M. A simple process for lignin nanoparticle preparation. *Green Chem.* **2016**, *18*, 1416–1422. [CrossRef]
26. Frangville, C.; Rutkevičius, M.; Richter, A.P.; Velev, O.D.; Stoyanov, S.D.; Paunov, V.N. Fabrication of environmentally biodegradable lignin nanoparticles. *ChemPhysChem* **2012**, *13*, 4235–4243. [CrossRef] [PubMed]
27. Qian, Y.; Deng, Y.; Qiu, X.; Li, H.; Yang, D. Formation of uniform colloidal spheres from lignin, a renewable resource recovered from pulping spent liquor. *Green Chem.* **2014**, *16*, 2156–2163. [CrossRef]
28. Qian, Y.; Zhang, Q.; Qiu, X.; Zhu, S. CO_2-responsive diethylaminoethyl-modified lignin nanoparticles and their application as surfactants for CO_2/N_2-switchable Pickering emulsions. *Green Chem.* **2014**, *16*, 4963–4968. [CrossRef]
29. Yiamsawas, D.; Baier, G.; Thines, E.; Landfester, K.; Wurm, F.R. Biodegradable lignin nanocontainers. *RSC Adv.* **2014**, *4*, 11661–11663. [CrossRef]
30. Gilca, I.A.; Popa, V.I.; Crestini, C. Obtaining lignin nanoparticles by sonication. *Ultrason. Sonochem.* **2015**, *23*, 369–375. [CrossRef]
31. Tortora, M.; Cavalieri, F.; Mosesso, P.; Ciaffardini, F.; Melone, F.; Crestini, C. Ultrasound driven assembly of lignin into microcapsules for storage and delivery of hydrophobic molecules. *Biomacromolecules* **2014**, *15*, 1634–1643. [CrossRef]
32. Nair, S.S.; Sharma, S.; Pu, Y.; Sun, Q.; Pan, S.; Zhu, J.Y.; Deng, Y.; Ragauskas, A.J. High shear homogenization of lignin to nanolignin and thermal stability of nanolignin-polyvinyl alcohol blends. *ChemSusChem* **2014**, *7*, 3513–3520. [CrossRef]
33. Yearla, S.R.; Padmasree, K. Preparation and characterisation of lignin nanoparticles: Evaluation of their potential as antioxidants and UV protectants. *J. Exp. Nanosci.* **2016**, *11*, 289–302. [CrossRef]
34. Richter, A.P.; Bharti, B.; Armstrong, H.B.; Brown, J.S.; Plemmons, D.A.; Paunov, V.N.; Stoyanov, S.D.; Velev, O.D. Synthesis and characterization of biodegradable lignin nanoparticles with tunable surface properties. *Langmuir* **2016**, *32*, 6468–6477. [CrossRef] [PubMed]
35. Ago, M.; Huan, S.; Borghei, M.; Raula, J.; Kauppinen, E.; Rojas, O. High-throughput synthesis of lignin particles (∼30 nm to ∼2 µm) via aerosol flow reactor: Size fractionation and utilization in Pickering emulsions. *ACS Appl. Mater. Interfaces* **2016**, *8*, 23302–23310. [CrossRef]
36. Beisl, S.; Miltner, A.; Friedl, A. Lignin from Micro- to Nanosize: Production Methods. *Int. J. Mol. Sci.* **2017**, *18*, 1244. [CrossRef] [PubMed]
37. Roth, S.; Spiess, A.C. Laccases for biorefinery applications: A critical review on challenges and perspectives. *Bioproc. Biosyst. Eng.* **2015**, *38*, 2285–2313. [CrossRef] [PubMed]
38. Munk, L.; Sitarz, A.K.; Kalyani, D.C.; Mikkelsen, J.D.; Meyer, A.S. Can laccases catalyze bond cleavage in lignin? *Biotechnol. Adv.* **2015**, *33*, 13–24. [CrossRef] [PubMed]
39. Mattinen, M.-L.; Valle-Delgado, J.J.; Leskinen, T.; Anttila, T.; Riviere, G.; Sipponen, M.; Paananen, A.; Lintinen, K.; Kostiainen, K.; Österberg, M. Enzymatically and chemically oxidized lignin nanoparticles for biomaterial applications. *Enzyme Microb. Technol.* **2018**, *111*, 48–56. [CrossRef]
40. Mohammadinejad, R.; Karimi, S.; Iravani, S.; Varma, R.S. Plant-derived nanostructures: Types and applications. *Green Chem.* **2016**, *18*, 20–52. [CrossRef]
41. Pan, K.; Zhong, Q. Organic Nanoparticles in Foods: Fabrication, Characterization and Utilization. *Annu. Rev. Food Sci. Technol.* **2016**, *7*, 245–266. [CrossRef] [PubMed]

42. Leskinen, T.; Witos, J.; Valle-Delgado, J.J.; Lintinen, K.; Kostiainen, M.A.; Wiedmer, S.K.; Österberg, M.; Mattinen, M.-L. Adsorption of Proteins on Colloidal Lignin Particles for Advanced Biomaterials. *Biomacromolecules* **2017**, *18*, 2767–2776. [CrossRef] [PubMed]
43. Richter, A.P.; Brown, J.S.; Bharti, B.; Wang, A.; Gangwal, S.; Houck, K.; Cohen, E.; Hubal, A.; Paunov, V.N.; Stoyanov, S.D.; et al. An environmentally benign antimicrobial nanoparticle based on a silver-infused lignin core. *Nat. Nanotechnol.* **2015**, *10*, 817–823. [CrossRef]
44. Goffin, A.J.; Rajadas, J.; Fuller, G.G. Interfacial Flow Processing of Collagen. *Langmuir* **2010**, *26*, 3514–3521. [CrossRef]
45. Tenzer, S.; Docter, D.; Kuharev, J.; Musyanovych, A.; Fetz, V.; Hecht, R.; Schlenk, F.; Fischer, D.; Kiouptsi, K.; Reinhardt, C.; et al. Rapid formation of plasma protein corona critically affects nanoparticle pathophysiology. *Nat. Nanotechnol.* **2013**, *8*, 772–781. [CrossRef]
46. Niku-Paavola, M.; Karhunen, E.; Salola, P.; Raunio, V. Ligninolytic enzymes of the white-rot-fungus *Phlebia radiate*. *Biochem. J.* **1988**, *254*, 877–884. [CrossRef]
47. Rittstieg, K.; Suurnäkki, A.; Suortti, T.; Kruus, K.; Guebitz, G.; Buchert, J. Investigations on the laccase-catalyzed polymerization of lignin model compounds using size-exclusion HPLC. *Enzyme Microb. Technol.* **2002**, *31*, 403–410. [CrossRef]
48. Lantto, R.; Puolanne, E.; Kalkkinen, N.; Buchert, J.; Autio, K. Enzyme-aided modification of chicken-breast myofibril proteins: Effect of laccase and transglutaminase on gelation and thermal stability. *J. Agric. Food Chem.* **2005**, *53*, 9231–9237. [CrossRef] [PubMed]
49. Valle-Delgado, J.J.; Johansson, L.-S.; Österberg, M. Bioinspired lubricating films of cellulose nanofibrils and hyaluronic acid. *Colloids Surf. B Biointerfaces* **2016**, *138*, 86–93. [CrossRef]
50. Salas, C.; Rojas, O.J.; Lucia, L.A.; Hubbe, M.A.; Genzer, J. On the surface interactions of proteins with lignin. *ACS Appl. Mater. Interfaces* **2013**, *5*, 199–206. [CrossRef] [PubMed]
51. Johannsmann, D.; Mathauer, K.; Wegner, G.; Knoll, W. Viscoelastic properties of thin films probed with a quartz-crystal resonator. *Phys. Rev. B* **1992**, *46*, 7808–7815. [CrossRef]
52. Sipponen, M.H.; Pihlajaniemi, V.; Sipponen, S.; Pastinen, O.; Laakso, S. Autohydrolysis and aqueous ammonia extraction of wheat straw: Effect of treatment severity on yield and structure of hemicellulose and lignin. *RSC Adv.* **2014**, *4*, 23177–23184. [CrossRef]
53. Sader, J.E.; Chon, J.W.; Mulvaney, P. Calibration of rectangular atomic force microscope cantilevers. *Rev. Sci. Instrum.* **1999**, *70*, 3967–3969. [CrossRef]
54. Nugroho, R.W.N.; Harjumäki, R.; Zhang, X.; Lou, Y.-R.; Yliperttula, M.; Valle-Delgado, J.J.; Österberg, M. Quantifying the interactions between biomimetic biomaterials—Collagen I, collagen IV, laminin 521 and cellulose nanofibrils—By colloidal probe microscopy. *Colloids Surf. B Biointerfaces* **2019**, *173*, 571–580. [CrossRef]
55. Butt, H.; Cappella, B.; Kappl, M. Force measurements with the atomic force microscope: Technique, interpretation and applications. *Surf. Sci. Rep.* **2005**, *59*, 1–152. [CrossRef]
56. Verwey, E. Theory of the stability of lyophobic colloids. *J. Phys. Chem.* **1947**, *51*, 631–636. [CrossRef]
57. Assemi, S.; Nalaskowski, J.; Johnson, W.P. Direct force measurements between carboxylate-modified latex microspheres and glass using atomic force microscopy. *Colloid Surf. A Physicochem. Eng. Asp.* **2006**, *286*, 70–77. [CrossRef]
58. Bowen, W.R.; Hilal, N.; Lovitt, R.W.; Wright, C.J. Direct measurement of interactions between adsorbed protein layers using an atomic force microscope. *J. Colloid Interface Sci.* **1998**, *197*, 348–352. [CrossRef]
59. Schmidt, S.; Madaboosi, N.; Uhlig, K.; Köhler, D.; Skirtach, A.; Duschl, C.; Möhwald, H.; Volodkin, D.V. Control of Cell Adhesion by Mechanical Reinforcement of Soft Polyelectrolyte Films with Nanoparticles. *Langmuir* **2012**, *28*, 7249–7257. [CrossRef]
60. Bye, C.N. Casein and mixed protein adhesives. In *Handbook of Adhesives*; Skeist, I., Ed.; Van Nostrand Reinold: New York, NY, USA, 1990; pp. 135–152. ISBN 978-1-4613-0671-9.
61. Mazia, D. Adhesion of cells to surfaces coated with polylysine. Applications to electron microscopy. *J. Cell Biol.* **1975**, *66*, 198–200.
62. Gu, Z.; Yang, Z.; Wang, L.; Zhou, H.; Jimenez-Cruz, C.A.; Zhou, R. The role of basic residues in the adsorption of blood proteins onto the graphene surface. *Sci. Rep.* **2015**, *5*, 10873–10884. [CrossRef]
63. Van de Pas, D.; Hickson, A.; Donaldson, L.; Lloyd-Jones, G.; Tamminen, T.; Fernyhough, A.; Mattinen, M.-L. Characterization of fractionated lignins polymerized by fungal laccases. *BioResources* **2011**, *6*, 1105–1121.

64. Figueiredo, P.; Lintinen, K.; Kiriazis, A.; Hynninen, V.; Liu, V.; Ramos, T.B.; Rahikkala, A.; Correia, A.; Kohout, T.; Sarmento, B.; et al. In vitro evaluation of biodegradable lignin-based nanoparticles for drug delivery and enhanced antiproliferation effect in cancer cells. *Biomaterials* **2017**, *121*, 97–108. [CrossRef]
65. Monogioudi, E. *Enzymatic Cross-Linking of β-Casein and Its Impact on Digestibility and Allergenicity*; University of Helsinki: Helsinki, Finland, 18 January 2011; ISBN 978-951-38-7421-6.
66. Berglin, M.; Delage, L.; Potin, P.; Vilter, H.; Elwing, H. Enzymatic Cross-Linking of a Phenolic Polymer Extracted from the Marine Alga Fucus serratus. *Biomacromolecules* **2004**, *5*, 2376–2383. [CrossRef]
67. Boström, M.; Williams, D.; Ninham, B. Specific ion effects: Why DLVO theory fails for biology and colloid systems. *Phys. Rev. Lett.* **2001**, *87*, 168103–168107. [CrossRef]
68. Kim, J.-H.; Kim, H.; Choi, Y.; Lee, D.S.; Kim, J.; Yi, G.-R. Colloidal Mesoporous Silica Nanoparticles as Strong Adhesives for Hydrogels and Biological Tissues. *ACS Appl. Mater. Interfaces* **2017**, *9*, 31469–31477. [CrossRef]
69. Shin, K.; Choi, J.W.; Ko, G.; Baik, S.; Kim, D.; Park, O.K.; Lee, K.; Cho, H.R.; Han, S.I.; Lee, S.H.; et al. Multifunctional nanoparticles as a tissue adhesive and an injectable marker for image-guided procedures. *Nat. Commun.* **2017**, *8*, 15807–15819. [CrossRef]
70. Pradyawong, S.; Qi, G.; Li, N.; Sun, X.S.; Wang, D. Adhesion properties of soy protein adhesives enhanced by biomass lignin. *Int. J. Adhes. Adhes.* **2017**, *75*, 66–73. [CrossRef]
71. Luo, J.; Yuan, C.; Zhang, W.; Li, J.; Gao, Q.; Chen, H. An eco-friendly wood adhesive from soy protein and lignin: Performance properties. *RSC Adv.* **2015**, *5*, 100849–100855. [CrossRef]
72. Aracri, E.; Blanco, C.D.; Tzanov, T. An enzymatic approach to develop a lignin-based adhesive for wool floor coverings. *Green Chem.* **2014**, *16*, 2597–2603. [CrossRef]
73. Kai, D.; Tan, M.J.; Chee, P.L.; Chua, Y.K.; Yap, Y.L.; Loh, X.J. Towards lignin-based functional materials in a sustainable world. *Green Chem.* **2016**, *18*, 1175–1200. [CrossRef]
74. Didaskalou, C.; Buyuktiryaki, S.; Kecili, R.; Fonte, C.P.; Szekely, G. Valorisation of agricultural waste with an adsorption/nanofiltration hybrid process: From materials to sustainable process design. *Green Chem.* **2017**, *19*, 3116–3125. [CrossRef]
75. Ashok, R.P.B.; Oinas, P.; Lintinen, K.; Sarwar, G.; Kostiainen, M.A.; Österberg, M. Techno-economic assessment for the large-scale production of colloidal lignin particles. *Green Chem.* **2018**, *20*, 4911–4919. [CrossRef]
76. Tian, D.; Hu, J.; Bao, J.; Chandra, R.P.; Saddler, J.N.; Lu, C. Lignin valorization: Lignin nanoparticles as high-value bio-additive for multifunctional nanocomposites. *Biotechnol. Biofuels* **2017**, *10*, 192–203. [CrossRef]
77. García, J.L.; Pans, G.; Phanopoulos, C. Use of lignin in polyurethane-based structural wood adhesives. *J. Adhes.* **2018**, *94*, 814–828. [CrossRef]
78. Kalami, S.; Arefmanesh, M.; Master, E.; Nejad, M. Replacing 100% of phenol in phenolic adhesive formulations with lignin. *J. Appl. Polym. Sci.* **2017**, *134*, 45124–45133. [CrossRef]

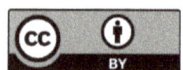

© 2018 by the authors. Licensee MDPI, Basel, Switzerland. This article is an open access article distributed under the terms and conditions of the Creative Commons Attribution (CC BY) license (http://creativecommons.org/licenses/by/4.0/).

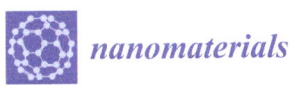

Review

Plasma and Nanomaterials: Fabrication and Biomedical Applications

Nagendra Kumar Kaushik [1,*], Neha Kaushik [2], Nguyen Nhat Linh [1], Bhagirath Ghimire [1], Anchalee Pengkit [1], Jirapong Sornsakdanuphap [1], Su-Jae Lee [2,*] and Eun Ha Choi [1,*]

1. Plasma Bioscience Research Center, Applied Plasma Medicine Center, Department of Electrical and Biological Physics, Kwangwoon University, Seoul 01897, Korea; nhatlinhusth@gmail.com (N.N.L.); ghimirebhagi@hotmail.com (B.G.); un_chaleep@hotmail.com (A.P.); jirakwangwoon@gmail.com (J.S.)
2. Department of Life Science, Hanyang University, Seoul 04763, Korea; neha.bioplasma@gmail.com
* Correspondence: kaushik.nagendra@kw.ac.kr (N.K.K.); sj0420@hanyang.ac.kr (S.-J.L.); ehchoi@kw.ac.kr (E.H.C.)

Received: 17 December 2018; Accepted: 8 January 2019; Published: 14 January 2019

Abstract: Application of plasma medicine has been actively explored during last several years. Treating every type of cancer remains a difficult task for medical personnel due to the wide variety of cancer cell selectivity. Research in advanced plasma physics has led to the development of different types of non-thermal plasma devices, such as plasma jets, and dielectric barrier discharges. Non-thermal plasma generates many charged particles and reactive species when brought into contact with biological samples. The main constituents include reactive nitrogen species, reactive oxygen species, and plasma ultra-violets. These species can be applied to synthesize biologically important nanomaterials or can be used with nanomaterials for various kinds of biomedical applications to improve human health. This review reports recent updates on plasma-based synthesis of biologically important nanomaterials and synergy of plasma with nanomaterials for various kind of biological applications.

Keywords: plasma; nanomaterials; nanomaterial synthesis; plasma liquid Interactions; non-thermal plasma; biomedical applications

1. Introduction

In recent years, nanomaterials have received great attention due to their exclusive characteristics compared to their bulk counterparts. With extremely small size and high surface area, nanomaterials demonstrate great biological activities in the human body. Nanomaterials play crucial roles in biomedicine, with a wide range of applications such as drug delivery, cancer therapy or bioimaging. Nevertheless, our current understanding of nanomaterials' behaviors in human health is still inadequate. Previous reports have claimed that nanomaterials could induce dangerous effects in living organisms. A reasonable explanation for this concern is that conventional chemical approaches for nanomaterial synthesis require toxic oxidants or reductants, which are essential for nanoparticle formation and stabilization. Therefore, an alternative toxic-chemical-free synthesis is important for nanotechnology development for biomedical applications. Currently, plasma technology is gaining great attention as a prominent "green" synthesis method for nanomaterials, due to its distinguishing properties when compared to solid, liquid and gas phase synthesis approaches. Furthermore, the combination of nanomaterials and plasma in biomedical applications demonstrates several synergistic effects and better treatment efficiency. A schematic diagram showing the synergistic relationship among plasmas, nanomaterials and their biomedical applications is shown in Figure 1. The use of plasmas for biomedical applications has been explored in various ways in the last few decades and have shown promising effects. The uses of nanomaterials in biomedical applications are also well known. Recently, synergistic effects of nanomaterials and cold plasmas in biomedical applications have been discovered. In this article, a review on the relationship between plasma and nanomaterials is presented. A brief description of non-thermal atmospheric pressure plasmas is included in Section 2. In Section 3, the synthesis of nanomaterials using different types of plasma is summarized. Section 4 focuses on the current advances related to the synergistic effects of plasma and nanomaterials in biomedical applications.

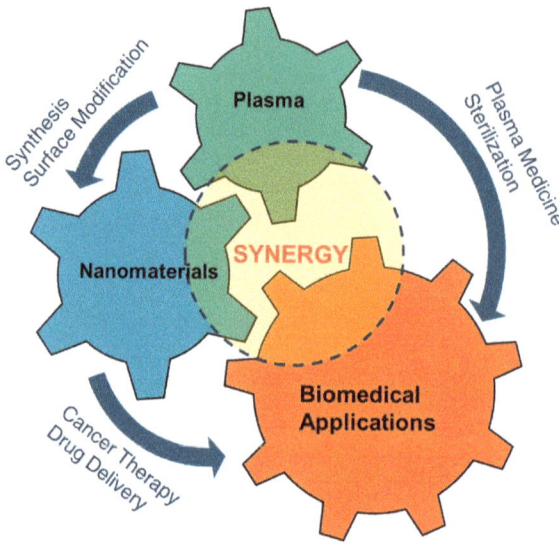

Figure 1. The synergistic relationship among plasmas, nanomaterials and their biomedical applications.

2. Overview of Non-Thermal Atmospheric Pressure Plasmas and Their Characteristics

Physical plasmas are ionized gases which generally contain electrons, ions, neutrals, excited species, electric field, reactive species, UV photons, etc. They exist naturally in the universe or can be generated within the laboratory environment in the earth. Production of plasma within the laboratories can be performed through dissociation of gas molecules with electrical energy confined between two electrodes. This type of plasma can be produced at low pressure, as well as at atmospheric pressure. Plasmas at low pressures (such as inductively coupled plasmas, plasma torches) are generated inside vacuum chambers and are much suitable for the uniform treatment of objects. They are also called thermal or quasi-equilibrium low-temperature plasmas, as the temperatures of light and heavy species are almost the same. At atmospheric pressures, plasmas (such as atmospheric pressure plasma jet discharges, dielectric barrier discharges (DBD)) could be generated by ionizing a gas between two narrow electrodes at ambient environment and no expensive vacuum equipment is required. Atmospheric pressure plasmas are also called non-thermal or non-equilibrium plasmas, as the electron temperature is much higher than ions or gas species and the temperature of gas species remains close to room temperature. Both thermal and non-thermal plasmas can be used for the synthesis of nanomaterials.

2.1. Non-Thermal Atmospheric Pressure Plasma Sources

Non-thermal atmospheric pressure plasmas generated at atmospheric conditions can be utilized for the synthesis of nanomaterials. Several types of plasma devices, such as DBD plasma or plasma jet, can be used for combinational treatments with nanomaterials [1]. The discharge generated in the ambient environment can be used for the modification of the surface properties of the materials through electrons, ions, excited species, reactive species, UVs, etc., generated through the plasma. An overview of non-thermal atmospheric pressure plasma sources and the reactive species generated by them is presented in this section.

2.1.1. Dielectric Barrier Discharge (DBD)

DBD is generated between two metal electrodes, where one electrode is connected to the high voltage power supply, and the other one is grounded. A dielectric material is placed in front of one (or both) metal electrode in order to prevent arcing. This is also known as silent or atmospheric-pressure-glow discharge [2], and was described for the first time by Ernst Werner von Siemens in 1857 [3]. Recent understandings of the physics of DBD have given rise to several improved forms of DBD-based devices. A schematic diagram of two common DBD-based devices are shown in Figure 2a,b. Both devices are constructed in a coplanar configuration, and the electrodes are fabricated above a dielectric material like glass. A protective layer made up of MgO or Al_2O_3 is used above the electrodes for the prevention of hydration and the promotion of long-term operation of the device. If one part of the coplanar electrode system is connected to a high-voltage power supply and the other part is grounded, it is known as surface DBD plasma (Figure 2a) [4]. Here, the material to be treated is placed below the plasma generation region. Because of the use of coplanar electrodes that are separated by a micrometer gap, the surface DBD plasma can be generated under normal atmospheric conditions (even without gas flow). On the other hand, if all the coplanar electrodes are connected to the high-voltage power supply and the target material acts as the ground electrode (with a high capacity of charge storage) such that the plasma generated in between the high voltage and the target is utilized for the modification of nanomaterial, it is known as floating electrode DBD plasma (FE-DBD) [5], as schematically shown in Figure 2b. Both types of plasma sources generate plasma over a wide area and can be used for the synthesis of nanomaterials.

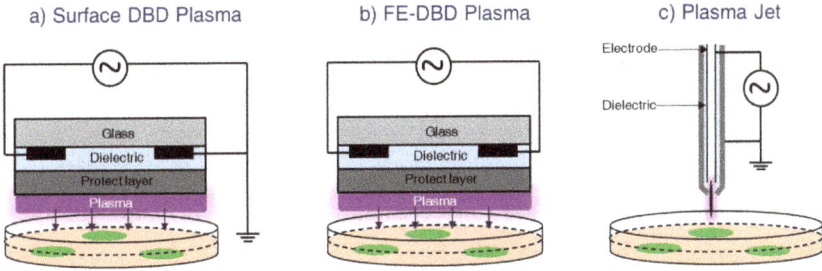

Figure 2. Typical structures of non-thermal DBD plasma and plasma jet devices at atmospheric pressure. (**a**) Surface DBD plasma; (**b**) FE-DBD plasma; and (**c**) plasma jet.

2.1.2. Plasma Jet

The plasma jet is an improved design of DBD. It was designed in order to extend the plasma plume at a long distance away from the discharge region, enabling the remote treatment of the sample. Extensive research works have been performed on the design of plasma jets for biomedical applications [6–8]. A schematic diagram of the plasma jet is as shown in Figure 2c. It consists of a high-voltage needle electrode and a ground electrode separated by a dielectric material. An inert gas flow (normally helium, argon, etc.) is maintained through the needle electrode in order to facilitate the breakdown process. Plasma is generated between the high-voltage and the ground electrodes with the help of working gases. Because of the high gas flow rate, the plasma constituents, including the short-lived reactive species, are carried towards the remote region, which is several centimeters from the discharge region. The temperature of the plasma carried to the remote region is close to room temperature and can be used for the surface modification/synthesis of nanomaterials.

2.2. Reactive Species Induced by Non-Thermal Atmospheric Pressure Plasmas and Their Applications

Plasma-synthesized nanomaterials can be used for various kinds of biological applications and for improving human health. The key to this application lies in the variety of reactive oxygen and nitrogen species (RONS) generated by the non-thermal atmospheric pressure plasma sources [9–14]. Plasma liquid interactions play a great role in the formation of nanomaterials as the chemistry of liquid is altered by the plasma generated RONS. The major RONS formed during plasma-liquid interactions include superoxide, hydroxyl radical, singlet oxygen, nitric oxide, ozone, hydrogen peroxide, etc. [15,16]. The densities of these species generated in plasma discharges are very high and have been tabulated in Table 1. Energetic electrons, heavy ions and UV photons present in the discharge may be responsible for enhancing the formation of these reactive species.

Table 1. Typical relative concentrations of various charged and neutral species generated by non-thermal DBD plasma in gas phase [17–20].

Plasma Generated Species	Density (cm^{-3})
Superoxide (O_2^-)	10^{10}–10^{12}
Hydroxyl (OH$^\bullet$)	10^{15}–10^{17}
Hydrogen Peroxide (H_2O_2)	10^{14}–10^{16}
Singlet Oxygen ($^1O_2$)	10^{14}–10^{16}
Ozone (O_3)	10^{15}–10^{17}
Nitric Oxide (NO)	10^{13}–10^{14}
Electrons (e$^-$)	10^{9}–10^{11}
Positive ions (M$^+$)	10^{10}–10^{12}

Few reported possible reactions for plasma–liquid interactions are given in Figure 3. There are many possibilities by which plasma-generated reactive species can have a direct or indirect effect on nanomaterial synthesis in aqueous medium. Some can have a direct effect, and some can react to form more stable long-lived reactive species, which can also have activity against biological samples. H_2O_2 is one of the most stable reactive species that can be generated from various other reactive species such as ·OH and superoxide [21–23]. Even though ·OH has a short lifetime, our group postulates that plasma-initiated UV may propagate into the aqua solution to result in the photolysis of water molecules for the production of ·OH even to or inside the cells [24]. Oehmigen et al. (2011) suggested most of the possible reactions for plasma gas/liquid interactions as shown in Figure 3. Plasma can not only be applied for surface modification, sterilization of medical equipment, antimicrobial, dermatology (including wound healing), etc. but also for cancer treatment by an endoscopic or branched organ targeting treatment technology [25].

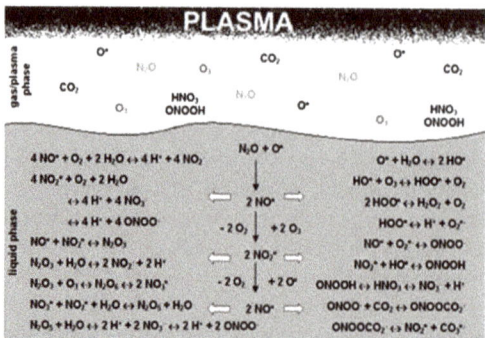

Figure 3. Possible reaction channels of plasma/gas–liquid interactions. With permission from Ref. [26] Copyright 2011 Wiley (Plasma Processes and Polymers 2011, 8, 904–913, DOI: 10.1002/ppap.201000099).

In a recent report, Laroussi et al. demonstrated the effectiveness of a low-temperature atmospheric-pressure plasma pencil on human T-cell leukemia cells [27]. Numerous other reports have explored the efficiency of cold plasmas on various types of cancer and normal cell lines [28–49]. Various types of non-thermal plasmas offer the ability to deliver ROS directly or indirectly into living tissues, implying its feasibility as an innovative device for use in cancer therapy by endoscopic or branched organ targeting treatment technology [50–52]. Some types of plasma devices, such as DBD plasmas or plasma jets, can be used for the combinational treatments with nanomaterials [1]. Recently, many groups have used the plasma jet device in combination with nanomaterials for antimicrobial and anticancer activities.

Although, a comparatively new field in medicine, the use of non-thermal atmospheric plasmas on tumor cells has attracted a great deal of attention [53]. The outcomes of several research groups have increased the hope that non-thermal plasmas could be an interesting new therapy alternative in cancer treatment. Much emerging evidence strongly indicates that cold plasma treatment could abolish the tumor cells without damaging the normal counterparts [33,54,55]. Numerous in vitro studies support the concept of the non-thermal plasma selectivity for many types of cancer cells, including breast cancer cells [55,56], melanoma cells [42,57], skin cancer cells [58], colon carcinoma cells [58], ovarian cancer cells [59], glioblastoma cells [60–62], and blood cancer cells [63]. A better understanding of biological pathways or mechanisms of plasma-mediated apoptosis, including its selectivity, will help to introduce it as a novel tool for application in anticancer treatment as illustrated in Figure 4.

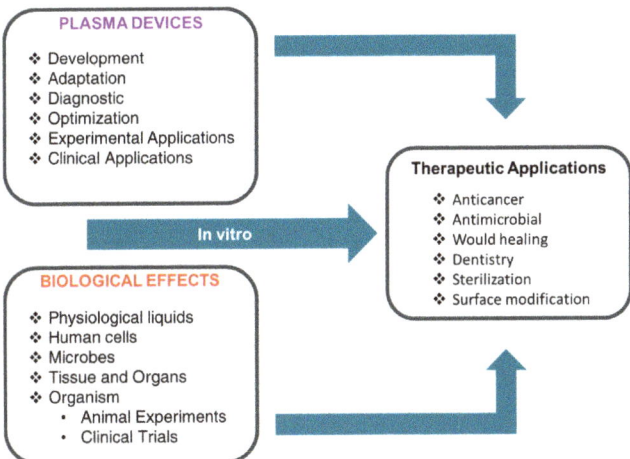

Figure 4. Plasma as reliable and safe therapeutic device for biomedical applications. For safe plasma clinical application, plasma devices and in vitro biological effects must be optimized.

3. Application of Plasma for the Synthesis and Modification of Nanomaterials

Nanomaterials for biomedical applications have been receiving a great deal of attention due to their unique physical and chemical properties. Noble metals, transition metals and alloys, semiconductors and carbon-based nanomaterials are among the most prominent materials in biomedical applications, including cancer therapy, bioimaging, drug delivery, tissue engineering, etc. [64–69]. Nevertheless, the most common strategy for nanomaterials fabrication is chemical synthesis, which involves dangerous and toxic chemical compounds as oxidizing/reducing agents. Thus, there is a need to develop alternative "green" approaches to control the toxicity of nanomaterials.

Plasma technology has been widely used in the fabrication of nanomaterials [70], especially low-pressure techniques such as Plasma-Enhanced Chemical Vapor Deposition (PE-CVD) and Sputtering. In contrast with low-pressure plasma, atmospheric plasma technology also can be used for the synthesis of nanomaterials while functioning in ambient room condition. Due to the advantages of operating in air, atmospheric plasma can produce a high quantity of RONS, which can directly reduce metal ions in liquid to form metal nanoparticles (NPs), without the presence of any additional reducing agents (Figure 5). Thus, this method is also considered a "green" method for the fabrication of nanomaterials towards applications in biomedical research. Herein, we summarize recent advances on the fabrication of nanomaterials by plasma.

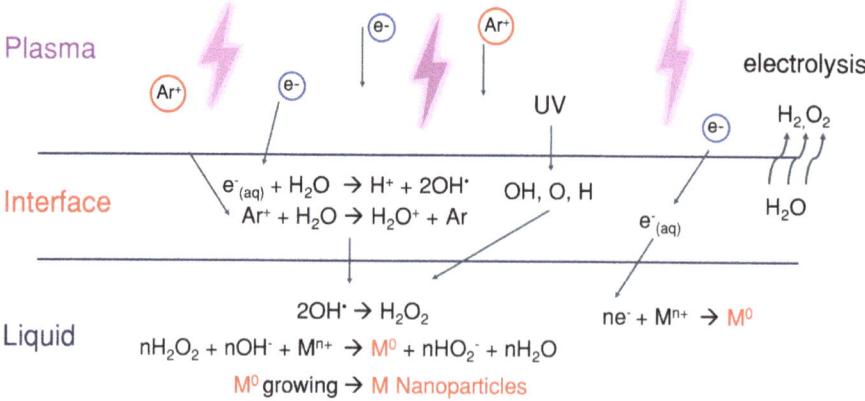

Figure 5. A schematic illustration of the metal ion reduction, diffusion and nucleation at the plasma-liquid interface. The reduction reactions can occur in liquid medium by either solvated plasma-induced electron or plasma induced reactive species.

3.1. Noble Metal Nanomaterials

Noble metals like Au, Ag, Pt and Pd possess high resistance to oxidation and corrosion in moist conditions and have been used in jewelry and currency since ancient times. In contrast to the bulk materials, the noble metals in nanometer size demonstrate unique physical properties, including the surface plasmon resonance phenomenon. Surface plasmon is an evanescent electromagnetic wave at the metal surface caused by free electron oscillation under light irradiation. Due to this property, Au and Ag NPs have been utilized in a great number of applications, such as Surface-Enhanced Raman Scattering, biosensors for biological processes, nanomedicine, chemical oxidation reactions, etc. The plasma synthesis of Ag nanomaterials was first reported in 1999, through arc discharge generated over a solution of $NaNO_3$ with silver electrodes; one was over the solution and another was immersed in the solution [71]. In 2005 Koo et al. reported the formation of PtNPs by exposing to H_2/He gas plasma on the solution of H_2PtCl_6 [72]. Since then, materials scientists have focused on the production of NPs by using plasma over liquid system.

As pioneers in the field of plasma synthesis, Sankaran and his group attributed the Au and Ag NP formation to the electron reduction Au and Ag ions provided by plasma either in anodic dissolution or the pristine metal salts [73,74]. A simple microplasma setup was employed for the study, and microplasma was generated between the surface of a liquid solution and a stainless-steel capillary (0.7 mm distance) with the help of inert gas (helium) at a flow rate of 25 sccm. The internal diameter of the metal capillary was less than 1 mm, and it was connected to the ground through a 100 kΩ resistor. A high-voltage DC (up to 2 kV) was applied to a counter metal foil (Au or Ag) electrode immersed few millimeters away from metal capillary and a current of 0–5 mA sustained the microplasma. Under the plasma discharge, the metal dissolution occurred at the metal foils surface, followed by the formation of metal NPs in liquid phase. Instead of metal foils, aqueous solutions of $HAuCl_4$ or $AgNO_3$ with different concentrations (from 0.05 to 1 mM) can also be used as a precursor for the synthesis of Au and Ag NPs with the same experimental setup. Electrons were injected into the liquid solution from the plasma, thus inducing plasma–liquid electrochemistry for the synthesis of nanomaterials [75]. The electrons were injected in the solution and induced the reduction of Au salt, forming Au^0 atoms, followed by the diffusion and aggregation to form NPs. The gas velocity of 25 sccm supposed to limit the interaction of the plasma with the surrounding air and study is focused on the influence of negatively charged species. With the above experimental setup, the microplasma processing was performed for 10 min, at which point the solution changed its color from transparent to purple, indicating the formation of Au NPs. This was verified by Transmission Electron Microscopy and a UV-visible absorption spectrum with resonance peak at 539 nm. The resonance peak wavelength and bandwidth depend on the size of the Au NPs [76]. The bandwidth also depends on the distribution of Au NPs. The size and distribution of Au NPs is usually determined by the concentration of $HAuCl_4$ solution. The colloidal Au NPs produced in this way were short-lived after processing. The stability can vary between 6 h and several months, depending on several conditions, such as storage conditions, precursor concentration and the processing current, even without using any surfactants [77]. A quantitative study for Au and Ag NPs synthesis by microplasma was also reported recently [78]. The mechanism of dissociative electron attachment and Au NP formation was also discussed. At the counter electrode, due to very high applied voltage, a large number of positive ions (e.g., H^+) are produced, causing a lower pH and increased conductivity. These positive ions can participate in the overall liquid chemistry or recombine with other species at the plasma–liquid interface. A range of species, including e^-, $OH^\bullet$, OH^-, O^-, H^-, etc., are produced at the plasma–liquid interface, and they can lead to dissociative Electron Attachment reactions (Figure 5). The most dominant reactive channel at the liquid interface is:

$$H_2O + e^-_{gas} \rightarrow H^- + OH^\bullet \tag{1}$$

If the electrons are solvated in liquid, the subsequent reaction inside the solution will occur:

$$H_2O + e^-_{aq} \rightarrow H^- + OH^\bullet \tag{2}$$

The subsequent cascaded chemistry could lead to the formation of hydrogen peroxide from either $OH^\bullet$ or OH^- [79]. This could happen as follows:

$$2OH^\bullet \rightarrow H_2O_2 \tag{3}$$

$$2OH^\bullet \rightarrow H_2O_2 + 2e^-_{aq} \tag{4}$$

When the Au^{3+} ion precursor is added to the solution, the formation of Au^0 metal particles in the solution will occur as:

$$[AuCl_4]^{3+} + 3e^-_{aq} \rightarrow Au^0 + 4Cl^- \tag{5}$$

Recently, Mariotti et al. demonstrated a continuous droplet flow plasma reactor for the synthesis of Au NPs. This method belongs to the most efficient and highest yielding of the reported methods for Au NPs synthesis [80]. Plasma interactions, ionic liquids, and molten salts are also very efficient approaches for nanomaterial synthesis. Ionic liquids possess several advantages over water solutions, such as low vapor pressure and non-volatility. Nanoparticles synthesized using plasma-ionic liquid systems do not require stabilizers due to their electrostatic stability. Synthesis of Au-Ag NPs by sputtering in plasma-ionic liquid systems has been reported previously [81,82]. The selection of ionic liquids based on low vapor pressure can facilitate highly efficient sputtering. In another reported work, evaporation of metal ions is also used for the synthesis of some NPs [83,84]. In this experiment, a metal wire was immersed in solution and acted as cathode while another inert Pt metal mesh used as anode. Evaporated cathode material moved to the solution surface and cooled down, finally being quenched in the solution, leading to formation of NPs. The amount and size of NPs depended on the applied voltage and electrolyte solution type. A bimetallic Ag/Pt can also be produced after 30 s of pulse plasma discharge between Ag cathode and Pt anode in solution of sodium dodecylsulfonate and sodium chloride. In addition to using chemical systems, physical sputtering by argon plasma was also used to produce Au/Ag and Au/Pd NPs. Nevertheless, the main drawback of ionic liquid-based systems is the relatively low solubility of metal ions compared to water-based systems. Another disadvantage is that ionic liquid decomposition by plasma can contaminate the nanomaterials. The reducing species produced by plasma moves more easily in water solution than ionic liquid. However, there are many possibilities in the field of ionic liquids development that can address all these critical issues in plasma-ionic liquid systems for the synthesis of nanomaterials.

3.2. Transition Metals and Alloys

The magnetic materials family is a large and compelling subject among biomedical researchers due to the attractive super paramagnetic property. This essential property offers many opportunities for biomedical applications, such as magnetic resonance imaging, drug delivery and biomedicine. Plasma-based systems are being considered as cost-efficient and high-speed production methods for metal NPs. For instance, carbon-encapsulated NPs demonstrated low toxicity on A549 cells, which is lung fibroblast. A simple pulse discharge plasma produced between the tips of two Fe rods has been used to synthesize the iron carbide NPs, encapsulated by graphite sheets [85,86]. Other materials, such as Fe_2O_3 [87] and carbon-encapsulated Co, Ni and Fe [88,89] NPs, have been fabricated from an aqueous solution of cationic surfactant and ethanol.

Many researchers have also studied inert material-coated iron oxide formation. Recently, silica-coated iron oxide was formed by using non-transferred arc plasma at atmospheric pressure, with a low degree of agglomeration [90]. In this study, there are 2 types of reactors—the hot wall reactor and the cold wall reactor—that are used to cause variations in the temperature gradient during the experimental period. In conclusion, silica-coated iron oxide NPs can be prepared by using non-transferred arc plasma at atmospheric pressure with $Fe(CO)_5$ and TEOS as the precursors. The synthesized particles mainly have Fe_3O_4 as a core particle and are covered by an amorphous external layer with a size on the order of 100 nm for cold wall reactors and below 20 nm in the case of hot wall reactors, with uniform size distribution.

Formation of metallic oxide by plasma–liquid interactions is also a simple process because of the presence of strong oxidizing species. An AC plasma was used to produce CuO NPs [91]. The plasma was generated between the Cu filaments, and another Cu filament was immersed in $NaNO_3$ solutions. The reactive species generated by plasma–liquid interaction reduced Cu ions to form CuO NPs. ZnO NPs can also be produced by plasma, which was generated between Zn wire and Pt wire mesh immersed in aqueous solution of K_2CO_3. The median electrical power input led to the formation of flower-like ZnO NPs.

Plasma–liquid interaction can also be used for production of alloy NPs [92,93]. Alloying of nanomaterials is one of the strategies for stabilizing NPs. FePt NPs were synthesized by using the displacement reaction. Argon plasma was used on $FeCl_2$ solution to produce Fe NPs, and then $PtCl_2$ was added to the molten solution, in which the Fe NPs were dissolved and produced. Pure FePt NPs were obtained by optimizing the ratio of $FeCl_2$ to $PtCl_2$ and plasma discharge doses. The synthesis of $CoPt_3$, CoPt, SmCo NPs can also be carried out using the same method. A recent work by the Mariotti group also proved that Co_3O_4 NPs can also be obtained by microplasma discharged in absolute ethanol [94].

3.3. Non-Metal Nanomaterials

Silicon-based NPs have been used in biomedical applications because of their high specific surface areas and great chemical and mechanical stability. Great efforts have been made to synthesize this family of materials using plasma technology. In 2005, Sankaran et al. reported a continuous-flow atmospheric-pressure microdischarge reactor for photoluminescent silicon NPs [95]. Silicon NPs with a size of a few nanometers were successfully fabricated, and they exhibited photoluminescence at 420 nm with an impressive quantum yield of 30%. The particles also remained stable under ambient conditions for several months. Surface engineering of silicon nanocrystals (Si-NCs) with a special focus on photovoltaic applications was also studied by Mariotti et al. using microplasma processing [96]. Si-NCs with a diameter below 5 nm exhibited quantum confinement properties and could be applied in third-generation photovoltaic solar cells with high efficiency, low cost and limited environmental footprint. It is believed that plasma-induced liquid chemistry offers the opportunity for surface engineering and industrial scaling. Surface engineering of silicon nanocrystals was performed in ethanol solution. Nickel was used as a capillary, diamond carbon rod acted as a counter electrode, and argon gas was employed for plasma generation. After 20 min of microplasma processing, the photoluminescence properties were observed to have improved. Also, microplasma processing preserved the photoluminescence properties of Si-NCs for several days. These results have not been achieved with standard electrochemistry. A detailed study of the cause of the photoluminescence properties was performed by Fourier transform infrared analysis. This revealed that Si-NCs under microplasma processing undergo surface modification, whereby Si-H bonds and other surface terminations are removed and mostly replaced with Si-O-R terminations, promoting surface reconstruction at the outer layer. Also, the efficiency of the microplasma-processed Si-NCs device increased over the full spectral range. Recently, researchers have also made efforts to synthesize Ge and Si quantum dots by using a plasma-ionic liquid system [97].

Carbon-related nanomaterials such as multiwall carbon nanotubes, carbon nanohorns, carbon NPs, etc., are prominent advanced materials due to their exceptional physical properties, such as high conductivity, strength, stiffness, and toughness. Recently, many researchers have used plasma discharge to form carbon-related nanomaterials in liquids. Nanodiamond formation by using microplasma operated in a gaseous phase of Ar/H2/ethanol has been reported [98]. Nowadays, carbon nanotubes have been intensely and extensively researched, because they have very unique and attractive physical and electrical properties, including high electrical conductivity, extraordinary mechanical strength, and thermal and chemical stability. Therefore, it is a promising material for versatile applications in the near future. In particular, it can be applied for optical and biomedical devices, as well as various sensors. In a recent work, vertically aligned multi-walled carbon nanotubes were prepared with a diameter of less than 80 nm and uniform thickness of 16 µm, by employing microwave plasma torch with a high-speed process of only 60–120 s [99]. Carbon-encapsulated magnetic materials were also obtained by plasma as described in the previous section [88].

Table 2 summarizes current advances of several nanomaterials synthesized by plasma technologies. In the future, the main focus of plasma-induced synthesis of nanomaterials should be on the improvement of several essential factors, such as controlled synthesis, oxidation prevention, impurity and industrial scale production. More detailed studies need to implement for synthesis and diagnostic for application of nanomaterials in biomedicine and other applications.

Table 2. Summary of nanomaterials synthesized by plasma technologies.

Materials	Methods	Average Size	References
Ag Nanowire	Arc Plasma	5–15 nm (diameter) <100 nm length	[71]
Pt NPs	RF Plasma	2 nm	[72]
Au NPs, Ag NPs	Microplasma	8 nm–10 nm	[73,74,77,78]
Au NPs	Microplasma	4.4 nm	[80]
Au NPs	Sputter	5.5 nm	[81]
Au-Ag Alloy	Sputter	2.6–6.0 nm	[82]
Ag Nanopowder	Wire explosion	20–200 nm	[83]
Au, Ag, Ti, Ni Nanoball	Plasma electrolysis	10 nm	[84]

Table 2. Cont.

Materials	Methods	Average Size	References
FeC NPs	Plasma in liquid ethanol	5–600 nm	[85]
FeC Nanocapsule	Plasma in liquid ethanol	10–20 nm	[86]
Fe_3O_4	Pulsed Plasma in liquid	19 nm	[87]
Fe NPs	Pulsed Plasma in liquid	35 nm	[88]
Ni NPs	Pulsed Plasma in liquid	26 nm	[88]
Co NPs	Pulsed Plasma in liquid	20 nm	[88]
Fe@C NPs	Pulsed Plasma in liquid	32 nm	[89]
Ni@C NPs	Pulsed Plasma in liquid	40 nm	[89]
Fe_3O_4@Si	Arc Plasma	20 nm	[90]
CuO nanorods	Arc Plasma	14–16 nm	[91]
Cu NPs	Arc Plasma	30–50 nm	[91]
Cu_2O NPs	Arc Plasma	4–10 nm	[91]
FePt NPs	Microplasma	Less the 100 nm	[92]
Co_3O_4 NPs	Microplasma	2–5 nm	[94]
Si NPs	Microplasma	1–3 nm	[95]
Nanodiamond	Microplasma	3 nm	[98]
Multiwalled-Carbon Nanotubes	Microwave Plasma	80 nm (diameter)	[99]

4. Plasma and Nanomaterial Combination Treatment on Cells and Microbes

Non-thermal plasma can directly or indirectly kill cancer cells. Use of conjugated or un-conjugated NPs can increase the specificity and efficiency of treatment. There are many reports in which researchers use antibody-conjugated NPs to enhance cell death and reduce the cell viability of cancer cells. In future, this combination technology could become a feasible therapeutic technology against various kinds of cancers or tumors.

In cancer treatment, it is very important to induce cell death specifically in cancer tissue or mass. However, plasma cannot efficiently distinguish between normal and cancer tissue. Recently, researchers used Au NPs (which are harmless to the human body at low doses) conjugated with antibody (which targets overexpressed proteins on or in cancer cells). Choi et al. used Au NPs conjugated with antibody against epidermal growth receptor (EGFR) [45]. EGFR protein is overexposed in many types of cancer cells, more specifically in oral cancer cells. They used low doses of air plasma (9.2 J/cm^2 for 30 s) with anti-EGFR antibody-conjugated Au NPs to selectively kill oral cancer cells. Morphology was changed from a spindle shape to a round shape, cell shrinkage and membrane rupture were observed in oral cancer cells treated with plasma plus conjugated Au NPs. However, the whole mechanism for this combination treatment is still not known, and has to be elucidated in the future.

The research group of Prof Michael Keider and Jonathan H. Sherman demonstrated the synergistic effect of Au NPs and cold plasma on glioblastoma (brain cancer) cancer cells [100]. They revealed that the synergistic effect between Au NPs and atmospheric pressure cold plasma is dependent on the concentration of Au NPs. Au NPs significantly increase cell death by 30% in glioblastoma cell line with the same plasma dosage. They concluded that intracellular reactive oxygen species accumulation results in the oxidative stress, which further changes the intracellular pathways, and also increases damage to protein, DNA and lipid molecules. These studies showed that synergy has great potential to improve cancer therapy and reduce the harm to normal cells.

Researchers also targeted NEU (human epidermal growth factor receptor 2) protein, which is frequently overexpressed on the cell membrane of skin cancer (melanoma) cells. They used anti-NEU antibody-conjugated Au NPs in this recent study. These nanoparticles were selectively uptaken by skin cancer cells rather than normal keratinocyte. Both cancers, as well as normal cells, were treated by non-thermal atmospheric pressure plasma after the addition of conjugated Au NPs. This combination treatment selectively enhanced the death rate of skin cancer cells significantly rather than normal keratinocyte cells. This selective skin cancer cell death is may be due to selective destruction of NEU protein and a downstream effect of NEU [101].

Recently, non-thermal atmospheric pressure plasma with Au NPs was also used for killing microbes. Non-thermal plasma efficiently kills oral bacteria on agar plates; however, it has less effect on the tooth surface. Therefore, researchers used 30-nm Au NPs to enhance the killing effect of non-thermal on oral bacteria (*Streptococcus mutans*) on the tooth. Non-thermal plasma treatment alone decreased viability by 5 log of *S. mutans* in vitro; however, plasma treatment of bacteria on tooth surface exhibited only a 3-log reduction in viability. When they added Au NPs to the bacteria, plasma treatment also showed a 5-log reduction in the viability of bacteria, while Au NPs alone did not show any antibacterial effect. The morphological examination by transmission electron microscopy showed that plasma treatment only perforated the bacterial cell walls; however, combination treatment with plasma and Au NPs caused significant cell damage, causing loss of intracellular components from many bacterial cells [102].

Our group has also reported the synergistic effect of PEG-coated Au NPs (PEG-Au NPs) and non-thermal plasma on epithelial-mesenchymal transition (EMT) and the maintenance of cancer stem cells (CSC) on solid cancer cells. The results showed that co-treatment with PEG-GNP and non-thermal plasma inhibited growth in cancer cells by altering the PI3K/AKT signaling axis. This non-thermal plasma and PEG-Au NP co-treatment reversed EMT in tumor cells by altering signaling proteins, resulting in the upregulation of epithelial markers such as E-cadherin and down-regulation of N-Cadherin, Slug and Zeb-1. It was also shown that this co-treatment also inhibited tumor growth by decreasing mesenchymal markers in tumor xenograft mice models. This kind of combination treatment also inhibited sphere formation and the self-renewal capacity of glioma-like stem cells [103,104].

In another recent report, the synergistic cytotoxicity of Au NPs and non-thermal plasma showed enhanced endocytosis and trafficking to the lysosomal compartment as well as temporarily increased membrane permeability. This report contributes knowledge to the mechanism of combination effects of non-thermal plasma and NPs and indicates a technology for possible drug delivery systems. It is demonstrated that the rates of Au NPs uptake and total amount accumulated in solid cancer cells are significantly enhanced after exposure to 75 kV non-thermal plasma generated by DBD. Chemical effects induced by direct and indirect exposure to non-thermal plasma appear the dominant mediator of enhanced uptake [105]. They also showed that Au NPs and non-thermal co-treatment caused many divots across the glioma cell membrane, making it more porous. In contrast, there was no significant effect or NP uptake in astrocyte (E6/E7) cells, and there was no change in the cell membrane morphology. These studies prove that plasma-based nano-drug delivery technology is safe and effective against solid tumors [106].

To maximize the preferential killing of melanoma cells non-thermal plasma is used with Au NPs tagged with antibodies targeting phosphorylated FAK (p-FAK). Combined treatment also showed the minimum effect against HaCaT keratinocyte cells. After co-treatment on melanoma cells, signaling molecules such as FAK, p-paxillin, and NEU were reduced with treatment. Therefore, it is suggested that these kinds of co-treatment strategies are effective and selective against melanomas [107]. Recently core-shell NPs were synthesized via co-axial electrospraying. Biocompatible poly (lactic-*co*-glycolic acid) was used as the polymer shell to encapsulate anti-cancer treatment. In vitro studies demonstrated the synergistic effect of these core-shell NPs and non-thermal plasma for inhibition of breast cancer cell growth when compared to each treatment alone. Non-thermal plasma induced down-regulation of metastasis-related gene expression (VEGF, MTDH, MMP9, and MMP2) and facilitated drug-loaded nanoparticle uptake, which could be an important breakthrough minimizing drug resistance, a major problem in cancer chemotherapy [108].

Iron NPs 50 nm in size were also used for combination treatment with non-thermal plasma against human breast adenocarcinoma cells. Findings showed that the combination of plasma and iron NPs inhibited the viability of cancer cells significantly. Molecular analysis demonstrated that the combination treatment induced shifting the *BAX/BCL-2* ratio in favor of apoptosis [109]. Table 3 summarizes recent updates on plasma and nanomaterials combination for cancer treatment.

Table 3. Recent updates on plasma and nanomaterial combination treatment against cancers.

Published Year	Cancer Type	Plasma Device	Nanomaterial	Reference
2014	Glioblastoma	Plasma jet	Au NPs	[100]
2015	Melanoma	Surface type air plasma	Anti-NEU-Au NPs	[101]
2017, 2016	Glioblastoma	Surface DBD air plasma	PEG-Au NPs	[103,104]
2018	Glioblastoma	DBD plasma	Au NPs	[105]
2015	Glioblastoma	Plasma jet	Au NPs	[106]
2017, 2009	Melanoma	DBD Plasma	Anti-FAK-Au NPs	[35,107]
2016	Breast Cancer	Cold atmospheric plasma	Fluorouracil loaded core-shell NPs	[108]
2016	Breast Cancer	Plasma jet	Iron NPs	[109]
2015	Colorectal Cancer	Plasma jet	Au NPs	[110]
2017	Lung Cancer	DBD plasma	Epidermal growth factor conjugated Au NPs	[111]

In addition, cold plasmas are widely used as treatment tools for biomaterial surfaces, such as polymers, metals, alloys, ceramics, and composites [112]. The plasma treatment is capable to activate or functionalize the material surfaces and also produces several exclusive properties compared to other chemical and physical methods. Due to the low penetration capability, plasma can only be able to modify very few thin layers of the surface with a thickness of a hundred nanometers. Thus, the surface properties can be altered, in order to enhance the biocompatibility and bio-functionalization, which are vital parameters towards practical applications of synthetic biomaterials. In general, plasma-modified biomaterials possess great potential for the applications in dentistry, tissue engineering or drug delivery. For instance, metal NPs with antimicrobial or bactericide properties can be incorporated or coated on the surfaces of implants by plasma modification techniques. Plasma treatment also can change the surface roughness and increase the hydrophilicity of biodegradable polymers, thus improve the cell affinity and cell adhesion of these materials. Moreover, plasma surface modification can promote the attachment, loading, and release of drug molecules in porous biomaterials.

Recently, Rosales et al. have reported the effect of plasma surface modification on antibacterial properties of Cu NPs [113]. The surface of Cu NPs was functionalized with polyacrylic acid, polyacrylonitrile, or polymethyl methacrylate by utilizing the radiofrequency plasma reactor to enhance the biocompatibility. During the plasma polymerization, the simultaneous removal of CuO upper layers on the surface of Cu NPs was observed. The polymer layers also acted as protecting layers, preventing Cu NPs being oxidized. The coating polymer films on Cu NPs were thin enough for the copper ions to easily diffuse through the coating layer and subsequently interact with bacteria. The antibacterial properties of the Cu NPs were not significantly affected by the plasma modification. They demonstrated outstanding antibacterial property against Gram-positive bacteria (*P. aeruginosa*). The plasma polymerization-coated Cu NPs also possessed significantly lower toxicity to normal human cells as compared to pristine copper NPs.

Titanium biomaterials are frequently used in medical and dental sciences. Titanium dental implants have promising potentials as the replacements of missing teeth. However, there are chances of failure in dental implants after surgeries in extraction sockets. Atmospheric pressure plasma treatment can be used to soft tissue around titanium dental implant abutments surface without causing topological changes. The topology and chemistry of titanium implants are important factors for osseointegration. A preliminary research work in this field studied the cellular attachment and differentiation of titanium nanotubes treated by air or nitrogen non-thermal atmospheric pressure plasma jets [114]. After plasma treatment the ostogenic properties were improved without any change in topographical morphology. In addition, plasma treatment of nanotubes further increased hydrophilicity, as well as modifying the surfaces. It was demonstrated that cellular activity and in vitro osseointegration were significantly enhanced on plasma-treated titanium nanotube.

Another example is Poly(lactide-*co*-glycolide) or PLGA NPs, which can be applied for sustained delivery of proteins for nervous tissue repair. However, sterilization of protein-loaded PLGA is a challenging task, due to the possibility of reducing the activity of proteins. Recently, researchers from Drexel University reported sterilization of protein-loaded PLGA NPs by using indirect plasma treatment [115]. They used plasma-treated water and PBS for sterilization of NPs and proteins. Plasma-treated water showed no morphological changes to the NPs. They concluded that treatment of particles in plasma-treated PBS is effective for decontaminating particles, as well as in maintaining protein activity; thus, is possible to apply it for nervous tissue repair therapy.

5. Summary and Future Prospectives

Great efforts have been carried out over the last few decades focusing on the synergistic effects of non-thermal plasma and nanomaterials towards applications in biomedical science. The combination of these two emerging research fields typically refers to two different strategies. The first is the synthesis of nanomaterials using non-thermal plasma, which has been proved as a simple, effective, low-cost and, furthermore, clean method. It can eliminate the consumption of toxic chemical components during the fabrication of nanomaterials, which are typically used in other conventional methods, such as chemical and physical synthesis technologies. Thus, the toxicity of plasma-synthesized nanomaterials is relatively lower, making them become more appropriate for biomedical practical applications. Depending on the structures of the nanomaterials, the RONS induced by plasma can be encapsulated inside the materials; hence, their live-time and travel distance will increase. These two parameters are vital problems that non-thermal plasma technology has been dealing with, in order to enhance effectiveness. The second is the combination of plasma and post-synthesized nanomaterials. Under non-thermal plasma treatment, the cell membranes can be open or enlarged, therefore increasing the cell permeation. Consequently, nanomaterials can easily penetrate through cell membranes. In addition, the low selectivity property of non-thermal plasma can be compensated by nanomaterials, which are generally functionalized for specific targets.

This review briefly summarizes recent progress in the combination of plasma and nanomaterials. Important challenges remain for the utilization of this interdisciplinary field in the future. The understanding of plasma and nanomaterials interactions, in both synthesis and post-synthesis are still inadequate. Due to the presence of a variety of species, electric field and radiation, non-equilibrium chemistry processes between plasma and nanomaterials are exceptionally complex and difficult to control. The homogeneity of the desired nanostructures by plasma synthesis is limited, compared to other methods. Thus, further studies are required to understand the natures and extending the use of plasma and nanomaterials combination, not only limited to biomedical, but also many other biological applications. In addition, plasma-assisted nano-drug delivery systems are potential subjects for future biomedical researches. This advanced technology can be utilized in clinical and aesthetic purposes.

Author Contributions: Conceptualization, N.K.K., N.K., A.P., B.G., J.S. and N.N.L.; Resources, N.K.K., S.J.L.; E.H.C.; Writing—original draft preparation, N.K.K., N.K., A.P., B.G., J.S. and N.N.L.; Writing—review and editing, N.K.K., N.K., A.P., B.G., J.S. and N.N.L.; Supervision, N.K.K., S.J.L. and E.H.C.; Funding acquisition, N.K.K., E.H.C.

Funding: This work was supported by a grant from the National Research Foundation of Korea (NRF), which is funded by the Korean Government, Ministry of Science, ICT and Future Planning (MSIP) NRF-2016K1A4A3914113; NRF-2016R1C1B2010851 and also by the Ministry of trade; industry & energy grant No. 20131610101840. This work is also funded by Kwangwoon University in 2018-19.

Conflicts of Interest: The authors declare no conflict of interest.

Abbreviations

List of repeated acronyms:

UV	ultra-violet
DBD	dielectric barrier discharge
FE-DBD	floating electrode dielectric barrier discharge
RONS	reactive oxygen and nitrogen species
ROS	reactive oxygen species
OH	hydroxyl radical
O_2^-	super oxide

H_2O_2	hydrogen peroxide
$^1O_2$	singlet oxygen
O_3	ozone
E^-	electron
M^+	positive ion
NPs (Au NPs, Cu NPs, Fe NPs, etc.)	Nanoparticles (Gold nanoparticles, Copper nanoparticles, Iron nanoparticles, etc.)
NCs	nanocrystals
Ar	argon
EMT	epithelial-mesenchymal transition
PEG-GNP	Polyethyleneglycol coated gold Nanoparticles

References

1. Kong, M.G.; Keidar, M.; Ostrikov, K. Plasmas meet nanoparticles-where synergies can advance the frontier of medicine. *J. Phys. D Appl. Phys.* **2011**, *44*. [CrossRef]
2. Eliasson, B.; Kogelschatz, U. Nonequilibrium volume plasma chemical processing. *IEEE Trans. Plasma Sci.* **1991**, *19*, 1063–1077. [CrossRef]
3. Eliasson, B.; Kogelschatz, U. Modeling and applications of silent discharge plasmas. *IEEE Trans. Plasma Sci.* **1991**, *19*, 309–323. [CrossRef]
4. Li, Y.; Kang, M.H.; Uhm, H.S.; Lee, G.J.; Choi, E.H.; Han, I. Effects of atmospheric-pressure non-thermal bio-compatible plasma and plasma activated nitric oxide water on cervical cancer cells. *Sci. Rep.* **2017**, *7*, 1–9. [CrossRef]
5. Fridman, G.; Peddinghaus, M.; Ayan, H.; Fridman, A.; Balasubramanian, M.; Gutsol, A.; Brooks, A.; Friedman, G. Blood coagulation and living tissue sterilization by floating-electrode dielectric barrier discharge in air. *Plasma Chem. Plasma Process.* **2006**, *26*, 425–442. [CrossRef]
6. Lu, X.; Laroussi, M.; Puech, V. On atmospheric-pressure non-equilibrium plasma jets and plasma bullets. *Plasma Sources Sci. Technol.* **2012**, *21*, 034005. [CrossRef]
7. Ghimire, B.; Lamichhane, P.; Lim, J.S.; Min, B.; Paneru, R.; Weltmann, K.D.; Choi, E.H. An atmospheric pressure plasma jet operated by injecting natural air. *Appl. Phys. Lett.* **2018**, *113*. [CrossRef]
8. Winter, J.; Brandenburg, R.; Weltmann, K.D. Atmospheric pressure plasma jets: An overview of devices and new directions. *Plasma Sources Sci. Technol.* **2015**, *24*. [CrossRef]
9. Von Woedtke, T.; Reuter, S.; Masur, K.; Weltmann, K.D. Plasmas for medicine. *Phys. Rep.* **2013**, *530*, 291–320. [CrossRef]
10. Park, G.Y.; Park, S.J.; Choi, M.Y.; Koo, I.G.; Byun, J.H.; Hong, J.W.; Sim, J.Y.; Collins, G.J.; Lee, J.K. Atmospheric-pressure plasma sources for biomedical applications. *Plasma Sources Sci. Technol.* **2012**, *21*. [CrossRef]
11. Laroussi, M. Low-Temperature Plasmas for Medicine? *IEEE Trans. Plasma Sci.* **2009**, *37*, 714–725. [CrossRef]
12. Laroussi, M.; Fridman, A.; Satava, R.M. Editorial. *Plasma Process. Polym.* **2008**, *5*, 501–502. [CrossRef]
13. Laroussi, M.; Lu, X. Room-temperature atmospheric pressure plasma plume for biomedical applications. *Appl. Phys. Lett.* **2005**, *87*, 113902. [CrossRef]
14. Kaushik, N.; Kaushik, N.K.; Kim, C.H.; Choi, E.H. Oxidative Stress and Cell Death Induced in U-937 Human Monocytic Cancer Cell Line by Non-Thermal Atmospheric Air Plasma Soft Jet. *Sci. Adv. Mater.* **2014**, *6*, 1740–1751. [CrossRef]
15. Ghimire, B.; Sornsakdanuphap, J.; Hong, Y.J.; Uhm, H.S.; Weltmann, K.D.; Choi, E.H. The effect of the gap distance between an atmospheric-pressure plasma jet nozzle and liquid surface on OH and N_2 species concentrations. *Phys. Plasmas* **2017**, *24*. [CrossRef]
16. Kaushik, N.K.; Ghimire, B.; Li, Y.; Adhikari, M.; Veerana, M.; Kaushik, N.; Jha, N.; Adhikari, B.; Lee, S.; Masur, K.; et al. Biological and medical applications of plasma- activated media, water and solutions. *Biol. Chem.* **2019**, *400*, 39–62. [CrossRef] [PubMed]
17. Kalghatgi, S.; Kelly, C.M.; Cerchar, E.; Torabi, B.; Alekseev, O.; Fridman, A.; Friedman, G.; Azizkhan-Clifford, J. Cerchar Effects of non-thermal plasma on mammalian cells. *PLoS ONE* **2011**, *6*, e16270. [CrossRef]
18. Fridman, A. *Plasma Chemistry*; Cambridge University Press: Cambridge, UK, 2008; ISBN 9780521847353.

19. Fridman, A.A.; Kennedy, L.A. *Plasma Physics and Engineering*; Taylor & Francis: New York, NY, USA, 2004.
20. Kogelschatz, U.; Eliasson, B.; Egli, W. From ozone generators to flat television screens: History and future potential of dielectric-barrier discharges. *Pure Appl. Chem.* **1999**, *71*. [CrossRef]
21. Desmet, T.; Morent, R.; De Geyter, N.; Leys, C.; Schacht, E.; Dubruel, P. Nonthermal Plasma Technology as a Versatile Strategy for Polymeric Biomaterials Surface Modification: A Review. *Biomacromolecules* **2009**, *10*, 2351–2378. [CrossRef]
22. Lukes, P.; Dolezalova, E.; Sisrova, I.; Clupek, M. Aqueous-phase chemistry and bactericidal effects from an air discharge plasma in contact with water: Evidence for the formation of peroxynitrite through a pseudo-second-order post-discharge reaction of H_2O_2 and HNO_2. *Plasma Sources Sci. Technol.* **2014**, *23*. [CrossRef]
23. Takamatsu, T.; Uehara, K.; Sasaki, Y.; Miyahara, H.; Matsumura, Y.; Iwasaki, A.; Ito, N.; Azuma, T.; Kohno, M.; Okino, A. Investigation of reactive species using various gas plasmas. *RSC Adv.* **2014**, *4*, 39901–39905. [CrossRef]
24. Kim, Y.H.; Hong, Y.J.; Baik, K.Y.; Kwon, G.C.; Choi, J.J.; Cho, G.S.; Uhm, H.S.; Kim, D.Y.; Choi, E.H. Measurement of reactive hydroxyl radical species inside the biosolutions during non-thermal atmospheric pressure plasma jet bombardment onto the solution. *Plasma Chem. Plasma Process.* **2014**, *34*, 457–472. [CrossRef]
25. Weltmann, K.; Woedtke, T. von Campus PlasmaMed—From Basic Research to Clinical Proof. *IEEE Trans. Plasma Sci.* **2011**, *39*, 1015–1025. [CrossRef]
26. Oehmigen, K.; Winter, J.; Hähnel, M.; Wilke, C.; Brandenburg, R.; Weltmann, K.-D.; von Woedtke, T. Estimation of Possible Mechanisms of Escherichia coli Inactivation by Plasma Treated Sodium Chloride Solution. *Plasma Process. Polym.* **2011**, *8*, 904–913. [CrossRef]
27. Barekzi, N.; Laroussi, M. Dose-dependent killing of leukemia cells by low-temperature plasma. *J. Phys. D Appl. Phys.* **2012**, *45*. [CrossRef]
28. Arjunan, K.P.; Friedman, G.; Fridman, A.; Clyne, A.M. Non-thermal dielectric barrier discharge plasma induces angiogenesis through reactive oxygen species. *J. R. Soc. Interface* **2012**, *9*, 147–157. [CrossRef] [PubMed]
29. Arndt, S.; Wacker, E.; Li, Y.-F.; Shimizu, T.; Thomas, H.M.; Morfill, G.E.; Karrer, S.; Zimmermann, J.L.; Bosserhoff, A.-K. Cold atmospheric plasma, a new strategy to induce senescence in melanoma cells. *Exp. Dermatol.* **2013**, *22*, 284–289. [CrossRef]
30. Kaushik, N.K.; Kim, Y.H.; Han, Y.G.; Choi, E.H. Effect of jet plasma on T98G human brain cancer cells. *Curr. Appl. Phys.* **2013**, *13*, 176–180. [CrossRef]
31. Kaushik, N.K.; Uhm, H.; Ha Choi, E. Micronucleus formation induced by dielectric barrier discharge plasma exposure in brain cancer cells. *Appl. Phys. Lett.* **2012**, *100*, 84102. [CrossRef]
32. Kaushik, N.; Kumar, N.; Kim, C.H.; Kaushik, N.K.; Choi, E.H. Dielectric Barrier Discharge Plasma Efficiently Delivers an Apoptotic Response in Human Monocytic Lymphoma. *Plasma Process. Polym.* **2014**, *11*, 1175–1187. [CrossRef]
33. Keidar, M.; Walk, R.; Shashurin, A.; Srinivasan, P.; Sandler, A.; Dasgupta, S.; Ravi, R.; Guerrero-Preston, R.; Trink, B. Cold plasma selectivity and the possibility of a paradigm shift in cancer therapy. *Br. J. Cancer* **2011**, *105*, 1295–1301. [CrossRef] [PubMed]
34. Kim, C.-H.; Bahn, J.H.; Lee, S.-H.; Kim, G.-Y.; Jun, S.-I.; Lee, K.; Baek, S.J. Induction of cell growth arrest by atmospheric non-thermal plasma in colorectal cancer cells. *J. Biotechnol.* **2010**, *150*, 530–538. [CrossRef] [PubMed]
35. Kim, G.C.; Park, S.R.; Kim, G.J.; Lee, J.K.; Jeon, S.M.; Seo, H.J.; Iza, F. Air plasma coupled with antibody-conjugated nanoparticles: A new weapon against cancer. *J. Phys. D Appl. Phys.* **2009**, *42*, 5. [CrossRef]
36. Ma, Y.; Ha, C.S.; Hwang, S.W.; Lee, H.J.; Kim, G.C.; Lee, K.-W.; Song, K. Non-Thermal Atmospheric Pressure Plasma Preferentially Induces Apoptosis in p53-Mutated Cancer Cells by Activating ROS Stress-Response Pathways. *PLoS ONE* **2014**, *9*, e91947. [CrossRef] [PubMed]
37. Partecke, L.I.; Evert, K.; Haugk, J.; Doering, F.; Normann, L.; Diedrich, S.; Weiss, F.-U.; Evert, M.; Huebner, N.O.; Guenther, C.; et al. Tissue tolerable plasma (TTP) induces apoptosis in pancreatic cancer cells in vitro and in vivo. *BMC Cancer* **2012**, *12*, 473. [CrossRef] [PubMed]
38. Schlegel, J.; Köritzer, J.; Boxhammer, V. Plasma in cancer treatment. *Clin. Plasma Med.* **2013**, *1*, 2–7. [CrossRef]
39. Thiyagarajan, M.; Gonzales, X.F.; Anderson, H. Regulated cellular exposure to non-thermal plasma allows preferentially directed apoptosis in acute monocytic leukemia cells. *Stud. Health Technol. Inform.* **2013**, *184*, 436–442. [PubMed]

40. Brulle, L.; Vandamme, M.; Ries, D.; Martel, E.; Robert, E.; Lerondel, S.; Trichet, V.; Richard, S.; Pouvesle, J.-M.; Le Pape, A. Effects of a non thermal plasma treatment alone or in combination with gemcitabine in a MIA PaCa$_2$-luc orthotopic pancreatic carcinoma model. *PLoS ONE* **2012**, *7*, e52653. [CrossRef]
41. Volotskova, O.; Hawley, T.S.; Stepp, M.A.; Keidar, M. Targeting the cancer cell cycle by cold atmospheric plasma. *Sci. Rep.* **2012**, *2*, 636. [CrossRef]
42. Zucker, S.N.; Zirnheld, J.; Bagati, A.; DiSanto, T.M.; Des Soye, B.; Wawrzyniak, J.A.; Etemadi, K.; Nikiforov, M.; Berezney, R. Preferential induction of apoptotic cell death in melanoma cells as compared with normal keratinocytes using a non-thermal plasma torch. *Cancer Biol. Ther.* **2012**, *13*, 1299–1306. [CrossRef]
43. Bundscherer, L.; Wende, K.; Ottmuller, K.; Barton, A.; Schmidt, A.; Bekeschus, S.; Hasse, S.; Weltmann, K.-D.; Masur, K.; Lindequist, U. Impact of non-thermal plasma treatment on MAPK signaling pathways of human immune cell lines. *Immunobiology* **2013**, *218*, 1248–1255. [CrossRef] [PubMed]
44. Chang, J.W.; Kang, S.U.; Shin, Y.S.; Kim, K.I.; Seo, S.J.; Yang, S.S.; Lee, J.-S.; Moon, E.; Lee, K.; Kim, C.-H. Non-thermal atmospheric pressure plasma inhibits thyroid papillary cancer cell invasion via cytoskeletal modulation, altered MMP-2/-9/uPA activity. *PLoS ONE* **2014**, *9*, e92198. [CrossRef] [PubMed]
45. Choi, B.-B.; Choi, Y.-S.; Lee, H.-J.; Lee, J.-K.; Kim, U.-K.; Kim, G.-C. Nonthermal Plasma-Mediated Cancer Cell Death; Targeted Cancer Treatment. *J. Therm. Sci. Technol.* **2012**, *7*, 399–404. [CrossRef]
46. Fridman, G.; Shereshevsky, A.; Jost, M.M.; Brooks, A.D.; Fridman, A.; Gutsol, A.; Vasilets, V.; Friedman, G. Floating electrode dielectric barrier discharge plasma in air promoting apoptotic behavior in Melanoma skin cancer cell lines. *Plasma Chem. Plasma Process.* **2007**, *27*, 163–176. [CrossRef]
47. Haertel, B.; Volkmann, F.; von Woedtke, T.; Lindequist, U. Differential sensitivity of lymphocyte subpopulations to non-thermal atmospheric-pressure plasma. *Immunobiology* **2012**, *217*, 628–633. [CrossRef] [PubMed]
48. Kalghatgi, S.; Kelly, C.; Cerchar, E.; Azizkhan-Clifford, J. Selectivity of non-thermal atmospheric-pressure microsecond-pulsed dielectric barrier discharge plasma induced apoptosis in tumor cells over healthy cells. *Plasma Med.* **2011**, *1*, 249–263. [CrossRef]
49. Kang, S.U.; Cho, J.-H.; Chang, J.W.; Shin, Y.S.; Kim, K.I.; Park, J.K.; Yang, S.S.; Lee, J.-S.; Moon, E.; Lee, K.; et al. Nonthermal plasma induces head and neck cancer cell death: The potential involvement of mitogen-activated protein kinase-dependent mitochondrial reactive oxygen species. *Cell Death Dis.* **2014**, *5*, e1056. [CrossRef]
50. Robert, E.; Vandamme, M.; Brullé, L.; Lerondel, S.; Le Pape, A.; Sarron, V.; Riès, D.; Darny, T.; Dozias, S.; Collet, G.; et al. Perspectives of endoscopic plasma applications. *Clin. Plasma Med.* **2013**, *1*, 8–16. [CrossRef]
51. Zuo, X.; Wei, Y.; Wei Chen, L.; Dong Meng, Y. Non-equilibrium atmospheric pressure microplasma jet: An approach to endoscopic therapies. *Phys. Plasmas* **2013**, *20*, 83507. [CrossRef]
52. Kim, J.Y.; Wei, Y.; Li, J.; Foy, P.; Hawkins, T.; Ballato, J.; Kim, S.-O. Single-cell-level microplasma cancer therapy. *Small* **2011**, *7*, 2291–2295. [CrossRef]
53. Ratovitski, E.A.; Cheng, X.; Yan, D.; Sherman, J.H.; Canady, J.; Trink, B.; Keidar, M.; Ratovitski, E.A.; Cheng, X.; Yan, D.; et al. Anti-cancer therapies of 21st century: Novel approach to treat human cancers using cold atmospheric plasma. *Plasma Process. Polym.* **2014**, *11*, 1128–1137. [CrossRef]
54. Panngom, K.; Baik, K.Y.; Nam, M.K.; Han, J.H.; Rhim, H.; Choi, E.H. Preferential killing of human lung cancer cell lines with mitochondrial dysfunction by nonthermal dielectric barrier discharge plasma. *Cell Death Dis.* **2013**, *4*, e642. [CrossRef] [PubMed]
55. Wang, M.; Holmes, B.; Cheng, X.; Zhu, W.; Keidar, M.; Zhang, L.G. Cold atmospheric plasma for selectively ablating metastatic breast cancer cells. *PLoS ONE* **2013**, *8*, e73741. [CrossRef] [PubMed]
56. Xu, X.; Dai, X.; Xiang, L.; Cai, D.; Xiao, S.; Ostrikov, K. Quantitative assessment of cold atmospheric plasma anti-cancer efficacy in triple-negative breast cancers. *Plasma Process. Polym.* **2018**, *15*, 1800052. [CrossRef]
57. Zirnheld, J.L.; Zucker, S.N.; DiSanto, T.M.; Berezney, R.; Etemadi, K. Nonthermal Plasma Needle: Development and Targeting of Melanoma Cells. *IEEE Trans. Plasma Sci.* **2010**, *38*, 948–952. [CrossRef]
58. Georgescu, N.; Lupu, A.R. Tumoral and Normal Cells Treatment With High-Voltage Pulsed Cold Atmospheric Plasma Jets. *IEEE Trans. Plasma Sci.* **2010**, *38*, 1949–1955. [CrossRef]
59. Iseki, S.; Nakamura, K.; Hayashi, M.; Tanaka, H.; Kondo, H.; Kajiyama, H.; Kano, H.; Kikkawa, F.; Hori, M. Selective killing of ovarian cancer cells through induction of apoptosis by nonequilibrium atmospheric pressure plasma. *Appl. Phys. Lett.* **2012**, *100*, 113702. [CrossRef]
60. Kaushik, N.K.; Attri, P.; Kaushik, N.; Choi, E.H. A preliminary study of the effect of DBD plasma and osmolytes on T98G brain cancer and HEK non-malignant cells. *Molecules* **2013**, *18*, 4917–4928. [CrossRef]

61. Kaushik, N.; Uddin, N.; Sim, G.B.; Hong, Y.J.; Baik, K.Y.; Kim, C.H.; Lee, S.J.; Kaushik, N.K.; Choi, E.H. Responses of solid tumor cells in DMEM to reactive oxygen species generated by non-thermal plasma and chemically induced ROS systems. *Sci. Rep.* **2015**, *5*, 8587. [CrossRef]
62. Kaushik, N.K.; Kaushik, N.; Park, D.; Choi, E.H. Altered antioxidant system stimulates dielectric barrier discharge plasma-induced cell death for solid tumor cell treatment. *PLoS ONE* **2014**, *9*, e103349. [CrossRef]
63. Kaushik, N.; Lee, S.J.; Choi, T.G.; Baik, K.Y.; Uhm, H.S.; Kim, C.H.; Kaushik, N.K.; Choi, E.H. Non-thermal plasma with 2-deoxy-D-glucose synergistically induces cell death by targeting glycolysis in blood cancer cells. *Sci. Rep.* **2015**, *5*, 8726. [CrossRef]
64. Tang, Y.; Ke, X. Advances of mesoporous silica nanoparticles as drug delivery system. *J. China Pharm. Univ.* **2012**, *43*, 567–572. [CrossRef]
65. Khan, Z.U.H.; Khan, A.; Chen, Y.; Shah, N.S.; Muhammad, N.; Khan, A.U.; Tahir, K.; Khan, F.U.; Murtaza, B.; Hassan, S.U.; et al. Biomedical applications of green synthesized Nobel metal nanoparticles. *J. Photochem. Photobiol. B Biol.* **2017**, *173*, 150–164. [CrossRef] [PubMed]
66. Tran, N.; Webster, T.J. Magnetic nanoparticles: Biomedical applications and challenges. *J. Mater. Chem.* **2010**, *20*, 8760–8767. [CrossRef]
67. Dasari Shareena, T.P.; McShan, D.; Dasmahapatra, A.K.; Tchounwou, P.B. A Review on Graphene-Based Nanomaterials in Biomedical Applications and Risks in Environment and Health. *Nano-Micro Lett.* **2018**, *10*, 1–34. [CrossRef] [PubMed]
68. Muhulet, A.; Miculescu, F.; Voicu, S.I.; Schütt, F.; Thakur, V.K.; Mishra, Y.K. Fundamentals and scopes of doped carbon nanotubes towards energy and biosensing applications. *Mater. Today Energy* **2018**, *9*, 154–186. [CrossRef]
69. Mishra, Y.K.; Adelung, R. ZnO tetrapod materials for functional applications. *Mater. Today* **2018**, *21*, 631–651. [CrossRef]
70. Ostrikov, K.; Neyts, E.C.; Meyyappan, M. Plasma nanoscience: From nano-solids in plasmas to nano-plasmas in solids. *Adv. Phys.* **2013**, *62*, 113–224. [CrossRef]
71. Zhou, Y.; Yu, S.H.; Cui, X.P.; Wang, C.Y.; Chen, Z.Y. Formation of Silver Nanowires by a Novel Solid-Liquid Phase Arc Discharge Method. *Chem. Mater.* **1999**, *11*, 545–546. [CrossRef]
72. Koo, I.G.; Lee, M.S.; Shim, J.H.; Ahn, J.H.; Lee, W.M. Platinum nanoparticles prepared by a plasma-chemical reduction method. *J. Mater. Chem.* **2005**, *15*, 4125–4128. [CrossRef]
73. Richmonds, C.; Sankaran, R.M. Plasma-liquid electrochemistry: Rapid synthesis of colloidal metal nanoparticles by microplasma reduction of aqueous cations. *Appl. Phys. Lett.* **2008**, *93*, 91–94. [CrossRef]
74. Chiang, W.H.; Richmonds, C.; Sankaran, R.M. Continuous-flow, atmospheric-pressure microplasmas: A versatile source for metal nanoparticle synthesis in the gas or liquid phase. *Plasma Sources Sci. Technol.* **2010**, *19*, 34011. [CrossRef]
75. Rumbach, P.; Bartels, D.M.; Sankaran, R.M.; Go, D.B. The solvation of electrons by an atmospheric-pressure plasma. *Nat. Commun.* **2015**, *6*, 1–6. [CrossRef] [PubMed]
76. Garcia, M.A. Surface plasmons in metallic nanoparticles: Fundamentals and applications. *J. Phys. D Appl. Phys.* **2011**, *44*, 283001. [CrossRef]
77. Zhou, M.; Wang, B.; De Vos, C.; Baneton, J.; Li, L.; Weng, J.; Patel, J.; Němcová, L.; Maguire, P.; Graham, W.G.; et al. Synthesis of surfactant-free electrostatically stabilized gold nanoparticles by plasma-induced liquid chemistry. *Nanotechnology* **2013**, *24*. [CrossRef]
78. De Vos, C.; Baneton, J.; Witzke, M.; Dille, J.; Godet, S.; Gordon, M.J.; Sankaran, R.M.; Reniers, F.; De Vos, C.; Baneton, J.; et al. A comparative study of the reduction of silver and gold salts in water by a cathodic microplasma electrode. *J. Phys. D Appl. Phys.* **2017**, *50*. [CrossRef]
79. Milosavljevic, B.H.; Micic, O.I. Solvated electron reactions in water-alcohol solutions. *J. Phys. Chem.* **1978**, *82*, 1359–1362. [CrossRef]
80. Maguire, P.; Rutherford, D.; Macias-Montero, M.; Mahony, C.; Kelsey, C.; Tweedie, M.; Pérez-Martin, F.; McQuaid, H.; Diver, D.; Mariotti, D. Continuous In-Flight Synthesis for On-Demand Delivery of Ligand-Free Colloidal Gold Nanoparticles. *Nano Lett.* **2017**, *17*, 1336–1343. [CrossRef]
81. Torimoto, T.; Okazaki, K.; Kiyama, T.; Hirahara, K.; Tanaka, N.; Kuwabata, S. Sputter deposition onto ionic liquids: Simple and clean synthesis of highly dispersed ultrafine metal nanoparticles. *Appl. Phys. Lett.* **2006**, *89*, 243117. [CrossRef]

82. Okazaki, K.; Kiyama, T.; Hirahara, K.; Tanaka, N.; Kuwabata, S.; Torimoto, T. Single-step synthesis of gold–silver alloy nanoparticles in ionic liquids by a sputter deposition technique. *Chem. Commun.* **2008**, 691–693. [CrossRef]
83. Cho, C.; Choi, Y.W.; Kang, C.; Lee, G.W. Effects of the medium on synthesis of nanopowders by wire explosion process. *Appl. Phys. Lett.* **2007**, *91*, 141501. [CrossRef]
84. Toriyabe, Y.; Watanabe, S.; Yatsu, S.; Shibayama, T.; Mizuno, T. Controlled formation of metallic nanoballs during plasma electrolysis. *Appl. Phys. Lett.* **2007**, *91*, 41501. [CrossRef]
85. Sergiienko, R.; Shibata, E.; Akase, Z.; Suwa, H.; Nakamura, T.; Shindo, D. Carbon encapsulated iron carbide nanoparticles synthesized in ethanol by an electric plasma discharge in an ultrasonic cavitation field. *Mater. Chem. Phys.* **2006**, *98*, 34–38. [CrossRef]
86. Sergiienko, R.; Shibata, E.; Akase, Z.; Suwa, H.; Shindo, D.; Nakamura, T. Synthesis of Fe-filled carbon nanocapsules by an electric plasma discharge in an ultrasonic cavitation field of liquid ethanol. *J. Mater. Res.* **2006**, *21*, 2524–2533. [CrossRef]
87. Kelgenbaeva, Z.; Omurzak, E.; Takebe, S.; Abdullaeva, Z.; Sulaimankulova, S.; Iwamoto, C.; Mashimo, T. Magnetite Nanoparticles Synthesized Using Pulsed Plasma in Liquid. *Jpn. J. Appl. Phys.* **2013**, *52*, 11NJ02. [CrossRef]
88. Abdullaeva, Z.; Omurzak, E.; Iwamoto, C.; Ganapathy, H.S.; Sulaimankulova, S.; Liliang, C.; Mashimo, T. Onion-like carbon-encapsulated Co, Ni, and Fe magnetic nanoparticles with low cytotoxicity synthesized by a pulsed plasma in a liquid. *Carbon N. Y.* **2012**, *50*, 1776–1785. [CrossRef]
89. Abdullaeva, Z.; Omurzak, E.; Iwamoto, C.; Ihara, H.; Ganapathy, H.S.; Sulaimankulova, S.; Koinuma, M.; Mashimo, T. Pulsed Plasma Synthesis of Iron and Nickel Nanoparticles Coated by Carbon for Medical Applications. *Jpn. J. Appl. Phys.* **2013**, *52*, 01AJ01. [CrossRef]
90. Kim, D.-W.; Kim, T.-H.; Choi, S.; Kim, K.-S.; Park, D.-W. Preparation of silica coated iron oxide nanoparticles using non-transferred arc plasma. *Adv. Powder Technol.* **2012**, *23*, 701–707. [CrossRef]
91. Yao, W.-T.; Yu, S.-H.; Zhou, Y.; Jiang, J.; Wu, Q.-S.; Zhang, L.; Jiang, J. Formation of uniform CuO nanorods by spontaneous aggregation: Selective synthesis of CuO, Cu_2O, and Cu nanoparticles by a solid-liquid phase arc discharge process. *J. Phys. Chem. B* **2005**, *109*, 14011–14016. [CrossRef]
92. Tokushige, M.; Yamanaka, T.; Matsuura, A.; Nishikiori, T.; Ito, Y. Synthesis of Magnetic Nanoparticles (Fe and FePt) by Plasma-Induced Cathodic Discharge Electrolysis. *IEEE Trans. Plasma Sci.* **2009**, *37*, 1156–1160. [CrossRef]
93. Tokushige, M.; Nishikiori, T.; Ito, Y. Formation of Fine Ni Nanoparticle by Plasma-Induced Cathodic Discharge Electrolysis Using Rotating Disk Anode. *J. Electrochem. Soc.* **2010**, *157*, e162–e166. [CrossRef]
94. Ni, C.; Carolan, D.; Rocks, C.; Hui, J.; Fang, Z.; Padmanaban, D.B.; Ni, J.-P.; Xie, D.-T.; Maguire, P.; Irvine, J.; et al. Microplasma-assisted electrochemical synthesis of Co_3O_4 nanoparticles in absolute ethanol for energy applications. *Green Chem.* **2018**, 18–20. [CrossRef]
95. Sankaran, R.M.; Holunga, D.; Flagan, R.C.; Giapis, K.P. Synthesis of blue luminescent Si nanoparticles using atmospheric-pressure microdischarges. *Nano Lett.* **2005**, *5*, 537–541. [CrossRef] [PubMed]
96. Švrček, V.; Mariotti, D.; Kondo, M. Microplasma-induced surface engineering of silicon nanocrystals in colloidal dispersion. *Appl. Phys. Lett.* **2010**, *97*, 23–26. [CrossRef]
97. von Brisinski, N.S.; Höfft, O.; Endres, F. Plasma electrochemistry in ionic liquids: From silver to silicon nanoparticles. *J. Mol. Liq.* **2014**, *192*, 59–66. [CrossRef]
98. Kumar, A.; Ann Lin, P.; Xue, A.; Hao, B.; Khin Yap, Y.; Sankaran, R.M. Formation of nanodiamonds at near-ambient conditions via microplasma dissociation of ethanol vapour. *Nat. Commun.* **2013**, *4*, 2618. [CrossRef] [PubMed]
99. Majzlíková, P.; Sedláček, J.; Prášek, J.; Pekárek, J.; Svatoš, V.; Bannov, A.G.; Jašek, O.; Synek, P.; Eliáš, M.; Zajíčková, L.; et al. Sensing properties of multiwalled carbon nanotubes grown in MW plasma torch: Electronic and electrochemical behavior, gas sensing, field emission, IR absorption. *Sensors* **2015**, *15*, 2644–2661. [CrossRef]
100. Cheng, X.; Murphy, W.; Recek, N.; Yan, D.; Cvelbar, U.; Vesel, A.; Mozetič, M.; Canady, J.; Keidar, M.; Sherman, J.H. Synergistic effect of gold nanoparticles and cold plasma on glioblastoma cancer therapy. *J. Phys. D Appl. Phys.* **2014**, *47*. [CrossRef]

101. Nanoparticles, G.; Choi, B.B.; Kim, M.S.; Song, K.W.; Kim, U.K.; Hong, J.W.; Lee, H.J.; Kim, G.C. Targeting NEU Protein in Melanoma Cells with Non-Thermal Atmospheric Pressure Plasma and Gold Nanoparticles. *J. Biomed. Nanotechnol.* **2015**, *11*, 900–905. [CrossRef]
102. Park, S.R.; Lee, H.W.; Hong, J.W.; Lee, H.J.; Kim, J.Y.; Choi, B.B.-R.; Kim, G.C.; Jeon, Y.C. Enhancement of the killing effect of low-temperature plasma on Streptococcus mutans by combined treatment with gold nanoparticles. *J. Nanobiotechnol.* **2014**, *12*, 29. [CrossRef]
103. Kaushik, N.K.N.; Kaushik, N.K.N.; Yoo, K.C.; Uddin, N.; Kim, J.S.; Lee, S.J.; Choi, E.H. Low doses of PEG-coated gold nanoparticles sensitize solid tumors to cold plasma by blocking the PI3K/AKT-driven signaling axis to suppress cellular transformation by inhibiting growth and EMT. *Biomaterials* **2016**, *87*, 118–130. [CrossRef] [PubMed]
104. Kaushik, N.K.; Kaushik, N.; Yoo, K.C.; Uddin, N.; Kim, J.S.; Lee, S.J.; Choi, E.H. Data on combination effect of PEG-coated gold nanoparticles and non-thermal plasma inhibit growth of solid tumors. *Data Br.* **2016**, *9*, 318–323. [CrossRef] [PubMed]
105. He, Z.; Liu, K.; Manaloto, E.; Casey, A.; Cribaro, G.P.; Byrne, H.J.; Tian, F.; Barcia, C.; Conway, G.E.; Cullen, P.J.; et al. Cold Atmospheric Plasma Induces ATP-Dependent Endocytosis of Nanoparticles and Synergistic U373MG Cancer Cell Death. *Sci. Rep.* **2018**, *8*, 5298. [CrossRef] [PubMed]
106. Cheng, X.; Rajjoub, K.; Sherman, J.; Canady, J.; Recek, N.; Yan, D.; Bian, K.; Murad, F.; Keidar, M. Cold Plasma Accelerates the Uptake of Gold Nanoparticles Into Glioblastoma Cells. *Plasma Process. Polym.* **2015**, *12*, 1364–1369. [CrossRef]
107. Choi, B.B.R.; Choi, J.H.; Hong, J.W.; Song, K.W.; Lee, H.J.; Kim, U.K.; Kim, G.C. Selective killing of melanoma cells with non-thermal atmospheric pressure plasma and p-FAK antibody conjugated gold nanoparticles. *Int. J. Med. Sci.* **2017**, *14*, 1101–1109. [CrossRef] [PubMed]
108. Zhu, W.; Lee, S.-J.; Castro, N.J.; Yan, D.; Keidar, M.; Zhang, L.G. Synergistic Effect of Cold Atmospheric Plasma and Drug Loaded Core-shell Nanoparticles on Inhibiting Breast Cancer Cell Growth. *Sci. Rep.* **2016**, *6*, 21974. [CrossRef] [PubMed]
109. Jalili, A.; Irani, S.; Mirfakhraie, R. Combination of cold atmospheric plasma and iron nanoparticles in breast cancer: Gene expression and apoptosis study. *Oncol. Targets Ther.* **2016**, *9*, 5911–5917. [CrossRef]
110. Irani, S.; Shahmirani, Z.; Atyabi, S.M.; Mirpoor, S. Induction of growth arrest in colorectal cancer cells by cold plasma and gold nanoparticles. *Arch. Med. Sci.* **2015**, *11*, 1286–1295. [CrossRef] [PubMed]
111. Kim, W.; Na, K.Y.; Lee, K.H.; Lee, H.W.; Lee, J.K.; Kim, K.T. Selective uptake of epidermal growth factor-conjugated gold nanoparticle (EGF-GNP) facilitates non-Thermal plasma (NTP)-mediated cell death. *Sci. Rep.* **2017**, *7*, 1–9. [CrossRef]
112. Cheruthazhekatt, S.; Černák, M.; Slavíček, P.; Havel, J. Gas plasmas and plasma modified materials in medicine. *J. Appl. Biomed.* **2010**, *8*, 55–66. [CrossRef]
113. Navarro-Rosales, M.; Ávila-Orta, C.A.; Neira-Velázquez, M.G.; Ortega-Ortiz, H.; Hernández-Hernández, E.; Solís-Rosales, S.G.; España-Sánchez, B.L.; Gónzalez-Morones, P.; Jímenez-Barrera, R.M.; Sánchez-Valdes, S.; et al. Effect of Plasma Modification of Copper Nanoparticles on their Antibacterial Properties. *Plasma Process. Polym.* **2014**, *11*, 685–693. [CrossRef]
114. Seo, H.Y.; Kwon, J.-S.; Choi, Y.-R.; Kim, K.-M.; Choi, E.H.; Kim, K.-N. Cellular Attachment and Differentiation on Titania Nanotubes Exposed to Air- or Nitrogen-Based Non-Thermal Atmospheric Pressure Plasma. *PLoS ONE* **2014**, *9*, e113477. [CrossRef] [PubMed]
115. Coleman, J.; Yost, A.; Goren, R.; Fridman, G.; Lowman, A. Nonthermal Atmospheric Pressure Plasma Decontamination of Protein-Loaded Biodegradable Nanoparticles for Nervous Tissue Repair. *Plasma Med.* **2011**, *1*, 215–230. [CrossRef]

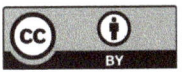

© 2019 by the authors. Licensee MDPI, Basel, Switzerland. This article is an open access article distributed under the terms and conditions of the Creative Commons Attribution (CC BY) license (http://creativecommons.org/licenses/by/4.0/).

MDPI
St. Alban-Anlage 66
4052 Basel
Switzerland
Tel. +41 61 683 77 34
Fax +41 61 302 89 18
www.mdpi.com

Nanomaterials Editorial Office
E-mail: nanomaterials@mdpi.com
www.mdpi.com/journal/nanomaterials

www.ingramcontent.com/pod-product-compliance
Lightning Source LLC
LaVergne TN
LVHW070235100526
838202LV00015B/2133